P9-CFY-246

SCHWARTZ'S PRINCIPLES OF SURGERY

ABSITE and Board Review

NOTICE

Medicine is an ever-changing science. As new research and clinical experience broaden our knowledge, changes in treatment and drug therapy are required. The editors and the publisher of this work have checked with sources believed to be reliable in their efforts to provide information that is complete and generally in accord with the standards accepted at the time of publication. However, in view of the possibility of human error or changes in medical sciences, neither the editors nor the publisher nor any other party who has been involved in the preparation or publication of this work warrants that the information contained herein is in every respect accurate or complete, and they disclaim all responsibility for any errors or omissions or for the results obtained from use of the information contained in this work. Readers are encouraged to confirm the information contained herein with other sources. For example and in particular, readers are advised to check the product information sheet included in the package of each drug they plan to administer to be certain that the information contained in this work is accurate and that changes have not been made in the recommended dose or in the contraindications for administration. This recommendation is of particular importance in connection with new or infrequently used drugs.

SCHWARTZ'S PRINCIPLES OF SURGERY

ABSITE and Board Review

Ninth Edition

Edited by

F. Charles Brunicardi, MD, FACS
DeBakey/Bard Professor and Chairman, Michael E. DeBakey Department of Surgery, Baylor College of Medicine, Houston, Texas

Associate Editors

Mary L. Brandt, MD, FACS
Professor and Vice Chair, Michael E. DeBakey Department of Surgery, Baylor College of Medicine, Houston, Texas

Dana K. Andersen, MD, FACS
Professor and Vice Chair, Department of Surgery, Johns Hopkins School of Medicine, Surgeon-in-Chief, Johns Hopkins Bayview Medical Center, Baltimore, Maryland

Timothy R. Billiar, MD, FACS
George Vance Foster Professor and Chairman of Surgery, Department of Surgery, University of Pittsburgh School of Medicine, Pittsburgh, Pennsylvania

David L. Dunn, MD, PhD, FACS
Vice President for Health Sciences, State University of New York, Buffalo, New York

John G. Hunter, MD, FACS
Mackenzie Professor and Chair, Department of Surgery, Oregon Health and Science University, Portland, Oregon

Jeffrey B. Matthews, MD, FACS
Dallas B. Phemister Professor and Chairman, Department of Surgery, University of Chicago, Chicago, Illinois

Raphael E. Pollock, MD, PhD, FACS
Head, Division of Surgery, Professor and Chairman, Department of Surgical Oncology, Senator A. M. Aiken, Jr., Distinguished Chair, The University of Texas M. D. Anderson Cancer Center, Houston, Texas

McGraw Hill Medical

New York Chicago San Francisco Lisbon London Madrid Mexico City
Milan New Delhi San Juan Seoul Singapore Sydney Toronto

Schwartz's Principles of Surgery: ABSITE and Board Review, Ninth Edition

Copyright © 2011, 2007, by The McGraw-Hill Companies, Inc. All rights reserved. Printed in the United States of America. Except as permitted under the United States Copyright Act of 1976, no part of this publication may be reproduced or distributed in any form or by any means, or stored in a data base or retrieval system, without the prior written permission of the publisher.

3 4 5 6 7 8 9 0 QVR/QVR 14 13 12

ISBN 978-0-07-160636-3
MHID 0-07-160636-X

This book was set in Minion Pro by Thomson Digital.
The editors were Anne M. Sydor and Christie Naglieri.
The production supervisor was Catherine Saggese.
Project management was provided by Aakriti Kathuria, Thomson Digital.
The index was prepared by Thomson Digital.
Quad/Graphics was printer and binder.

This book was printed on acid-free paper.

Library of Congress Cataloging-in-Publication Data

Schwartz's principles of surgery : ABSITE and board review / edited by
F. Charles Brunicardi ; associate editors, Mary L. Brandt ... [et al.]. — 9th ed.
p. ; cm.
Other title: Principles of surgery
Rev. ed. of: Schwartz's principles of surgery : self-assessment and board review. 8th ed. 2006.
Should be used in conjunction with the 9th ed. of Schwartz's principles of surgery.
Includes bibliographical references and index.
ISBN 978-0-07-160636-3 (softcover : alk. paper)
1. Surgery—Examinations, questions, etc. I. Schwartz, Seymour I., 1928- II. Brunicardi, F. Charles. III. Schwartz's principles of surgery. IV. Schwartz's principles of surgery : self-assessment and board review. V. Title: Principles of surgery.
[DNLM: 1. Surgical Procedures, Operative—Examination Questions. WO 18.2 S399 2011]
RD31.P882 2011
617.0076—dc22

2010010630

McGraw-Hill books are available at special quantity discounts to use as premiums and sales promotions or for use in corporate training programs. To contact a representative, please e-mail us at bulksales@mcgraw-hill.com.

CONTENTS

INTRODUCTION

This ninth edition of Principles of Surgery: ABSITE and Board Review, edited by F. Charles Brunicardi and colleagues, follows the same convenient side-by-side question and answer format introduced in its last printing, but has been extensively updated with new questions pulled directly from the pages of the new ninth edition of Schwartz's Principles of Surgery textbook. Designed primarily for residents in preparation for the American Board of Surgery (ABS) Qualifying, In-Training, and Certifying Examinations, it is also a capable recertification tool for board-certified surgeons.

Within each chapter questions have been subdivided into two categories: Basic Science and Clinical. The side-by-side placement of questions and answers allows the reader to engage in more efficient study and expedited self-assessment. In order to maintain the integrity of the practice test the user is urged to cover the right-hand column of the page to conceal the answer column until review. The style of questioning used mimics that of the ABS board examinations. Additionally, adjacent to each question is the answer, a paragraph-length explanation, and a specific page number reference should the user require a more extensive review of the topic.

This book consists of 1,142 multiple-choice questions that are representative of the major areas covered in the ninth edition of *Principles of Surgery* by Brunicardi and associates. Among the additions to this review are two new chapters: Accreditation Council for Graduate Medical Core Competencies and Ethics, Palliative Care and Care at the End of Life.

ACKNOWLEDGMENTS

Since the last edition, this PreTest has been expanded to include new questions for every chapter while also retaining viable questions from the eighth edition. The editors would like to recognize the enormous effort of Mary L. Brandt, M.D., F.A.C.P., who created many of the new questions and for her invaluable assistance in proofreading and fact-checking. We also acknowledge the essential and valuable contribution of Katie Elsbury, who worked with Dr. Brandt, the editors, the publisher, and me during each step of the editorial process.

F. Charles Brunicardi, M.D., F.A.C.S.

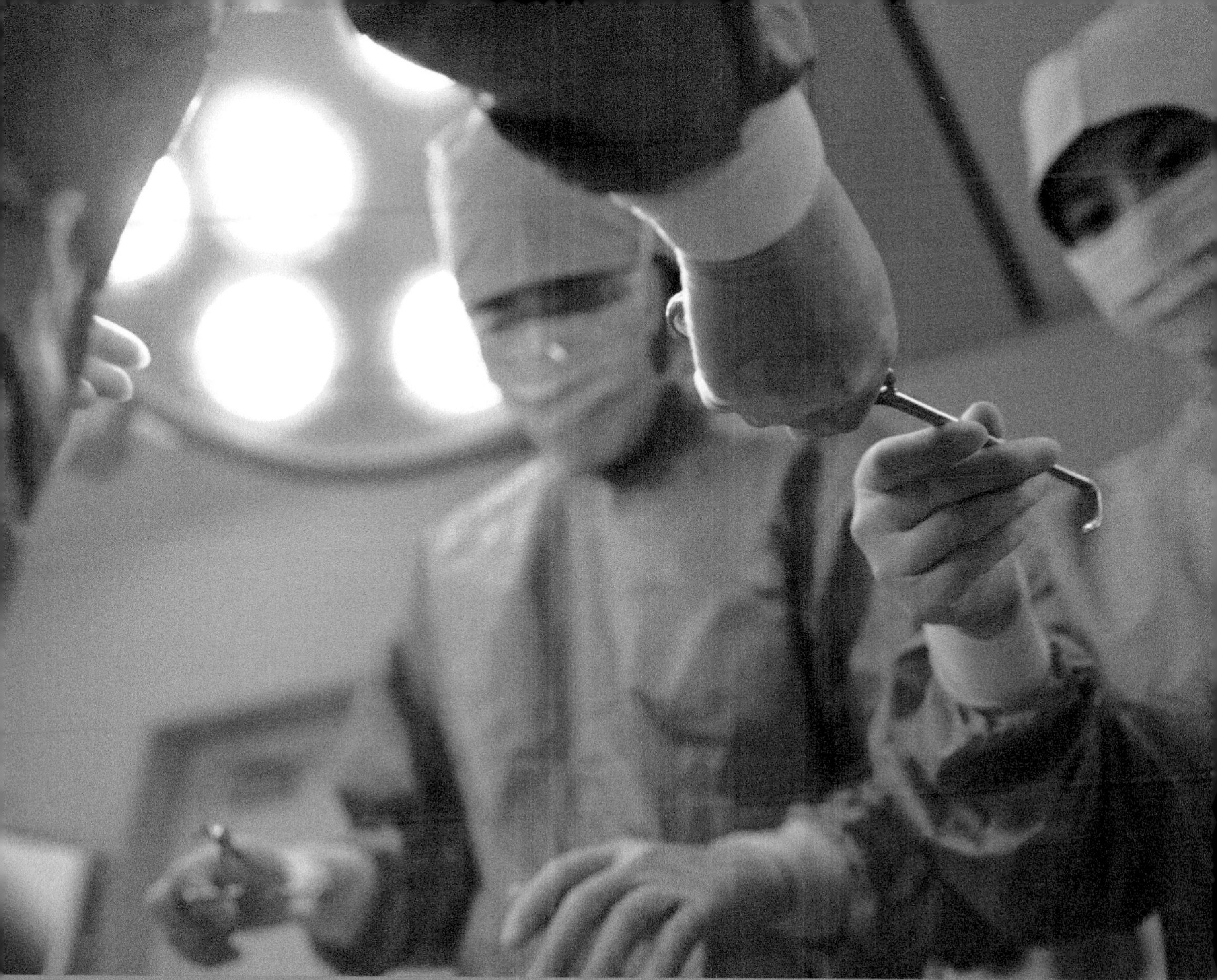

PART I

Basic Considerations

CHAPTER 1

Accreditation Council for Graduate Medical Education Core Competencies

1. Learning by presenting errors at a morbidity and mortality conference is a part of which of the following ACGME core competencies?
   A. Patient care
   B. Medical knowledge
   C. Practice-based learning and improvement
   D. System-based practice

Answer: C

Practice-based learning and improvement involves a cycle of four steps: identify areas for improvement, engage in learning, apply the new knowledge and skills to a practice, and check for improvement.... In residency training, the simplest example of practice-based learning is the surgical morbidity and mortality conference. This conference traditionally allows for in-depth discussions of surgical cases and adverse patient outcomes. Complications are categorized (preventable, probably preventable, possibly preventable, and unpreventable) and areas of improvement are identified. (See Schwartz 9th ed., p. 6, and Table 1-1.)

TABLE 1-1 Accreditation Council for Graduate Medical Education core competencies

Core Competency	Description
Patient care	To be able to provide compassionate and effective health care in the modern-day health care environment
Medical knowledge	To effectively apply current medical knowledge in patient care and to be able to use medical tools (i.e., PubMed) to stay current in medical education
Practice-based learning and improvement	To critically assimilate and evaluate information in a systematic manner to improve patient care practices
Interpersonal and communication skills	To demonstrate sufficient communication skills that allow for efficient information exchange in physician-patient interactions and as a member of a health care team
Professionalism	To demonstrate the principles of ethical behavior (i.e., informed consent, patient confidentiality) and integrity that promote the highest level of medical care
Systems-based practice	To acknowledge and understand that each individual practice is part of a larger health care delivery system and to be able to use the system to support patient care

2. Which of the following are mandated by the Residency Review Committee of the ACGME?
   A. One-on-one teaching with attending surgeons
   B. Surgical skills laboratory
   C. Departmental library with Internet access
   D. Morning report

Answer: B

Having recognized the importance of incorporating simulation training into today's residency, the Residency Review Committee (RRC) mandated that all surgery programs be required to have a surgical skills laboratory by July 2008 to maintain their accreditation. One-on-one teaching as well as conferences such as morning report occur in almost all surgical training programs. They are not, however, specifically mandated by the RRC. Although access to information, both printed and digital, is required, it is not mandated that this be provided by the department. (See Schwartz 9th ed., p. 5.)

3. Lawsuits and sentinel events most often are the result of
   A. Inadequate medical knowledge
   B. Substandard patient care
   C. Poor interpersonal and communication skills
   D. Unprofessional behavior

Answer: C

Studies reveal that physicians with good communication and interpersonal skills have improved patient outcomes and are subject to less medical litigation. In support of this, a root cause analysis by the Joint Commission identified breakdown in communication as the leading cause of wrong-site operations and other sentinel events. (See Schwartz 9th ed., p. 8.)

4. Which of the following is one of the three principles of the ACS Code of Professional Conduct?
   A. Dedication to the patient's welfare, independent of administrative forces
   B. Reasonable reimbursement for testifying as an expert witness
   C. Accepting patients, regardless of ability to pay
   D. Referring patients to other doctors when conflicts do not allow the surgeon to continue to care for the patient

Answer: A

The ACS endorsed the Charter of Medical Professionalism as its Code of Professional Conduct in 2002. This model of professionalism is based on three principles. First, the physician should be dedicated to the patient's welfare. This should supersede all financial, societal, and administrative forces. Second, the physician should have respect for the patient's autonomy. This entails being honest and providing the patient with all the necessary information to make an informed decision. Third, the medical profession should promote justice in the health care system by removing discrimination due to any societal barriers. (See Schwartz 9th ed., p. 9.)

CHAPTER 2

Systemic Response to Injury and Metabolic Support

BASIC SCIENCE QUESTIONS

1. The vagus nerve mediates which of the following in the setting of systemic inflammation?
   A. Enhanced gut motility
   B. Decreased protein production by the liver
   C. Decreased IL-10 production
   D. Increased heart rate to increase cardiac output

Answer: A

The vagus nerve exerts several homeostatic influences, including enhancing gut motility, reducing heart rate, and regulating inflammation. Central to this pathway is the understanding of neurally controlled anti-inflammatory pathways of the vagus nerve. Parasympathetic nervous system activity transmits vagus nerve efferent signals primarily through the neurotransmitter acetylcholine. This neurally mediated anti-inflammatory pathway allows for a rapid response to inflammatory stimuli and also for the potential regulation of early proinflammatory mediator release, specifically tumor necrosis factor (TNF). Vagus nerve activity in the presence of systemic inflammation may inhibit cytokine activity and reduce injury from disease processes such as pancreatitis, ischemia and reperfusion, and hemorrhagic shock. This activity is primarily mediated through nicotinic acetylcholine receptors on immune mediator cells such as tissue macrophages. Furthermore, enhanced inflammatory profiles are observed after vagotomy, during stress conditions. (See Schwartz 9th ed., p. 17.)

2. Cytokines are which type of hormone?
   A. Polypeptide
   B. Amino acid
   C. Fatty acid
   D. Carbohydrate

Answer: A

Cytokines are polypeptide hormones. Humans release hormones in several chemical categories, including polypeptides (e.g., cytokines, glucagon, and insulin), amino acids (e.g., epinephrine, serotonin, and histamine), and fatty acids (e.g., glucocorticoids, prostaglandins, and leukotrienes). There are no carbohydrate hormones. (See Schwartz 9th ed., p. 17.)

3. Which of the following is a function of heat shock proteins?
   A. Binding of autologous proteins to improve ligand binding
   B. Induction of the white cell oxidative burst
   C. Binding to capillary endothelium to prevent fluid extravasation
   D. Stabilization of membranes to prevent cell lysis

Answer: A

Heat shock proteins (HSPs) are a group of intracellular proteins that are increasingly expressed during times of stress, such as burn injury, inflammation, and infection. HSPs participate in many physiologic processes, including protein folding and protein targeting. The formation of HSPs requires gene induction by the heat shock transcription factor. HSPs bind both autologous and foreign proteins and thereby function as intracellular chaperones for ligands such as bacterial DNA and endotoxin. HSPs are presumed to protect cells from the deleterious effects of traumatic stress and, when released by damaged cells, alert the immune system of the tissue damage. (See Schwartz 9th ed., p. 20.)

4. Which of the following is an eicosanoid?
   A. Tumor necrosis factor (TNF)
   B. Arachidonic acid
   C. Thromboxane
   D. IL-10

Answer: C

Thromboxane is an eicosanoid. Arachidonic acid is one of two precursors of the eicosanoids. TNF and IL-10 are cytokines. Eicosanoids are derived primarily by oxidation of the membrane phospholipid arachidonic acid (eicosatetraenoic acid) and are composed of subgroups, including prostaglandins, prostacyclins, hydroxyeicosatetraenoic acids (HETEs), thromboxanes, and leukotrienes. The synthesis of arachidonic acid from phospholipids requires the enzymatic activation of phospholipase A_2 (Fig. 2-1). Products of the COX pathway include all of the prostaglandins and thromboxanes. The lipoxygenase pathway generates leukotrienes and HETE.... Eicosanoids are produced primarily through two major pathways: (1) with arachidonic acid (omega-6 fatty acid) as substrate and (2) eicosapentaenoic acid (omega-3 fatty acid) as substrate. (See Schwartz 9th ed., p. 22.)

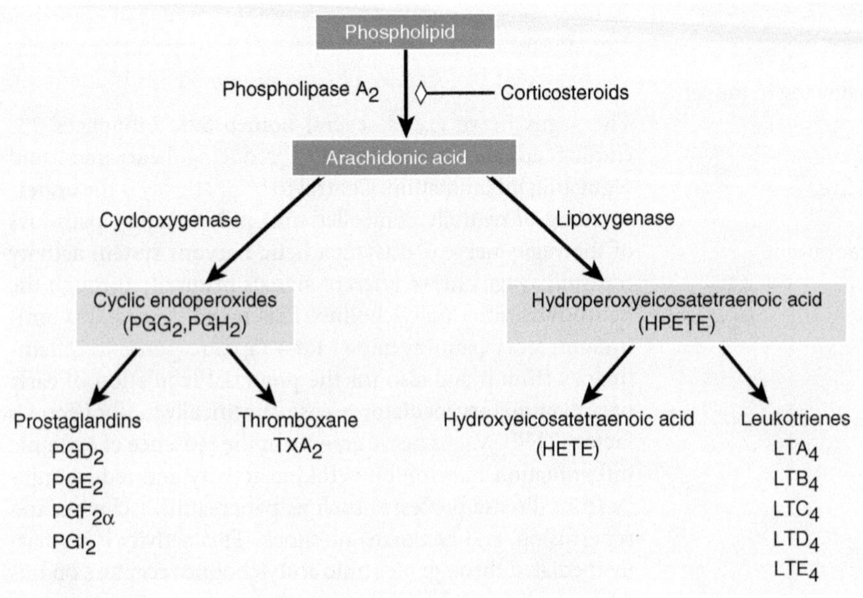

FIG. 2-1. Schematic diagram of arachidonic acid metabolism. LT = leukotriene; PG = prostaglandin; TXA_2 = thromboxane A_2.

5. Omega-3 fatty acids have which of the following effects on the inflammatory response?
   A. Increased inflammatory response
   B. Decreased inflammatory response
   C. Delayed inflammatory response
   D. No effect on the inflammatory response

Answer: B

Omega-3 fatty acids have specific anti-inflammatory effects, including inhibition of NF-B activity, TNF release from hepatic Kupffer cells, as well as leukocyte adhesion and migration. The anti-inflammatory effects of omega-3 fatty acids on chronic autoimmune diseases such as rheumatoid arthritis, psoriasis, and lupus have been documented in both animals and humans. In experimental models of sepsis, omega-3 fatty acids inhibit inflammation, ameliorate weight loss, increase small bowel perfusion, and may increase gut barrier protection. In human studies, omega-3 supplementation is associated with decreased production of TNF, interleukin-1β, and interleukin-6 by endotoxin stimulated monocytes. In a study of surgical patients, preoperative supplementation with omega-3 fatty acid was associated with reduced need for mechanical ventilation, decreased hospital length of stay, and decreased mortality with a good safety profile. (See Schwartz 9th ed., p. 22.)

6. Which of the following are known effects of tumor necrosis factor (TNF)?
   A. Decreases catabolic response
   B. Promotes insulin entry into cells
   C. Enhances the expression of eicosanoids
   D. Delays activation of the coagulation pathway

Answer: C

Tumor necrosis factor alpha (TNF) is a cytokine that is rapidly mobilized in response to stressors such as injury and infection, and is a potent mediator of the subsequent inflammatory response. TNF is primarily synthesized by macrophages, monocytes, and T cells, which are abundant in peritoneum and splanchnic tissues. Although the circulating half-life of TNF is brief, the activity of TNF elicits many metabolic and immunomodulatory activities. TNF stimulates muscle breakdown and cachexia through increased catabolism, insulin resistance, and redistribution of amino acids to hepatic circulation as fuel substrates. In addition, TNF also mediates coagulation activation, cell migration, and macrophage phagocytosis, and enhances the expression of adhesion molecules, prostaglandin E_2, platelet-activating factor, glucocorticoids, and eicosanoids. (See Schwartz 9th ed., p. 24.)

7. Which of the following are adhesion molecules (i.e., cells that mediate leukocyte to endothelial adhesion)?
   A. Platelet activating factor
   B. L-selectin
   C. Transforming growth factor beta (TGF-β)
   D. Tumor necrosis factor (TNF)

Answer: B

There are 4 families of adhesions molecules: selectins, immunoglobulins, Beta (CD18) integrins, and Beta (CD29) integrins. L-selectin is a member of the selectin family of adhesion molecules. Platelet activating factor is a phospholipid which mediates leukocyte function but does not contribute to adhesion. TGF-β is a polypeptide growth factor which is upregulated in some malignant tumors. TNF is a cytokine which is upregulated in inflammatory conditions, but which does not play a role in adhesion of leukocytes to endothelium (Table 2-1). (See Schwartz 9th ed., p. 33.)

TABLE 2-1 Molecules that mediate leukocyte-endothelial adhesion, categorized by family

Adhesion Molecule	Action	Origin	Inducers of Expression	Target Cells
Selectins				
L-selectin	Fast rolling	Leukocytes	Native	Endothelium, platelets, eosinophils
P-selectin	Slow rolling	Platelets and endothelium	Thrombin, histamine	Neutrophils, monocytes
E-selectin	Very slow rolling	Endothelium	Cytokines	Neutrophils, monocytes, lymphocytes
Immunoglobulins				
ICAM-1	Firm adhesion/transmigration	Endothelium, leukocytes, fibroblasts, epithelium	Cytokines	Leukocytes
ICAM-2	Firm adhesion	Endothelium, platelets	Native	Leukocytes
VCAM-1	Firm adhesion/transmigration	Endothelium	Cytokines	Monocytes, lymphocytes
PECAM-1	Adhesion/transmigration	Endothelium, platelets, leukocytes	Native	Endothelium, platelets, leukocytes
β_2-(CD18) Integrins				
CD18/11a	Firm adhesion/transmigration	Leukocytes	Leukocyte activation	Endothelium
CD18/11b (Mac-1)	Firm adhesion/transmigration	Neutrophils, monocytes, natural killer cells	Leukocyte activation	Endothelium
CD18/11c	Adhesion	Neutrophils, monocytes, natural killer cells	Leukocyte activation	Endothelium
β_1-(CD29) Integrins				
VLA-4	Firm adhesion/transmigration	Lymphocytes, monocytes	Leukocyte activation	Monocytes, endothelium, epithelium

ICAM-1 = intercellular adhesion molecule-1; ICAM-2 = intercellular adhesion molecule-2; Mac-1 = macrophage antigen 1; PECAM-1 = platelet-endothelial cell adhesion molecule-1; VCAM-1 = vascular cell adhesion molecule-1; VLA-4 = very late antigen-4.

8. The primary physiologic effect of nitric oxide (NO) is
   A. Increased platelet adhesion
   B. Increased leukocyte-endothelial adhesion
   C. Increased microthrombosis
   D. Increased smooth muscle relaxation

Answer: D

Nitric oxide (NO) was initially known as *endothelium-derived relaxing factor* due to its effect on vascular smooth muscle and has important functions in both physiologic and pathologic control of vascular tone. Normal vascular smooth muscle relaxation is maintained by a constant output of NO and subsequent activation of soluble quanylyl cyclase. NO also can reduce microthrombosis by reducing platelet adhesion and aggregation (Fig. 2-2). NO easily traverses cell membranes and has a short half-life of a few seconds and is oxidized into nitrate and nitrite. NO is constitutively expressed by endothelial cells; however, inducible NO synthase, which is normally not expressed, is upregulated in response to inflammatory stimuli, which increases NO production. Increased NO is detectable in septic shock and in response to TNF, IL-1, IL-2, and hemorrhage. NO mediates hypotension observed during septic shock; however, a clinical trial of a nonselective NOS inhibitor showed increased organ dysfunction and mortality. (See Schwartz 9th ed., p. 33.)

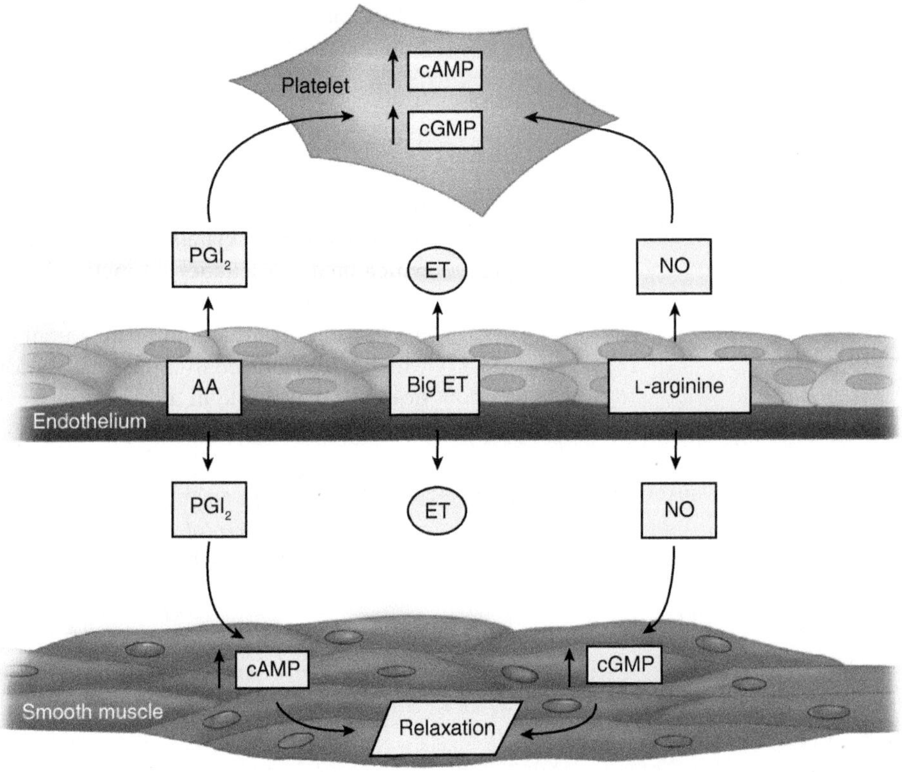

FIG. 2-2. Endothelial interaction with smooth muscle cells and with intraluminal platelets. Prostacyclin (prostaglandin I_2, or PGI_2) is derived from arachidonic acid (AA), and nitric oxide (NO) is derived from L-arginine. The increase in cyclic adenosine monophosphate (cAMP) and cyclic guanosine monophosphate (cGMP) results in smooth muscle relaxation and inhibition of platelet thrombus formation. Endothelins (ETs) are derived from "big ET," and they counter the effects of prostacyclin and NO.

9. Prostacyclin has which of the following effects in systemic inflammation?
   A. Inhibition of platelet aggregation
   B. Vasoconstriction
   C. Increased adhesion molecules
   D. Decreased cardiac output

Answer: A

Prostacyclin is a member of the eicosanoid family and is primarily produced by endothelial cells. Prostacyclin is an effective vasodilator and also inhibits platelet aggregation. During systemic inflammation, endothelial prostacyclin expression is impaired, and thus the endothelium favors a more procoagulant profile. Prostacyclin therapy during sepsis has been shown to reduce the levels of cytokines, growth factors, and adhesion molecules through a cAMP-dependent pathway. In clinical trials, prostacyclin infusion is associated with increased cardiac output, splanchnic blood flow, and oxygen delivery and consumption with no significant decrease in mean arterial pressure. However, further study is required before the widespread use of prostacyclin is recommended. (See Schwartz 9th ed., p. 33.)

10. How many calories per day are required to maintain basal metabolism in a healthy adult?
    A. 10-15 kcal/kg/day
    B. 20-25 kcal/kg/day
    C. 30-35 kcal/kg/day
    D. 40-45 kcal/kg/day

Answer: B

To maintain basal metabolic needs (i.e., at rest and fasting), a normal healthy adult requires approximately 22 to 25 kcal/kg per day drawn from carbohydrate, lipid, and protein sources. (See Schwartz 9th ed., p. 34.)

11. The primary source of calories during acute starvation (<5 days fasting) is
    A. Fat
    B. Muscle (protein)
    C. Glycogen
    D. Ketone bodies

Answer: A

In the healthy adult, principal sources of fuel during short-term fasting (<5 days) are derived from muscle protein and body fat, with fat being the most abundant source of energy. (See Schwartz 9th ed., p. 34.)

12. Which of the following is the primary fuel source in prolonged starvation?
    A. Fat
    B. Muscle (protein)
    C. Glycogen
    D. Ketone bodies

Answer: D

In prolonged starvation, systemic proteolysis is reduced to approximately 20 g/d and urinary nitrogen excretion stabilizes at 2 to 5 g/d (Fig. 2-3). This reduction in proteolysis reflects the adaptation by vital organs (e.g., myocardium, brain, renal cortex, and skeletal muscle) to using ketone bodies as their principal fuel source. In extended fasting, ketone bodies become an important fuel source for the brain after 2 days and gradually become the principal fuel source by 24 days. (See Schwartz 9th ed., p. 35.)

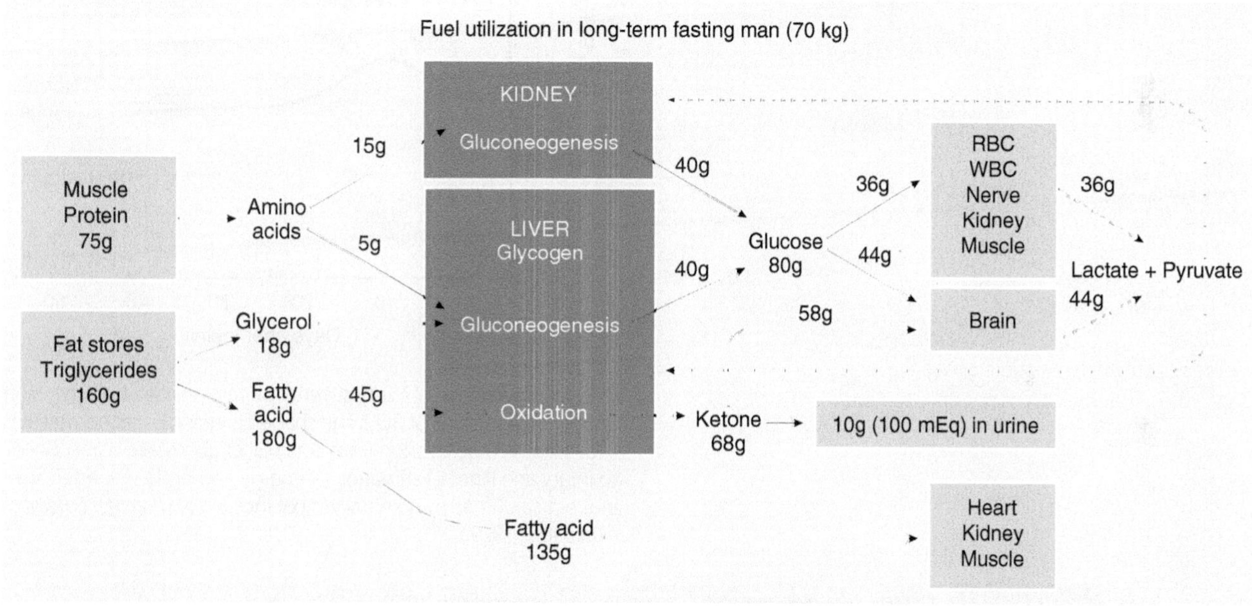

FIG. 2-3. Fuel utilization in extended starvation. Liver glycogen stores are depleted, and there is adaptive reduction in proteolysis as a source of fuel. The brain uses ketones for fuel. The kidneys become important participants in gluconeogenesis. RBC = red blood cell; WBC = white blood cell. (Adapted with permission from Cahill GF: Starvation in man. *N Engl J Med* 282:668, 1970. Copyright © Massachusetts Medical Society. All rights reserved.)

13. Which of the following is the primary fuel source after acute injury?
    A. Fat
    B. Muscle (protein)
    C. Glycogen
    D. Ketone bodies

Answer: A

Lipids are not merely nonprotein, noncarbohydrate fuel sources that minimize protein catabolism in the injured patient. Lipid metabolism potentially influences the structural integrity of cell membranes as well as the immune response during systemic inflammation. Adipose stores within the body (triglycerides) are the predominant energy source (50 to 80%) during critical illness and after injury. Fat mobilization (lipolysis) occurs mainly in response to catecholamine stimulus of the hormone-sensitive triglyceride lipase. Other hormonal influences which potentiate lipolysis include adrenocorticotropic hormone (ACTH), catecholamines, thyroid hormone, cortisol, glucagon, growth hormone release, reduction in insulin levels, and increased sympathetic stimulus. (See Schwartz 9th ed., p. 36.)

14. Sepsis increases metabolic needs by approximately what percentage?
    A. 25%
    B. 50%
    C. 75%
    D. 100%

Answer: B

Sepsis increases metabolic needs to approximately 150-160% of resting energy expenditure, or 50% above normal. The magnitude of metabolic expenditure appears to be directly proportional to the severity of insult, with thermal injuries and severe infections having the highest energy demands (Fig. 2-4). The increase in energy expenditure is mediated in part by sympathetic activation and catecholamine release, which has been replicated by the administration of catecholamines to healthy human subjects. (See Schwartz 9th ed., p. 36, and Table 2-2.)

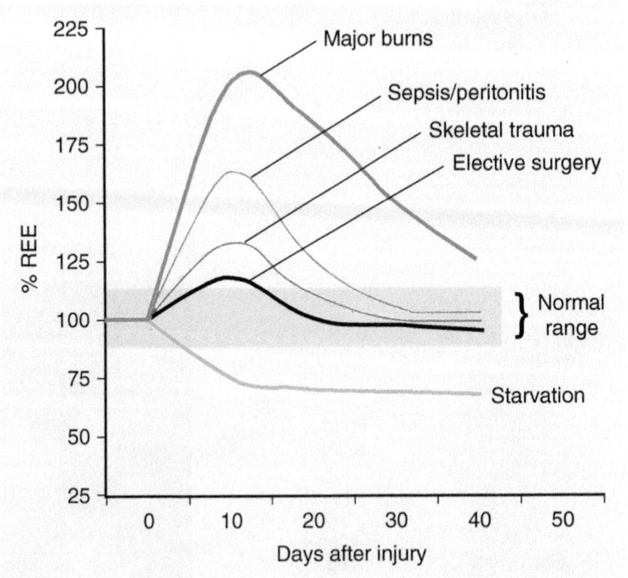

FIG. 2-4. Influence of injury severity on resting metabolism (resting energy expenditure, or REE). The shaded area indicates normal REE. (Adapted with permission from Long CL et al: Metabolic response to injury and illness: Estimation of energy and protein needs from indirect calorimetry and nitrogen balance. *JPEN J Parenter Enteral Nutr* 3:452, 1979.)

TABLE 2-2 Caloric adjustments above basal energy expenditure (BEE) in hypermetabolic conditions

Condition	kcal/kg per Day	Adjustment above BEE	Grams of Protein/kg per Day	Nonprotein Calories: Nitrogen
Normal/moderate malnutrition	25–30	1.1	1.0	150:1
Mild stress	25–30	1.2	1.2	150:1
Moderate stress	30	1.4	1.5	120:1
Severe stress	30–35	1.6	2.0	90–120:1
Burns	35–40	2.0	2.5	90–100:1

15. What is the most abundant amino acid in the human body?
    A. Leucine
    B. Tyrosine
    C. Glutamine
    D. Alanine

Answer: C

Glutamine is the most abundant amino acid in the human body, comprising nearly two thirds of the free intracellular amino acid pool. Of this, 75% is found within the skeletal muscles. In healthy individuals, glutamine is considered a nonessential amino acid, because it is synthesized within the skeletal muscles and the lungs. Glutamine is a necessary substrate for nucleotide synthesis in most dividing cells and hence provides a major fuel source for enterocytes. It also serves as an important fuel source for immunocytes such as lymphocytes and macrophages, and is a precursor for glutathione, a major intracellular antioxidant. (See Schwartz 9th ed., p. 46.)

1. A patient presents to the emergency room with a temperature of 39° C, a heart rate of 115, and a respiratory rate of 25. There are no localizing symptoms and the work-up does not reveal any specific source for the fever. Which of the following best describes this patient's condition?
   A. Infection
   B. SIRS
   C. Sepsis
   D. Septic shock

Answer: B

This patient meets the criteria for SIRS. Because there is no identifiable source for the condition, the criteria for infection and sepsis have not been met. Septic shock is sepsis with cardiovascular collapse (Table 2-3). (See Schwartz 9th ed., p. 16.)

TABLE 2-3 Clinical spectrum of infection and systemic inflammatory response syndrome (SIRS)

Term	Definition
Infection	Identifiable source of microbial insult
SIRS	Two or more of following criteria are met: Temperature ≥38°C (100.4°F) or ≤36°C (96.8°F) Heart rate ≥90 beats per minute Respiratory rate ≥20 breaths per minute or $Paco_2$ ≤32 mmHg or mechanical ventilation White blood cell count ≥12,000/μL or ≤4000/μL or ≥10% band forms
Sepsis	Identifiable source of infection + SIRS
Severe sepsis	Sepsis + organ dysfunction
Septic shock	Sepsis + cardiovascular collapse (requiring vasopressor support)

$Paco_2$ = partial pressure of arterial carbon dioxide.

2. Cortisol is elevated in response to severe injury. How long can this response persist in a patient with a significant burn?
   A. 2 days
   B. 1 week
   C. 1 month
   D. 3 months

Answer: C

Cortisol is a glucocorticoid steroid hormone released by the adrenal cortex in response to ACTH. Cortisol release is increased during times of stress and may be chronically elevated in certain disease processes. For example, burn-injured patients may exhibit elevated levels for 4 weeks. (See Schwartz 9th ed., p. 18.)

3. Which of the following can be used to mitigate cortisol effects on wound healing?
   A. Vitamin A
   B. Vitamin B1
   C. Vitamin C
   D. Vitamin E

Answer: A

Wound healing also is impaired, because cortisol reduces transforming growth factor beta (TGF-β) and insulin-like growth factor I (IGF-I) in the wound. This effect can be partially ameliorated by the administration of vitamin A. (See Schwartz 9th ed., p. 18.)

4. Which of the following is found in patients with adrenal insufficiency?
   A. Hyperglycemia
   B. Hyperkalemia
   C. Hypercalcemia
   D. Hypernatremia

Answer: B

Laboratory findings in adrenal insufficiency include hypoglycemia from decreased gluconeogenesis, hyponatremia from impaired renal tubular sodium resorption, and hyperkalemia from diminished kaliuresis. Calcium levels are not typically affected by adrenal insufficiency. (See Schwartz 9th ed., p. 19.)

5. Overfeeding (RQ >1.0) in a critically ill patient can result in
   A. Pancreatitis
   B. Increased risk of infection
   C. Atelectasis
   D. Increased risk of DVT

Answer: B

Excess glucose from overfeeding, as reflected by RQs >1.0, can result in conditions such as glucosuria, thermogenesis, and conversion to fat (lipogenesis). Excessive glucose administration results in elevated carbon dioxide production, which may be deleterious in patients with suboptimal pulmonary function, as well as hyperglycemia, which may contribute to infectious risk and immune suppression.... Overfeeding may contribute to clinical deterioration via increased oxygen consumption, increased carbon dioxide production and prolonged need for ventilatory support, fatty liver, suppression of leukocyte function, hyperglycemia, and increased risk of infection. (See Schwartz 9th ed., p. 38.)

6. Which of the following is the initial enteral formula for the majority of surgical patients?
   A. Low-residue isotonic formula
   B. Elemental formula
   C. Calorie dense formula
   D. High protein formula

Answer: A

Most low-residue isotonic formulas provide a caloric density of 1.0 kcal/mL, and approximately 1500 to 1800 mL are required to meet daily requirements. These low-osmolarity compositions provide baseline carbohydrates, protein, electrolytes, water, fat, and fat soluble vitamins (some do not have vitamin K) and typically have a nonprotein-calorie:nitrogen ratio of 150:1. These contain no fiber bulk and therefore leave minimum residue. These solutions usually are considered to be the standard or first-line formulas for stable patients with an intact gastrointestinal tract. (See Schwartz 9th ed., p. 42.)

7. Which nutrient is proportionally increased in "pulmonary failure" enteral formula?
   A. Carbohydrate
   B. Protein
   C. Fat
   D. Vitamins

Answer: C

In pulmonary-failure formulas, fat content is usually increased to 50% of the total calories, with a corresponding reduction in carbohydrate content. The goal is to reduce carbon dioxide production and alleviate ventilation burden for failing lungs. (See Schwartz 9th ed., p. 43.)

8. Which vitamin is not present in commercially prepared intravenous vitamin preparations and, therefore, must be supplemented in a patient receiving TPN?
   A. Vitamin A
   B. Vitamin D
   C. Vitamin E
   D. Vitamin K

Answer: D

Intravenous vitamin preparations also should be added to parenteral formulas. Vitamin deficiencies are rare occurrences if such preparations are used. In addition, because vitamin K is not part of any commercially prepared vitamin solution, it should be supplemented on a weekly basis. (See Schwartz 9th ed., p. 45.)

9. New onset of glucose intolerance in a TPN dependent patient can be due to
   A. Zinc deficiency
   B. Copper deficiency
   C. Chromium deficiency
   D. Manganese deficiency

Answer: C

The most frequent presentation of trace mineral deficiencies is the eczematoid rash developing both diffusely and at intertriginous areas in zinc deficient patients. Other rare trace mineral deficiencies include a microcytic anemia associated with copper deficiency, and glucose intolerance presumably related to chromium deficiency. The latter complications are seldom seen except in patients receiving parenteral nutrition for extended periods. The daily administration of commercially available trace mineral supplements will obviate most such problems. Manganese deficiency is extremely rare and poorly described but may be associated with poor wound healing. (See Schwartz 9th ed., p. 45.)

10. Which of the following is a potential physiologic effect of anabolism (positive nitrogen balance)?
   A. Glycosuria
   B. Metabolic acidosis
   C. Hypercalcemia
   D. Hypermagnesemia

Answer: A

Glycosuria can result from hypokalemia. Since potassium is the most abundant intracellular anion, anabolism requires a large shift of potassium into the new cells, leading to serum hypokalemia.

Potassium is essential to achieve positive nitrogen balance and replace depleted intracellular stores. In addition, a significant shift of potassium ion from the extracellular to the intracellular space may take place because of the large glucose infusion, with resultant hypokalemia, metabolic alkalosis, and poor glucose utilization. In some cases as much as 240 mEq of potassium ion daily may be required. Hypokalemia may cause glycosuria, which would be treated with potassium, not insulin. Thus, before giving insulin, the serum potassium level must be checked to avoid exacerbating the hypokalemia. Magnesium tends to follow potassium—in this setting hypomagnesemia would be expected, not hypermagnesemia. Serum calcium levels should not be significantly affected by anabolism. (See Schwartz 9th ed., p. 46.)

CHAPTER 3

Fluid and Electrolyte Management of the Surgical Patient

BASIC SCIENCE QUESTIONS

1. What percentage of body weight is made up of water?
   A. 10-20%
   B. 30-40%
   C. 50-60%
   D. 70-80%

Answer: C

Water constitutes approximately 50 to 60% of total body weight. In an average young adult male 60% of total body weight is TBW, whereas in an average young adult female it is 50%. The lower percentage of TBW in females correlates with a higher percentage of adipose tissue and lower percentage of muscle mass. Estimates of percentage of TBW should be adjusted downward approximately 10 to 20% for obese individuals and upward by 10% for malnourished individuals. (See Schwartz 9th ed., pp 51 & 52.)

2. Which of the following is the largest fluid compartment in the body?
   A. Plasma
   B. Central spinal fluid
   C. Interstitial fluid
   D. Intracellular fluid

Answer: D

Intracellular fluid is the largest fluid compartment in the body and makes up approximately 40% of total body weight (Fig. 3.1). Extracellular fluid, which is composed of plasma and interstitial fluid, makes up 20% of body weight. Central spinal fluid is a very small fluid compartment, composed mostly of plasma. (See Schwartz 9th ed., p 52; See Fig. 3-1.)

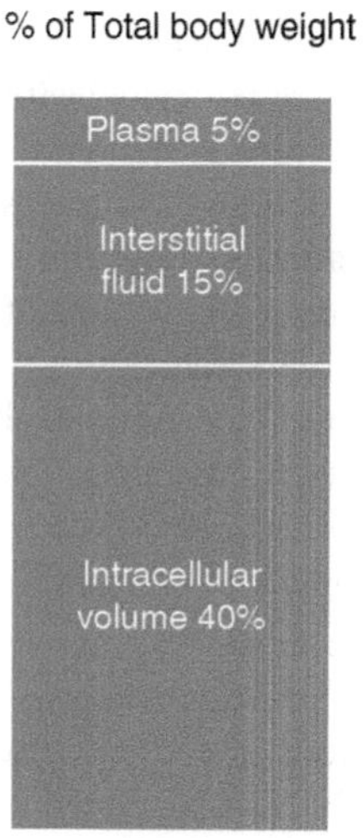

Volume of TBW	Male (70 kg)	Female (60 kg)
Extracellular volume	14,000 mL	10,000 mL
Plasma	3500 mL	2500 mL
Interstitial	10,500 mL	7500 mL
Intracellular volume	28,000 mL	20,000 mL
	42,000 mL	30,000 mL

FIG. 3-1. Functional body fluid compartments. TBW = total body water.

3. Which of the following is the cation present in largest amounts in intracellular fluid?
   A. Sodium
   B. Chloride
   C. Potassium
   D. Calcium

Answer: C

Potassium is the most common cation present in intracellular fluid (Fig. 3-2). Sodium is the most common cation present in extracellular fluid (plasma and interstitial fluid). Calcium is virtually absent in intracellular fluid, and is present only in small amounts in extracellular fluid. Chloride is an anion. (See Schwartz 9th ed., p 52; See Fig. 3-2.)

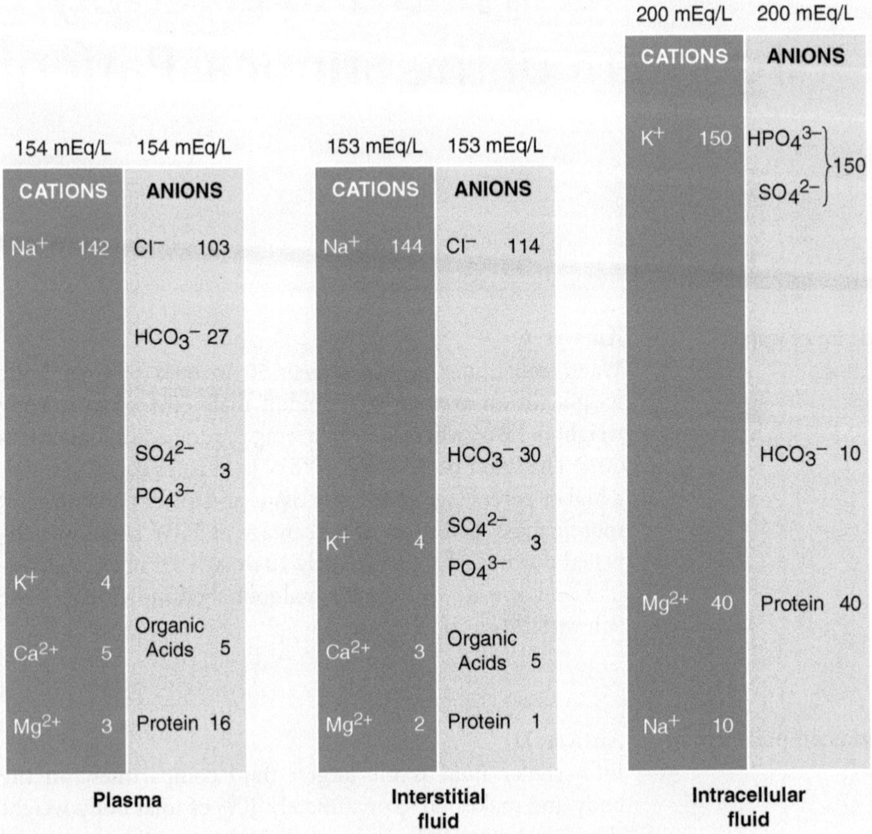

FIG. 3-2. Chemical composition of body fluid compartments.

CLINICAL QUESTIONS

1. If 1 liter of 0.9% NaCl solution is given intravenously, how much will be distributed to the interstitial space?
   A. 100 cc
   B. 250 cc
   C. 400 cc
   D. 750 cc

Answer: D

Sodium is confined to the extracellular fluid (ECF) compartment, and because of its osmotic and electrical properties, it remains associated with water. Therefore, sodium-containing fluids are distributed throughout the ECF and add to the volume of both the intravascular and interstitial spaces. Although the administration of sodium-containing fluids expands the intravascular volume, it also expands the interstitial space by approximately three times as much as the plasma.

One liter of normal saline will be distributed 3:1 to the interstitial space. Therefore, 750 ml will be distributed to the interstitial space and 250 ml will remain in the intravascular volume. (See Schwartz 9th ed., p 53.)

2. What is the approximate serum osmolality for a patient with the following laboratory findings?
   Na 130   Cl 94   K 5.2 CO_2 14   Glucose 360
   BUN 84   Creatinine 3.2
   A. 270
   B. 290
   C. 310
   D. 330

Answer: C

The principal determinants of osmolality are the concentrations of sodium, glucose, and urea (blood urea nitrogen, or BUN): Calculated serum osmolality = 2 sodium + (glucose/18) + (BUN/2.8)

For this patient: $(130 \times 2) + (360 / 18) + (84 / 2.8) = 260 + 20 + 30 = 310$ (See Schwartz 9th ed., p 53.)

3. A patient develops a high output fistula following abdominal surgery. The fluid is sent for evaluation with the following results: Na 135 K 5 Cl 70. Which of the following is the most likely source of the fistula?
   A. Stomach
   B. Small bowel
   C. Pancreas
   D. Biliary tract

Answer: C
The composition of pancreatic secretions is marked by a high level of bicarbonate (HCO_3^-). (Table 3-1) In this example, the patient has a total of 140 mEq of cation (Na + K) and only 70 mEq of anion (Cl). The remaining 70 mEq (to balance the 140 mEq of cation) must be bicarbonate. (See Schwartz 9th ed., p 54, and Table 3-1.)

TABLE 3-1 Composition of GI secretions

Type of Secretion	Volume (mL/24 h)	Na (mEq/L)	K (mEq/L)	Cl (mEq/L)	HCO_3^- (mEq/L)
Stomach	1000–2000	60–90	10–30	100–130	0
Small intestine	2000–3000	120–140	5–10	90–120	30–40
Colon	—	60	30	40	0
Pancreas	600–800	135–145	5–10	70–90	95–115
Bile	300–800	135–145	5–10	90–110	30–40

4. Which of the following diagnoses would be most likely in a patient who presents with normovolemic hyponatremia?
   A. Syndrome of inappropriate anti-diuretic hormone secretion (SIADH)
   B. High output renal failure
   C. Water toxicity
   D. GI losses

Answer: A
Water toxicity would be associated with hypervolemia. Primary renal disease and GI losses would be expected to result in hypovolemia (Fig. 3-3). A normal volume status in the setting of hyponatremia should prompt an evaluation for a syndrome of inappropriate secretion of ADH. (See Schwartz 9th ed., p 56; See Fig. 3-3A.)

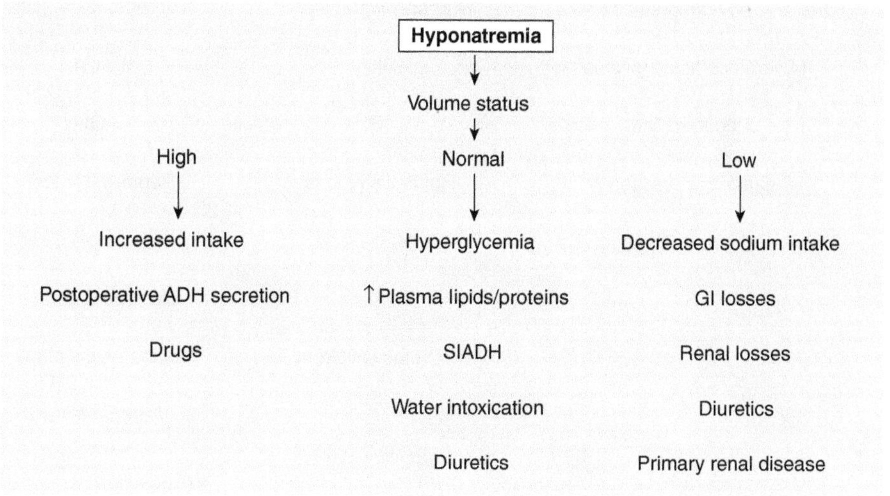

FIG. 3-3A. "ADH = anti-diuretic hormone; SIADH = syndrome of inappropriate secretion of anti-diuretic hormone."

5. A patient is admitted with a glucose of 500 and a sodium of 151. Which of the following is the best approximation of the patient's actual serum sodium level?
   A. 157
   B. 151
   C. 145
   D. 138

Answer: A
Hyponatremia also can be seen with an excess of solute relative to free water, such as with untreated hyperglycemia or mannitol administration. Glucose exerts an osmotic force in the extracellular compartment, causing a shift of water from the intracellular to the extracellular space. Hyponatremia therefore can be seen when the effective osmotic pressure of the extracellular compartment is normal or even high. When hyponatremia in the presence of hyperglycemia is being evaluated, the corrected sodium concentration should be calculated as follows: For every 100-mg/dL increment in plasma glucose above normal, the plasma sodium should decrease by 1.6 mEq/L.

For this patient, a serum glucose of 500 is roughly 400 mg above normal. To correct for the elevated serum glucose, multiply $4 \times 1.6 = 6.4$. This value can be added to 151 to obtain a corrected serum sodium of 157.4. (See Schwartz 9th ed., p 55.)

6. Which of the following is the most likely diagnosis in a patient with a serum sodium of 152 mEq/L, a urine sodium concentration of >20 mEq/L, and a urine osmolality of >300 mOsm/L?
   A. Syndrome of inappropriate anti-diuretic hormone (SIADH)
   B. Diabetes insipidus
   C. Renal tubular disease
   D. Cushing's syndrome

Answer: D

Hypernatremia results from either a loss of free water or a gain of sodium in excess of water. Like hyponatremia, it can be associated with an increased, normal, or decreased extracellular volume (see Fig. 3-3B). Hypervolemic hypernatremia usually is caused either by iatrogenic administration of sodium-containing fluids, including sodium bicarbonate, or mineralocorticoid excess as seen in hyperaldosteronism, Cushing's syndrome, and congenital adrenal hyperplasia. Urine sodium concentration is typically >20 mEq/L and urine osmolarity is >300 mOsm/L. (See Schwartz 9th ed., p 56.)

This patient has hypernatremia, urinary sodium excretion >20mEq/L and elevated urinary osmolality, which are all suggestive of sodium retention.

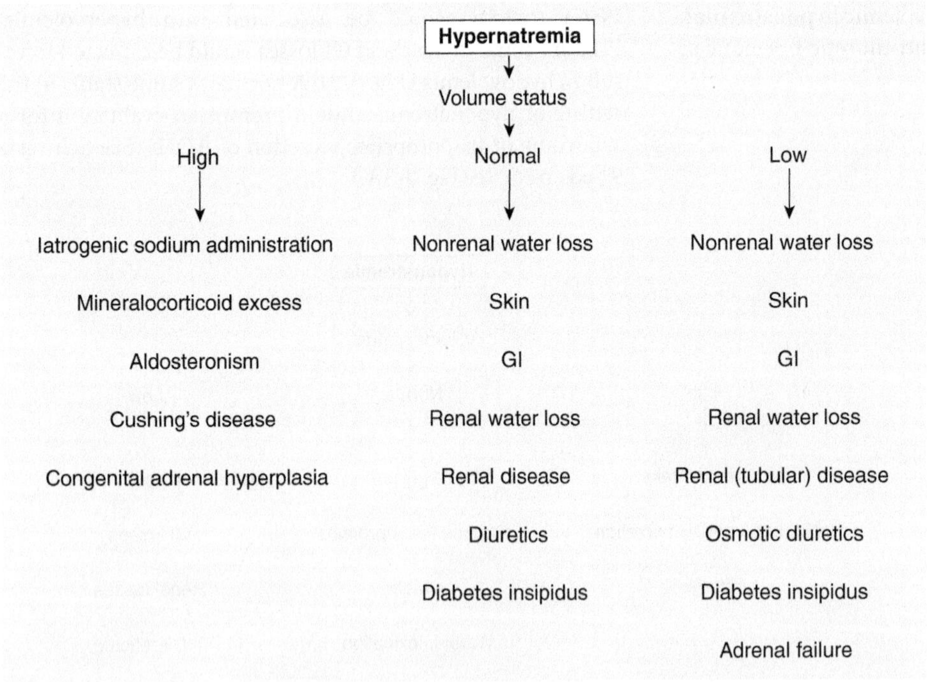

FIG. 3-3B. Differential diagnosis of hypernatremia

7. Which of the following can contribute to hyperkalemia in patients with renal insufficiency?
   A. Loop diuretics
   B. Aspirin
   C. Calcium channel blockers
   D. Nonsteroidal anti-inflammatory drugs (NSAIDs)

Answer: D

A number of medications can contribute to hyperkalemia, particularly in the presence of renal insufficiency, including potassium-sparing diuretics, angiotensinconverting enzyme inhibitors, and NSAIDs. (See Schwartz 9th ed., p 56.) Loop diuretics would tend to contribute to hypokalemia. Aspirin and calcium channel blockers have no significant effect on potassium levels.

8. Which of the following would cause decreased deep tendon reflexes?
   A. Hypokalemia
   B. Hypomagnesemia
   C. Hypocalcemia
   D. Hypoglycemia

Answer: A

Hypokalemia causes decreased deep tendon reflexes. Hypomagnesemia and hypocalcemia cause increased deep tendon reflexes. Hypoglycemia has no effect on deep tendon reflexes. (See Schwartz 9th ed., p 57.)

9. Which of the following is an early ECG change seen in hyperkalemia?
   A. Prolonged PR interval
   B. Sine wave formation
   C. Peaked T waves
   D. Flattened P wave

Answer: C

Although all of the listed findings are associated with hyperkalemia, peaked T waves are the first ECG change seen in most patients.

ECG changes that may be seen with hyperkalemia include high peaked T waves (early), widened QRS complex, flattened P wave, prolonged PR interval (first-degree block), sine wave formation, and ventricular fibrillation. (See Schwartz 9th ed., p 57.)

10. A postoperative patient with a potassium of 2.9 is given 1 mEq/kg replacement with KCl (potassium chloride). Repeat tests after the replacement show the serum K to be 3.0. The most likely diagnosis is
    A. Hypomagnesemia
    B. Hypocalcemia
    C. Metabolic acidosis
    D. Metabolic alkalosis

Answer: A

In cases in which potassium deficiency is due to magnesium depletion, potassium repletion is difficult unless hypomagnesemia is first corrected. (See Schwartz 9th ed., p 57.)

Alkalosis will change serum potassium (a decrease in 0.3 mEq/L for every 0.1 increase in pH above normal). This is not enough to explain the lack of response to repletion in the patient. Metabolic acidosis would not decrease potassium. Calcium does not play a role in potassium metabolism.

11. What is the actual serum calcium level in a patient with an albumin of 2.0 and a serum calcium level of 6.6?
    A. 6.6
    B. 7.4
    C. 8.2
    D. 9.9

Answer: C

When total serum calcium levels are measured, the albumin concentration must be taken into consideration: Adjust total serum calcium down by 0.8 mg/dL for every 1-g/dL decrease in albumin. (See Schwartz 9th ed., p 57.)

$0.8 \times 2 = 1.6 + 6.6 = 8.2$

12. Which of the following is a cause of acute hypophosphatemia?
    A. Chronic ingestion of magnesium containing laxatives
    B. Insulin coma
    C. Refeeding syndrome
    D. Rhabdomyolosis

Answer: C

Acute hypophosphatemia is usually caused by an intracellular shift of phosphate in association with respiratory alkalosis, insulin therapy, refeeding syndrome, and hungry bone syndrome. Clinical manifestations of hypophosphatemia usually are absent until levels fall significantly. In general, symptoms are related to adverse effects on the oxygen availability of tissue and to a decrease in high-energy phosphates and can be manifested as cardiac dysfunction or muscle weakness.

Refeeding syndrome occurs when excess calories are given to a starved person (anorexia). Refeeding syndrome is a potentially lethal condition that can occur with rapid and excessive feeding of patients with severe underlying malnutrition due to starvation, alcoholism, delayed nutritional support, anorexia nervosa, or massive weight loss in obese patients. With refeeding, a shift in metabolism from fat to carbohydrate substrate stimulates insulin release, which results in the cellular uptake of electrolytes, particularly phosphate, magnesium, potassium, and calcium. (See Schwartz 9th ed., p 64.)

Magnesium containing laxatives can cause hypermagnesemia in patients with renal failure but does not affect phosphorous levels.

Patients with insulin coma (hypoglycemia) are not at risk for hypophosphatemia. However, hypophosphatemia is common in diabetic ketoacidosis.

Rhabdomyolosis is associated with hyperkalemia and hyperphosphatemia.

13. Hypomagnesemia clinically resembles which of the following?
    A. Hypoglycemia
    B. Hypokalemia
    C. Hypophosphatemia
    D. Hypocalcemia

Answer: D

The magnesium ion is essential for proper function of many enzyme systems. Depletion is characterized by neuromuscular and central nervous system hyperactivity. Symptoms are similar to those of calcium deficiency, including hyperactive reflexes, muscle tremors, tetany, and positive Chvostek's and Trousseau's signs (see Table 3-2). Severe deficiencies can lead to delirium and seizures. A number of ECG changes also can occur and include prolonged QT and PR intervals, ST-segment depression, flattening or inversion of P waves, torsades de pointes, and arrhythmias. Hypomagnesemia is important not only because of its direct effects on the nervous system but also because it can produce hypocalcemia and lead to persistent hypokalemia. When hypokalemia or hypocalcemia coexists with hypomagnesemia, magnesium should be aggressively replaced to assist in restoring potassium or calcium homeostasis. (See Schwartz 9th ed., p 58.)

TABLE 3-2 Clinical manifestations of abnormalities in potassium, magnesium, and calcium levels

	Increased Serum Levels		
System	**Potassium**	**Magnesium**	**Calcium**
GI	Nausea/vomiting, colic, diarrhea	Nausea/vomiting	Anorexia, nausea/vomiting, abdominal pain
Neuromuscular	Weakness, paralysis, respiratory failure	Weakness, lethargy, decreased reflexes	Weakness, confusion, coma, bone pain
Cardiovascular	Arrhythmia, arrest	Hypotension, arrest	Hypertension, arrhythmia, polyuria
Renal	—	—	Polydipsia
	Decreased Serum Levels		
System	**Potassium**	**Magnesium**	**Calcium**
GI	Ileus, constipation	—	—
Neuromuscular	Decreased reflexes, fatigue, weakness, paralysis	Hyperactive reflexes, muscle tremors, tetany, seizures	Hyperactive reflexes, paresthesias, carpopedal spasm, seizures
Cardiovascular	Arrest	Arrhythmia	Heart failure

14. A patient presents obtunded to the ER with the following labs:

    Na 130   Cl 105   K 3.2 HCO_3 15

    Which of the following is the most likely diagnosis?
    A. GI losses
    B. Lactic acidosis
    C. Methanol ingestion
    D. Renal failure

Answer: A

This is a normal anion gap acidosis. Lactic acidosis, methanol ingestion, and renal failure are all associated with an increased anion gap. (See Schwartz 9th ed., p 58; See Table 3-3.)

Evaluation of a patient with a low serum bicarbonate level and metabolic acidosis includes determination of the anion gap (AG), an index of unmeasured anions.

$$AG = (Na) - (Cl + HCO_3)$$

The normal AG is <12 mmol/L and is due primarily to the albumin effect, so that the estimated AG must be adjusted for albumin (hypoalbuminemia reduces the AG). Corrected AG = actual AG − [2.5(4.5 − albumin)].

Metabolic acidosis with an increased AG occurs either from ingestion of exogenous acid such as from ethylene glycol, salicylates, or methanol, or from increased endogenous acid production of the following:

- Hydroxybutyrate and acetoacetate in ketoacidosis
- Lactate in lactic acidosis
- Organic acids in renal insufficiency

TABLE 3-3 Etiology of metabolic acidosis

Increased Anion Gap Metabolic Acidosis
Exogenous acid ingestion
Ethylene glycol
Salicylate
Methanol
Endogenous acid production
Ketoacidosis
Lactic acidosis
Renal insufficiency
Normal Anion Gap
Acid administration (HCl)
Loss of bicarbonate
GI losses (diarrhea, fistulas)
Ureterosigmoidoscopy
Renal tubular acidosis
Carbonic anhydrase inhibitor

15. Which of the following is the best choice to replace isotonic (serum) fluid loss?
  A. D_5 ¼ NS with 20 mEq KCl/liter
  B. D_5 ½ NS with 20 mEq KCl/liter
  C. 3% saline solution
  D. Lactated Ringer's

Answer: D

Lactated Ringer's best approximates serum electrolytes and would be the fluid of choice to replace isotonic serum fluid loss. (See Schwartz 9th ed., p 60; See Table 3-4.)

TABLE 3-4 Electrolyte solutions for parenteral administration

	Electrolyte Composition (mEq/L)						
Solution	**Na**	**Cl**	**K**	**HCO_3^-**	**Ca**	**Mg**	**mOsm**
Extracellular fluid	142	103	4	27	5	3	280–310
Lactated Ringer's	130	109	4	28	3		273
0.9% Sodium chloride	154	154					308
D_5 0.45% Sodium chloride	77	77					407
D_5W							253
3% Sodium chloride	513	513					1026

D_5 = 5% dextrose; D_5W = 5% dextrose in water.

16. Which of the following should be the first treatment administered to a patient with a potassium level of 6.3 and flattened P waves on their ECG?
  A. Kayexalate
  B. Insulin and glucose
  C. Calcium gluconate
  D. Inhaled albuterol

Answer: C

Treatment options for symptomatic hyperkalemia are listed in Table 3-5. The goals of therapy include reducing the total body potassium, shifting potassium from the extracellular to the intracellular space, and protecting the cells from the effects of increased potassium. For all patients exogenous sources of potassium should be removed, including potassium supplementation in IV fluids and enteral and parenteral solutions. Potassium can be removed from the body using a cation-exchange resin such as Kayexalate that binds potassium in exchange for sodium. It can be administered either orally, in alert patients, or rectally. Immediate measures also should include attempts to shift potassium intracellularly with glucose and bicarbonate infusion. Nebulized albuterol (10 to 20 mg) may also be used. Use of glucose alone will cause a rise in insulin secretion, but in the acutely ill this response may be blunted, and therefore both glucose and insulin may be necessary. Circulatory overload and hypernatremia may result from the administration of Kayexalate and bicarbonate, so care should be exercised when administering these agents to patients with fragile cardiac function. When ECG changes are present, calcium chloride or calcium gluconate (5 to 10 mL of 10% solution) should be administered immediately to counteract the myocardial effects of hyperkalemia. Calcium infusion should be used cautiously in patients receiving digitalis, because digitalis toxicity may be precipitated. All of the aforementioned measures are temporary, lasting from 1 to approximately 4 hours. Dialysis should be considered in severe hyperkalemia when conservative measures fail. (See Schwartz 9th ed., p 60, and Table 3-5.)

TABLE 3-5 Treatment of symptomatic hyperkalemia

Potassium removal
Kayexalate
Oral administration is 15–30 g in 50–100 mL of 20% sorbitol
Rectal administration is 50 g in 200 mL of 20% sorbitol
Dialysis
Shift potassium
Glucose 1 ampule of D_{50} and regular insulin 5–10 units IV
Bicarbonate 1 ampule IV
Counteract cardiac effects
Calcium gluconate 5–10 mL of 10% solution

D_{50} = 50% dextrose.

17. The approximate IV rate for maintenance fluids for a 50-kg patient would be
    A. 75 ml/hr
    B. 90 ml/hr
    C. 105 ml/hr
    D. 120 ml/hr

For the first 0 to 10 kg	Give 100 mL/kg per day
For the next 10 to 20 kg	Give an additional 50 mL/kg per day
For weight >20 kg	Give an additional 20 mL/kg per day

Answer: B

Once the daily total is established, dividing by 24 will give an approximate hourly rate. Alternatively, dividing by 25 (instead of 24) gives a rapid approximate rate. In other words, the hourly IV rate will be

4 ml/kg/hour for the 1st 10 kg
2 ml/kg/hour for the 2nd 10 kg
1 ml/kg/hour for each kg >20 kg

In this example, $4 \times 10 = 40$ (for the 1st 10 kg), $2 \times 10 = 20$ (for the 2nd 10 kg), and $1 \times 30 = 30$ (for the remaining kg). $40 + 20 + 30 = 90$ ml/hr. (The number if one divides by 24 instead of 25 is 87.5 ml/hr.) (See Schwartz 9th ed., p 63.)

CHAPTER 4

Hemostasis, Surgical Bleeding, and Transfusion

BASIC SCIENCE QUESTIONS

1. What percentage of platelets can be sequestered in the spleen?
   A. 15%
   B. 30%
   C. 45%
   D. 60%

Answer: B

Platelets are anucleate fragments of megakaryocytes. The normal circulating number of platelets ranges between 150,000 and 400,000/μL. Up to 30% of circulating platelets may be sequestered in the spleen. (See Schwartz 9th ed., p 68.)

2. Which of the following is required for platelet adherence to exposed areas of an injured vessel?
   A. Prothrombin
   B. von Willebrand factor
   C. Glycoprotein IX
   D. Prostaglandin GI_2

Answer: B

Platelets do not normally adhere to each other or to the vessel wall but can form a plug that aids in cessation of bleeding when vascular disruption occurs. Injury to the intimal layer in the vascular wall exposes subendothelial collagen to which platelets adhere. This process requires von Willebrand's factor (vWF), a protein in the subendothelium that is lacking in patients with von Willebrand's disease. The vWF binds to glycoprotein I/IX/V on the platelet membrane. After adhesion, platelets initiate a release reaction that recruits other platelets from the circulating blood to seal the disrupted vessel. Up to this point, this process is known as *primary hemostasis.*

Prothrombin initiates the common phase of the coagulation cascade, which occurs after primary hemostasis.

Prostaglandin GI is a vasodilator and inhibits platelet aggregation. (See Schwartz 9th ed., p 68.)

3. Which of the following drugs irreversibly inhibits platelet COX (cyclo-oxygenase)?
   A. Ibuprofen
   B. Clopidogrel
   C. Aspirin
   D. Celebrex

Answer: C

Arachidonic acid released from the platelet membranes is converted by COX to prostaglandin $G_2(PGG_2)$ and then to prostaglandin $H_2(PGH_2)$, which, in turn, is converted to TXA_2. TXA_2 has potent vasoconstriction and platelet aggregation effects. Arachidonic acid may also be shuttled to adjacent endothelial cells and converted to prostacyclin (PGI_2), which is a vasodilator and acts to inhibit platelet aggregation. Platelet COX is irreversibly inhibited by aspirin and reversibly blocked by NSAIDs but is not affected by COX-2 inhibitors.

Ibuprofen is a nonsteroidal anti-inflammatory drug (NSAID) and reversibly affects platelet COX.

Both aspirin and clopidogrel irreversibly inhibit platelet function, clopidogrel through selective irreversible inhibition of ADP-induced platelet aggregation and aspirin through irreversible acetylation of platelet prostaglandin synthase.

Celebrex is a COX-2 inhibitor and therefore does not affect platelet COX. (See Schwartz 9th ed., p 68.)

4. An abnormal aPTT (partial thromboplastin time) is associated with an abnormality in which portion of the clotting mechanism?
   A. Platelet aggregation
   B. Intrinsic pathway
   C. Extrinsic pathway
   D. Coagulation (clot formation)

Answer: B

One convenient feature of depicting the coagulation cascade with two merging arms is that commonly used laboratory tests segregate abnormalities of clotting to one of the two arms (Table 4-1). An elevated activated partial thromboplastin time (aPTT) is associated with abnormal function of the intrinsic arm of the cascade, whereas an elevated prothrombin time (PT) is associated with the extrinsic arm. (See Schwartz 9th ed., p 69.)

TABLE 4-1 Coagulation factors tested by the PT and the aPTT

PT	aPTT
VII	XII
X	High molecular weight kininogen
V	Prekallikrein
II (prothrombin)	XI
Fibrinogen	IX
	VIII
	X
	V
	II
	Fibrinogen

aPTT = activated partial thromboplastin time; PT = prothrombin time.

5. Patients with factor V Leiden are predisposed to thrombosis because they have a genetic mutation in factor V which
   A. Leads to inadequate production of factor V
   B. Leads to overproduction of factor V
   C. Leads to an inability to inactivate factor V
   D. Leads to an inability to activate factor V

Answer: C

A third major mechanism of inhibition of thrombin formation is the protein C system. On its formation, thrombin binds to thrombomodulin and activates protein C to activated protein C (APC), which then forms a complex with its cofactor, protein S, on a phospholipid surface. The APC–protein S complex cleaves factors Va and VIIIa so they are no longer able to participate in the formation of tissue factor–VIIa or prothrombinase complexes. Of interest is an inherited form of factor V that carries a genetic mutation, called *factor V Leiden*, that is resistant to cleavage by APC and thus remains active (procoagulant). Patients with factor V Leiden are predisposed to venous thromboembolic events. (See Schwartz 9th ed., p 70.)

CLINICAL QUESTIONS

1. A patient with hemophilia has a factor level of 8%. This is considered to be
   A. Mild hemophilia
   B. Moderately severe hemophilia
   C. Severe hemophilia
   D. Extremely severe hemophilia

Answer: A

Hemophilia A and hemophilia B are inherited as sex-linked recessive disorders with males being affected almost exclusively. The clinical severity of hemophilia A and hemophilia B depends on the measurable level of factor VIII or factor IX in the patient's plasma. Plasma factor levels <1% of normal are considered severe disease, factor levels between 1 and 5% moderately severe, and levels of 5 to 30% mild disease. Patients with severe hemophilia have severe spontaneous bleeds, frequently into joints, which leads to crippling arthropathies. Intramuscular hematomas, retroperitoneal hematomas, and GI, genitourinary, and retropharyngeal bleeding are added clinical sequelae seen with severe disease. Intracranial bleeding and bleeding from the tongue or lingual frenulum may be life-threatening with severe disease. Patients with moderately severe hemophilia have less spontaneous bleeding but are likely to bleed severely after trauma or surgery. Those with mild disease do not bleed spontaneously and frequently have only minor bleeding after major trauma or surgery. Because platelet function is normal in individuals with hemophilia, patients may not bleed immediately after an injury or minor surgery because they have a normal response with platelet activation and formation of a platelet plug. At times, the diagnosis of hemophilia is not made in these patients until after their first minor procedure (e.g., tooth extraction or tonsillectomy). (See Schwartz 9th ed., p 71.)

2. Which of the following is the best choice to prepare a patient with type 1 von Willebrand's disease for surgery?
   A. Recombinant (pure) factor XIII
   B. von Willebrand factor
   C. Factor XIII
   D. Desmopressin

Answer: D

von Willebrand's disease (vWD), the most common congenital bleeding disorder, is characterized by low levels of factor VIII. It is an autosomal dominant disorder, and the primary defect is a low level of vWF, a large glycoprotein responsible for carrying factor VIII and platelet adhesion. The latter is important for normal platelet adhesion to exposed subendothelium and for aggregation under high-shear conditions. Patients with vWD have bleeding that is characteristic of platelet disorders (i.e., easy bruising and mucosal bleeding). Menorrhagia is common in women. vWD is classified into three types. Type I is a partial quantitative deficiency, type II is a qualitative defect, and type III is total deficiency. One treatment for vWD is an intermediate-purity factor VIII concentrate such as Humate-P that contains vWF as well as factor VIII. The second treatment strategy is desmopressin acetate, which raises endogenous vWF levels by triggering release of the factor from endothelial cells. Desmopressin acetate is used once a day because time is needed for synthesis of new stores of vWF within the endothelial cells. Historically, patients with type I disease have been found to respond well to desmopressin acetate. Type II patients may respond, depending on the particular defect. Type III patients are usually unresponsive. (See Schwartz 9th ed., p 71.)

3. Hemophilia C is caused by a deficiency of
   A. Factor VIII
   B. Factor IX
   C. Factor X
   D. Factor XI

Answer: D

Factor XI deficiency, an autosomal recessive inherited condition sometimes referred to as *hemophilia C*, is more prevalent in the Ashkenazi Jewish population. Spontaneous bleeding is rare, but bleeding may occur after surgery, trauma, or invasive procedures. Patients with factor XI deficiency who present with bleeding or for whom surgery is planned and who are known to have bled previously are treated with fresh-frozen plasma (FFP). Each milliliter of plasma contains 1 unit of factor XI activity, so the volume needed depends on the patient's baseline level, the desired level, and the plasma volume. Recombinant factor VIIa treatment has been used successfully in children with severe factor XI deficiency who require major operations such as open heart surgery. Desmopressin acetate also may be useful in the prevention of surgical bleeding in these patients. (See Schwartz 9th ed., pp 71-72.)

4. Factor XIII deficiency most commonly presents as
   A. Severe intraoperative bleeding
   B. Delayed bleeding after injury or surgery
   C. Spontaneous hemarthrosis
   D. Spontaneous gastrointestinal bleeding

Answer: B
Congenital factor XIII deficiency, originally recognized by François Duckert in 1960, is a rare autosomal recessive disease usually associated with a severe bleeding diathesis. The male:female ratio is 1:1. Although acquired factor XIII deficiency has been described in association with hepatic failure, inflammatory bowel disease, and myeloid leukemia, the only significant association with bleeding in children is the inherited deficiency. Bleeding typically is delayed, because clots form normally but are susceptible to fibrinolysis. Umbilical stump bleeding is characteristic, and there is a high risk of intracranial bleeding. Spontaneous abortion is usual in women with factor XIII deficiency unless they receive replacement therapy. Replacement can be accomplished with FFP, cryoprecipitate, or a factor XIII concentrate. Levels of 1 to 2% are usually adequate for hemostasis. (See Schwartz 9th ed., p 72.)

5. Bleeding in patients with thrombasthenia is treated with
   A. Factor V
   B. Factor VII
   C. Fresh frozen plasma transfusion
   D. Platelet transfusion

Answer: D
Thrombasthenia or Glanzmann thrombasthenia is a rare genetic platelet disorder, inherited in an autosomal recessive pattern, in which the platelet glycoprotein IIb/IIIa complex is either lacking or present but dysfunctional. This defect leads to faulty platelet aggregation and subsequent bleeding. The disorder was first described by Dr. Eduard Glanzmann in 1918. Bleeding in thrombasthenic patients must be treated with platelet transfusions. (See Schwartz 9th ed., p 72.)

6. Bleeding in patients with the Bernard-Soulier syndrome is treated with
   A. Factor V
   B. Factor VII
   C. Fresh frozen plasma transfusion
   D. Platelet transfusion

Answer: D
The Bernard-Soulier syndrome, caused by a defect in the glycoprotein Ib/IX/V receptor for vWF, is necessary for platelet adhesion to the subendothelium. Transfusion of normal platelets is required to treat bleeding in these patients. (See Schwartz 9th ed., p 72.)

7. A patient with partial albinism and a bleeding disorder most likely has
   A. von Willebrand's disease
   B. Hemophilia C
   C. Dense granule deficiency
   D. Factor XIII deficiency

Answer: C
The most common intrinsic platelet defect is storage pool disease. It involves loss of dense granules [storage sites for ADP, adenosine triphosphate (ATP), Ca^{2+}, and inorganic phosphate] and α-granules. Dense granule deficiency is the most prevalent of these. It may be an isolated defect or occur with partial albinism in the Hermansky-Pudlak syndrome. Bleeding is variable, depending on the severity of the granule defect. Bleeding is caused by the decreased release of ADP from these platelets.... Patients with mild bleeding as a consequence of a form of storage pool disease can be treated with desmopressin acetate. It is likely that the high levels of vWF in the plasma after desmopressin acetate administration somehow compensate for the intrinsic platelet defect. With more severe bleeding, platelet transfusion is required. (See Schwartz 9th ed., p 72.)

8. First line therapy in an adult with idiopathic thrombocytopenia purpura includes
   A. Retuximab
   B. Splenectomy
   C. IV immunoglobulin
   D. Desmopressin

Answer: C
First line therapy for ITP in adults is corticosteroids and IV immunoglobulin. Splenectomy is second line therapy. Desmopressin is not used in the treatment of ITP. (See Schwartz 9th ed., pp 72-73, and Table 4-2.)

TABLE 4-2 Management of idiopathic thrombocytopenic purpura (ITP) in adults

First Line

a. Corticosteroids: The majority of patients respond, but only a few long term.

b. IV immunoglobulin: Indicated with clinical bleeding, along with platelet transfusion, and when condition is steroid unresponsive. Response is rapid but transient.

c. Anti-D immunoglobulin: Active only in Rh-positive patients before splenectomy. Response is transient.

Second Line

a. Splenectomy: Open or laparoscopic. Criteria include severe thrombocytopenia, high risk of bleeding, and continued need for steroids. Treatment failure may be due to retained accessory splenic tissue.

Third Line

a. Patients for whom first- and second-line therapies fail are considered to have chronic ITP. The objective in this subset of patients is to maintain the platelet count $>20\text{–}30 \times 10^9/L$ and to minimize side effects of medications.

b. Rituximab, an anti-CD20 monoclonal antibody: Acts by eliminating B cells.

c. Alternative medications producing mixed results and a limited response: Danazol, cyclosporine A, dapsone, azathioprine, and vinca alkaloids.

d. Thrombopoietic agents: A new class of drugs for patients with impaired production of platelets rather than accelerated destruction of platelets. Second-generation drugs still in clinical trials include AMG531 and eltrombopag.

9. The diagnosis of heparin-induced thrombocytopenia is made by
   A. >20% fall in platelet count
   B. Positive serotonin release assay
   C. Platelets <25,000 with clinical bleeding
   D. Prolonged aPTT

Answer: B

Heparin-induced thrombocytopenia (HIT) is a form of drug induced immune thrombocytopenia. It is an immunologic disorder in which antibodies against PF4 formed during exposure to heparin affect platelet activation and endothelial function with resultant thrombocytopenia and intravascular thrombosis. The platelet count typically begins to fall 5 to 7 days after heparin has been started, but if it is a re-exposure, the decrease in count may occur within 1 to 2 days. HIT should be suspected if the platelet count falls to <100,000/μL or if it drops by 50% from baseline in a patient receiving heparin. Although HIT is more common with full-dose unfractionated heparin (1 to 3%), it also can occur with prophylactic doses or with low molecular weight heparins. Interestingly, approximately 17% of patients receiving unfractionated heparin and 8% of those receiving low molecular weight heparin develop antibodies against PF4, yet a much smaller percentage develop thrombocytopenia and even fewer clinical HIT. In addition to the mild to moderate thrombocytopenia, this disorder is characterized by a high incidence of thrombosis, which may be arterial or venous. Importantly, the absence of thrombocytopenia in these patients does not preclude the diagnosis of HIT.

The diagnosis of HIT may be made by using either a serotonin release assay or an enzyme-linked immunosorbent assay (ELISA). The serotonin release assay is highly specific but not sensitive, so that a positive test result supports the diagnosis but a negative result does not exclude HIT. On the other hand, the ELISA has a low specificity, so although a positive ELISA result confirms the presence of anti–heparin-PF4, it does not help in the diagnosis of clinical HIT. A negative ELISA result, however, essentially rules out HIT. (See Schwartz 9th ed., p 73.)

10. In addition to stopping the heparin, a patient with heparin-induced thrombocytopenia (HIT) should be treated with
A. Lepirudin
B. Low molecular weight heparin
C. Warfarin
D. Aspirin

Answer: A
The initial treatment of suspected HIT is to stop heparin and begin an alternative anticoagulant. Stopping heparin without adding another anticoagulant is not adequate to prevent thrombosis in this setting. Alternative anticoagulants are primarily thrombin inhibitors. Those available in the United States are lepirudin, argatroban, and bivalirudin. In Canada and Europe, danaparoid also is available. Danaparoid is a heparinoid that has approximately 20% cross reactivity with HIT antibodies in vitro but a much lower cross reactivity in vivo. Because of warfarin's early induction of a hypercoagulable state, only once full anticoagulation with an alternative agent has been accomplished and the platelet count has begun to recover should warfarin be instituted. (See Schwartz 9th ed., p 73.)

11. The most effective treatment for bleeding secondary to thrombotic thrombocytopenic purpura is
A. Platelet transfusion
B. Desmopressin
C. Emergency splenectomy
D. Plasmapheresis

Answer: D
In thrombotic thrombocytopenic purpura (TTP), large vWF molecules interact with platelets, which leads to activation. These large molecules result from inhibition of a metalloproteinase enzyme, ADAMTS13, which cleaves the large vWF molecules. TTP is classically characterized by thrombocytopenia, microangiopathic hemolytic anemia, fever, and renal and neurologic signs or symptoms. The finding of schistocytes on a peripheral blood smear aids in the diagnosis. The most effective treatment for TTP is plasmapheresis, although plasma infusion also has been attempted. A recent study comparing these two modalities reported a higher relapse rate and a higher mortality with plasma infusions. Platelet transfusions are contraindicated. Additionally, rituximab, a monoclonal antibody against the CD20 protein on B lymphocytes, has shown promise as an immunomodulatory therapy directed against acquired TTP, which in the majority of cases is autoimmune mediated. (See Schwartz 9th ed., p 73.)

12. In a 70-kg patient, transfusion of 1 unit of platelets should raise the circulating platelet count by approximately
A. 10,000
B. 20,000
C. 30,000
D. 40,000

Answer: A
One unit of platelet concentrate contains approximately 5.5×10^{10} platelets and would be expected to increase the circulating platelet count by approximately 10,000/μL in the average 70-kg person. (See Schwartz 9th ed., p 74.)

13. Which of the following is a common initiating event for disseminated intravascular coagulation (DIC)?
A. Spider bite
B. Depressed skull fracture
C. Type A influenza
D. Amniotic fluid embolization

Answer: D
The presence of an underlying condition that predisposes a patient to DIC is required for the diagnosis. Specific injuries include central nervous system injuries with embolization of brain matter, fractures with embolization of bone marrow, and amniotic fluid embolization. Embolized materials are potent thromboplastins that activate the DIC cascade. Additional causes include malignancy, organ injury (such as severe pancreatitis), liver failure, certain vascular abnormalities (such as large aneurysms), snakebites, illicit drugs, transfusion reactions, transplant rejection, and sepsis. DIC frequently accompanies sepsis and may be associated with multiple organ failure. (See Schwartz 9th ed., p 74.)

14. A patient with a prolonged aPTT and deep venous thrombosis should be evaluated for which of the following conditions?
   A. Heparin-induced thrombocytopenia
   B. Thrombotic thrombocytopenic purpura
   C. Antiphospholipid syndrome
   D. Protein C deficiency

Answer: C
Among the most common acquired disorder of coagulation inhibition is the antiphospholipid syndrome (APLS), in which the lupus anticoagulant and anticardiolipin antibodies are present. These antibodies may be associated with either venous or arterial thrombosis, or both. In fact, patients who show recurrent thrombosis should be evaluated for APLS. The presence of antiphospholipid antibodies is very common in patients with systemic lupus erythematosus but also may be seen in association with rheumatoid arthritis and Sjögren's syndrome. There are also individuals who have no autoimmune disorders but develop transient antibodies in response to infections or who develop drug-induced APLS. The hallmark of APLS is a prolonged aPTT in vitro but an increased risk of thrombosis in vivo. (See Schwartz 9th ed., p 75.)

15. Which of the following would increase the effect of warfarin and require a decrease in the dose given for anticoagulation?
   A. Barbiturates
   B. Corticosteroids
   C. Cephalosporins
   D. Oral contraceptive pills

Answer: C
Cephalosporins are among the agents that can increase the effect of warfarin. (See Schwartz 9th ed., p 76, and Table 4-3.)

TABLE 4-3 Medications that can alter warfarin dosing

↓ Warfarin effect ↑ Warfarin requirements	Barbiturates, oral contraceptives, estrogen-containing compounds, corticosteroids, adrenocorticotropic hormone
↑ Warfarin effect ↓ Warfarin requirements	Phenylbutazone, clofibrate, anabolic steroids, L-thyroxine, glucagons, amiodarone, quinidine, cephalosporins

16. A patient on chronic warfarin therapy presents with acute appendicitis. INR is 1.4. Which of the following is the most appropriate management?
   A. Proceed immediately with surgery without stopping the warfarin
   B. Stop the warfarin, give fresh frozen plasma, and proceed with surgery
   C. Stop the warfarin and proceed with surgery in 8-12 hours
   D. Stop the warfarin and proceed with surgery in 24-36 hours

Answer: A
Surgical intervention may prove necessary in patients receiving anticoagulation therapy. Increasing experience suggests that surgical treatment can be undertaken without discontinuing the anticoagulant program, depending on the procedure being performed. Furthermore, the risk of thrombotic complications may be increased when anticoagulation therapy is discontinued abruptly. When the aPTT is <1.3 times the control value in a patient receiving heparin or when the INR is <1.5 in a patient taking warfarin, reversal of anticoagulation therapy may not be necessary. However, meticulous surgical technique is mandatory, and the patient must be observed closely throughout the postoperative period. (See Schwartz 9th ed., p 76.)

17. Which of the following devices is most advantageous for hemostasis during a thyroidectomy?
   A. Monopolar electrocautery
   B. Bipolar electrocautery
   C. Harmonic scalpel
   D. Argon coagulator

Answer: C
The Harmonic scalpel is an instrument that cuts and coagulates tissue via vibration at 55 kHz. The device converts electrical energy into mechanical motion. The motion of the blade causes collagen molecules within the tissue to become denatured, forming a coagulum. No significant electrical current flows through the patient. The instrument has proved advantageous in performing thyroidectomy, hemorrhoidectomy, and transsection of the short gastric veins during splenectomy, and in transecting hepatic parenchyma.

Heat achieves hemostasis by denaturation of protein that results in coagulation of large areas of tissue. With cautery, heat is transmitted from the instrument by conduction directly to the tissue. When electrocautery is used, heating occurs by induction from an alternating current source. (See Schwartz 9th ed., p 77.)

18. Which topical anticoagulating agent is best for use in patients with a coagulopathy?
    A. Gelfoam
    B. Fibrin sealant
    C. Thrombostat (topical thrombin)
    D. Surgiceal

Answer: B

Thrombin-derivative products direct the conversion of fibrinogen to fibrin, aiding in clot formation. Thrombin takes advantage of natural physiologic processes, thereby avoiding foreign body or inflammatory reactions, and the wound bed is not disturbed.

Fibrin sealants are prepared from cryoprecipitate (homologous or synthetic) and have the advantage of not promoting inflammation or tissue necrosis. The sealant is administered using a dual syringe compartment system. In one compartment is fibrinogen, factor XIII, fibronectin, and fibrinolysis inhibitors. The second compartment contains thrombin and calcium chloride. The use of fibrin glue is particularly helpful in patients who have received heparin or who have deficiencies in coagulation (e.g., hemophilia or von Willebrand's disease).

Purified gelatin solution can be prepared into several vehicles, including powders, sponges or foams, and sheets or films. Gelatin is hygroscopic, absorbing many times its weight in water or liquid. It is effectively metabolized and degraded by proteinases in the wound bed over a period of 4 to 6 weeks. Gelfoam provides effective hemostasis for operative fields with diffuse small-vessel oozing. Thrombin may be applied to this vehicle to boost hemostasis. Gelatin is relatively inexpensive, readily available, pliable, and easy to handle. Although relatively inert, the implanted gelatin can serve as a nidus for infection. (See Schwartz 9th ed., p 77, and Table 4-4.)

TABLE 4-4 Common hemostatic agents

Hemostatic Agent	Manufacturer	Cost	Comments
Thrombin Products			
Floseal	Baxter	$1500 per 6 pack/5 mL	Disseminated intravascular coagulation may result from intravascular exposure. Solution soaked in gauze or injected over wound bed, forming attachment.
Thrombostat	Parke-Davis	$56–60/5000–10,000 vial	
Thrombin-JMI	King Pharmaceuticals	$285/10,000 units	
Fibrin Sealant			
Tisseel	Baxter	$135/2 mL	Useful in skin grafts or anticoagulated patients. Crosseal contains no aprotinin, reduces anaphylaxis risk.
Crosseal	Johnson & Johnson	$100–150/1 mL	
Gelatin Agents			
Gelfoam	Pfizer	$90/1 g	Forms hydrated meshwork to promote clotting. Can swell. May cause granulomatous reaction.
Surgifoam	Johnson & Johnson	$8–14/gelatin square	

19. What percent of the population is Rh negative?
    A. 5%
    B. 15%
    C. 25%
    D. 35%

Answer: B

Rh-negative recipients should receive transfusions only of Rh-negative blood. However, this group represents only 15% of the population. Therefore, the administration of Rh-positive blood is acceptable if Rh-negative blood is not available. However, Rh-positive blood should not be transfused to Rh-negative females who are of childbearing age. (See Schwartz 9th ed., p 78.)

20. What is the maximum number of units of blood that can be autologously donated for elective surgery as long as the patient's hemoglobin is >11 gm?
    A. A single donation can be made 2-3 weeks before surgery
    B. 2 donations can be made 2 and 4 weeks before surgery
    C. 3 donations can be made, 1 week apart, starting 4 weeks before surgery
    D. 5 donations can be made, 3-4 days apart, starting 6 weeks before surgery

Answer: D

The use of autologous transfusion is growing. Up to 5 units can be collected for subsequent use during elective procedures. Patients can donate blood if their hemoglobin concentration exceeds 11 g/dL or if the hematocrit is >34%. The first procurement is performed 40 days before the planned operation and the last one is performed 3 days before the operation. Donations can be scheduled at intervals of 3 to 4 days. Administration of recombinant human erythropoietin accelerates generation of red blood cells and allows for more frequent harvesting of blood. (See Schwartz 9th ed., p 78.)

21. When should cryoprecipitate be given to a patient needing a massive transfusion of packed RBCs?
    A. 1 unit of cryoprecipitate should be given for each unit of PRBCs
    B. 10 units of cryoprecipitate should be given for each unit of PRBCs
    C. After 6 units of PRBCs, cryoprecipitate should be given if the serum fibrinogen level is <100 mg/dl
    D. Never, fresh frozen plasma will provide the necessary factors

Answer: C

(See Schwartz 9th ed., p 80, and Table 4-5.)

TABLE 4-5	Component therapy administration during massive transfusion
Fresh-frozen plasma (FFP)	As soon as the need for massive transfusion is recognized. For every 6 units of red blood cells (RBCs), give 6 units of FFP (1:1 ratio).
Platelets	For every 6 units of RBCs and plasma, give one 6-pack of platelets. Six random-donor platelet packs = 1 apheresis platelet unit. Keep platelet counts >100,000 μ/L during active hemorrhage control.
Cryoprecipitate	After first 6 units of RBCs, check fibrinogen level. If ≤100 mg/dL, give 20 units of cryoprecipitate (2 g fibrinogen). Repeat as needed, depending on fibrinogen level.

22. Which of the following best assesses clot strength?
    A. Clinical history
    B. Thrombin levels
    C. Ivy bleeding time
    D. Thromboelastogram (TEG)

Answer: D

TEG measures the viscoelastic properties of blood as it is induced to clot in a low-shear environment (resembling sluggish venous flow). The patterns of change in shear elasticity allow the kinetics of clot formation and growth as well as the strength and stability of the formed clot to be determined. The strength and stability data provide information about the ability of the clot to perform the work of hemostasis, whereas the kinetic data determine the adequacy of quantitative factors available for clot formation.

The usefulness of TEG has been sufficiently documented in general surgery, cardiac surgery, urologic surgery, obstetrics, pediatrics, and liver transplantation. It is the only test measuring all dynamic steps of clot formation until eventual clot lysis or retraction. Its role in evaluating coagulopathic patients is still being investigated. (See Schwartz 9th ed., p 84.)

CHAPTER 5

Shock

BASIC SCIENCE QUESTIONS

1. The initiating event in shock is
   A. Hypotension
   B. Decreased cardiac output
   C. Decreased oxygen delivery
   D. Cellular energy deficit

Answer: D

Regardless of etiology, the initial physiologic responses in shock are driven by tissue hypoperfusion and the developing cellular energy deficit. This imbalance between cellular supply and demand leads to neuroendocrine and inflammatory responses, the magnitude of which is usually proportional to the degree and duration of shock. (See Schwartz 9th ed., p. 91, and Fig. 5-1.)

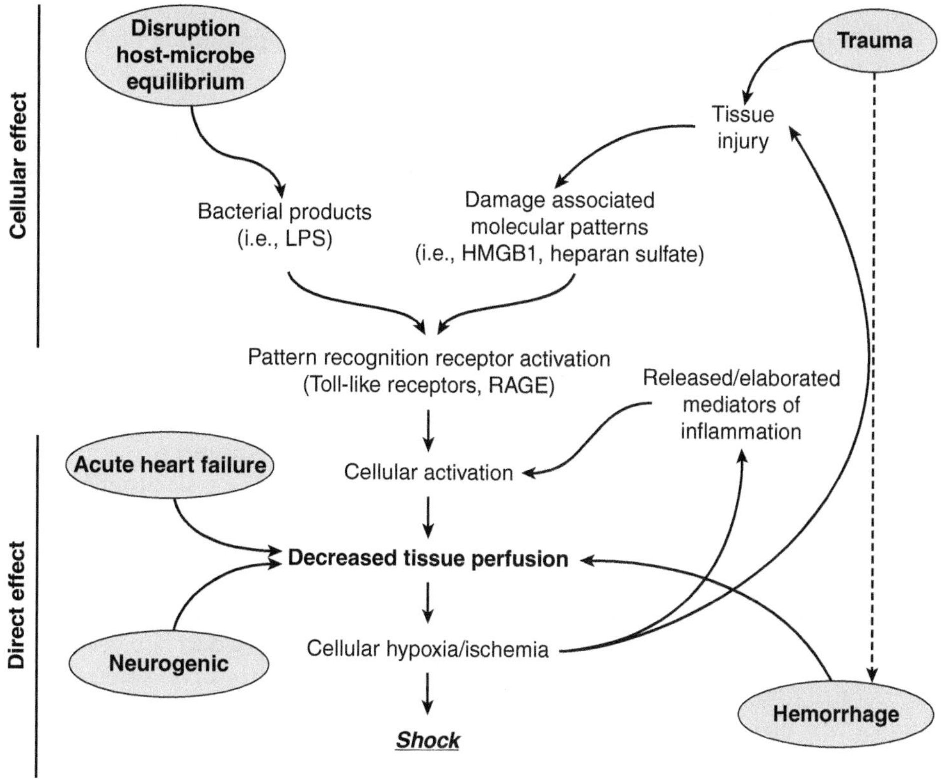

FIG. 5-1. Pathways leading to decreased tissue perfusion and shock. Decreased tissue perfusion can result directly from hemorrhage/hypovolemia, cardiac failure, or neurologic injury. Decreased tissue perfusion and cellular injury can then result in immune and inflammatory responses. Alternatively, elaboration of microbial products during infection or release of endogenous cellular products from tissue injury can result in cellular activation to subsequently influence tissue perfusion and the development of shock. HMGB1 = high mobility group box 1; LPS = lipopolysaccharide; RAGE = receptor for advanced glycation end products.

2. Which of the following can initiate afferent impulses to the CNS which triggers the neuroendocrine response of shock?
   A. Severe alkalosis
   B. Hypothermia
   C. Hyperthermia
   D. Hyperglycemia

Answer: B

Afferent impulses transmitted from the periphery are processed within the central nervous system (CNS) and activate the reflexive effector responses or efferent impulses. These effector responses are designed to expand plasma volume, maintain peripheral perfusion and tissue O_2 delivery, and restore homeostasis. The afferent impulses that initiate the body's intrinsic adaptive responses and converge in the CNS originate from a variety of sources. The initial inciting event usually is loss of circulating blood volume. Other stimuli that can produce the neuroendocrine response include pain, hypoxemia, hypercarbia, acidosis, infection, change in temperature, emotional arousal, or hypoglycemia. The sensation of pain from injured tissue is transmitted via the spinothalamic tracts, resulting in activation of the hypothalamic-pituitary-adrenal axis, as well as activation of the autonomic nervous system (ANS) to induce direct sympathetic stimulation of the adrenal medulla to release catecholamines. (See Schwartz 9th ed., p. 93.)

3. Vasoconstriction is one of the initial physiologic responses to hypovolemic shock. This is mediated by
   A. Activation of alpha adrenergic receptors on the arterioles
   B. Downregulation of alpha adrenergic receptors on the arterioles
   C. Activation of beta adrenergic receptors on the arterioles
   D. Downregulation of beta adrenergic receptors on the arterioles

Answer: A

Direct sympathetic stimulation of the peripheral circulation via the activation of alpha$_1$-adrenergic receptors on arterioles induces vasoconstriction and causes a compensatory increase in systemic vascular resistance and blood pressure. (See Schwartz 9th ed., p. 93.)

4. Anti-diuretic hormone (ADH) is secreted in response to shock and remains elevated for approximately 1 week. Which of the following is seen as a result of this increased level of ADH?
   A. Decreased water permeability in the distal tubule
   B. Increased sodium loss in the distal tubule
   C. Mesenteric vasoconstriction
   D. Mesenteric vasodilation

Answer: C

The pituitary also releases vasopressin or ADH in response to hypovolemia, changes in circulating blood volume sensed by baroreceptors and left atrial stretch receptors, and increased plasma osmolality detected by hypothalamic osmoreceptors. Epinephrine, angiotensin II, pain, and hyperglycemia increase production of ADH. ADH levels remain elevated for about 1 week after the initial insult, depending on the severity and persistence of the hemodynamic abnormalities. ADH acts on the distal tubule and collecting duct of the nephron to increase water permeability, decrease water and sodium losses, and preserve intravascular volume. Also known as *arginine vasopressin*, ADH acts as a potent mesenteric vasoconstrictor, shunting circulating blood away from the splanchnic organs during hypovolemia. This may contribute to intestinal ischemia and predispose to intestinal mucosal barrier dysfunction in shock states. Vasopressin also increases hepatic gluconeogenesis and increases hepatic glycolysis. (See Schwartz 9th ed., p. 94.)

5. Hypoxia at the cellular level decreases ATP production (also called dysoxia). This results in
   A. Changes in intracellular calcium signaling
   B. Increased cell membrane potential
   C. Increased intracellular pH
   D. Increased number of mitochondria

Answer: A

The majority of ATP is generated in our bodies through aerobic metabolism in the process of oxidative phosphorylation in the mitochondria. This process is dependent on the availability of O_2 as a final electron acceptor in the electron transport chain. As O_2 tension within a cell decreases, there is a decrease in oxidative phosphorylation, and the generation of ATP slows. When O_2 delivery is so severely impaired such that oxidative phosphorylation cannot be sustained, the state is termed *dysoxia*. When oxidative phosphorylation is insufficient, the cells shift to anaerobic metabolism and glycolysis to generate ATP. This occurs via the breakdown of cellular glycogen stores to pyruvate. Although glycolysis is a rapid process, it is not efficient, allowing for the production of only 2 mol of ATP from 1 mol of glucose. This is compared to complete oxidation of 1 mol of glucose that produces 38 mol of ATP. Additionally, under hypoxic conditions in anaerobic metabolism, pyruvate is converted into lactate, leading to an intracellular metabolic acidosis. There are numerous consequences secondary to these metabolic changes. The depletion of ATP potentially influences all ATP dependent cellular processes. This includes maintenance of cellular membrane potential, synthesis of enzymes and proteins, cell signaling, and DNA repair mechanisms. Decreased intracellular pH also influences vital cellular functions such as normal enzyme activity, cell membrane ion exchange, and cellular metabolic signaling. These changes also will lead to changes in gene expression within the cell. Furthermore, acidosis leads to changes in calcium metabolism and calcium signaling. Compounded, these changes may lead to irreversible cell injury and death. (See Schwartz 9th ed., p. 95.)

6. Toll-like receptors play a role in the "danger signaling" pathway which modulates the immune response to injury. Stimulation of these receptors is by molecules released from
   A. The pituitary
   B. The adrenal medulla
   C. Macrophages
   D. Damaged cells

Answer: D

Only recently has it been realized that the release of intracellular products from damaged and injured cells can have paracrine and endocrine-like effects on distant tissues to activate the inflammatory and immune responses. This hypothesis, which was first proposed by Matzinger, is known as *danger signaling*. Under this novel paradigm of immune function, endogenous molecules are capable of signaling the presence of danger to surrounding cells and tissues. These molecules that are released from cells are known as *damage associated molecular patterns* (DAMPs, Table 5-1). DAMPs are recognized by cell surface receptors to effect intracellular signaling that primes and amplifies the immune response. These receptors are known as *pattern recognition receptors (PRRs)* and include the Toll-like receptors (TLRs) and the receptor for advanced glycation end products. Interestingly, TLRs and PRRs were first recognized for their role in signaling as part of the immune response to the entry of microbes and their secreted products into a normally sterile environment. (See Schwartz 9th ed., p. 95.)

TABLE 5-1 Endogenous damage associated molecular pattern molecules
Hyaluronan oligomers
Heparan sulfate
Extra domain A of fibronectin
Heat shock proteins 60, 70, Gp96
Surfactant Protein A
b-Defensin 2
Fibrinogen
Biglycan
High mobility group box 1
Uric acid
Interleukin-1a
S-100s
Nucleolin

7. Which of the following cytokines is released immediately after major injury?
   A. IL-10
   B. IL-2
   C. TNF-alpha
   D. TNF-beta

Answer: C

Tumor necrosis factor alpha (TNF-α) was one of the first cytokines to be described, and is one of the earliest cytokines released in response to injurious stimuli. Monocytes, macrophages, and T cells release this potent proinflammatory cytokine. TNF-α levels peak within 90 minutes of stimulation and return frequently to baseline levels within 4 hours. Release of TNF-α may be induced by bacteria or endotoxin, and leads to the development of shock and hypoperfusion, most commonly observed in septic shock. Production of TNF-α also may be induced following other insults, such as hemorrhage and ischemia. TNF-α levels correlate with mortality in animal models of hemorrhage. In contrast, the increase in serum TNF-α levels reported in trauma patients is far less than that seen in septic patients. Once released, TNF-α can produce peripheral vasodilation, activate the release of other cytokines, induce procoagulant activity, and stimulate a wide array of cellular metabolic changes. During the stress response, TNF-α contributes to the muscle protein breakdown and cachexia. (See Schwartz 9th ed., p. 96.)

8. Which of the following is an anti-inflammatory cytokine?
   A. IL-1
   B. IL-6
   C. IL-8
   D. IL-10

Answer: D

IL-10 is an anti-inflammatory cytokine. IL-1, 6, and 8 are proinflammatory cytokines. (See Schwartz 9th ed., p. 96, and Table 5-2.)

TABLE 5-2 Inflammatory mediators of shock

Proinflammatory	Anti-Inflammatory
Interleukin-1a/b	Interleukin-4
Interleukin-2	Interleukin-10
Interleukin-6	Interleukin-13
Interleukin-8	Prostaglandin E_2
Interferon	TGFb
TNF	
PAF	

PAF = platelet activating factor; TGFb = transforming growth factor beta; TNF = tumor necrosis factor.

9. Which of the following best describes the hemodynamic response to neurogenic shock?
   A. Increased cardiac index, unchanged venous capacitance
   B. Increased cardiac index, decreased venous capacitance
   C. Variable change in cardiac index (can increase or decrease), increased venous capacitance
   D. Variable change in cardiac index (can increase or decrease), decreased venous capacitance

Answer: A

(See Schwartz 9th ed., p. 93, and Table 5-3.)

- Increased cardiac index, unchanged venous capacitance is seen in neurogenic shock
- Increased cardiac index, decreased venous capacitance is most most commonly associated with in septic shock
- Variable change in cardiac index (can increase or decrease), increased venous capacitance is most likely seen in cardiogenic shock
- Variable change in cardiac index (can increase or decrease), decreased venous capacitance = septic shock

TABLE 5-3 Hemodynamic responses to different types of shock

Type of Shock	Cardiac Index	SVR	Venous Capacitance	CVP/PCWP	Svo_2	Cellular/Metabolic Effects
Hypovolemic	↓	↑	↓	↓	↓	Effect
Septic	↑↑	↓	↑	↑↓	↑↓	Cause
Cardiogenic	↓↓	↑↑	→	↑	↓	Effect
Neurogenic	↑	↓	→	↓	↓	Effect

The hemodynamic responses are indicated by arrows to show an increase (↑), severe increase (↑↑), decrease (↓), severe decrease (↓↓), varied response (↑↓), or little effect (→). CVP = central venous pressure; PCWP = pulmonary capillary wedge pressure; Svo_2 = mixed venous oxygen saturation; SVR = systemic vascular resistance.

10. What percentage of the blood volume is normally in the splanchnic circulation?
   A. 10%
   B. 20%
   C. 30%
   D. 40%

Answer: B

Most alterations in cardiac output in the normal heart are related to changes in preload. Increases in sympathetic tone have a minor effect on skeletal muscle beds but produce a dramatic reduction in splanchnic blood volume, which normally holds 20% of the blood volume. (See Schwartz 9th ed., p. 94.)

1. Which of the following can be used to indirectly estimate the oxygen debt incurred during shock?
   A. Arterial pH
   B. Arteriolar-alveolar O_2 gradient
   C. Base deficit
   D. Serum bicarbonate

Answer: C

Hypoperfused cells and tissues experience what has been termed *oxygen debt*, a concept first proposed by Crowell in 1961. The O_2 debt is the deficit in tissue oxygenation over time that occurs during shock. When O_2 delivery is limited, O_2 consumption can be inadequate to match the metabolic needs of cellular respiration, creating a deficit in O_2 requirements at the cellular level. The measurement of O_2 deficit uses calculation of the difference between the estimated O_2 demand and the actual value obtained for O_2 consumption. Under normal circumstances, cells can "re-pay" the O_2 debt during reperfusion. The magnitude of the O_2 debt correlates with the severity and duration of hypoperfusion. Surrogate values for measuring O_2 debt include base deficit and lactate levels. (See Schwartz 9th ed., p. 95.)

2. A 70-kg -man with a laceration to the brachial artery loses a total of 800 mL of blood. What ACS (American College of Surgeons) class of hemorrhage would this represent?
   A. Class I hemorrhage
   B. Class II hemorrhage
   C. Class III hemorrhage
   D. Class IV hemorrhage

Answer: B

Blood volume in an adult can roughly be calculated as 70 ml per kg. Therefore, this patient would have a blood volume of 4900 ml (hence the estimate that an adult male has a blood volume of approximately 5 liters). 800 mL is 16.3% of the estimated total blood volume, which would make this a Class II hemorrhage.

Loss of up to 15% of the circulating volume (700 to 750 mL for a 70-kg patient) may produce little in terms of obvious symptoms, while loss of up to 30% of the circulating volume (1.5 L) may result in mild tachycardia, tachypnea, and anxiety. Hypotension, marked tachycardia [i.e., pulse greater than 110 to 120 beats per minute (bpm)], and confusion may not be evident until more than 30% of the blood volume has been lost; loss of 40% of circulating volume (2 L) is immediately life threatening, and generally requires operative control of bleeding (Table 5-4). (See Schwartz 9th ed., p. 99.)

TABLE 5-4 Classification of hemorrhage

	Class			
Parameter	**I**	**II**	**III**	**IV**
Blood loss (mL)	<750	750–1500	1500–2000	>2000
Blood loss (%)	<15	15–30	30–40	>40
Heart rate (bpm)	<100	>100	>120	>140
Blood pressure	Normal	Orthostatic	Hypotension	Severe hypotension
CNS symptoms	Normal	Anxious	Confused	Obtunded

bpm = beats per minute; CNS = central nervous system.

3. A patient arrives in the ER following a motor vehicle accident with multiple injuries. Hypotension in this patient is defined as systolic blood pressure less than
   A. 110
   B. 90
   C. 70
   D. 50

Answer: A

Recent data in trauma patients suggest that a systolic blood pressure (SBP) of less than 110 mmHg is a clinically relevant definition of hypotension and hypoperfusion based upon an increasing rate of mortality below this pressure (Fig. 5-2). (See Schwartz 9th ed., p. 99.)

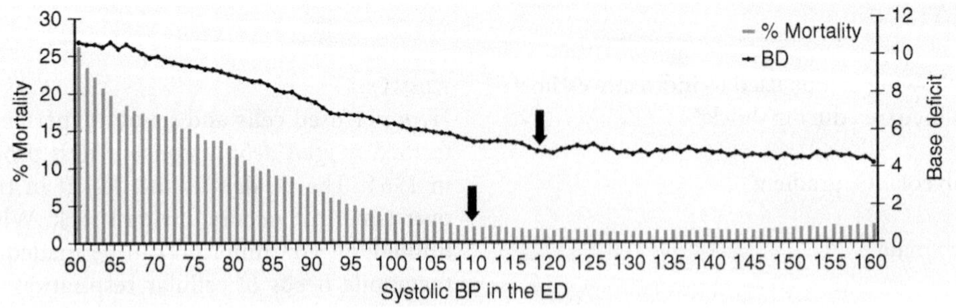

FIG. 5-2. The relationship between systolic blood pressure and mortality in trauma patients with hemorrhage. These data suggest that a systolic blood pressure of less than 110 mmHg is a clinically relevant definition of hypotension and hypoperfusion based upon an increasing rate of mortality below this pressure. Base deficit (BD) is also shown on this graph. ED = emergency department. (Reproduced with permission from Eastridge BJ, Salinas J, McManus JG, et al: Hypotension begins at 110 mmHg: Redefining "hypotension" with data. *J Trauma* 63:291; discussion 297, 2007.)

4. 2 hours following major surgery with significant blood loss, a patient has a base deficit of –6. This would be classified as
   A. Mild base deficit
   B. Moderate base deficit
   C. Severe base deficit
   D. Extremely severe base deficit

Answer: B

Davis and colleagues stratified the extent of base deficit into mild (–3 to –5 mmol/L), moderate (–6 to –9 mmol/L), and severe (less than –10 mmol/L), and from this established a correlation between base deficit upon admission with transfusion requirements, the development of multiple organ failure, and death. (See Schwartz 9th ed., p. 99.)

5. The probability of death for a patient with a base deficit of –6 is approximately
   A. 5%
   B. 15%
   C. 25%
   D. 35%

Answer: C

The probability of death after blunt trauma can be estimated based on logistic regression analysis as described by Siegel. (*Arch Surg* 125:498, 1990). The LD_{50} for base deficit is approximately –11.8. The predicted mortality for a patient with a base deficit of –6 is approximately 25%. (See Schwartz 9th ed., p. 100.)

6. In a patient with ongoing hemorrhage, the risk of death increases 1%
   A. Every 3 minutes in the ER
   B. Every 10 minutes in the ER
   C. Every 30 minutes in the ER
   D. Every 60 minutes in the ER

Answer: A

Control of ongoing hemorrhage is an essential component of the resuscitation of the patient in shock.... Patients who fail to respond to initial resuscitative efforts should be assumed to have ongoing active hemorrhage from large vessels and require prompt operative intervention. Based on trauma literature, patients with ongoing hemorrhage demonstrate increased survival if the elapsed time between the injury and control of bleeding is decreased. Although there are no randomized controlled trials, retrospective studies provide compelling evidence in this regard. To this end, Clarke and colleagues demonstrated that trauma patients with major injuries isolated to the abdomen requiring emergency laparotomy had an increased probability of death with increasing length of time in the emergency department than patients who were in the emergency department for 90 minutes or less. This probability increased approximately 1% for each 3 minutes in the emergency department. (See Schwartz 9th ed., p. 100.)

7. A 24-year-old arrives at the emergency department (ED) with multiple stab wounds to the abdomen, severe blunt trauma to the head (GCS 10), and a systolic blood pressure of 80 mm Hg. An appropriate goal for resuscitation in the ED would be a systolic blood pressure of
   A. 80–90 mm Hg
   B. 90–100 mm Hg
   C. 100–110 mm Hg
   D. 110–120 mm Hg

Answer: A

Reasonable conclusions in the setting of uncontrolled hemorrhage include: Any delay in surgery for control of hemorrhage increases mortality; with uncontrolled hemorrhage attempting to achieve normal blood pressure may increase mortality, particularly with penetrating injuries and short transport times; a goal of SBP of 80 to 90 mmHg may be adequate in the patient with penetrating injury; and profound hemodilution should be avoided by early transfusion of red blood cells. For the patient with blunt injury, where the major cause of death is a closed head injury, the increase in mortality with hypotension in the setting of brain injury must be avoided. In this setting, a SBP of 110 mmHg would seem to be more appropriate. (See Schwartz 9th ed., p. 101.)

8. An INR of 1.5 on arrival to the intensive care unit (ICU) is associated with what probability of death?
   A. INR is not predictive of outcome
   B. 10%
   C. 20%
   D. 30%

Answer: C

Fresh frozen plasma (FFP) should also be transfused in patients with massive bleeding or bleeding with increases in prothrombin or activated partial thromboplastin 1.5 times greater than control. Civilian trauma data show that severity of coagulopathy early after ICU admission is predictive of mortality (Fig. 5-3). (See Schwartz 9th ed., p. 101.)

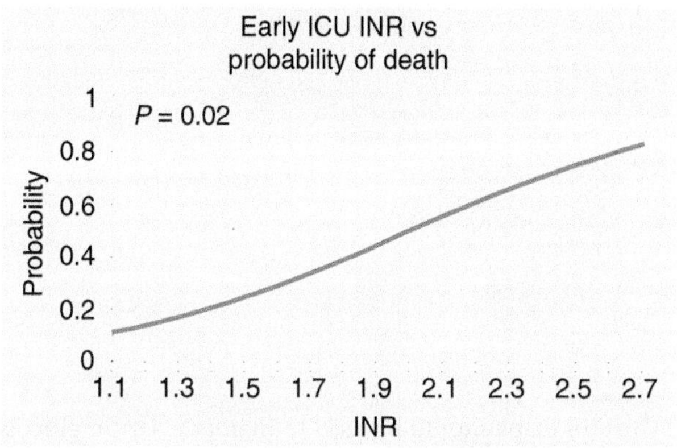

FIG. 5-3. The relationship between coagulopathy and mortality in trauma patients. Civilian trauma data show that severity of coagulopathy as determined by an increasing International Normalized Ratio (INR) early after intensive care unit (ICU) admission is predictive of mortality. (Reproduced with permission from Gonzalez EA, Moore FA, Holcomb JB, et al: Fresh frozen plasma should be given earlier to patients requiring massive transfusion. *J Trauma* 62:112, 2007.)

9. In a patient requiring massive transfusion, 1 unit of FFP (fresh frozen plasma) should be given for every
   A. 1.5 units of PRBCs (1 to 1.5 ratio FFP:PRBC)
   B. 3 units of PRBCs (1 to 3 ratio FFP:PRBC)
   C. 6 units of PRBCs (1 to 6 ratio FFP:PRBC)
   D. 8 units of PRBCs (1 to 8 ratio FFP:PRBC)

Answer: A

Evolving data suggest, more liberal transfusion of FFP in bleeding patients, but the clinical efficacy of FFP requires further investigation. Recent data collected from a U.S. Army combat support hospital in patients who received massive transfusion of packed red blood cells (>10 units in 24 hours) suggest, that a high plasma to RBC ratio (1:1.4 units) was independently associated with improved survival (Fig. 5-4). (See Schwartz 9th ed., p. 101.)

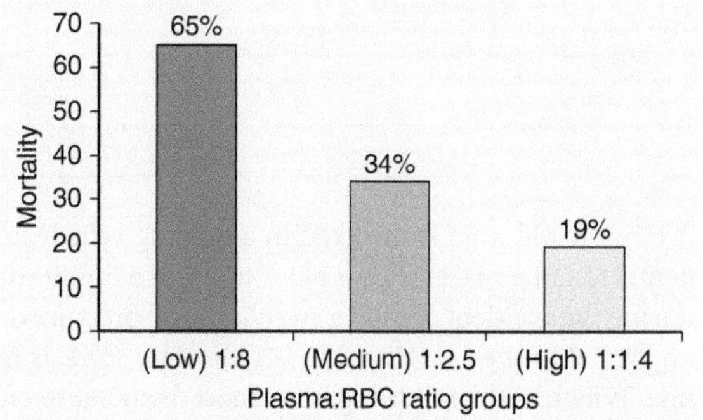

FIG. 5-4. Increasing ratio of transfusion of fresh frozen plasma to red blood cells improves outcome of trauma patients receiving massive transfusions. RBC = red blood cell. (Reproduced with permission from Borgman MA, Spinella PC, Perkins JG, et al: The ratio of blood products transfused affects mortality in patients receiving massive transfusions at a combat support hospital. *J Trauma* 63:805, 2007.)

10. Shock following severe carbon monoxide poisoning is most commonly
    A. Hypovolemic shock
    B. Neurogenic shock
    C. Cardiogenic shock
    D. Vasodilatory shock

Answer: D

The most frequently encountered form of vasodilatory shock is septic shock. Other causes of vasodilatory shock include hypoxic lactic acidosis, carbon monoxide poisoning, decompensated and irreversible hemorrhagic shock, terminal cardiogenic shock, and postcardiotomy shock (Table 5-5). Thus, vasodilatory shock seems to represent the final common pathway for profound and prolonged shock of any etiology. (See Schwartz 9th ed., p. 102.)

TABLE 5-5 Causes of septic and vasodilatory shock
Systemic response to infection
Noninfectious systemic inflammation
Pancreatitis
Burns
Anaphylaxis
Acute adrenal insufficiency
Prolonged, severe hypotension
Hemorrhagic shock
Cardiogenic shock
Cardiopulmonary bypass
Metabolic
Hypoxic lactic acidosis
Carbon monoxide poisoning

11. Insulin drips should be used to maintain serum glucose in nondiabetic, critically ill patients at levels between
    A. 80 and 110 mg/dL
    B. 100 and 150 mg/dL
    C. 120 and 200 mg/dL
    D. 150 and 250 mg/dL

Answer: A

Hyperglycemia and insulin resistance are typical in critically ill and septic patients, including patients without underlying diabetes mellitus. A recent study reported significant positive impact of tight glucose management on outcome in critically ill patients. The two treatment groups in this randomized, prospective study were assigned to receive intensive insulin therapy (maintenance of blood glucose between 80 and 110 mg/dL) or conventional treatment (infusion of insulin only if the blood glucose level exceeded 215 mg/dL, with a goal between 180 and 200 mg/dL). The mean morning glucose level was significantly higher in the conventional treatment as compared to the intensive insulin therapy group (153 vs. 103 mg/dL). Mortality in the intensive insulin treatment group (4.6%) was significantly lower than in the conventional treatment group (8.0%), representing a 42% reduction in mortality. This reduction in mortality was most notable in the patients requiring longer than 5 days in the ICU. Furthermore, intensive insulin therapy reduced episodes of septicemia by 46%, reduced duration of antibiotic therapy, and decreased the need for prolonged ventilatory support and renal replacement therapy. (See Schwartz 9th ed., p. 103.)

12. A 62-year-old man is involved in a moving vehicle accident. He suffered significant blunt trauma to the sternum during the accident. He has a systolic blood pressure of 95 on arrival to the ER. His CVP is 15 and his CXR is normal. Which of the following is the most likely cause of his hypotension?
    A. Cardiac contusion
    B. Spinal cord injury
    C. Myocardial infarction
    D. Intra-abdominal hemorrhage

Answer: C

Relatively few patients with blunt cardiac injury will develop cardiac pump dysfunction. Those who do generally exhibit cardiogenic shock early in their evaluation. Therefore, establishing the diagnosis of blunt cardiac injury is secondary to excluding other etiologies for shock and establishing that cardiac dysfunction is present.

Both spinal cord injury and hemorrhage would result in a low CVP. (See Schwartz 9th ed., p. 106.)

13. A patient unresponsive to catecholamines after an acute myocardial infarction is placed on amrinone. Which of the following is a common side effect of amrinone?
    A. Neutropenia
    B. Anemia
    C. Thrombocytopenia
    D. Bone marrow failure

Answer: C
The phosphodiesterase inhibitors amrinone and milrinone may be required on occasion in patients with resistant cardiogenic shock. These agents have long half-lives and induce thrombocytopenia and hypotension, and use is reserved for patients unresponsive to other treatment. (See Schwartz 9th ed., p. 106.)

14. A 72-year-old woman suffered an acute MI and, 12 hours later, is in cardiogenic shock. Which of the following is the best treatment for this patient?
    A. Inotropic support until stabilized then PTCA (percutaneous transluminal coronary angiography)
    B. Immediate PTCA with stenting, if feasible
    C. Immediate PTCA to define anatomy followed by coronary artery bypass
    D. None of the above

Answer: B
Current guidelines of the American Heart Association recommend percutaneous transluminal coronary angiography for patients with cardiogenic shock, ST elevation, left bundle-branch block, and age less than 75 years. Early definition of coronary anatomy and revascularization is the pivotal step in treatment of patients with cardiogenic shock from acute MI. When feasible, percutaneous transluminal coronary angioplasty (generally with stent placement) is the treatment of choice. Coronary artery bypass grafting seems to be more appropriate for patients with multiple vessel disease or left main coronary artery disease. (See Schwartz 9th ed., p. 106.)

15. An unconscious patient with a systolic BP of 80 and a HR of 80 most likely has
    A. Cardiogenic shock
    B. Hemorrhagic shock
    C. Neurogenic shock
    D. Obstructive shock

Answer: C
Sympathetic input to the heart, which normally increases heart rate and cardiac contractility, and input to the adrenal medulla, which in-creases catecholamine release, may also be disrupted [with spinal cord injury], preventing the typical reflex tachycardia that occurs with hypovolemia.

The classic description of neurogenic shock consists of decreased blood pressure associated with bradycardia (absence of reflexive tachycardia due to disrupted sympathetic discharge), warm extremities (loss of peripheral vasoconstriction), motor and sensory deficits indicative of a spinal cord injury, and radiographic evidence of a vertebral column fracture. (See Schwartz 9th ed., pp. 107-108.)

CHAPTER 6

Surgical Infections

BASIC SCIENCE QUESTIONS

1. Which of the following is a critical component of the initial response to bacterial contamination of the peritoneal cavity?
   A. Macrophage upregulation
   B. Platelet adherence
   C. Phagocytosis by PMNs
   D. Opsonization

Answer: A

Microbes also immediately encounter a series of host defense mechanisms that reside within the vast majority of tissues of the body. These include resident macrophages and low levels of complement (C) proteins and immunoglobulins (Ig, antibodies). Resident macrophages secrete a wide array of substances in response to the above-mentioned processes, some of which appear to regulate the cellular components of the host defense response. Macrophage cytokine synthesis is upregulated. Secretion of tumor necrosis factor alpha (TNF-α), of interleukins (IL)-1β, 6, and 8; and of interferongamma (INF-γ) occurs within the tissue milieu, and, depending on the magnitude of the host defense response, the systemic circulation. Concurrently, a counterregulatory response is initiated consisting of binding proteins (TNF-BP), cytokine receptor antagonists (IL-1ra), and anti-inflammatory cytokines (IL-4 and IL-10). The interaction of microbes with these first-line host defenses leads to microbial opsonization (C1q, C3bi, and IgFc), phagocytosis, and both extracellular (C5b6-9 membrane attack complex) and intracellular microbial destruction (phagocytic vacuoles). Concurrently, the classic and alternate complement pathways are activated both via direct contact with and via IgM > IgG binding to microbes, leading to the release of a number of different complement protein fragments (C3a, C4a, C5a) that are biologically active, acting to markedly enhance vascular permeability. Bacterial cell wall components and a variety of enzymes that are expelled from leukocyte phagocytic vacuoles during microbial phagocytosis and killing act in this capacity as well. (See Schwartz 9th ed., p. 116.)

2. Severe sepsis is differentiated from sepsis by
   A. A history of premorbid conditions such as diabetes
   B. Positive blood cultures for bacteria or fungus
   C. Acute organ failure such as renal insufficiency
   D. Prolonged arterial hypotension

Answer: C

SIRS caused by infection is termed *sepsis* and is mediated by the production of a cascade of proinflammatory mediators produced in response to exposure to microbial products. *Severe sepsis* is characterized as sepsis (defined above) combined with the presence of new-onset organ failure. Severe sepsis is the most common cause of death in noncoronary critical care units, with a mortality rate of 51 cases/100,000 population per year in 2003. *Septic shock* is a state of acute circulatory failure identified by the presence of persistent arterial hypotension (systolic blood pressure <90 mmHg) despite adequate fluid resuscitation, without other identifiable causes. Septic shock is the most severe manifestation of infection, occurring in approximately 40% of patients with severe sepsis; it has an attendant mortality rate of 45 to 60%. (See Schwartz 9th ed., pp. 116-117, and Fig. 6-1.)

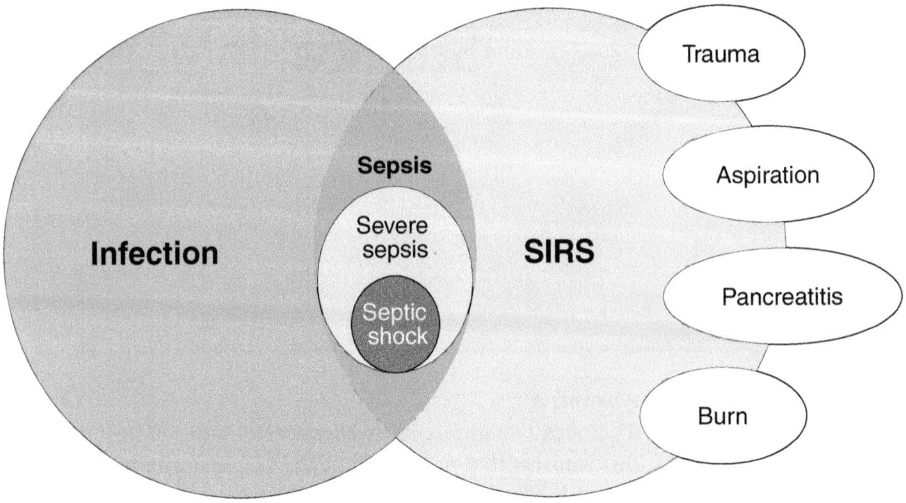

FIG. 6-1. Relationship between infection and systemic inflammatory response syndrome (SIRS). Sepsis is the presence of both infection and the systemic inflammatory response, shown here as the intersection of these two areas. Other conditions may cause SIRS as well (trauma, aspiration, etc.). Severe sepsis (and septic shock) are both subsets of sepsis.

CLINICAL QUESTIONS

1. Which of the following antifungal agents is associated with decreased cardiac contractility?
   A. Liposomal amphotericin B
   B. Itraconozole
   C. Voriconozole
   D. Caspofungin

Answer: B

Itraconozole is associated with decreased cardiac contractility. Liposomal amphotericin B primarily has renal toxicity. Voriconozole can cause visual disturbances (Table 6-1). (See Schwartz 9th ed., p. 118.)

TABLE 6-1 Antifungal agents and their characteristics

Antifungal	Advantages	Disadvantages	Approximate Daily Cost
Amphotericin B	Broad-spectrum, inexpensive	Renal toxicity, premeds, IV only	\$11
Liposomal amphotericin B	Broad-spectrum	Expensive, IV only, renal toxicity	\$600
Azoles			
Fluconazole	IV and PO availability	Narrow-spectrum, drug interactions	\$21 (IV), <\$1 (PO)
Itraconazole	IV and PO availability	Narrow-spectrum, no CSF penetration, drug interactions, decreased cardiac contractility	\$200 (IV), \$3 (PO)
Posaconazole	Broad-spectrum, zygomycete activity	PO only	\$100
Voriconazole	IV and PO availability, broad-spectrum	IV diluent accumulates in renal failure, visual disturbances	\$200 (IV), \$70 (PO)
Echinocandins			
Anidulafungin, caspofungin, micafungin	Broad-spectrum	IV only, poor CNS penetration	\$100–250

CSF = cerebrospinal fluid.

2. Which of the following is the most effective dosing of antibiotics in a patient undergoing elective colon resection?
   A. A single dose given within 30 min prior to skin incision
   B. A single dose given at the time of skin incision
   C. A single preoperative dose + 24 hours of postoperative antibiotics
   D. A single preoperative dose + 48 hours of postoperative antibiotics

Answer: A

By definition, prophylaxis is limited to the time before and during the operative procedure; in the vast majority of cases only a single dose of antibiotic is required, and only for certain types of procedures (see Surgical Site Infections below). However, patients who undergo complex, prolonged procedures in which the duration of the operation exceeds the serum drug half-life should receive an additional dose or doses of the antimicrobial agent. *Nota bene:* There is no evidence that administration of postoperative doses of an antimicrobial agent provides additional benefit, and this practice should be discouraged, as it is costly and is associated with increased rates of microbial drug resistance. (See Schwartz 9th ed., p. 119.)

3. The antibiotic of choice in a penicillin allergic patient undergoing a cholecystectomy for acute cholecystitis is
   A. Ertepenem
   B. Ceftriaxone
   C. Vancomycin + Metronidazole
   D. Fluoroquinolone + Metronidazole

Answer: D

Fluoroquinolone plus either metronidazole or clindamycin (for anaerobic coverage) is indicated in penicillin allergic patients undergoing biliary tract surgery with active infection (Table 6-2). (See Schwartz 9th ed., p. 119.)

TABLE 6-2 Prophylactic use of antibiotics

Site	Antibiotic	Alternative (e.g., penicillin allergic)
Cardiovascular surgery	Cefazolin, cefuroxime	Vancomycin
Gastroduodenal area	Cefazolin, cefotetan, cefoxitin, ampicillin-sulbactam	Fluoroquinolone
Biliary tract with active infection (e.g., cholecystitis)	Ampicillin-sulbactam, ticarcillin-clavulanate, piperacillin-tazobactam	Fluoroquinolone plus clindamycin or metronidazole
Colorectal surgery, obstructed small bowel	Cefazolin plus metronidazole, ertapenem, ticarcillin-clavulanate, piperacillin-tazobactam	Gentamicin or fluoroquinolone plus clindamycin or metronidazole
Head and neck	Cefazolin	Aminoglycoside plus clindamycin
Neurosurgical procedures	Cefazolin	Vancomycin
Orthopedic surgery	Cefazolin, ceftriaxone	Vancomycin
Breast, hernia	Cefazolin	Vancomycin

4. Appropriate duration of antibiotic therapy for most patients with bacterial peritonitis from perforated appendicitis is
   A. 3-5 days
   B. 7-10 days
   C. 14-21 days
   D. >21 days

Answer: A

The majority of studies examining the optimal duration of antibiotic therapy for the treatment of polymicrobial infection have focused on patients who develop peritonitis. Cogent data exist to support the contention that satisfactory outcomes are achieved with 12 to 24 hours of therapy for penetrating GI trauma in the absence of extensive contamination, 3 to 5 days of therapy for perforated or gangrenous appendicitis, 5 to 7 days of therapy for treatment of peritoneal soilage due to a perforated viscus with moderate degrees of contamination, and 7 to 14 days of therapy to adjunctively treat extensive peritoneal soilage (e.g., feculent peritonitis) or that occurring in the immunosuppressed host.

In the later phases of postoperative antibiotic treatment of serious intra-abdominal infection, the absence of an elevated WBC count, lack of band forms of PMNs on peripheral smear, and lack of fever [<38.6°C (100.5°F)] provide close to complete assurance that infection has been eradicated. Under these circumstances, antibiotics can be discontinued with impunity. (See Schwartz 9th ed., p. 122.)

5. Which of the following is NOT a risk factor for developing a surgical site infection (SSI)?
   A. Radiation exposure
   B. Recent surgery
   C. Prolonged hospitalization
   D. Infancy

Answer: D

Infancy is not a risk factor for developing a SSI (Table 6-3). (See Schwartz 9th ed., p. 123.)

TABLE 6-3 Risk factors for development of surgical site infections

Patient factors
Older age
Immunosuppression
Obesity
Diabetes mellitus
Chronic inflammatory process
Malnutrition
Peripheral vascular disease
Anemia
Radiation

(continued)

TABLE 6-3 (continued)
Chronic skin disease
Carrier state (e.g., chronic Staphylococcus carriage)
Recent operation
Local factors
Poor skin preparation
Contamination of instruments
Inadequate antibiotic prophylaxis
Prolonged procedure
Local tissue necrosis
Hypoxia, hypothermia
Microbial factors
Prolonged hospitalization (leading to nosocomial organisms)
Toxin secretion
Resistance to clearance (e.g., capsule formation)

6. Which of the following best estimates the risk of a surgical site infection (SSI) in a patient undergoing an elective low anterior colon resection?
   A. 1-5%
   B. 2-10%
   C. 10-25%
   D. >25%

Answer: C

The expected infection rate in colorectal surgery (clean/contaminated) is 9.4 to 25%.

Clean/contaminated wounds (class II) include those in which a hollow viscus such as the respiratory, alimentary, or genitourinary tracts with indigenous bacterial flora is opened under controlled circumstances without significant spillage of contents. Interestingly, while elective colorectal cases have classically been included as class II cases, a number of studies in the last decade have documented higher SSI rates (9 to 25%). One study identified two thirds of infections presenting after discharge from hospital, highlighting the need for careful follow-up of these patients. Infection is also more common in cases involving entry into the rectal space. (See Schwartz 9th ed., p. 123, and Table 6-4.)

TABLE 6-4 Wound class, representative procedures, and expected infection rates

Wound Class	Examples of Cases	Expected Infection Rates
Clean (class I)	Hernia repair, breast biopsy	1.0–5.4%
Clean/contaminated (class II)	Cholecystectomy, elective GI surgery (not colon)	2.1–9.5%
Clean/contaminated (class II)	Colorectal surgery	9.4–25%
Contaminated (class III)	Penetrating abdominal trauma, large tissue injury, enterotomy during bowel obstruction	3.4–13.2%
Dirty (class IV)	Perforated diverticulitis, necrotizing soft tissue infections	3.1–12.8%

7. Which of the following is NOT one of the components of the PIRO staging system for sepsis?
   A. Pre-existing medical conditions
   B. Nature and extent of the infection
   C. Remedy (type of antibiotics given previously)
   D. Organ dysfunction

Answer: C

The PIRO Staging System stratifies patients based on their predisposing conditions (P), the nature and extent of the infection (I), the nature and magnitude of the host response (R), and the degree of concomitant organ dysfunction (O). Current definitions using this system are listed in Table 6-5. Published trials using this classification system have confirmed the validity of this concept. Further investigation is ongoing to evaluate the clinical utility of this scheme. (See Schwartz 9th ed., p. 117.)

TABLE 6-5 PIRO classification scheme

Domain	Means of Classification
Predisposition	Premorbid illness that affects probability of survival (e.g., immunosuppression, age, genetics)
Insult (infection)	Type of infecting organisms, location of disease, intervention (source control)
Response	SIRS, other signs of sepsis, presence of shock, tissue markers (e.g., C-reactive protein, IL-6)
Organ dysfunction	Organ dysfunction as a number of failing organs or composite score

IL-6 = interleukin-6; SIRS = systemic inflammatory response syndrome.

8. The most common cause of hepatic abscess in the United States is
   A. GI infection with entoameoba histolytica
   B. Pylephlebitis from appendicitis
   C. Biliary tract procedures
   D. Primary bacterial infection after septicemia

Answer: C

Hepatic abscesses are rare, currently accounting for approximately 15 per 100,000 hospital admissions in the United States. Pyogenic abscesses account for approximately 80% of cases, the remaining 20% being equally divided among parasitic and fungal forms. Formerly, pyogenic liver abscesses were caused by pylephlebitis due to neglected appendicitis or diverticulitis. Today, manipulation of the biliary tract to treat a variety of diseases has become a more common cause, although in nearly 50% of patients no cause is identified. (See Schwartz 9th ed., p. 125.)

9. Which of the following has been shown to decrease the rate of pancreatic abscess in patients with necrotizing pancreatitis?
   A. Prophylactic antibiotics
   B. Frequent imaging with percutaneous sampling of new fluid collections
   C. Enteral nutrition
   D. Parenteral nutrition

Answer: C

Current care of patients with severe acute pancreatitis includes staging with dynamic, contrast-enhanced helical CT scan with 3-mm tomographs to determine the extent of pancreatic necrosis, coupled with the use of one of several prognostic scoring systems. Patients who exhibit significant pancreatic necrosis (grade greater than C, Fig. 6-2) should be carefully monitored in the ICU and undergo follow-up CT examination. A recent change in practice has been the elimination of the routine use of prophylactic antibiotics for prevention of infected pancreatic necrosis. Early results were promising; however, several randomized multicenter trials have failed to show benefit and three meta-analyses have confirmed this finding. In two small studies, enteral feedings initiated early, using nasojejunal feeding tubes placed past the ligament of Treitz, have been associated with decreased development of infected pancreatic necrosis, possibly due to a decrease in gut translocation of bacteria. Recent guidelines support the practice of enteral alimentation in these patients, with the addition of parenteral nutrition if nutritional goals cannot be met by tube feeding alone. (See Schwartz 9th ed., p. 126.)

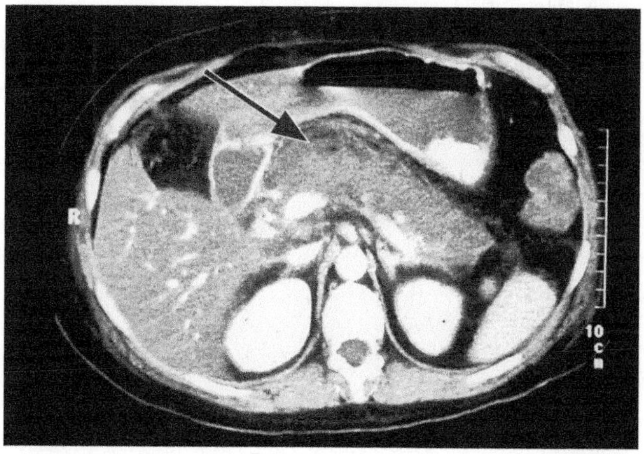

FIG. 6-2. Contrast-enhanced computed tomographic scan of pancreas with severe pancreatic necrosis. Note lack of IV contrast within the boggy pancreatic bed (*large black arrow*).

10. Which of the following is most suggestive of a necrotizing soft tissue infection and would mandate immediate surgical exploration?
    A. A small amount of grayish, cloudy fluid from a wound
    B. Red, swollen extremity which is tender to palpation
    C. Soft tissue infection with a fever >104°
    D. Induration with pitting edema on the trunk

Answer: A

All of the above are suggestive of soft-tissue infection and may, in the appropriate clinical scenario, support surgical exploration. Since time from onset of symptoms to surgical debridement is one of the most critical factors in determination of outcome, the clinician should be willing to explore a potentially-affected area without a definitive diagnosis. Careful examination should be undertaken for an entry site such as a small break or sinus in the skin from which grayish, turbid semipurulent material ("dishwater pus") can be expressed, as well as for the presence of skin changes (bronze hue or brawny induration), blebs, or crepitus. The patient often develops pain at the site of infection that appears to be out of proportion to any of the physical manifestations. Any of these findings mandates immediate surgical intervention, which should consist of exposure and direct visualization of potentially infected tissue (including deep soft tissue, fascia, and underlying muscle) and radical resection of affected areas. (See Schwartz 9th ed., p. 127.)

11. The appropriate duration of antibiotic therapy for nosocomial urinary tract infection is
    A. 3-5 days
    B. 7-10 days
    C. 21 days
    D. Until the patient is asymptomatic and the urinalysis is normal

Answer: A

The presence of a postoperative UTI should be considered based on urinalysis demonstrating WBCs or bacteria, a positive test for leukocyte esterase, or a combination of these elements. The diagnosis is established after more than 10^4 CFU/mL of microbes are identified by culture techniques in symptomatic patients, or more than 10^5 CFU/mL in asymptomatic individuals. Treatment for 3 to 5 days with a single antibiotic that achieves high levels in the urine is appropriate. Postoperative surgical patients should have indwelling urinary catheters removed as quickly as possible, typically within 1 to 2 days, as long as they are mobile. (See Schwartz 9th ed., p. 127.)

12. Surgeons should receive an immunization to protect them from infection with
    A. Hepatitis A
    B. Hepatitis B
    C. Hepatitis C
    D. Human Immunodeficiency Virus

Answer: B

Hepatitis B virus (HBV) is a DNA virus that affects only humans. Primary infection with HBV generally is self-limited (~6% of those infected are over 5 years of age), but can progress to a chronic carrier state. Death from chronic liver disease or hepatocellular cancer occurs in roughly 30% of chronically infected persons. Surgeons and other health care workers are at high risk for this blood-borne infection and should receive the HBV vaccine; children are routinely vaccinated in the United States. This vaccine has contributed to a significant decline in the number of new cases of HBV per year in the United States, from approximately 27,000 new cases in 1984 to 4700 new cases in 2006. In the postexposure setting, hepatitis B immune globulin confers approximately 75% protection from HBV infection.

There are no immunizations available for hepatitis C or HIV. Hepatitis A infection results in a self-limited disease that does not result in chronic infection or chronic liver disease. Hepatitis A infection is spread by the fecal-oral route and indicated groups for vaccination include children between 1 and -2 years of age and travelers to countries where endemic Hepatitis A is present. The magnitude of risk for transmission of Hepatitis A infection to health care workers is low, and does not justify routine immunization. (See Schwartz 9th ed., p. 130.)

13. The typical CXR finding in anthrax is
    A. Bilateral fluffy infiltrates
    B. Pneumothorax
    C. Cavitating lesions, primarily in the upper lobes
    D. Widened mediastinum and pleural effusions

Answer: D

Inhalational anthrax develops after a 1- to 6-day incubation period, with nonspecific symptoms including malaise, myalgia, and fever. Over a short period of time, these symptoms worsen, with development of respiratory distress, chest pain, and diaphoresis. Characteristic chest roentgenographic findings include a widened mediastinum and pleural effusions. A key aspect in establishing the diagnosis is eliciting an exposure history. Rapid antigen tests are currently under development for identification of this gram-positive rod. Drugs such as cephalosporins and trimethoprimsulfamethoxazole are not active against this agent. Postexposure prophylaxis consists of administration of either ciprofloxacin or doxycycline. (See Schwartz 9th ed., p. 130.)

CHAPTER 7

Trauma

CLINICAL QUESTIONS

1. What are the "ABCs" of the primary survey?
   A. Assess (stability of patient), Begin (treatment), Cervical spine (don't forget to stabilize the cervical spine)
   B. Airway, Breathing, Circulation
   C. Accident (history), Background (patient's past medical history), Community (family medical history)
   D. Assess, Begin (to treat), Complete (evaluation of all injuries)

Answer: B

The first step in patient management is performing the primary survey, the goal of which is to identify and treat conditions that constitute an immediate threat to life. The ATLS course refers to the primary survey as assessment of the 'ABCs' (*A*irway with cervical spine protection, *B*reathing, and *C*irculation). Although the concepts within the primary survey are presented in a sequential fashion, in reality they often proceed simultaneously. Life-threatening injuries must be identified (Table 7-1) and treated before advancing to the secondary survey. (See Schwartz 9th ed., pp 136-137.)

TABLE 7-1 Immediately life-threatening injuries to be identified during the primary survey

Airway
Airway obstruction
Airway injury
Breathing
Tension pneumothorax
Open pneumothorax
Flail chest with underlying pulmonary contusion
Circulation
Hemorrhagic shock
Massive hemothorax
Massive hemoperitoneum
Mechanically unstable pelvis fracture
Extremity losses
Cardiogenic shock
Cardiac tamponade
Neurogenic shock
Cervical spine injury
Disability
Intracranial hemorrhage/mass lesion

2. Which of the following would mandate elective intubation in a patient with a normal voice, normal oxygen saturation, and no respiratory distress?
   A. Airway bleeding
   B. Stab wound to the neck with mild swelling in the left lateral neck
   C. Localized right lateral subcutaneous emphysema
   D. Bilateral mandibular fracture

Answer: A

In general, patients who are conscious, do not show tachypnea, and have a normal voice do not require early attention to the airway. Exceptions are patients with penetrating injuries to the neck and an expanding hematoma; evidence of chemical or thermal injury to the mouth, nares, or hypopharynx; extensive subcutaneous air in the neck; complex maxillofacial trauma; or airway bleeding. Although these patients may initially have a satisfactory airway, it may become obstructed if soft tissue swelling, hematoma formation, or edema progresses. In these cases, elective intubation should be performed before evidence of airway compromise. Patients with stab wounds to the neck do not necessarily require elective intubation, nor do patients with localized subcutaneous emphysema. Bilateral mandibular fracture without airway compromise does not require intubation. (See Schwartz 9th ed., pp 136-137.)

3. What is the most common indication for intubation in a trauma patient?
   A. Altered mental status
   B. Inhalation injury
   C. Facial injury
   D. Cervical hematoma

Answer: A

Establishment of a definitive airway (i.e., endotracheal intubation) is indicated in patients with apnea; inability to protect the airway due to altered mental status; impending airway compromise due to inhalation injury, hematoma, facial bleeding, soft tissue swelling, or aspiration; and inability to maintain oxygenation. Altered mental status is the most common indication for intubation. Agitation or obtundation, often attributed to intoxication or drug use, may actually be due to hypoxia. (See Schwartz 9th ed., p 137.)

4. Which of the following trauma patients with airway compromise and failed endotracheal intubation should undergo emergency tracheostomy (rather than a cricothyroidotomy)?
   A. An 84-year-old male with blunt trauma to the neck
   B. A 65-year-old female with a stab wound to the submandibular region
   C. A 16-year-old male with a gunshot wound to the neck
   D. A 6-year-old female with a crush injury to the face

Answer: D

In patients under the age of 8, cricothyroidotomy is contraindicated due to the risk of subglottic stenosis, and tracheostomy should be performed.

Emergent tracheostomy is indicated in patients with laryngotracheal separation or laryngeal fractures, in whom cricothyroidotomy may cause further damage or result in complete loss of the airway. This procedure is best performed in the OR where there is optimal lighting and availability of more equipment (e.g., sternal saw). In these cases, often after a 'clothesline' injury, direct visualization and instrumentation of the trachea usually is done through the traumatic anterior neck defect or after a collar skin incision.

Cricothyroidotomy (Fig. 7-1) is performed through a generous vertical incision, with sharp division of the subcutaneous tissues and strap muscles. Visualization may be improved by having an assistant retract laterally on the neck incision using army-navy retractors. The cricothyroid membrane is verified by digital palpation through the space into the airway. The airway may be stabilized before incision of the membrane using a tracheostomy hook; the hook should be placed under the thyroid cartilage to elevate the airway. A 6.0 tracheostomy tube (maximum diameter in adults) is then advanced through the cricothyroid opening and sutured into place. (See Schwartz 9th ed., p 137.)

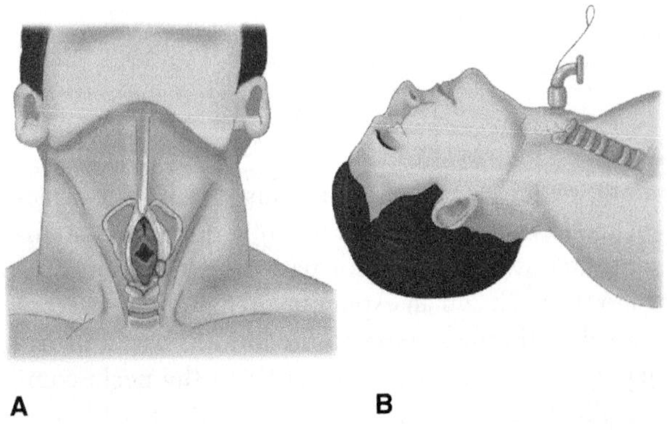

FIG. 7-1. Cricothyroidotomy is recommended for emergent surgical establishment of a patent airway. A vertical skin incision avoids injury to the anterior jugular veins, which are located just lateral to the midline. Hemorrhage from these vessels obscures vision and prolongs the procedure. When a transverse incision is made in the cricothyroid membrane, the blade of the knife should be angled inferiorly to avoid injury to the vocal cords. **A.** Use of a tracheostomy hook stabilizes the thyroid cartilage and facilitates tube insertion. **B.** A 6.0 tracheostomy tube or endotracheal tube is inserted after digital confirmation of airway access.

5. Which of the following is the most appropriate initial treatment of a sucking chest wound?
   A. Occlusive dressing taped on 3 out of 4 sides
   B. Chest tube placed through the wound, cover wound (and chest tube) with occlusive dressing
   C. Chest tube placed in a clear area, closure of the wound
   D. Closure of the wound, intubation of the patient, sedation

Answer: A

An open pneumothorax or 'sucking chest wound' occurs with full-thickness loss of the chest wall, permitting free communication between the pleural space and the atmosphere (Fig. 7-2). This compromises ventilation due to equilibration of atmospheric and pleural pressures, which prevents lung inflation and alveolar ventilation, and results in hypoxia and hypercarbia. Complete occlusion of the chest wall defect without a tube thoracostomy may convert an open pneumothorax to a tension pneumothorax. Temporary management of this injury includes covering the wound with an occlusive dressing that is taped on three sides. This acts as a flutter valve, permitting effective ventilation on inspiration while allowing accumulated air to escape from the pleural space on the untaped side, so that a tension pneumothorax is prevented. Definitive treatment requires closure of the chest wall defect and tube thoracostomy remote from the wound.

Placing the chest tube through the wound would increase infectious complications and would result in inadequate closure and healing of the wound. Closing the wound with a remotely placed chest tube is the definitive treatment, which is usually done in the operating room, rather than as initial treatment in the ED. Closing the wound without a chest tube could result in a tension pneumothorax and is contraindicated. (See Schwartz 9th ed., p 138.)

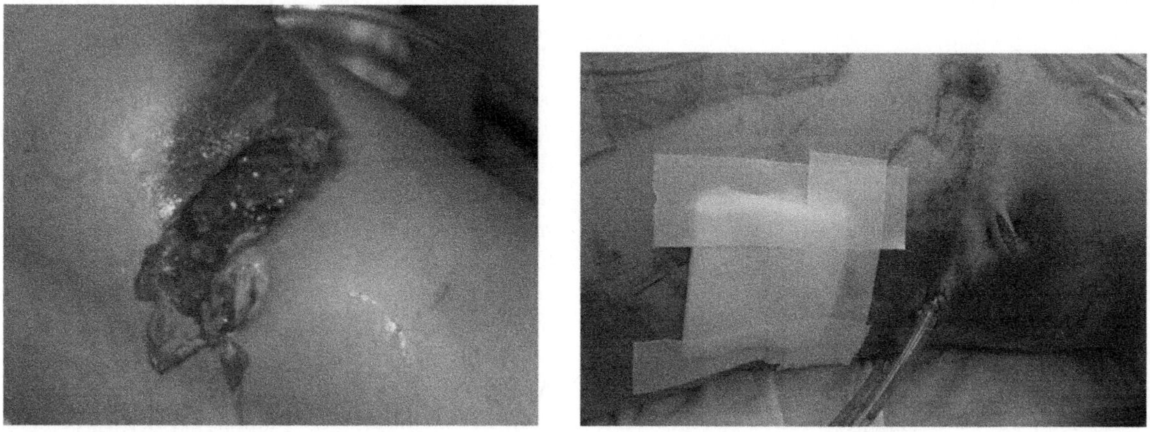

A B

FIG. 7-2. A. Full-thickness loss of the chest wall results in an open pneumothorax. B. The defect is temporarily managed with an occlusive dressing that is taped on three sides, which allows accumulated air to escape from the pleural space and thus prevents a tension pneumothorax. Repair of the chest wall defect and tube thoracostomy remote from the wound is definitive treatment.

6. A 4-year-old is brought hypotensive to the ED after an MVA. Peripheral IV access is attempted but is unsuccessful. The next best access is
   A. Cordis introducer in the internal jugular vein
   B. Single lumen subclavian venous catheter
   C. Double lumen femoral venous catheter
   D. Intraosseous catheter

Answer: D

In hypovolemic patients under 6 years of age, an intraosseous needle can be placed in the proximal tibia (preferred) or distal femur of an unfractured extremity (Fig. 7-3). Flow through the needle should be continuous and does not require pressure. All medications administered IV may be administered in a similar dosage intraosseously. Although safe for emergent use, the needle should be removed once alternative access is established to prevent osteomyelitis. A Cordis introducer would be excessively large for even central veins in a 4-year-old child. Both the single and double lumen catheters would be less effective than the interosseous for resuscitation. According to Poiseuille's law, the flow of liquid through a tube is proportional to the diameter and inversely proportional to the length; therefore, venous lines for volume resuscitation should be short with a large diameter. (See Schwartz 9th ed., p 139.)

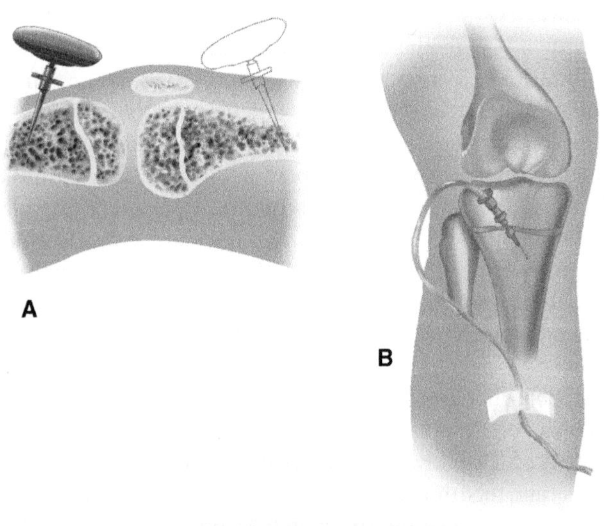

FIG. 7-3. Intraosseous infusions are indicated for children <6 years of age in whom one or two attempts at IV access have failed. **A.** The proximal tibia is the preferred location. Alternatively, the distal femur can be used if the tibia is fractured. **B.** The needle should be directed away from the epiphyseal plate to avoid injury. The position is satisfactory if bone marrow can be aspirated and saline can be easily infused without evidence of extravasation.

7. Which of the following is a life-threatening compromise to circulation and must be identified during the primary survey?
   A. Unstable pelvic fracture
   B. Pericardial effusion
   C. 40% pneumothorax
   D. Femoral artery injury

Answer: A

During the circulation section of the primary survey, four life-threatening injuries that must be identified are (a) massive hemothorax, (b) cardiac tamponade, (c) massive hemoperitoneum, and (d) mechanically unstable pelvic fractures. A pericardial effusion (without tamponade) is not immediately life threatening, nor is a pneumothorax or a peripheral arterial injury. (See Schwartz 9th ed., p 140.)

8. Which of the following is defined as a massive hemothorax?
   A. 1600 ml of intrathoracic blood in a 100-kg woman
   B. 900 m of intrathoracic blood in a 70-kg man
   C. 800 ml of intrathoracic blood in a 50-kg woman
   D. 200 ml of intrathoracic blood in a 20-kg boy

Answer: A

A massive hemothorax is defined as >1500 mL of blood or, in the pediatric population, one third of the patient's blood volume in the pleural space. Blood volume can be quickly estimated by multiplying body weight (in kg) $\times$ 70. So, the 20-kg child would have a total blood volume of 1400 ml. One third of his blood volume (the amount necessary to be classified as a massive hemothorax) would be 466 ml. (See Schwartz 9th ed., p 140.)

9. Which of the following is the best initial treatment for acute traumatic pericardial tamponade in a patient with a systolic blood pressure of 90 mmHg?
   A. Immediate ER thoracotomy with pericardiotomy and repair of the injury
   B. ER thoracoscopy for pericardial drainage
   C. Fluid resuscitation to stabilize blood pressure during transfer to the operating room for definitive repair
   D. Ultrasound guided placement of a pericardial catheter

Answer: D

Early in the course of tamponade, blood pressure and cardiac output will transiently improve with fluid administration. In patients with any hemodynamic disturbance, a pericardial drain is placed using ultrasound guidance (Fig. 7-4). Removing as little as 15 to 20 mL of blood will often temporarily stabilize the patient's hemodynamic status, prevent subendocardial ischemia and associated lethal arrhythmias, and allow transport to the OR for sternotomy. Pericardiocentesis is successful in decompressing tamponade in approximately 80% of cases; the majority of failures are due to the presence of clotted blood within the pericardium. Patients with a SBP <70 mmHg warrant emergency department thoracotomy (EDT) with opening of the pericardium to address the injury. Thoracoscopy is not considered a reasonable treatment for traumatic chest wounds with hypotension. This patient does not warrant an ER thoracotomy because the systolic BP is >70 mmHg. The best initial treatment is ultrasound guided placement of a pericardial catheter followed by transfer to the operating room for definite treatment. (See Schwartz 9th ed., pp 140-141.)

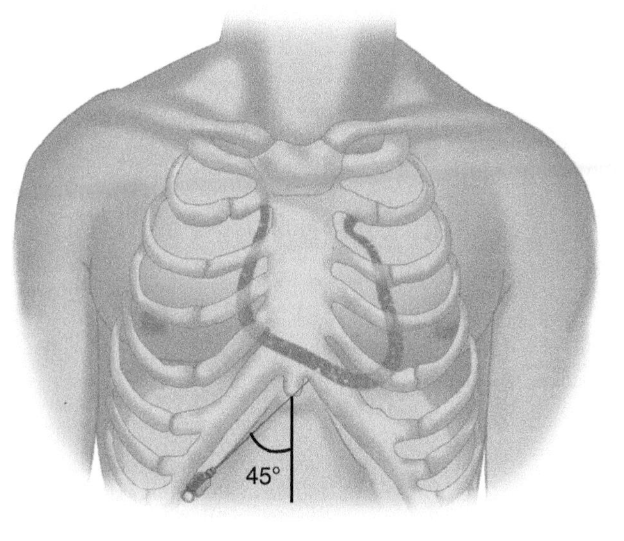

A

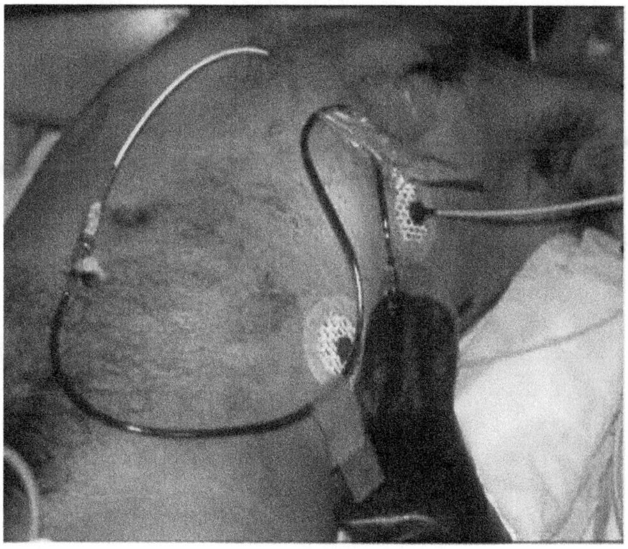

B

FIG. 7-4. Pericardiocentesis is indicated for patients with evidence of pericardial tamponade. A. Access to the pericardium is obtained through a subxiphoid approach, with the needle angled 45 degrees up from the chest wall and toward the left shoulder. B. Seldinger technique is used to place a pigtail catheter. Blood can be repeatedly aspirated with a syringe or the tubing may be attached to a gravity drain. Evacuation of unclotted pericardial blood prevents subendocardial ischemia and stabilizes the patient for transport to the operating room for sternotomy.

10. Which of the following is an indication for emergency department thoracotomy (EDT)?
    A. Witnessed cardiac arrest after a stab wound to the chest with 25 min of CPR
    B. Witnessed cardiac arrest after blunt trauma to the chest with 10 min of CPR
    C. Profound hypotension (systolic BP <70) following a stab wound to the chest
    D. Cardiac arrest in the ED following closed head injury

Answer: C

The utility of EDT has been debated for many years. Current indications are based on 30 years of prospective data (Table 7-2). EDT is associated with the highest survival rate after isolated cardiac injury; 35% of patients presenting in shock and 20% without vital signs (i.e., pulse or obtainable blood pressure) are resuscitated after isolated penetrating injury to the heart. For all penetrating wounds, survival rate is 15%. Conversely, patient outcome is poor when EDT is done for blunt trauma, with 2% survival among patients in shock and <1% survival among those with no vital signs. A is incorrect because there was more than 15 min of CPR following a penetrating injury. B is incorrect because there was more than 5 min of CPR following a blunt injury. D is incorrect; there is no indication for EDT after isolated head injury. (See Schwartz 9th ed., pp 140-142, and Fig. 7-5.)

TABLE 7-2	Current indications and contraindications for emergency department thoracotomy
Indications	
Salvageable postinjury cardiac arrest:	
Patients sustaining witnessed penetrating trauma with <15 min of prehospital CPR	
Patients sustaining witnessed blunt trauma with <5 min of prehospital CPR	
Persistent severe postinjury hypotension (SBP ≤60 mmHg) due to:	
Cardiac tamponade	
Hemorrhage—intrathoracic, intra-abdominal, extremity, cervical	
Air embolism	
Contraindications	
Penetrating trauma: CPR >15 min and no signs of life (pupillary response, respiratory effort, motor activity)	
Blunt trauma: CPR >5 min and no signs of life or asystole	

CPR = cardiopulmonary resuscitation; SBP = systolic blood pressure.

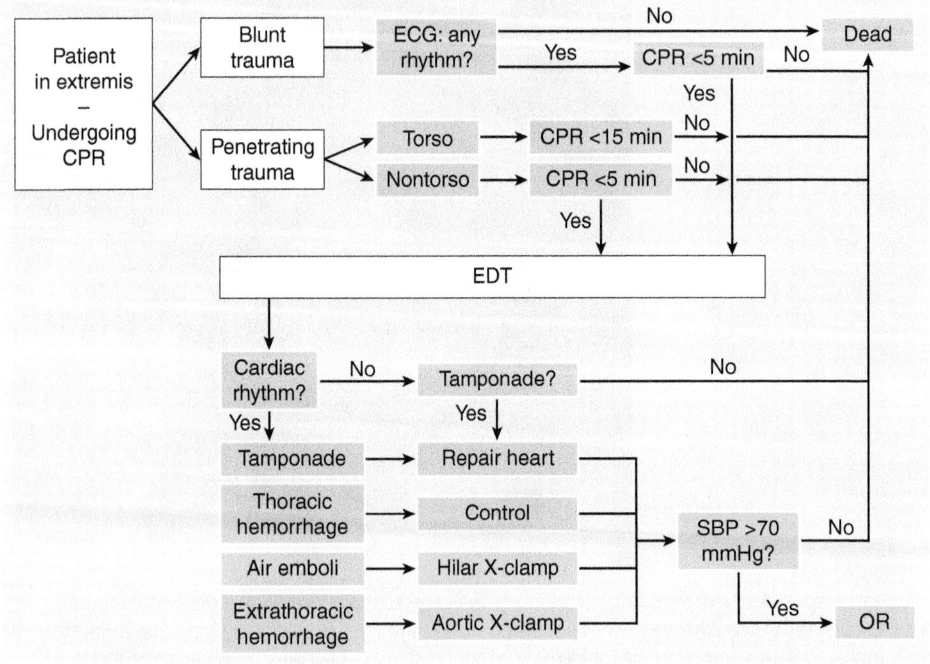

FIG. 7-5. Algorithm directing the use of emergency department thoracotomy (EDT) in the injured patient undergoing cardiopulmonary resuscitation (CPR). ECG = electrocardiogram; OR = operating room; SBP = systolic blood pressure.

11. Management of suspected blunt cardiac injury includes which of the following?
    A. Mandatory admission to an intensive care unit
    B. Cardiac catheterization
    C. Continuous monitoring if EKG abnormalities are noted
    D. Cardiac enzymes

Answer: C

Although as many as one third of patients sustaining significant blunt chest trauma experience blunt cardiac injury, few such injuries result in hemodynamic embarrassment. Patients with electrocardiographic (ECG) abnormalities or dysrhythmias require continuous ECG monitoring and antidysrhythmic treatment as needed. Unless myocardial infarction is suspected, there is no role for measurement of cardiac enzyme levels—they lack specificity and do not predict significant dysrhythmias. The patient with hemodynamic instability requires aggressive resuscitation and may benefit from the placement of a pulmonary artery catheter to optimize preload and guide inotropic support. Echocardiography may be indicated to exclude pericardial tamponade or valvular or septal injuries. It typically demonstrates right ventricular dyskinesia but is less helpful in titrating treatment and monitoring the response to therapy unless done repeatedly. Patients with refractory cardiogenic shock may require placement of an intra-aortic balloon pump to decrease myocardial work and enhance coronary perfusion. Admission to an intensive care unit is determined by whether or not there is need for continuous monitoring and/or any hemodynamic instability. It is not mandatory for all patients with blunt cardiac injury. Cardiac catheterization is not used in the diagnosis or treatment of blunt cardiac injury. Cardiac enzymes are not specific for blunt cardiac injury and do not help in the management of these patients. (See Schwartz 9th ed., p 143.)

12. A patient presents with stable vital signs and respiratory distress after a stab wound to the chest. Chest tubes are placed and an air leak is noted. The patient is electively intubated. The patient arrests after positive pressure ventilation is started. What is the most likely diagnosis?
    A. Unrecognized hemorrhage in the abdomen
    B. Tension pneumothorax
    C. Pericardial tamponade
    D. Air embolism

Answer: D

Air embolism is a frequently overlooked or undiagnosed lethal complication of pulmonary injury. Air emboli can occur after blunt or penetrating trauma, when air from an injured bronchus enters an adjacent injured pulmonary vein (bronchovenous fistula) and returns air to the left heart. Air accumulation in the left ventricle impedes diastolic filling, and during systole air is pumped into the coronary arteries, disrupting coronary perfusion. The typical case is a patient with a penetrating thoracic injury who is hemodynamically stable but experiences arrest after being intubated and placed on positive pressure ventilation. The patient should immediately be placed in Trendelenburg's position to trap the air in the apex of the left ventricle. Emergency thoracotomy is followed by cross-clamping of the pulmonary hilum on the side of the injury to prevent further introduction of air (Fig. 7-6). Air is aspirated from the apex of the left ventricle and the aortic root with an 18-gauge needle and 50-mL syringe. Vigorous massage is used to force the air bubbles through the coronary arteries; if this is unsuccessful, a tuberculin syringe may be used to aspirate air bubbles from the right coronary artery. Once circulation is restored, the patient should be kept in Trendelenburg's position with the pulmonary hilum clamped until the pulmonary venous injury is controlled operatively. (See Schwartz 9th ed., p 144.)

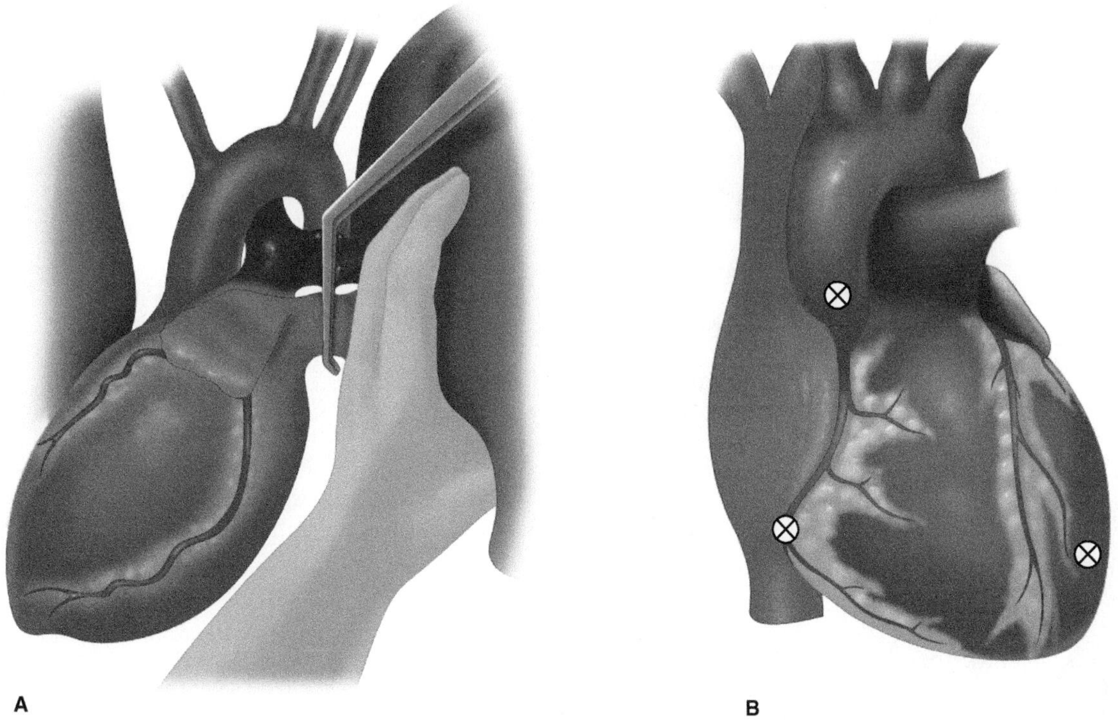

FIG. 7-6. **A.** A Satinsky clamp is used to clamp the pulmonary hilum to prevent further bronchovenous air embolism. **B.** Sequential sites of aspiration include the left ventricle, the aortic root, and the right coronary artery.

13. Which of the following is the expected blood loss in a patient with 6 rib fractures?
    A. 240 ml
    B. 480 ml
    C. 750 ml
    D. 1500 ml

Answer: C

For each rib fracture there is approximately 100 to 200 mL of blood loss; for tibial fractures, 300 to 500 mL; for femur fractures, 800 to 1000 mL; and for pelvic fractures, >1000 mL. Although no single injury may appear to cause a patient's hemodynamic instability, the sum of the injuries may result in life-threatening blood loss. (See Schwartz 9th ed., p 145.)

14. A 25-year-old man presents following blunt trauma to the abdomen. FAST exam shows injury to the spleen. His HR is 110, RR is 25 and he is mildly anxious. What percentage of his blood volume do you estimate he has lost?
    A. <15%
    B. 15-30%
    C. 30-40%
    D. >40%

Answer: B

He has class II hemorrhagic shock (based on his vital signs) with a loss of between 15% and 30% of his blood volume. (See Schwartz 9th ed., p 145, and Table 7-3.)

TABLE 7-3 Signs and symptoms of advancing stages of hemorrhagic shock

	Class I	Class II	Class III	Class IV
Blood loss (mL)	Up to 750	750–1500	1500–2000	>2000
Blood loss (%BV)	Up to 15%	15–30%	30–40%	>40%
Pulse rate	<100	>100	>120	>140
Blood pressure	Normal	Normal	Decreased	Decreased
Pulse pressure (mmHg)	Normal or increased	Decreased	Decreased	Decreased
Respiratory rate	14–20	20–30	30–40	>35
Urine output (mL/h)	>30	20–30	5–15	Negligible
CNS/mental status	Slightly anxious	Mildly anxious	Anxious and confused	Confused and lethargic

BV = blood volume; CNS = central nervous system.

15. A 40-year-old man is struck in the head. A CT scan is obtained, which is shown below. What is the diagnosis?
    A. Subdural hematoma
    B. Subarachnoid hemorrhage
    C. Intraparenchymal hemorrhage
    D. Epidural hematoma

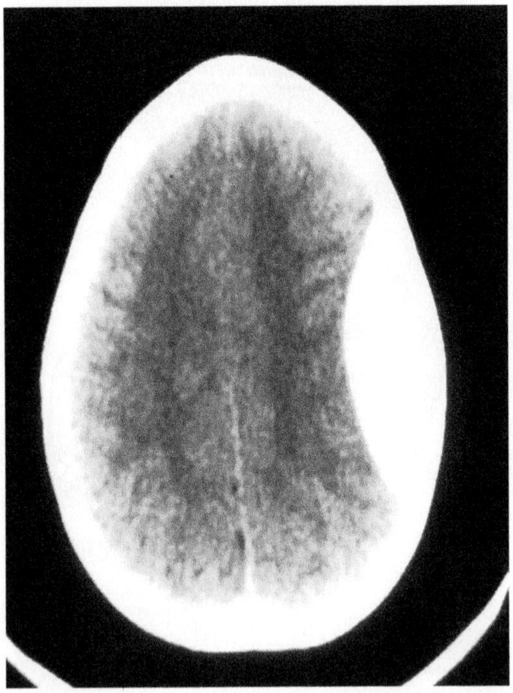

FIG. 7-7. Epidural hematoma. A distinctive convex shape on computed tomographic scan.

Answer: D

This is an epidural hematoma. Epidural hematomas have a distinctive convex shape on computed tomographic scan, whereas subdural hematomas are concave along the surface of the brain. (See Schwartz 9th ed., p 148, and Fig. 7-7.)

16. A 27-year-old man presents to the ED after receiving blows to the head. He opens his eyes with painful stimuli, is confused, and localizes to pain. What is his Glasgow Coma Score?
    A. 13
    B. 11
    C. 9
    D. 7

Answer: B

His score is 2 (eye) + 4 (verbal) + 5 (motor) = 11. (See Schwartz 9th ed., p 145, and Table 7-4.)

TABLE 7-4 Glasgow Coma Scale[a]

		Adults	Infants/Children
Eye opening	4	Spontaneous	Spontaneous
	3	To voice	To voice
	2	To pain	To pain
	1	None	None
Verbal	5	Oriented	Alert, normal vocalization
	4	Confused	Cries but consolable
	3	Inappropriate words	Persistently irritable
	2	Incomprehensible words	Restless, agitated, moaning
	1	None	None

(continued)

TABLE 7-4 (continued)

		Adults	Infants/Children
Motor response	6	Obeys commands	Spontaneous, purposeful
	5	Localizes pain	Localizes pain
	4	Withdraws	Withdraws
	3	Abnormal flexion	Abnormal flexion
	2	Abnormal extension	Abnormal extension
	1	None	None

[a]Score is calculated by adding the scores of the best motor response, best verbal response, and eye opening. Scores range from 3 (the lowest) to 15 (normal).

17. A 75-year-old woman presents to the ED following an MVA. She has decreased strength and sensation in her arms. She has normal strength and sensation in her legs. The most likely diagnosis is
    A. Brown-Séquard syndrome
    B. Anterior cord syndrome
    C. Central cord syndrome
    D. Posterior cord syndrome

Answer: C

There are several partial or incomplete spinal cord injury syndromes. Central cord syndrome usually occurs in older persons who experience hyperextension injuries. Motor function and pain and temperature sensation are preserved in the lower extremities but diminished in the upper extremities. Some functional recovery usually occurs but is often not a return to normal. Anterior cord syndrome is characterized by diminished motor function and pain and temperature sensation below the level of the injury, but position sensing, vibratory sensation, and crude touch are maintained. Prognosis for recovery is poor. Brown-Séquard syndrome is usually the result of a penetrating injury in which the right or left half of the spinal cord is transected. This rare lesion is characterized by the ipsilateral loss of motor function, proprioception, and vibratory sensation, whereas pain and temperature sensation are lost on the contralateral side. Posterior cord syndrome does not exist. (See Schwartz 9th ed., p 150.)

18. The appropriate treatment of an asymptomatic patient with a stab wound to Zone III of the neck is
    A. Observation
    B. CT of the neck
    C. Angiography
    D. Operative exploration

Answer: A

Zone III is the superior portion of the neck, above the angle of the mandible. Asymptomatic patients can be observed. Zone III injuries that are symptomatic should be evaluated with angiography and, if necessary, embolization of bleeding vessels. (See Schwartz 9th ed., pp 150-151, and Figs. 7-8 and 7-9.)

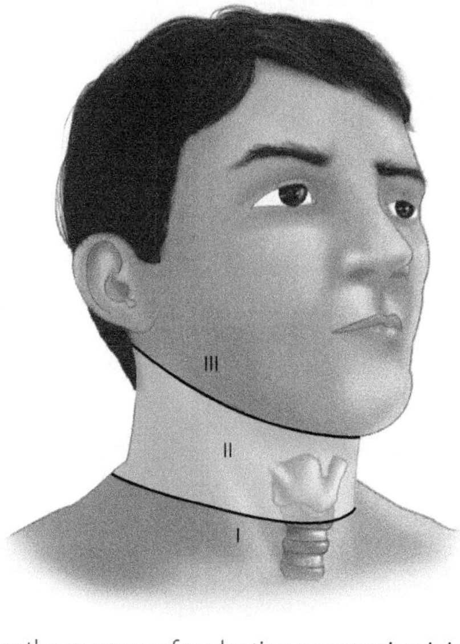

FIG. 7-8. For the purpose of evaluating penetrating injuries, the neck is divided into three zones. Zone I is up to the level of the cricoid and is also known as the *thoracic outlet*. Zone II is located between the cricoid cartilage and the angle of the mandible. Zone III is above the angle of the mandible.

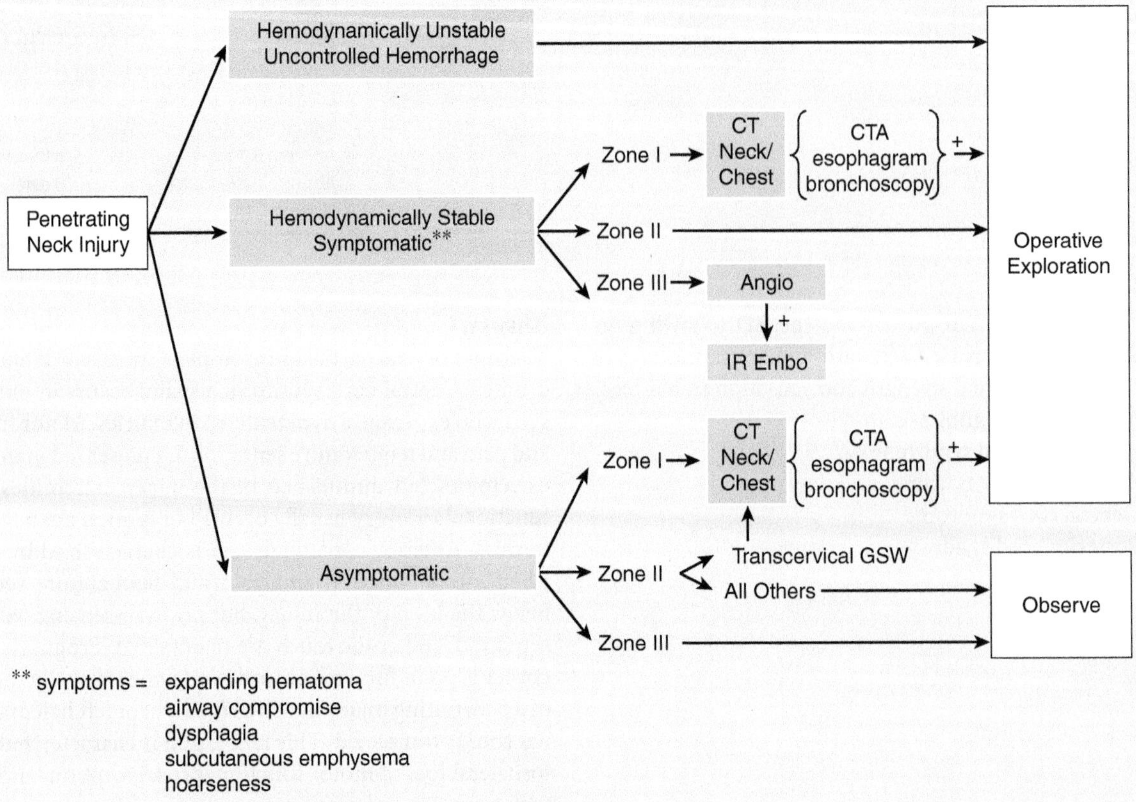

FIG. 7-9. Algorithm for the selective management of penetrating neck injuries. CT = computed tomography; CTA = computed tomographic angiography; GSW = gunshot wound; IR Embo = interventional radiology embolization.

19. Which of the following is an indication for CT of the chest to rule out a thoracic aortic injury?
    A. Left hemopneumothorax
    B. Respiratory distress with multiple rib fractures
    C. High speed head-on MVC with normal chest radiograph
    D. Left scapular pain

Answer: C

At least 7% of patients with a descending torn aorta have a normal chest radiograph. Therefore, screening spiral CT scanning is performed based on the mechanism of injury: high-energy deceleration motor vehicle collision with frontal or lateral impact, motor vehicle collision with ejection, falls of >25 ft, or direct impact (horse kick to chest, snowmobile or ski collision with tree). The CXR finding of a left apical cap is suggestive of a thoracic aortic injury. Multiple rib fractures or scapular pain alone are not suggestive of a thoracic aortic injury. (See Schwartz 9th ed., p 151, and Table 7-5.)

TABLE 7-5	Findings on chest radiograph suggestive of a descending thoracic aortic tear
1. Widened mediastinum	
2. Abnormal aortic contour	
3. Tracheal shift	
4. Nasogastric tube shift	
5. Left apical cap	
6. Left or right paraspinal stripe thickening	
7. Depression of the left main bronchus	
8. Obliteration of the aorticopulmonary window	
9. Left pulmonary hilar hematoma	

20. A 20-year-old young man presents with an left anterior 8th intercostal space stab wound. He is in no distress and a chest x-ray is normal. A diagnostic peritoneal lavage is perfomed and has a RBC count of 8,000/µl and a WBC count of 300/µl. Which of the following is the best treatment for this patient?
    A. Observation only
    B. CT scan
    C. Laparoscopy
    D. Exploratory Laparotomy

Answer: C

Occult injury to the diaphragm must be ruled out in patients with stab wounds to the lower chest. For patients undergoing DPL evaluation, laboratory value cutoffs are different for those with thoracoabdominal stab wounds and for those with standard anterior abdominal stab wounds (see Table 7-6). An RBC count of >10,000/µL is considered a positive finding and an indication for laparotomy; patients with a DPL RBC count between 1000/µL and 10,000/µL should undergo laparoscopy or thoracoscopy. (See Schwartz 9th ed., pp 153-155.)

TABLE 7-6 Criteria for "positive" finding on diagnostic peritoneal lavage

	Anterior Abdominal Stab Wounds	Thoracoabdominal Stab Wounds
Red blood cell count	>100,000/mL	>10,000/mL
White blood cell count	>500/mL	>500/mL
Amylase level	>19 IU/L	>19 IU/L
Alkaline phosphatase level	>2 IU/L	>2 IU/L
Bilirubin level	>0.01 mg/dL	>0.01 mg/dL

21. A 45-year-old, otherwise healthy woman presents after a moving vehicle accident. She is hemodynamically stable and with only minimal tenderness in her right upper quadrant. A FAST exam (focused abdominal sonographic test) is positive with fluid seen in the hepatorenal fossa and the pelvis. Which of the following is the next best step in her management?
    A. Observation only
    B. CT scan
    C. Laparoscopy
    D. Exploratory laparotomy

Answer: B

Patients with fluid on FAST examination, considered a 'positive FAST,' who do not have immediate indications for laparotomy and are hemodynamically stable undergo CT scanning to quantify their injuries. Injury grading using the American Association for the Surgery of Trauma grading scale (Table 7-7) is a key component of nonoperative management of solid organ injuries. Because of the risk of a solid organ injury, observation is not indication. If she has an isolated liver or spleen injury, the correct treatment is most likely observation; therefore, both laparoscopy and laparotomy would not be indicated. (See Schwartz 9th ed., pp 155-157, and Fig. 7-10.)

TABLE 7-7 American Association for the Surgery of Trauma grading scales for solid organ injuries

	Subcapsular Hematoma	Laceration
Liver Injury Grade		
Grade I	<10% of surface area	<1 cm in depth
Grade II	10–50% of surface area	1–3 cm
Grade III	>50% of surface area or >10 cm in depth	>3 cm
Grade IV	25–75% of a hepatic lobe	
Grade V	>75% of a hepatic lobe	
Grade VI	Hepatic avulsion	
Splenic Injury Grade		
Grade I	<10% of surface area	<1 cm in depth
Grade II	10–50% of surface area	1–3 cm
Grade III	>50% of surface area or >10 cm in depth	>3 cm
Grade IV	>25% devascularization	Hilum
Grade V	Shattered spleen Complete devascularization	

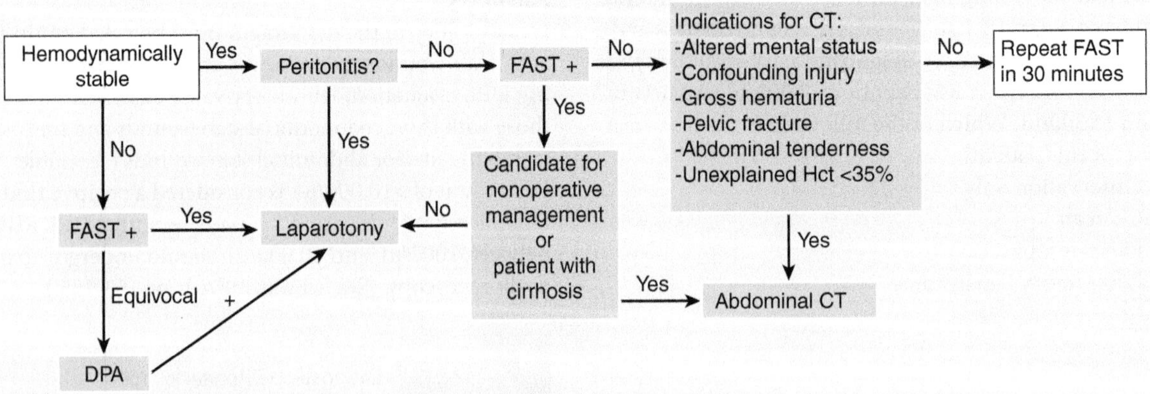

FIG. 7-10. Algorithm for the initial evaluation of a patient with suspected blunt abdominal trauma. CT = computed tomography; DPA = diagnostic peritoneal aspiration; FAST = focused abdominal sonography for trauma; Hct = hematocrit.

22. After CT scan, she is shown to have a liver laceration as shown below. There is a 4-cm laceration into the right lobe with a 10-cm subcapsular hematoma (see Fig. 7-11). What grade liver injury does she have?

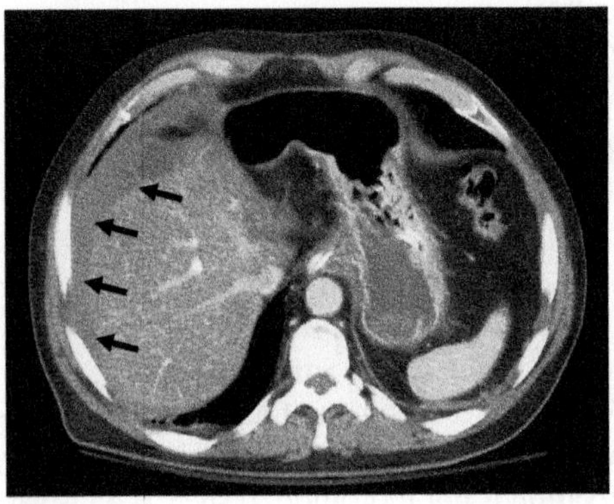

FIG. 7-11.

A. Grade I
B. Grade II
C. Grade III
D. Grade IV

Answer: C
Because she has a laceration >3 cm in depth, she has a Grade III liver injury. (See Schwartz 9th ed., p 157.)

23. A stable patient with a Grade III splenic laceration has the following laboratory results 2 hours after admission: Hg/Hct 8.7/29 Plt 70,000 INR 1.3.
A. No transfusions are indicated
B. Transfuse PRBCs only
C. Transfuse PRBCs and platelets
D. Transfuse PRBCs, platelets, and FFP

Answer: B
Although current critical care guidelines indicate that PRBC transfusion should occur once the patient's hemoglobin level is <7 g/dL, in the acute phase of resuscitation the end-point is 10 g/dL. Fresh-frozen plasma is transfused to keep the patient's International Normalized Ratio (INR) less than 1.5 and partial thromboplastin time (PTT) <45 seconds. Primary hemostasis relies on platelet adherence and aggregation to injured endothelium, and a platelet count of 50,000/μL is considered adequate if platelet function is normal. With massive transfusion, however, platelet dysfunction is common, and therefore a target of 100,000/μL is advocated. If fibrinogen levels drop below 100 mg/dL, cryoprecipitate should be administered. This patient, who is in the acute phase of resuscitation, should receive PRBCs because the Hg is less than 10. Because platelets are >50,000 and INR is <1.5, transfusions of platelets and/or FFP are not indicated. (See Schwartz 9th ed., p 158.)

24. Which of the following is an indication for operative intervention in a patient with an isolated duodenal hematoma?
    A. Hematoma >3 cm in diameter
    B. Total or near total occlusion of the duodenum by the hematoma
    C. Failure to resolve 10 days after admission
    D. Contained retroperitoneal leak

Answer: D

The majority of duodenal hematomas are managed nonoperatively with nasogastric suction and parenteral nutrition. Patients with suspected associated perforation, suggested by clinical deterioration or imaging with retroperitoneal free air or contrast extravasation, should undergo operative exploration. A marked drop in nasogastric tube output heralds resolution of the hematoma, which typically occurs within 2 weeks; repeat imaging to confirm these clinical findings is optional. If the patient shows no clinical or radiographic improvement within 3 weeks, operative evaluation is warranted. The size of the hematoma is not a criterion for operative intervention, nor is the degree of initial occlusion by the hematoma. Patients with persistent duodenal occlusion after 3 weeks should undergo operative exploration. Any sign of perforation is an indication for exploration. (See Schwartz 9th ed., p 179.)

25. Which of the following is an indication for a lower leg fasciotomy?
    A. >35-mmHg difference in diastolic pressure and the compartment pressure
    B. >35-mmHg difference in mean arterial pressure and the compartment pressure
    C. >25mmHg difference in systolic pressure and the compartment pressure
    D. >25-mmHg compartment pressure, regardless of blood pressure

Answer: A

In conscious patients with compartment syndrome, pain is the prominent symptom, and active or passive motion of muscles in the involved compartment increases the pain. Paresthesias may also be described. In the lower extremity, numbness between the first and second toes is the hallmark of early compartment syndrome in the exquisitely sensitive anterior compartment and its enveloped deep peroneal nerve. Progression to paralysis can occur, and loss of pulses is a late sign. In comatose or obtunded patients, the diagnosis is more difficult to secure. In patients with a compatible history and a tense extremity, compartment pressures should be measured with a handheld Stryker device. Fasciotomy is indicated in patients with a gradient of <35 mmHg (gradient = diastolic pressure − compartment pressure), ischemic periods of >6 hours, or combined arterial and venous injuries. In the absence of clinical signs such as pain and paresthesias, compartment pressures are used to determine the need for fasciotomy. The difference between the diastolic blood pressure and the compartment pressure is measured. Patients with a gradient >35 mmHg should undergo a fasciotomy. (See Schwartz 9th ed., p 185, and Fig. 7-12.)

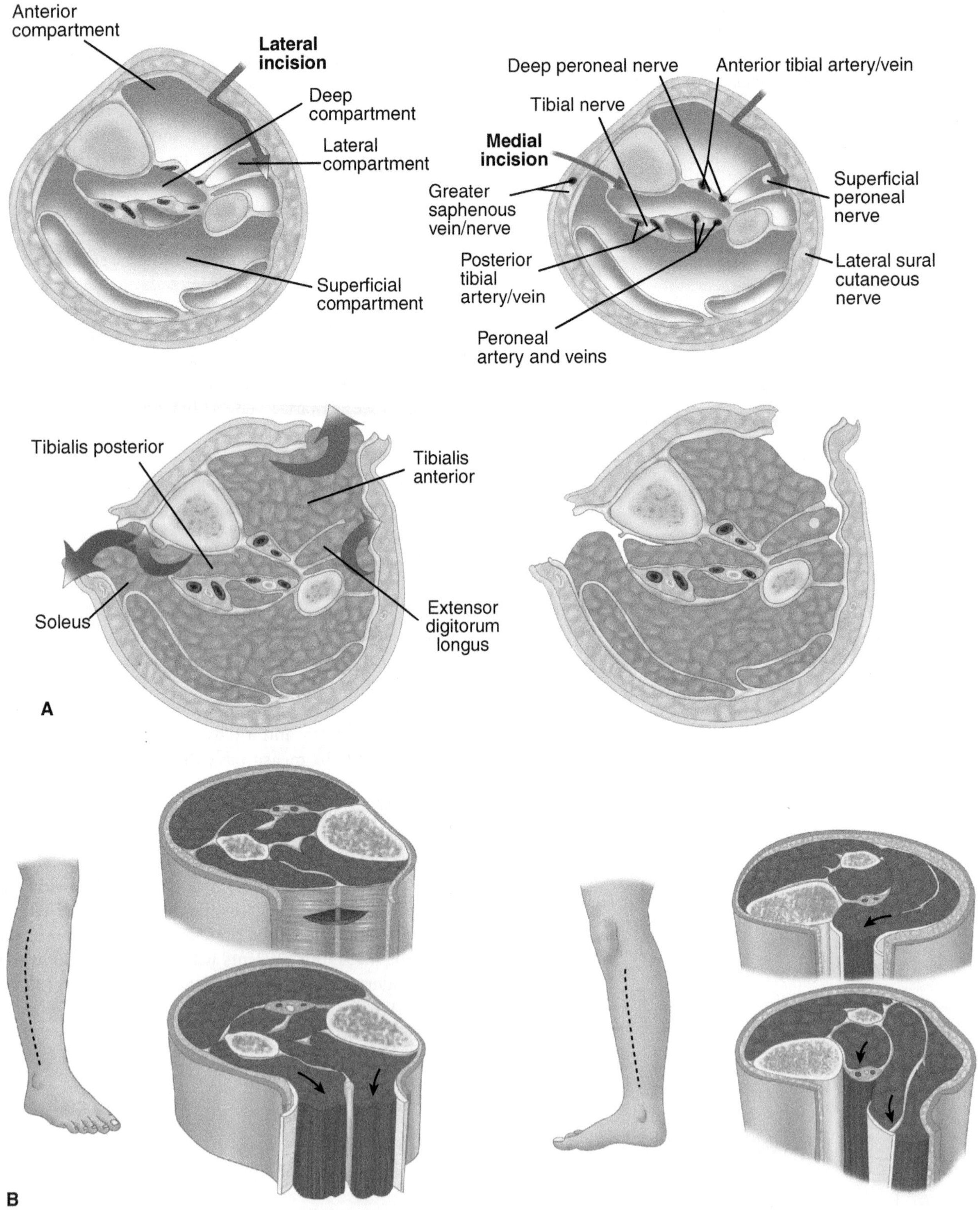

FIG. 7-12. A. The anterior and lateral compartments are approached from a lateral incision, with identification of the fascial raphe between the two compartments. Care must be taken to avoid the superficial peroneal nerve running along the raphe. B. To decompress the deep flexor compartment, which contains the tibial nerve and two of the three arteries to the foot, the soleus muscle must be detached from the tibia.

26. Which of the following bladder pressures is an absolute indication for a decompressive laparotomy?
    A. >5 mmHg
    B. >15 mmHg
    C. >25 mmHg
    D. >35 mmHg

Answer: D

Generally, no specific bladder pressure prompts therapeutic intervention, except when the pressure is >35 mmHg. Rather, emergent decompression is carried out when intra-abdominal hypertension reaches a level at which end-organ dysfunction occurs. Mortality is directly affected by decompression, with 60% mortality in patients undergoing presumptive decompression, 70% mortality in patients with a delay in decompression, and nearly uniform mortality in those not undergoing decompression. Abdominal hypertension is classified by grade, with Grade I (mild) being >10 mmHg (≥13 cm H_2O). Grade IV hypertension or >35 mmHg (≥48 cm H_2O) is an absolute indication for decompressive laparotomy. (See Schwartz 9th ed., p 188, Table 7-8 and Fig. 7-13.)

TABLE 7-8 Abdominal compartment syndrome grading system

	Bladder Pressure	
Grade	**mmHg**	**cm H_2O**
I	10–15	13–20
II	16–25	21–35
III	26–35	36–47
IV	>35	>48

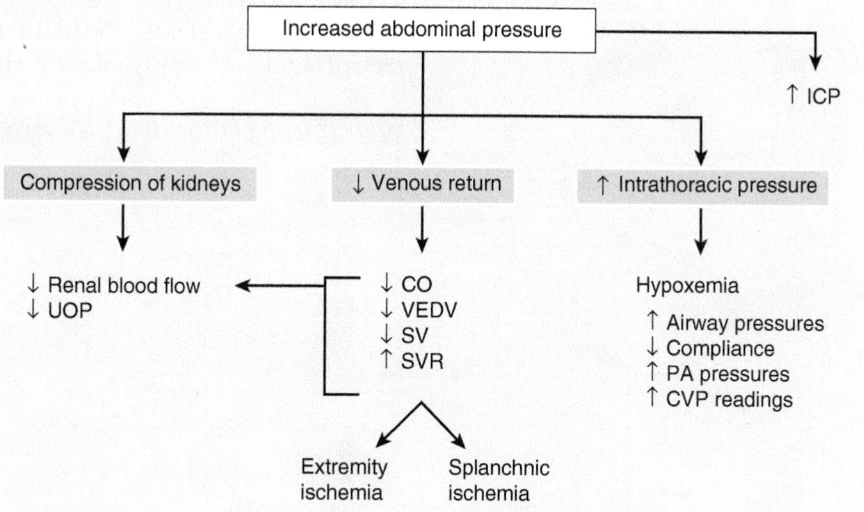

FIG. 7-13. Abdominal compartment syndrome is defined by the end organ sequelae of intra-abdominal hypertension. CO = cardiac output; CVP = central venous pressure; ICP = intracranial pressure; PA = pulmonary artery; SV = stroke volume; SVR = systemic vascular resistance; UOP = urine output; VEDV = ventricular end diastolic volume.

27. Which of the following is a normal physiologic change during pregnancy?
    A. Relative anemia
    B. Decrease in circulating blood volume
    C. Respiratory acidosis
    D. Bradycardia

Answer: A

Pregnancy results in physiologic changes that may impact postinjury evaluation (Table 7-9). Heart rate increases by 10 to 15 beats per minute during the first trimester and remains elevated until delivery. Blood pressure diminishes during the first two trimesters due to a decrease in systemic vascular resistance and rises again slightly during the third trimester (mean values: first = 105/60, second = 102/55, third = 108/67). Intravascular volume is increased by up to 8 L, which results in a relative anemia but also a relative hypervolemia. Consequently, a pregnant woman may lose 35% of her blood volume before exhibiting signs of shock. Pregnant patients have an increase in tidal volume and minute ventilation but a decreased functional residual capacity; this results in a diminished PCO_2 reading and respiratory alkalosis. Also, pregnant patients may desaturate more rapidly, particularly in the supine position and during intubation. Supplemental oxygen is always warranted in the trauma patient but is particularly critical in the injured pregnant patient, because the oxygen dissociation curve is shifted to the left for the fetus compared to the mother (i.e., small changes in maternal oxygenation result in larger changes for the fetus because the fetus is operating in the steep portions of the dissociation curve).

As noted earlier there is a relative anemia during pregnancy, but a hemoglobin level of <11 g/dL is considered abnormal. Additional hematologic changes include a moderate leukocytosis (up to 20,000 mm^3) and a relative hypercoagulable state due to increased levels of factors VII, VIII, IX, X, and XII and decreased fibrinolytic activity. (See Schwartz 9th ed., pp 190-191.)

TABLE 7-9 Physiologic effects of pregnancy
Cardiovascular
Increase in heart rate by 10–15 bpm
Decreased systemic vascular resistance resulting in:
(a) Increased intravascular volume
(b) Decreased blood pressure during the first two trimesters
Pulmonary
Elevated diaphragm
Increased tidal volume
Increased minute ventilation
Decreased functional residual capacity
Hematopoietic
Relative anemia
Leukocytosis
Hypercoagulability
(a) Increased levels of factors VII, VIII, IX, X, XII
(b) Decreased fibrinolytic activity
Other
Decreased competency of lower esophageal sphincter
Increased enzyme levels on liver function tests
Impaired gallbladder contractions
Decreased plasma albumin level
Decreased blood urea nitrogen and creatinine levels
Hydronephrosis and hydroureter

CHAPTER 8

Burns

BASIC SCIENCE QUESTIONS

1. The affinity of carbon monoxide for hemoglobin is
   A. 2-5 times greater than oxygen
   B. 20-50 times greater than oxygen
   C. 200-250 times greater than oxygen
   D. 2000-2500 times greater than oxygen

Answer: C
Another important contributor to early mortality in burns is carbon monoxide (CO) poisoning resulting from smoke inhalation. The affinity of CO for hemoglobin is approximately 200–250 times more than that of oxygen, which decreases the levels of normal oxygenated hemoglobin and can quickly lead to anoxia and death. Unexpected neurologic symptoms should raise the level of suspicion, and an arterial carboxyhemoglobin level must be obtained because pulse oximetry is falsely elevated. (See Schwartz 9th ed., p 198.)

2. A 100-kg patient with a 50% TBSA full thickness burn receives 10 L of 0.9% NaCl solution in transit to the hospital. His laboratory values 6 hours after the injury are likely to reflect which of the following:
   A. Acidosis
   B. Alkalosis
   C. Hypoxia
   D. Dilutional anemia

Answer: A
The most commonly used formula, the Parkland or Baxter formula, consists of 3 to 4 ml/kg per percent burned of Lactated Ringer's, of which half is given during the first 8 hours postburn, and the remaining half over the subsequent 16 hours. Given these large volumes of intravenous resuscitation fluid, Lactated Ringer's solution is preferred, because 0.9% NaCl results in hypernatremia and more importantly a hyperchloremic acidosis. (See Schwartz 9th ed., p 200.)

3. The topical antimicrobial agent mafenide acetate is most likely to cause which of the following complications:
   A. Methemoglobinemia
   B. Neutropenia
   C. Metabolic acidosis
   D. Nephrotoxicity

Answer: C
Mafenide acetate, either in cream or solution form, is an effective topical antimicrobial. It is effective even in the presence of eschar and can be used in both treating and preventing wound infections, and the solution form is an excellent antimicrobial for fresh skin grafts. The use of mafenide acetate may be limited by pain with application to partial-thickness burns. Mafenide is absorbed systemically and a major side effect is metabolic acidosis resulting from carbonic anhydrase inhibition. (See Schwartz 9th ed., p 202.)

CLINICAL QUESTIONS

1. Which of the following patients should be immediately referred to a burn center?
   A. A 20-year-old with a 12% partial thickness burn
   B. A 30-year-old with a major liver injury and a 15% partial thickness burn
   C. A 2% TBSA partial thickness burn to the anterior leg, crossing the knee
   D. A 10-year-old with a 7% partial thickness burn

Answer: A
All patients with a partial thickness burn >10% TBSA should be transferred to a burn center. A patient with a burn and other major trauma can be treated and stabilized in the trauma center first. Burns that involve the entire joint should be transferred to a burn center, but a small burn to the anterior surface of the knee would not necessarily mandate transfer. Children should be transferred if there are no personnel able to care for

them, but for a child with a 7% TBSA burn, this would not be mandatory. (See Schwartz 9th ed., p 198; See Table 8-1.)

TABLE 8-1 Guidelines for referral to a burn center
Partial-thickness burns greater than 10% TBSA
Burns involving the face, hands, feet, genitalia, perineum, or major joints
Third-degree burns in any age group
Electrical burns, including lightning injury
Chemical burns
Inhalation injury
Burn injury in patients with complicated pre-existing medical disorders
Patients with burns and concomitant trauma in which the burn is the greatest risk. If the trauma is the greater immediate risk, the patient may be stabilized in a trauma center before transfer to a burn center.
Burned children in hospitals without qualified personnel for the care of children
Burn injury in patients who will require special social, emotional, or rehabilitative intervention

TBSA = total body surface area.

2. Which of the following should prompt immediate, elective intubation in a patient with a major burn?
   A. Subjective dyspnea
   B. Singed nasal hair
   C. Perioral burns
   D. Oxygen saturation <96%

Answer: A
Perioral burns and singed nasal hairs are signs that the oral cavity and pharynx should be further evaluated for mucosal injury, but in themselves these physical findings do not indicate an upper airway injury. Signs of impending respiratory compromise may include a hoarse voice, wheezing, or stridor; subjective dyspnea is a particularly concerning symptom, and should trigger prompt elective endotracheal intubation. (See Schwartz 9th ed., p 197.)

3. Which of the following is indicated in a 46-year-old patient with a 22% TBSA partial thickness burn?
   A. Prophylactic 1st generation cephalosporin
   B. Prophylactic clindamycin
   C. Tetanus booster
   D. Tetanus toxoid

Answer: C
Patients with acute burn injuries should never receive prophylactic antibiotics. This intervention has been clearly demonstrated to promote development of fungal infections and resistant organisms and was abandoned in the mid-1980s. A tetanus booster should be administered in the emergency room. (See Schwartz 9th ed., p 198.)

4. A 4-year-old patient presents with a diffuse scald wound after being held in a hot tub of water. There are circumferential blisters present over the right leg (from hip to toes) and circumferential blistering over the lower left leg (from knee to toes). The right thigh, abdomen and back below the umbilicus, as well as the buttocks and perineum are red but without blisters. What is the total BSA burn?
   A. 25%
   B. 36%
   C. 46%
   D. 54%

Answer: A
The 'rule of nines' is a crude but quick and effective method of estimating burn size (Fig. 8-1). In adults, the anterior and posterior trunk each account for 18%, each lower extremity is 18%, each upper extremity is 9%, and the head is 9%. In children younger than 3 years old, the head accounts for a larger relative surface area and should be taken into account when estimating burn size. Diagrams such as the Lund and Browder chart give a more accurate accounting of the true burn size in children. The importance of an accurate burn size assessment cannot be overemphasized. Superficial or first-degree burns should not be included when calculating the percent of TBSA, and thorough cleaning of soot and debris is mandatory to avoid confusing areas of soiling with burns. Examination of referral data suggests that physicians inexperienced with burns tend to overestimate the size of small burns and underestimate the size of large burns, with potentially detrimental effects on pretransfer resuscitation.

If patient in question is over the age of 3; the adult estimates can be used. Only the areas of partial thickness (in this case, blistering) are used to calculate the burn area. The left leg is 18%, and the lower right leg should be slightly less than half of 18% (i.e., approximately 7-8%). (See Schwartz 9th ed., p 198.)

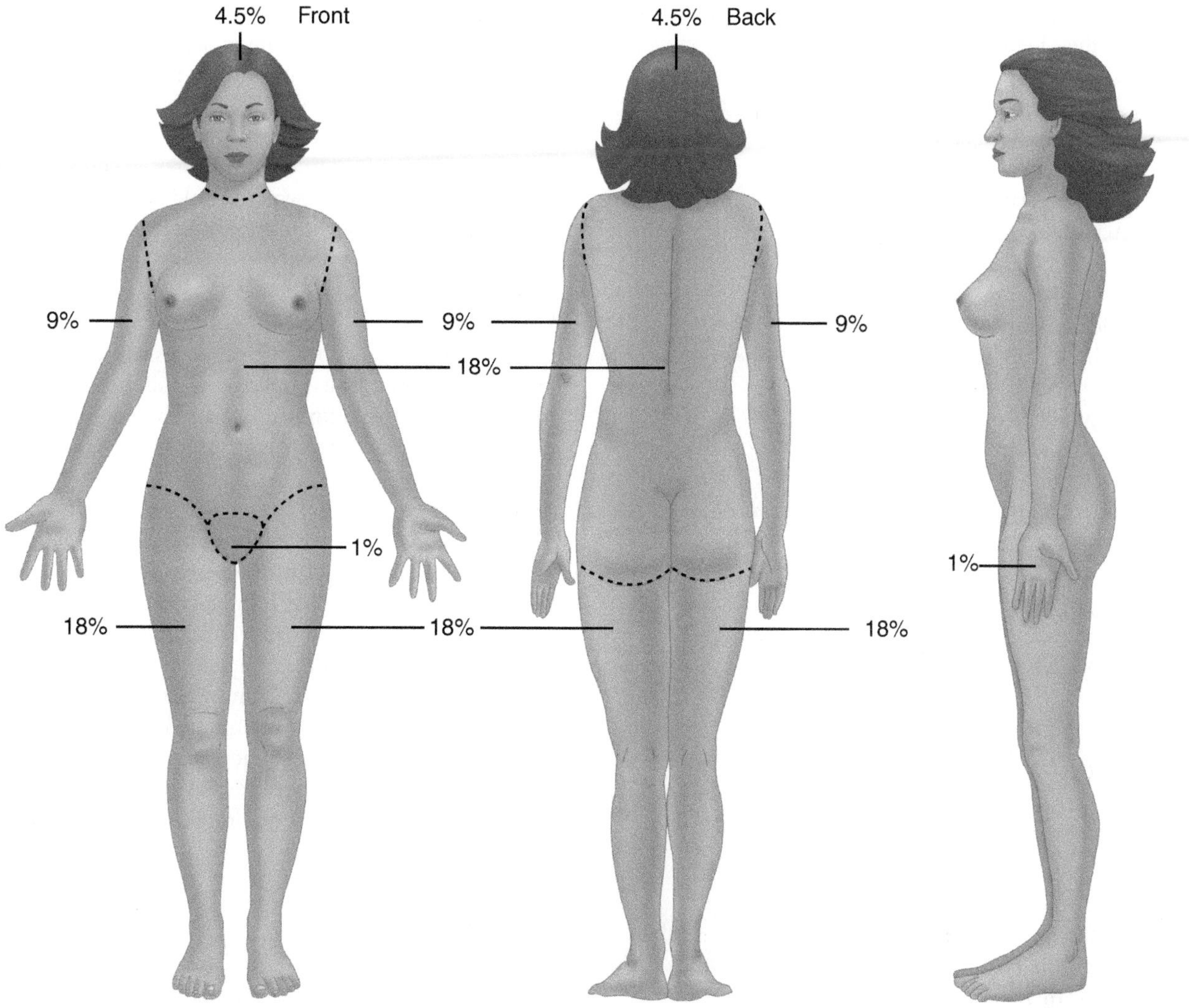

FIG. 8-1. The Rule of Nines can be used as a quick reference for estimating a patient's burn size by dividing the body into regions to which total body surface area is allocated in multiples of nine.

5. 100% inhaled oxygen decreases the half-life of carbon monoxide from 250 minutes to approximately
   A. 200 minutes
   B. 150 minutes
   C. 100 minutes
   D. 50 minutes

Answer: D

Administration of 100% oxygen is the gold standard for treatment of CO poisoning, and reduces the half-life of CO from 250 minutes in room air to 40 to 60 minutes. (See Schwartz 9th ed., p 198.)

6. Which of the following is used to treat severe hydrogen cyanide poisoning?
   A. Hydroxocobalamin
   B. Methylene blue
   C. Dialysis
   D. None of the above—there is no effective treatment

Answer: A

Hydrogen cyanide toxicity may also be a component of smoke inhalation injury. Afflicted patients may have a persistent lactic acidosis or S-T elevation on electrocardiogram (ECG). Cyanide inhibits cytochrome oxidase, which in turn inhibits cellular oxygenation. Treatment consists of sodium thiosulfate, hydroxocobalamin, and 100% oxygen. Sodium thiosulfate works by transforming cyanide into a nontoxic thiocyanate derivative; however, it works slowly and is not effective for acute therapy. Hydroxocobalamin quickly complexes with cyanide and is excreted by the kidney, and is recommended for immediate therapy. In the majority of patients, the lactic acidosis will resolve with ventilation and sodium thiosulfate treatment becomes unnecessary. (See Schwartz 9th ed., p 198.)

7. Most chemical burns require large volumes of water to remove the chemical. Which of the following chemical burns should be treated by careful wiping or sweeping of the skin, rather than water?
   A. Powdered form of lye
   B. Formic acid
   C. Hydrofluoric acid
   D. Acetic acid

Answer: A
Chemical burns are less common, but potentially are severe burns. The most important components of initial therapy are careful removal of the toxic substance from the patient and irrigation of the affected area with water for a minimum of 30 minutes. An exception to this is in cases of concrete powder or powdered forms of lye, which should be swept from the patient to avoid activating the aluminum hydroxide with water. (See Schwartz 9th ed., p 199.)

8. Formic acid burns are associated with
   A. Hemoglobinuria
   B. Rhabdomyolosis
   C. Hypocalemia
   D. Hypokalemia

Answer: A
The offending agents in chemical burns can be systemically absorbed and may cause specific metabolic derangements. Formic acid has been known to cause hemolysis and hemoglobinuria. (See Schwartz 9th ed., p 199.)

9. The agent most effective in treating hydrofluoric acid burns is
   A. Calcium
   B. Magnesium
   C. Vitamin K
   D. Vitamin A

Answer: A
Hydrofluoric acid is a particularly common offender due to its widespread industrial uses. Calcium-based therapies are the mainstay of treating hydrofluoric acid burns, with topical calcium gluconate applied to wounds, and subcutaneous or IV infiltration of calcium gluconate for systemic symptoms. Intra-arterial infusion of calcium gluconate may be effective in the most severe cases. Patients undergoing intra-arterial therapy need continuous cardiac monitoring. Persistent electrocardiac abnormalities or refractory hypocalcemia may signal the need for emergent excision of the burned areas. (See Schwartz 9th ed., p 199.)

10. The major improvement in burn survival in the 20th century can be attributed to the introduction of which of the following therapies:
    A. Antibiotics
    B. Central venous fluid resuscitation
    C. Nutritional support
    D. Early excision of the burn wound

Answer: D
The strategy of early excision and grafting in burned patients revolutionized survival outcomes in burn care. Not only did it improve mortality, but early excision decreased reconstruction surgery, improved hospital length of stay, and reduced costs of care. After the initial resuscitation is complete and the patient is hemodynamically stable, attention should be turned to excising the burn wound. Burn excision and wound coverage should ideally start within the first several days, and in larger burns, serial excisions can be performed as the patient's condition allows. (See Schwartz 9th ed., p 204.)

CHAPTER 9

Wound Healing

BASIC SCIENCE QUESTIONS

1. The peak number of fibroblasts in a healing wound occurs
   A. 2 days after injury
   B. 6 days after injury
   C. 15 days after injury
   D. 60 days after injury

Answer: B

(See Schwartz 9th ed., p 211, and See Figure. 9-1.)

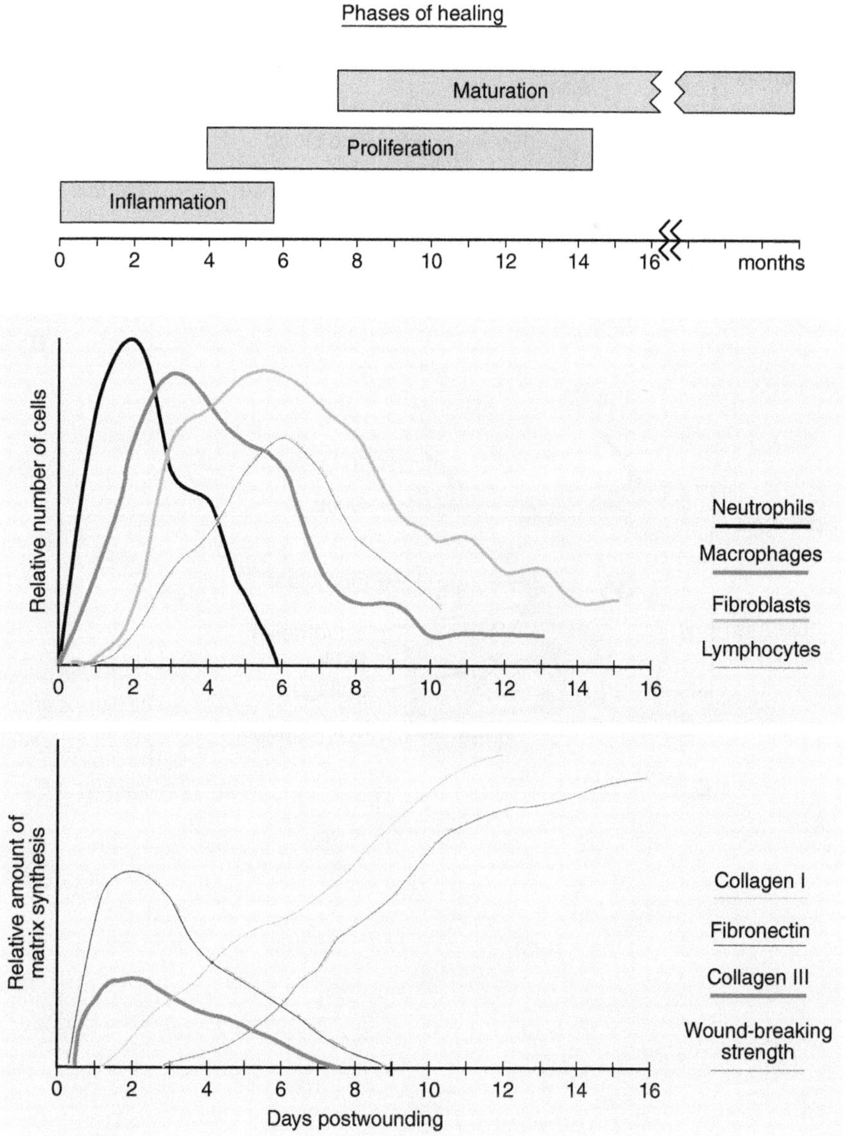

FIG. 9-1. The cellular, biochemical, and mechanical phases of wound healing.

2. Macrophages are present in the wound starting on the 4th day after injury until the wound is completely healed. The primary function of the macrophages in wound healing is
   A. Intracellular killing of bacteria
   B. Collagen production
   C. Activation of cell proliferation
   D. Modulation of the wound environment

Answer: C

The second population of inflammatory cells that invades the wound consists of macrophages, which are recognized as being essential to successful healing. Derived from circulating monocytes, macrophages achieve significant numbers in the wound by 48 to 96 hours postinjury and remain present until wound healing is complete. Macrophages, like neutrophils, participate in wound débridement via phagocytosis and contribute to microbial stasis via oxygen radical and nitric oxide synthesis (see Fig. 9-2C). The macrophage's most pivotal function is activation and recruitment of other cells via mediators such as cytokines and growth factors, as well as directly by cell–cell interaction and intercellular adhesion molecules. By releasing such mediators as TGFβ, vascular endothelial growth factor (VEGF), insulin-like growth factor, epithelial growth factor, and lactate, macrophages regulate cell proliferation, matrix synthesis, and angiogenesis. Macrophages also play a significant role in regulating angiogenesis and matrix deposition and remodeling (Table 9-1). Modulation of the wound environment is most likely performed by T lymphocytes in the wound. (See Schwartz 9th ed., p 211.)

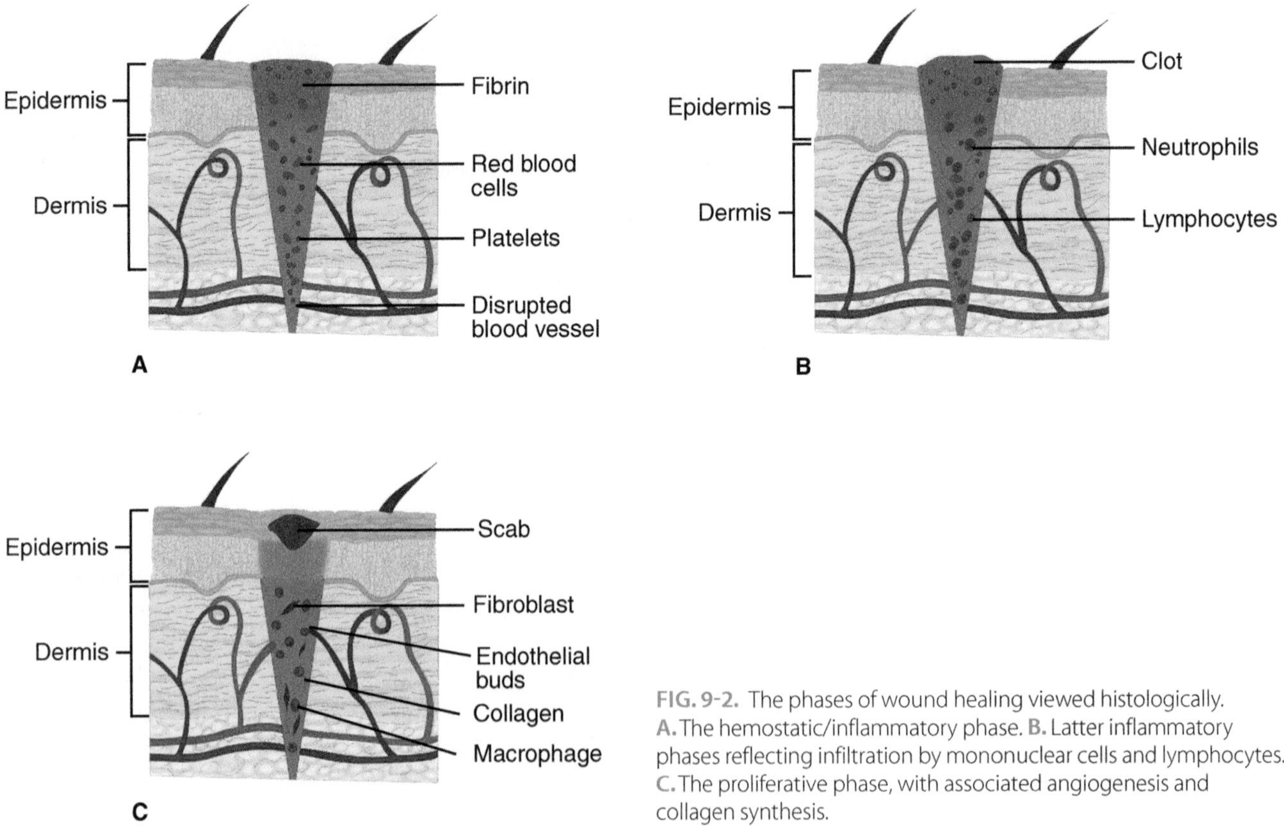

FIG. 9-2. The phases of wound healing viewed histologically. A. The hemostatic/inflammatory phase. B. Latter inflammatory phases reflecting infiltration by mononuclear cells and lymphocytes. C. The proliferative phase, with associated angiogenesis and collagen synthesis.

TABLE 9-1 Macrophage activities during wound healing	
Activity	**Mediators**
Phagocytosis	Reactive oxygen species Nitric oxide
Débridement	Collagenase, elastase
Cell recruitment and activation	Growth factors: PDGF, TGFβ, EGF, IGF Cytokines: TNF-α, IL-1, IL-6 Fibronectin
Matrix synthesis	Growth factors: TGFβ, EGF, PDGF Cytokines: TNF-α, IL-1, IFN-γ Enzymes: arginase, collagenase Prostaglandins Nitric oxide
Angiogenesis	Growth factors: FGF, VEGF Cytokines: TNF-α Nitric oxide

EGF = epithelial growth factor; FGF = fibroblast growth factor; IGF = insulin-like growth factor; IFN-γ = interferon-γ; IL = interleukin; PDGF = platelet-derived growth factor; TGFβ = transforming growth factor beta; TNF-α = tumor necrosis factor alpha; VEGF = vascular endothelial growth factor.

3. The first cells to migrate into a wound are
   A. Macrophages
   B. T lymphocytes
   C. PMNs
   D. Fibroblasts

Answer: C

PMNs are the first infiltrating cells to enter the wound site, peaking at 24 to 48 hours. Increased vascular permeability, local prostaglandin release, and the presence of chemotactic substances, such as complement factors, interleukin-1 (IL-1), tumor necrosis factor alpha (TNF-α), TGFβ, platelet factor 4, or bacterial products, all stimulate neutrophil migration. (See Schwartz 9th ed., p 210.)

4. There are 18 types of collagen in the human body. Which two are the most important in wound healing?
   A. Type I and III
   B. Type III and VIII
   C. Type II and X
   D. Type VI and XII

Answer: A

Although there are at least 18 types of collagen described, the main ones of interest to wound repair are types I and III. Type I collagen is the major component of extracellular matrix in skin. Type III, which is also normally present in skin, becomes more prominent and important during the repair process. (See Schwartz 9th ed., p 212.)

5. The tensile strength of a completely healed wound approaches the strength of uninjured tissue
   A. 2 weeks after injury
   B. 3 months after injury
   C. 12 months after injury
   D. Never

Answer: D

By several weeks postinjury the amount of collagen in the wound reaches a plateau, but the tensile strength continues to increase for several more months. Fibril formation and fibril cross-linking result in decreased collagen solubility, increased strength, and increased resistance to enzymatic degradation of the collagen matrix. Scar remodeling continues for many (6 to 12) months postinjury, gradually resulting in a mature, avascular, and acellular scar. The mechanical strength of the scar never achieves that of the uninjured tissue. (See Schwartz 9th ed., p 213.)

6. How long does re-epithelialization (i.e., complete repair of the external barrier) take in a well-approximated surgical wound?
   A. 2 days
   B. 1 week
   C. 2 weeks
   D. 1 month

Answer: A

Re-epithelialization is complete in less than 48 hours in the case of approximated incised wounds, but may take substantially longer in the case of larger wounds, in which there is a significant epidermal/dermal defect. If only the epithelium and superficial dermis are damaged, such as occurs in split-thickness skin graft donor sites or in superficial second-degree burns, then repair consists primarily of re-epithelialization with minimal or no fibroplasia and granulation tissue formation. (See Schwartz 9th ed., p 214.)

7. Which of the following is an important cytokine mediator of wound healing?
   A. TGFβ
   B. α–interferon
   C. Interleukin 12
   D. β–Defensin 2

Answer: A
TGFβ is a mediator of wound healing primarily by mediating angiogenesis (see Table 9-2). Alpha interferon, Interleukin 12 and Beta Defensin 2 do not play a major role in wound healing. (See Schwartz 9th ed., p 215.)

TABLE 9-2 Growth factors participating in wound healing

Growth Factor	Wound Cell Origin	Cellular and Biologic Effects
PDGF	Platelets, macrophages, monocytes, smooth muscle cells, endothelial cells	Chemotaxis: fibroblasts, smooth muscle, monocytes, neutrophils Mitogenesis: fibroblasts, smooth muscle cells Stimulation of angiogenesis Stimulation of collagen synthesis
FGF	Fibroblasts, endothelial cells, smooth muscle cells, chondrocytes	Stimulation of angiogenesis (by stimulation of endothelial cell proliferation and migration) Mitogenesis: mesoderm and neuroectoderm Stimulates fibroblasts, keratinocytes, chondrocytes, myoblasts
Keratinocyte growth factor	Keratinocytes, fibroblasts	Significant homology with FGF; stimulates keratinocytes
EGF	Platelets, macrophages, monocytes (also identified in salivary glands, duodenal glands, kidney, and lacrimal glands)	Stimulates proliferation and migration of all epithelial cell types
TGFα	Keratinocytes, platelets, macrophages	Homology with EGF; binds to EGF receptor Mitogenic and chemotactic for epidermal and endothelial cells
TGFβ (three isoforms: β_1, β_2, β_3)	Platelets, T lymphocytes, macrophages, monocytes, neutrophils	Stimulates angiogenesis TGFβ_1 stimulates wound matrix production (fibronectin, collagen glycosaminoglycans); regulation of inflammation TGFβ_3 inhibits scar formation
Insulin-like growth factors (IGF-I, IGF-II)	Platelets (IGF-I in high concentrations in liver; IGF-II in high concentrations in fetal growth); likely the effector of growth hormone action	Promote protein/extracellular matrix synthesis Increase membrane glucose transport
Vascular endothelial growth factor	Macrophages, fibroblasts, keratinocytes	Similar to PDGF Mitogen for endothelial cells (not fibroblasts) Stimulates angiogenesis
Granulocyte-macrophage colony-stimulating factor	Macrophage/monocytes, endothelial cells, fibroblasts	Stimulates macrophage differentiation/proliferation

EGF = epidermal growth factor; FGF = fibroblast growth factor; PDGF = platelet-derived growth factor; TGF = transforming growth factor.

8. The most common mode of inheritance of Ehlers-Danlos Syndrome is
   A. Autosomal dominant
   B. Autosomal recessive
   C. X-linked dominant
   D. X-linked recessive

Answer: A
Of the 10 types of Ehlers-Danlos syndrome, 6 are inherited with an autosomal dominant pattern, 2 are autosomal recessive, and 2 are X-linked recessive. (See Schwartz 9th ed., p 215, and Table 9-3.)

TABLE 9-3 Clinical, genetic, and biochemical aspects of Ehlers-Danlos subtypes

Type	Clinical Features	Inheritance	Biochemical Defect
I	Skin: soft, hyperextensible, easy bruising, fragile, atrophic scars; hypermobile joints; varicose veins; premature births	AD	Not known
II	Similar to type I, except less severe	AD	Not known
III	Skin: soft, not hyperextensible, normal scars; small and large joint hypermobility	AD	Not known
IV	Skin: thin, translucent, visible veins, normal scarring, no hyperextensibility; no joint hypermobility; arterial, bowel, and uterine rupture	AD	Type III collagen defect
V	Similar to type II	XLR	Not known
VI	Skin: hyperextensible, fragile, easy bruising; hypermobile joints; hypotonia; kyphoscoliosis	AR	Lysyl hydroxylase deficiency
VII	Skin: soft, mild hyperextensibility, no increased fragility; extremely lax joints with dislocations	AD	Type I collagen gene defect
VIII	Skin: soft, hyperextensible, easy bruising, abnormal scars with purple discoloration; hypermobile joints; generalized periodontitis	AD	Not known
IX	Skin: soft, lax; bladder diverticula and rupture; limited pronation and supination; broad clavicle; occipital horns	XLR	Lysyl oxidase defect with abnormal copper use
X	Similar to type II with abnormal clotting studies	AR	Fibronectin defect

AD = autosomal dominant; AR = autosomal recessive; XLR = X-linked recessive. Reproduced with permission from Phillips C, Wenstrup RJ: Biosynthetic and genetic disorders of collagen, in Cohen IK, Diegelmann RF, Linblad WJ (eds): *Wound Healing: Biochemical and Clinical Aspects*. Philadelphia: WB Saunders, 1992, p 152. Copyright © Elsevier.

9. Which of the following proteins is defective in patients with Marfan's syndrome?
   A. Collagen type I
   B. Fibrillin
   C. Lysyl hydroxylase
   D. Fibronectin

Answer: B

Patients with Marfan syndrome generally have tall stature, arachnodactyly, lax ligaments, myopia, scoliosis, pectus excavatum, and aneurysm of the ascending aorta. The genetic defect is in an extracellular protein, fibrillin, which is associated with elastic fibers. Patients who suffer from this syndrome also are prone to hernias. Surgical repair of a dissecting aneurysm is difficult, as the soft connective tissue fails to hold sutures. Skin may be hyperextensible, but shows no delay in wound healing. Abnormalities of collagen type III. Lysyl hydroxylase and fibronectin are seen in specific subtypes of Ehlers-Danlos syndrome. (See Schwartz 9th ed., p 216.)

10. Which of the following proteins is defective in patients with osteogenesis imperfecta (OI)?
   A. Collagen type I
   B. Fibrillin
   C. Lysyl hydroxylase
   D. Fibronectin

Answer: A

Characteristics of OI are brittle bones, osteopenia, low muscle mass, hernias, and ligament and joint laxity. OI is a result of a mutation in type I collagen. There are four major OI subtypes with mild to lethal manifestations. Patients experience dermal thinning and increased bruisability. Scarring is normal, and the skin is not hyperextensible. Surgery can be successful but difficult in these patients, as their bones fracture easily under minimal stress. Table 9-4 lists the various features associated with the clinical subtypes of OI. Type I collagen is also defective in one of the subtypes of Ehlers Danlos syndrome, as is fibronectin. Fibrillin is defective in Marfan's syndrome. (See Schwartz 9th ed., p 216.)

TABLE 9-4 Osteogenesis imperfecta: clinical and genetic features

Type	Clinical Features	Inheritance
I	Mild bone fragility, blue sclera	Dominant
II	"Prenatal lethal"; crumpled long bones, thin ribs, dark blue sclera	Dominant
III	Progressively deforming; multiple fractures; early loss of ambulation	Dominant/recessive
IV	Mild to moderate bone fragility; normal or gray sclera; mild short stature	Dominant

Reproduced with permission from Phillips C, Wenstrup RJ: Biosynthetic and genetic disorders of collagen, in Cohen IK, Diegelmann RF, Linblad WJ (eds): *Wound Healing: Biochemical and Clinical Aspects*. Philadelphia: WB Saunders, 1992, p 152. Copyright © Elsevier.

11. Which of the following components of wound healing is impaired in a child with acrodermatis enteropathica (AE)?
   A. Macrophage signaling
   B. Formation of granulation tissue
   C. Collagen deposition
   D. Collagen cross-linking

Answer: B

AE is an autosomal recessive disease of children that causes an inability to absorb sufficient zinc from breast milk or food. The AE mutation affects zinc uptake in the intestine by preventing zinc from binding to the cell surface and its translocation into the cell. Zinc deficiency is associated with impaired granulation tissue formation, as zinc is a necessary cofactor for DNA polymerase and reverse transcriptase, and its deficiency may impair healing due to inhibition of cell proliferation. AE is characterized by impaired wound healing as well as erythematous pustular dermatitis involving the extremities and the areas around the bodily orifices. Diagnosis is confirmed by the presence of an abnormally low blood zinc level (>100 mg/dL). Oral supplementation with 100 to 400 mg zinc sulfate orally per day is curative for impaired healing.

Zinc is the most well-known element in wound healing and has been used empirically in dermatologic conditions for centuries. It is essential for wound healing in animals and humans. There are more than 150 known enzymes for which zinc is either an integral part or an essential cofactor, and many of these enzymes are critical to wound healing. With zinc deficiency there is decreased fibroblast proliferation, decreased collagen synthesis, impaired overall wound strength, and delayed epithelialization. These defects are reversed by zinc supplementation. To date, no study has shown improved wound healing with zinc supplementation in patients who are not zinc deficient. (See Schwartz 9th ed., p 216.)

12. Which layer of the intestine has the greatest tensile strength (i.e. ability to hold sutures)?
    A. Serosa
    B. Muscularis
    C. Submucosa
    D. Mucosa

Answer: C

The submucosa is the layer that imparts the greatest tensile strength and greatest suture-holding capacity, a characteristic that should be kept in mind during surgical repair of the GI tract. Additionally, serosal healing is essential for quickly achieving a watertight seal from the luminal side of the bowel. The importance of the serosa is underscored by the significantly higher rates of anastomotic failure observed clinically in segments of bowel that are extraperitoneal and lack serosa (i.e., the esophagus and rectum). (See Schwartz 9th ed., p 216.)

13. Leaks from a bowel anastomosis most commonly occur 5 to 7 days after surgery. The reason is
    A. Delayed collagen deposition
    B. Increased collagenolysis
    C. Breakdown of the initial fibrin seal by intraluminal bacteria
    D. Increased macrophage migration from the peritoneum

Answer: B

Injuries to all parts of the GI tract undergo the same sequence of healing as cutaneous wounds. However, there are some significant differences (Table 9-5). Mesothelial (serosal) and mucosal healing can occur without scarring. The early integrity of the anastomosis is dependent on formation of a fibrin seal on the serosal side, which achieves watertightness, and on the suture-holding capacity of the intestinal wall, particularly the submucosal layer. There is a significant decrease in marginal strength during the first week due to an early and marked collagenolysis. The lysis of collagen is carried out by collagenase derived from neutrophils, macrophages, and intraluminal bacteria. Collagenase activity occurs early in the healing process, and during the first 3 to 5 days collagen breakdown far exceeds collagen synthesis. The integrity of the anastomosis represents equilibrium between collagen lysis, which occurs early, and collagen synthesis, which takes a few days to initiate (Fig. 9-3). (See Schwartz 9th ed., pp 216-217.)

TABLE 9-5 Comparison of wound healing in the gastrointestinal tract and skin

		GI Tract	Skin
Wound environment	pH	Varies throughout GI tract in accordance with local exocrine secretions.	Usually constant except during sepsis or local infection.
	Microorganisms	Aerobic and anaerobic, especially in the colon and rectum; problematic if they contaminate the peritoneal cavity.	Skin commensals rarely cause problems; infection usually results from exogenous contamination or hematogenous spread.
	Shear stress	Intraluminal bulk transit and peristalsis exert distracting forces on the anastomosis.	Skeletal movements may stress the suture line but pain usually acts as a protective mechanism preventing excess movement.
	Tissue oxygenation	Dependent on intact vascular supply and neocapillary formation.	Circulatory transport of oxygen as well as diffusion.
Collagen synthesis	Cell type	Fibroblasts and smooth muscle cells.	Fibroblasts.
	Lathyrogens	D-Penicillamine has no effect on collagen cross-linking.	Significant inhibition of cross-linking with decreased wound strength.
	Steroids	Contradictory evidence exists concerning their negative effect on GI healing; increased abscess in the anastomotic line may play a significant role.	Significant decrease in collagen accumulation.
Collagenase activity	—	Increased presence throughout GI tract after transection and reanastomosis; during sepsis excess enzyme may promote dehiscence by decreasing suture-holding capacity of tissue.	Not as significant a role in cutaneous wounds.
Wound strength	—	Rapid recovery to preoperative level.	Less rapid than GI tissue.
Scar formation	Age	Definite scarring seen in fetal wound sites.	Usually heals without scar formation in the fetus.

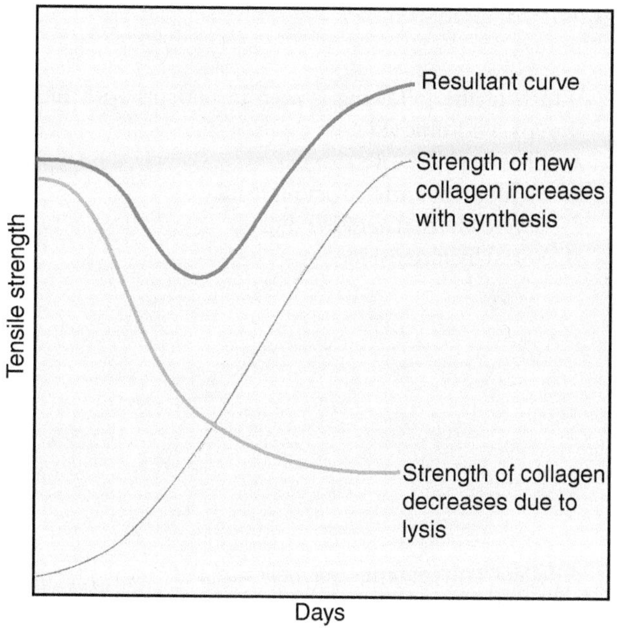

FIG. 9-3. Diagrammatic representation of the concept of GI wound healing as a fine balance between collagen synthesis and collagenolysis. The "weak" period when collagenolysis exceeds collagen synthesis can be prolonged or exacerbated by any factors that upset the equilibrium. (Reproduced with permission from Hunt TK, Van Winkle W Jr: Wound healing: normal repair, in Dunphy JE (ed): *Fundamentals of Wound Management in Surgery*. New York: Chirurgecom, Inc., 1976, p. 29.)

14. Supplementation with which of the following amino acids may improve wound healing?
    A. Glutamine
    B. Arginine
    C. Alanine
    D. Guanine

Answer: B

The possible role of single amino acids in enhanced wound healing has been studied for the last several decades. Arginine appears most active in terms of enhancing wound fibroplasia.... Studies have been carried out in healthy human volunteers to examine the effect of arginine supplementation on collagen accumulation. Young, healthy, human volunteers (aged 25 to 35 years) were found to have significantly increased wound collagen deposition after oral supplementation with either 30 g of arginine aspartate (17 g of free arginine) or 30 g of arginine HCl (24.8 g of free arginine) daily for 14 days. In a study of healthy older humans (aged 67 to 82 years), daily supplements of 30 g of arginine aspartate for 14 days resulted in significantly enhanced collagen and total protein deposition at the wound site when compared to controls given placebos. There was no enhanced DNA synthesis present in the wounds of the arginine-supplemented subjects, suggesting that the effect of arginine is not mediated by an inflammatory mode of action. In this study, arginine supplementation had no effect on the rate of epithelialization of a superficial skin defect. This further suggests that the main effect of arginine on wound healing is to enhance wound collagen deposition. (See Schwartz 9th ed., p 221.)

CLINICAL QUESTIONS

1. Which of the following is seen in patients with Ehlers-Danlos syndrome (EDS)?
   A. Elevated PT/PTT
   B. Spontaneous arteriovenous fistulae
   C. Severe internal hemorrhoids
   D. Portal hypertension

Answer: B
EDS is a group of 10 disorders that present as a defect in collagen formation. Characteristics include thin, friable skin with prominent veins, easy bruising, poor wound healing, abnormal scar formation, recurrent hernias, and hyperextensible joints. GI problems include bleeding, hiatal hernia, intestinal diverticulae, and rectal prolapse. Small blood vessels are fragile, making suturing difficult during surgery. Large vessels may develop aneurysms, varicosities, arteriovenous fistulas, or may spontaneously rupture. EDS must be considered in every child with recurrent hernias and coagulopathy, especially when accompanied by platelet abnormalities and low coagulation factor levels. Inguinal hernias in these children resemble those seen in adults.' (See Schwartz 9th ed., p 215.)

2. A patient with epidermolysis bullosa (EB) requires placement of a feeding gastrostomy due to esophageal erosions. What kind of dressing should be placed after surgery?
   A. None—leave the wound open to air
   B. Steri-strips, gauze, and atraumatic tape
   C. Tissue adhesive only
   D. Nonadhesive pad with circumferential bulky dressing

Answer: D
EB is classified into three major subtypes: EB simplex, junctional EB, and dystrophic EB. The genetic defect involves impairment in tissue adhesion within the epidermis, basement membrane, or dermis, resulting in tissue separation and blistering with minimal trauma. Characteristic features of EB are blistering and ulceration. Management of nonhealing wounds in patients with EB is a challenge, as their nutritional status is compromised because of oral erosions and esophageal obstruction. Surgical interventions include esophageal dilation and gastrostomy tube placement. Dermal incisions must be meticulously placed to avoid further trauma to skin. The skin requires nonadhesive pads covered by 'bulky' dressing to avoid blistering. (See Schwartz 9th ed., p 216.)

3. Which phase of healing is most affected by exogenous corticosteroids?
   A. Initial phase of cell migration and angiogenesis
   B. Proliferative phase
   C. Maturation
   D. Scar remodeling

Answer: A
Large doses or chronic usage of glucocorticoids reduce collagen synthesis and wound strength. The major effect of steroids is to inhibit the inflammatory phase of wound healing (angiogenesis, neutrophil and macrophage migration, and fibroblast proliferation) and the release of lysosomal enzymes. The stronger the anti-inflammatory effect of the steroid compound used, the greater the inhibitory effect on wound healing. Steroids used after the first 3 to 4 days postinjury do not affect wound healing as severely as when they are used in the immediate postoperative period. Therefore, if possible, their use should be delayed or, alternatively, forms with lesser anti-inflammatory effects should be administered. In addition to their effect on collagen synthesis, steroids also inhibit epithelialization and contraction and contribute to increased rates of wound infection, regardless of the time of administration. (See Schwartz 9th ed., p 220.)

4. Which of the following should be given to promote wound healing in patients receiving steroids?
   A. Vitamin A
   B. Vitamin B1
   C. Vitamin B2
   D. Vitamin C

Answer: A
Steroid-delayed healing of cutaneous wounds can be stimulated to epithelialize by topical application of vitamin A. Collagen synthesis of steroid-treated wounds also can be stimulated by vitamin A. (See Schwartz 9th ed., p 220.)

5. How long does protein calorie malnutrition need to be present in patients in order to affect wound healing?
   A. Days
   B. Weeks
   C. 1 month
   D. >3 months

Answer: A
Two additional nutrition-related factors warrant discussion. First, the degree of nutritional impairment need not be long-standing in humans, as opposed to the experimental situation. Thus, patients with brief preoperative illnesses or reduced nutrient intake in the period immediately preceding the injury or operative intervention will demonstrate impaired fibroplasias. Second, brief and not necessarily intensive nutritional intervention, either via the parenteral or enteral route, can reverse or prevent the decreased collagen deposition noted with malnutrition or with postoperative starvation. (See Schwartz 9th ed., p 221.)

6. A homeless, malnourished 48-year-old patient is admitted to the ICU after a severe blunt injury. A reasonable daily dose of vitamin C for this patient would be
   A. 60 mg
   B. 150 mg
   C. 400 mg
   D. ≥1 gm

Answer: D
Scurvy, or vitamin C deficiency, leads to a defect in wound healing, particularly via a failure in collagen synthesis and cross-linking. Biochemically, vitamin C is required for the conversion of proline and lysine to hydroxyproline and hydroxylysine, respectively. Vitamin C deficiency has also been associated with an increased incidence of wound infection, and if wound infection does occur, it tends to be more severe. These effects are believed to be due to an associated impairment in neutrophil function, decreased complement activity, and decreased walling-off of bacteria secondary to insufficient collagen deposition. The recommended dietary allowance is 60 mg daily. This provides a considerable safety margin for most healthy nonsmokers. In severely injured or extensively burned patients this requirement may increase to as high as 2g daily. There is no evidence that excess vitamin C is toxic; however, there is no evidence that supertherapeutic doses of vitamin C are of any benefit. (See Schwartz 9th ed., p 221.)

7. A previously healthy 18-year-old woman is involved in a housefire and is admitted with 60% deep partial thickness burns to the ICU. A reasonable daily dose of vitamin A for this patient would be
   A. 1000 mg
   B. 2500 mg
   C. 10,000 mg
   D. 25,000 mg

Answer: D
Vitamin A deficiency impairs wound healing, whereas supplemental vitamin A benefits wound healing in nondeficient humans and animals. Vitamin A increases the inflammatory response in wound healing, probably by increasing the lability of lysosomal membranes. There is an increased influx of macrophages, with an increase in their activation and increased collagen synthesis. Vitamin A directly increases collagen production and epidermal growth factor receptors when it is added in vitro to cultured fibroblasts. As mentioned in the section Steroids and Chemotherapeutic Drugs, supplemental vitamin A can reverse the inhibitory effects of corticosteroids on wound healing. Vitamin A also can restore wound healing that has been impaired by diabetes, tumor formation, cyclophosphamide, and radiation. Serious injury or stress leads to increased vitamin A requirements. In the severely injured patient, supplemental doses of vitamin A have been recommended. Doses ranging from 25,000 to 100,000 IU per day have been advocated. (See Schwartz 9th ed., p 222.)

8. The ideal time to administer prophylactic antibiotics to a patient undergoing a colon resection is
   A. 8 hours before surgery with a dose repeated at the time of incision
   B. 2 hours before surgery with a dose repeated at the time of incision
   C. 1 hour before surgery
   D. At the time of incision

Answer: C
Antibiotic prophylaxis is most effective when adequate concentrations of antibiotic are present in the tissues at the time of incision, and assurance of adequate preoperative antibiotic dosing and timing has become a significant hospital performance measure. Addition of antibiotics after operative contamination has occurred is clearly ineffective in preventing postoperative wound infections. (See Schwartz 9th ed., p 222.)

9. A 28-year-old patient with chronic granulomatous disease is scheduled for cystoscopy under general anesthesia. Which of the following tests should be obtained preoperatively?
   A. Pulmonary function test
   B. Echocardiogram
   C. Abdominal ultrasound
   D. EKG

Answer: A

Chronic granulomatous disease (CGD) comprises a genetically heterogeneous group of diseases in which the reduced nicotinamide adenine dinucleotide phosphate–dependent oxide enzyme is deficient. This defect impairs the intracellular killing of microorganisms, leaving the patient liable to infection by bacteria and fungi. Afflicted patients have recurrent infections and form granulomas, which can lead to obstruction of the gastric antrum and genitourinary tracts and poor wound healing. Surgeons become involved when the patient develops infectious or obstructive complications. The nitroblue tetrazolium reduction test is used to diagnose CGD. Normal neutrophils can reduce this compound, whereas neutrophils from affected patients do not, facilitating the diagnosis via a colorimetric test. Clinically, patients develop recurrent infections such as pneumonia, lymphadenitis, hepatic abscess, and osteomyelitis. Organisms most commonly responsible are *Staphylococcus aureus*, *Aspergillus*, *Klebsiella*, *Serratia*, or *Candida*. When CGD patients require surgery, a preoperative pulmonary function test should be considered because such patients are predisposed to obstructive and restrictive lung disease. Wound complications, mainly infection, are common. Sutures should be removed as late as possible because the wounds heal slowly. Abscess drains should be left in place for a prolonged period until the infection is completely resolved. (See Schwartz 9th ed., p 224.)

10. Which of the following should be performed in a patient with a suspected Marjolin ulcer?
   A. Hyperbaric therapy for 6 weeks
   B. Zinc supplementation
   C. Oral tetracycline for 6 weeks
   D. Biopsy

Answer: D

Malignant transformation of chronic ulcers can occur in any long-standing wound (Marjolin ulcer). Any wound that does not heal for a prolonged period of time is prone to malignant transformation. Malignant wounds are differentiated clinically from nonmalignant wounds by the presence of overturned wound edges. In patients with suspected malignant transformations, biopsy of the wound edges must be performed to rule out malignancy. Cancers arising de novo in chronic wounds include both squamous and basal cell carcinomas. (See Schwartz 9th ed., p 224.)

11. Which of the following is considered the most effective therapy for venous stasis ulcers?
   A. Supplemental vitamin A
   B. Topical antibiotic ointment
   C. Compression therapy
   D. Hyperbaric therapy

Answer: C

The cornerstone of treatment of venous ulcers is compression therapy, although the best method to achieve it remains controversial. Compression can be accomplished via rigid or flexible means. The most commonly used method is the rigid, zinc oxide–impregnated, nonelastic bandage. Others have proposed a four-layered bandage approach as a more optimal method of obtaining graduated compression. Wound care in these patients focuses on maintaining a moist wound environment, which can be achieved with hydrocolloids. Other, more modern approaches include use of vasoactive substances and growth factor application, as well as the use of skin substitutes. Most venous ulcers can be healed with perseverance and by addressing the venous hypertension. Unfortunately, recurrences are frequent in spite of preventative measures, largely because of patients' lack of compliance. (See Schwartz 9th ed., p 225.)

12. Which of the following is most likely to cause a diabetic ulcer?
    A. Uncontrolled hyperglycemia
    B. Large vessel ischemia (peripheral vascular disease)
    C. Small vessel ischemia
    D. Neuropathy

Answer: D
It is estimated that 60 to 70% of diabetic ulcers are due to neuropathy, 15 to 20% are due to ischemia, and another 15 to 20% are due to a combination of both. The neuropathy is both sensory and motor, and is secondary to persistently elevated glucose levels. The loss of sensory function allows unrecognized injury to occur from ill-fitting shoes, foreign bodies, or other trauma. The motor neuropathy or Charcot foot leads to collapse or dislocation of the interphalangeal or metatarsophalangeal joints, causing pressure on areas with little protection. There is also severe micro and macrovascular circulatory impairment. (See Schwartz 9th ed., p 225.)

13. A teenage, African American girl presents with large keloids on both earlobes 12 months following ear piercing. Which therapy should be added to surgical debulking of the lesions?
    A. None—surgical resection alone is sufficient as the initial therapy
    B. Intralesional corticosteroids
    C. Pressure earrings
    D. Radiation therapy

Answer: B
Excision alone of keloids is subject to a high recurrence rate, ranging from 45 to 100%. There are fewer recurrences when surgical excision is combined with other modalities such as intralesional corticosteroid injection, topical application of silicone sheets, or the use of radiation or pressure. Surgery is recommended for debulking large lesions or as second-line therapy when other modalities have failed. Silicone application is relatively painless and should be maintained for 24 hours a day for about 3 months to prevent rebound hypertrophy. It may be secured with tape or worn beneath a pressure garment. The mechanism of action is not understood, but increased hydration of the skin, which decreases capillary activity, inflammation, hyperemia, and collagen deposition, may be involved. Silicone is more effective than other occlusive dressings and is an especially good treatment for children and others who cannot tolerate the pain involved in other modalities.

Intralesional corticosteroid injections decrease fibroblast proliferation, collagen and glycosaminoglycan synthesis, the inflammatory process, and TGFβ levels. When used alone, however, there is a variable rate of response and recurrence, therefore steroids are recommended as first-line treatment for keloids and second-line treatment for HTSs if topical therapies have failed. Intralesional injections are more effective on younger scars. They may soften, flatten, and give symptomatic relief to keloids, but they cannot make the lesions disappear nor can they narrow wide HTSs. Success is enhanced when used in combination with surgical excision. Serial injections every 2 to 3 weeks are required. Complications include skin atrophy, hypopigmentation, telangiectasias, necrosis, and ulceration.

Although radiation destroys fibroblasts, it has variable, unreliable results and produces poor results with 10 to 100% recurrence when used alone. It is more effective when combined with surgical excision. The timing, duration, and dosage for radiation therapy are still controversial, but doses ranging from 1500 to 2000 rads appear effective. Given the risks of hyperpigmentation, pruritus, erythema, paresthesias, pain, and possible secondary malignancies, radiation should be reserved for adults with scars resistant to other modalities.

Pressure aids collagen maturation, flattens scars, and improves thinning and pliability. It reduces the number of cells in a given area, possibly by creating ischemia, which decreases tissue metabolism and increases collagenase activity. External compression is used to treat HTSs, especially after burns. Therapy must begin early, and a pressure between 24 and 30 mmHg must be achieved in order to exceed capillary pressure, yet preserve peripheral blood circulation. Garments should be worn for 23 to 24 hours a day for up to 1 or more years to avoid rebound hypertrophy. Scars older than 6 to 12 months respond poorly. (See Schwartz 9th ed., p 226.)

14. The risk of small bowel obstruction in the first 10 years after left colectomy is
   A. <5%
   B. 10%
   C. 20%
   D. 30%

Answer: D
Intra-abdominal adhesions are the most common cause (65 to 75%) of small bowel obstruction, especially in the ileum. Operations in the lower abdomen have a higher chance of producing small bowel obstruction. After rectal surgery, left colectomy, or total colectomy, there is an 11% chance of developing small bowel obstruction within 1 year, and this rate increases to 30% by 10 years. (See Schwartz 9th ed., p 227.)

15. Intra-abdominal adhesions can be decreased after laparotomy by
   A. Frequent irrigation to keep bowel surfaces moist
   B. Using antibiotic irrigation at the completion of the case
   C. Wrapping anastomoses in hyaluronic acid sheets prior to closure
   D. Using only monofilament sutures in abdominal wound closure

Answer: A
There are two major strategies for adhesion prevention or reduction. Surgical trauma is minimized within the peritoneum by careful tissue handling, avoiding desiccation and ischemia, and spare use of cautery, laser, and retractors. Fewer adhesions form with laparoscopic surgical techniques due to reduced tissue trauma. The second major advance in adhesion prevention has been the introduction of barrier membranes and gels, which separate and create barriers between damaged surfaces, allowing for adhesion-free healing. Modified oxidized regenerated cellulose and hyaluronic acid membranes or solutions have been shown to reduce adhesions in gynecologic patients, and have been investigated for their ability to prevent adhesion formation in patients undergoing bowel surgery. Wrapping of the bowel suture area or placement in the proximity of the anastomoses with these substances is, however, contraindicated due to an elevated risk of leak. (See Schwartz 9th ed., p 227.)

16. A healthy 20-year-old presents to the emergency room with a large, contaminated laceration that he received during a touch football game. Which of the following solutions should be used to irrigate this wound?
   A. Sterile water
   B. Normal saline
   C. Dilute iodine solution
   D. Dakin's solution

Answer: B
Irrigation to visualize all areas of the wound and remove foreign material is best accomplished with normal saline (without additives). High-pressure wound irrigation is more effective in achieving complete débridement of foreign material and nonviable tissues. Iodine, povidone-iodine, hydrogen peroxide, and organically based antibacterial preparations have all been shown to impair wound healing due to injury to wound neutrophils and macrophages, and thus should not be used. (See Schwartz 9th ed., p 228.)

17. Once the wound described above has been irrigated and débrided, which suture should be used to close the subcutaneous layer?
   A. Biologic absorbable monofilament (plain gut)
   B. Synthetic absorbable monofilament
   C. Absorbable braided
   D. None of the above

Answer: C
In general, the smallest suture required to hold the various layers of the wound in approximation should be selected in order to minimize suture-related inflammation. Nonabsorbable or slowly absorbing monofilament sutures are most suitable for approximating deep fascial layers, particularly in the abdominal wall. Subcutaneous tissues should be closed with braided absorbable sutures, with care to avoid placement of sutures in fat. Although traditional teaching in wound closure has emphasized multiple-layer closures, additional layers of suture closure are associated with increased risk of wound infection, especially when placed in fat. Drains may be placed in areas at risk of forming fluid collections. (See Schwartz 9th ed., p 228.)

18. An alginate dressing is best used in which of the following wounds?
    A. An open traumatic wound
    B. An open surgical wound
    C. An infected wound
    D. A partial thickness burn wound

Answer: B
Alginates are derived from brown algae and contain long chains of polysaccharides containing mannuronic and glucuronic acid. The ratios of these sugars vary with the species of algae used, as well as the season of harvest. Processed as the calcium form, alginates turn into soluble sodium alginate through ion exchange in the presence of wound exudates. The polymers gel, swell, and absorb a great deal of fluid. Alginates are being used when there is skin loss, in open surgical wounds with medium exudation, and on full-thickness chronic wounds. (See Schwartz 9th ed., p 229.)

19. Which of the following topical agents has been shown to improve healing in diabetic foot ulcers?
    A. Epithelial growth factor
    B. TGFβ
    C. Platelet derived growth factor BB
    D. Endothelial growth factor

Answer: C
At present, only platelet-derived growth factor BB (PDGF-BB) is currently approved by the Food and Drug Administration for treatment of diabetic foot ulcers. Application of recombinant human PDGF-BB in a gel suspension to these wounds increases the incidence of total healing and decreases healing time. Several other growth factors have been tested clinically and show some promise, but currently none are approved for use. A great deal more needs to be discovered about the concentration, temporal release, and receptor cell population before growth factor therapy is to make a consistent impact on wound healing. (See Schwartz 9th ed., p 231.)

CHAPTER 10

Oncology

BASIC SCIENCE QUESTIONS

1. What is the most common cancer in the world?
   A. Breast
   B. Gastric
   C. Lung
   D. Liver

Answer: C
Lung cancer is the leading cancer in the world, accounting for 1.35 million new cases and 1.15 million deaths per year. Breast cancer is now the second most common cause of cancer (1.15 million cases per year) followed by gastric cancer (934,000 cases), colorectal cancer (1.03 million cases), and liver cancer (626,000 case). (See Schwartz 9th ed., p. 237.)

2. Approximately how many people die of cancer annually in the United States?
   A. 100,000
   B. 500,000
   C. 2,000,000
   D. 5,000,000

Answer: B
In the year 2008, an estimated 1.44 million new cancer cases were diagnosed in the United States. In addition, over a million cases of basal and squamous cell carcinomas of the skin, 54,020 cases of melanoma in situ, and 67,770 cases of carcinoma in situ of the breast were predicted. Furthermore, an estimated 565,650 people were expected to die of cancer in the United States in the same year. Cancer deaths accounted for 23% of all deaths in the United States in 2005, second only to deaths from heart disease. (See Schwartz 9th ed., p. 236.)

3. The incidence of breast cancer is highest in developed nations with the exception of
   A. France
   B. England
   C. Japan
   D. Australia

Answer: C
The incidence of breast cancer is high in all of the most highly developed regions except Japan, including the United States and Canada, Australia, and Northern and Western Europe, ranging from 82.5 to 99.4 per 100,000 women per year. (See Schwartz 9th ed., p. 238.)

4. Which of the following is associated with an increased incidence of liver cancer?
   A. Salted food
   B. Infection with Hepatitis A
   C. Exposure to aflatoxin
   D. Helicobacter pylori

Answer: C
In contrast to colon cancers, 82% of liver cancers occur in developing countries. The incidence of liver cancer is especially high in China (37.9 per 100,000 men), whereas it is relatively low in North and South America and Europe (2.6 to 6.2 per 100,000 men). Worldwide, the major risk factors for liver cancer are infection with hepatitis B and C viruses and consumption of foods contaminated with aflatoxin. Hepatitis B immunization in children has recently been shown to reduce the incidence of liver cancer. (See Schwartz 9th ed., p. 238.)

5. Which of the following is NOT one of the six cell alterations that permit malignant growth to occur in cells?
   A. Self-sufficiency of growth signals
   B. Predisposition to apoptosis
   C. Angiogenesis
   D. Invasion and metastasis

Answer: B

Although there are >100 types of cancer, it has been proposed that there are six essential alterations in cell physiology that dictate malignant growth: self-sufficiency of growth signals, insensitivity to growth-inhibitory signals, evasion of apoptosis (programmed cell death), potential for limitless replication, angiogenesis, and invasion and metastasis (Fig. 10-1). (See Schwartz 9th ed., p. 239.)

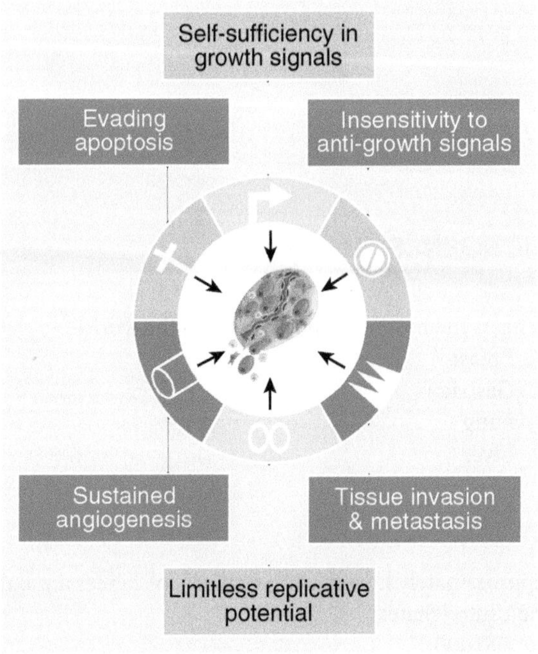

FIG. 10-1. Acquired capabilities of cancer. (Modified with permission from Hanahan D, Weinberg RA: The hallmarks of cancer. *Cell* 100:57, 2000. Copyright © Elsevier.)

6. Which of the following occurs in abnormally proliferating, transformed cells?
   A. Anchorage-dependent growth
   B. Immortalization
   C. Increased contact inhibition
   D. Increased cell-cell adherence

Answer: B

In normal cells, cell growth and proliferation are under strict control. In cancer cells, cells become unresponsive to normal growth controls, which leads to uncontrolled growth and proliferation. Human cells require several genetic changes for neoplastic transformation. Cell type–specific differences also exist for tumorigenic transformation. Abnormally proliferating, transformed cells outgrow normal cells in the culture dish (i.e., in vitro) and commonly display several abnormal characteristics. These include loss of contact inhibition (i.e., cells continue to proliferate after a confluent monolayer is formed); an altered appearance and poor adherence to other cells or to the substratum; loss of anchorage dependence for growth; immortalization; and gain of tumorigenicity (i.e., the ability to give rise to tumors when injected into an appropriate host). (See Schwartz 9th ed., p. 240.)

7. A "field effect" is best described as
   A. The effect of oncogene amplification in a cell on the adjacent cells
   B. The effect of loss of tumor-suppressor gene function in a cell on the adjacent cells
   C. Increased oncogene amplification or loss of tumor-suppressor gene function in a group of cells
   D. The effect of radiation on a tumor

Answer: C

Tumorigenesis is proposed to have three steps: initiation, promotion and progression. Initiating events such as gain of function of genes known as *oncogenes* or loss of function of genes known as *tumor-suppressor genes* may lead a single cell to acquire a distinct growth advantage. Although tumors usually arise from a single cell or clone, it is thought that sometimes not a single cell but rather a large number of cells in a target organ may have undergone the initiating genetic event; thus many normal-appearing cells may have an elevated malignant potential. This is referred to as a *field effect*. The initiating events are usually genetic and occur as deletions of tumor-suppressor genes or amplification of oncogenes. Subsequent events can lead to accumulations of additional deleterious mutations in the clone. (See Schwartz 9th ed., p. 240.)

8. Malignant cells are LEAST likely to be in which of the following stages of the cell cycle?
   A. S phase
   B. G_0 phase
   C. G_1 phase
   D. M phase

Answer: B

Malignant cells are cells that do not enter the G_0 stage (quiescent stage) after proliferation.

The proliferative advantage of tumor cells is a result of their ability to bypass quiescence. Cancer cells often show alterations in signal transduction pathways that lead to proliferation in response to external signals. Mutations or alterations in the expression of cell-cycle proteins, growth factors, growth factor receptors, intracellular signal transduction proteins, and nuclear transcription factors all can lead to disturbance of the basic regulatory mechanisms that control the cell cycle, allowing unregulated cell growth and proliferation. The cell cycle is divided into four phases (Fig. 10-2). During the synthetic or S phase, the cell generates a single copy of its genetic material, whereas in the mitotic or M phase, the cellular components are partitioned between two daughter cells. The G_1 and G_2 phases represent gap phases during which the cells prepare themselves for completion of the S and M phases, respectively. When cells cease proliferation, they exit the cell cycle and enter the quiescent state referred to as G_0. In human tumor cell-cycle regulators like INK4A, INK4B, and KIP1 are frequently mutated or altered in expression. These alterations underscore the importance of cell-cycle regulation in the prevention of human cancers. (See Schwartz 9th ed., p. 240.)

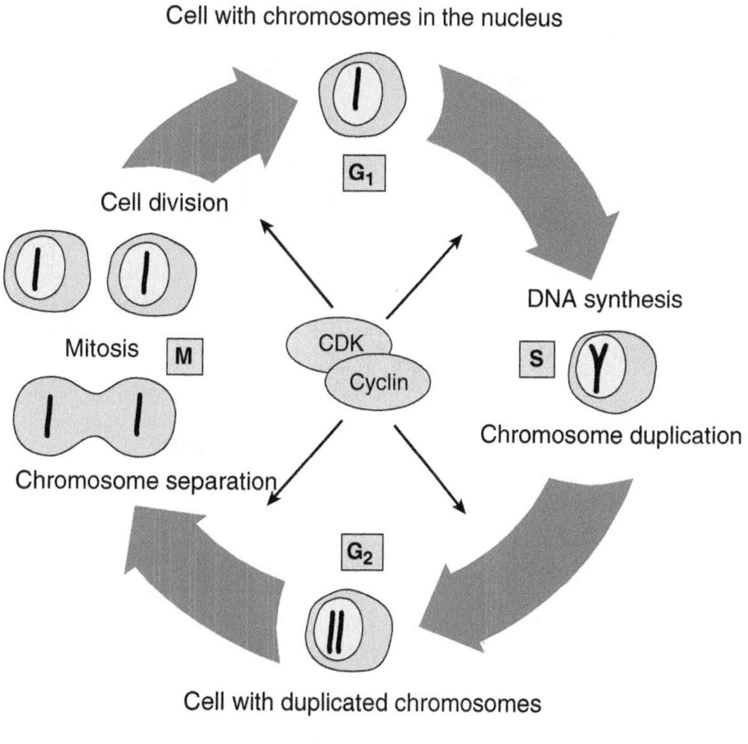

FIG. 10-2. Schematic representation of the phases of the cell cycle. Mitogenic growth factors can drive a quiescent cell from G_0 into the cell cycle. Once the cell cycle passes beyond the restriction point, mitogens are no longer required for progression into and through S phase. The DNA is replicated in S phase, and the chromosomes are condensed and segregated in mitosis. In early G_1 phase, certain signals can drive a cell to exit the cell cycle and enter a quiescent phase. Cell-cycle checkpoints have been identified in G_1, S, G_2, and M phases. CDK = cyclin-dependent kinase. (Adapted from Kastan M, Skapek S: Molecular biology of cancer: The cell cycle, in DeVita V, Hellman S, Rosenberg S (eds): *Cancer: Principles and Practice of Oncology*, 7th ed. Philadelphia: Lippincott Williams & Wilkins, 2005.)

9. Which of the following is a proto-oncogene that is activated to promote malignant growth by gene amplification?
   A. BRCA 1
   B. ras
   C. *HER2/neu*
   D. p53

Answer: C

Normal cellular genes that contribute to cancer when abnormal are called *oncogenes*. The normal counterpart of such a gene is referred to as a *proto-oncogene*. Oncogenes are usually designated by three-letter abbreviations, such as *myc* or *ras*. Oncogenes are further designated by the prefix "v-" for virus or "c-" for cell or chromosome, corresponding to the origin of the oncogene when it was first detected. Proto-oncogenes can be activated (show increased activity) or overexpressed (expressed at increased protein levels) by translocation (e.g., *abl*), promoter insertion (e.g., c-*myc*), mutation (e.g., *ras*), or amplification (e.g., *HER2/neu*). More than 100 oncogenes have been identified. (See Schwartz 9th ed., p. 241.)

10. HER2, also known as neu, is an oncogene that promotes malignant potential by
    A. Forming a hetrodimer with other EGFR members
    B. Increasing cell proliferation and growth
    C. Suppressing apoptosis
    D. All of the above

Answer: D

HER2 can interact with different members of the EGFR family and regulate mitogenic and survival signaling (Fig 10-3). (See Schwartz 9th ed., p. 242.)

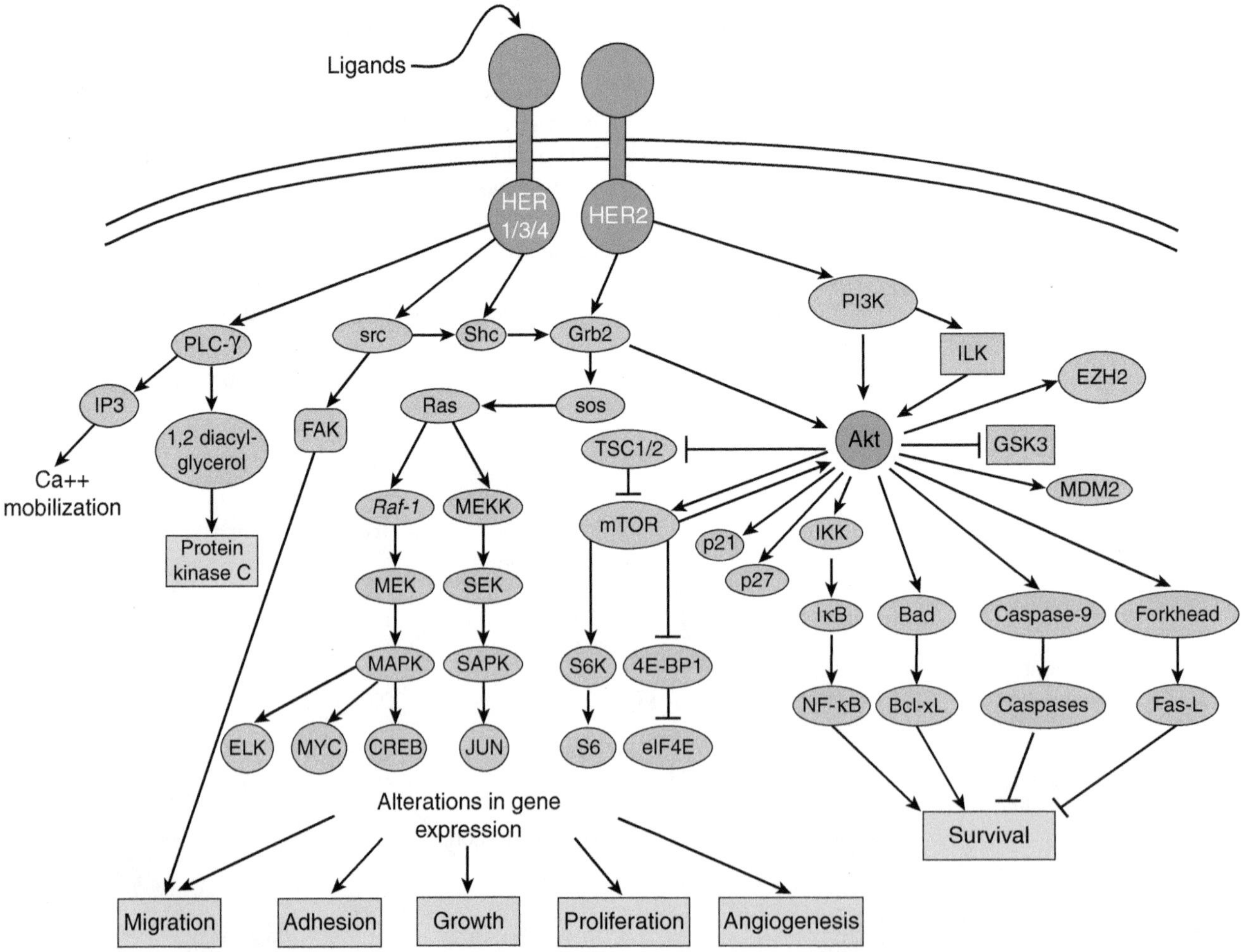

FIG. 10-3. Selected HER2 signaling pathways. HER2 can interact with different members of the HER family and activate mitogenic and antiapoptotic pathways. 4E-BP1 = eIF4E binding protein 1; CREB = cyclic adenosine monophosphate element binding; eIF4E = eukaryotic initiation factor 4E; EZH = enhancer of zeste homolog; FAK = focal adhesion kinase; Fas-L = Fas ligand; GSK3 = glycogen synthase kinase-3; HER = human epidermal growth receptor; IKK = IκB kinase; ILK= integrin-linked kinase; IP3 = inositol triphosphate; IκB = inhibitor of NF-κB; MAPK = mitogen-activated protein kinase; MDM2 = mouse double minute 2 homologue; MEK = mitogen-activated protein/extracellular signal regulated kinase kinase; MEKK = MEK kinase; mTOR = mammalian target of rapamycin; NF-κB = nuclear factor κB; PI3K = phosphoinositide-3 kinase; PLC-γ = phospholipase Cγ, SAPK = stress-activated protein kinase; SEK = SAPK/extracellular signal regulated kinase kinase; TSC = tuberous sclerosis complex. (Modified with permission from Meric-Bernstam F, Hung MC: Advances in targeting human epidermal growth factor receptor-2 signaling for cancer therapy. *Clin Cancer Res* 12:6326, 2006.)

11. What percentage of malignant tumors have activating mutations in one of the ras genes?
    A. 1%
    B. 5%
    C. 20%
    D. 70%

Answer: C

Approximately 20% of all tumors have activating mutations in one of the ras genes. The frequency of *ras* mutations varies widely by cancer type (e.g., 90% of pancreatic cancers, but <5% of breast cancers). Tumors that lack *ras* mutations, however, may undergo activation of the *ras* signaling pathway by other mechanisms, such as growth factor receptor activation, loss of GAP, or activation of *ras* effectors. (See Schwartz 9th ed., p. 243.)

12. Which of the following stimulates the extrinsic (death receptor) apoptotic pathway?
    A. Tumor necrosis factor
    B. DNA damage
    C. Release of cytochrome C from the mitochondria
    D. BcL-2 activcation

Answer: A

The effectors of apoptosis are a family of proteases called *caspases* (cysteine-dependent and aspartate-directed proteases). The initiator caspases (e.g., 8, 9, and 10), which are upstream, cleave the downstream executioner caspases (e.g., 3, 6, and 7) that carry out the destructive functions of apoptosis.

Two principal molecular pathways signal apoptosis by cleaving the initiator caspases with the potential for crosstalk: the mitochondrial pathway and the death receptor pathway. In the mitochondrial (or intrinsic) pathway, death results from the release of cytochrome c from the mitochondria.

The mitochondrial pathway can be stimulated by many factors, including DNA damage, reactive oxygen species, or the withdrawal of survival factors. The permeability of the mitochondrial membrane determines whether the apoptotic pathway will proceed. The Bcl-2 family of regulatory proteins includes proapoptotic proteins (e.g., Bax, Bad, and Bak) and antiapoptotic proteins (e.g., Bcl-2 and Bcl-xL). The activity of the Bcl-2 proteins is centered on the mitochondria, where they regulate membrane permeability.

The second principal apoptotic pathway is the death receptor pathway, sometimes referred to as the *extrinsic pathway*. Cell-surface death receptors include Fas/APO1/CD95, tumor necrosis factor receptor 1, and KILL-ER/DR5, which bind their ligands Fas-L, tumor necrosis factor (TNF), and TNF-related apoptosis-inducing ligand (TRAIL), respectively. When the receptors are bound by their ligands, they form a death-inducing signaling complex (DISC). (See Schwartz 9th ed., p. 243.)

13. Which of the following is INCORRECT?
    A. A feature of malignant cells is invasion
    B. In situ cancer lies above the basement membrane
    C. Invasion involves changes in adhesion, motility, and proteolysis of extracellular matrix
    D. E-cadherin molecules increase invasion

Answer: D

A feature of malignant cells is their ability to invade the surrounding normal tissue. Tumors in which the malignant cells appear to lie exclusively above the basement membrane are referred to as *in situ cancer*, whereas tumors in which the malignant cells are demonstrated to breach the basement membrane, penetrating into surrounding stroma, are termed *invasive cancer*. The ability to invade involves changes in adhesion, initiation of motility, and proteolysis of the extracellular matrix (ECM). Cell-to-cell adhesion in normal cells involves interactions between cell-surface proteins. Calcium adhesion molecules of the cadherin family (E-cadherin, P-cadherin, and N-cadherin) are thought to enhance the cells' ability to bind to one another and suppress invasion. (See Schwartz 9th ed., p. 244.)

14. Which of the following is NOT a gene associated with hereditary cancer
    A. FBN1
    B. CDH1
    C. HER2
    D. RET

Answer: A
FBN1 is the gene associated with Marfan's syndrome and is not associated with malignancy. CDH1, HER2, and RET are associated with hereditary cancers. (See Schwartz 9th ed., p. 247, and Table 10-1.)

TABLE 10-1 Genes associated with hereditary cancer

Gene	Location	Syndrome	Cancer Sites and Associated Traits
APC	17q21	Familial adenomatous polyposis (FAP)	Colorectal adenomas and carcinomas, duodenal and gastric tumors, desmoids, medulloblastomas, osteomas
BMPRIA	10q21-q22	Juvenile polyposis coli	Juvenile polyps of the GI tract, GI and colorectal malignancy
BRCA1	17q21	Breast-ovarian syndrome	Breast cancer, ovarian cancer, colon cancer, prostate cancer
BRCA2	13q12.3	Breast-ovarian syndrome	Breast cancer, ovarian cancer, colon cancer, prostate cancer, cancer of the gallbladder and bile duct, pancreatic cancer, gastric cancer, melanoma
p16; CDK4	9p21; 12q14	Familial melanoma	Melanoma, pancreatic cancer, dysplastic nevi, atypical moles
CDH1	16q22	Hereditary diffuse gastric cancer	Gastric cancer
hCHK2	22q12.1	Li-Fraumeni syndrome and hereditary breast cancer	Breast cancer, soft tissue sarcoma, brain tumors
hMLH1; hMSH2; hMSH6; PMS1; hPMS2	3p21; 2p22-21; 2p16; 2q31-33; 7p22	Hereditary nonpolyposis colorectal cancer	Colorectal cancer, endometrial cancer, transitional cell carcinoma of the ureter and renal pelvis, and carcinomas of the stomach, small bowel, ovary, and pancreas
MEN1	11q13	Multiple endocrine neoplasia type 1	Pancreatic islet cell cancer, parathyroid hyperplasia, pituitary adenomas
MET	7q31	Hereditary papillary renal cell carcinoma	Renal cancer
NF1	17q11	Neurofibromatosis type 1	Neurofibroma, neurofibrosarcoma, acute myelogenous leukemia, brain tumors
NF2	22q12	Neurofibromatosis type 2	Acoustic neuromas, meningiomas, gliomas, ependymomas
PTC	9q22.3	Nevoid basal cell carcinoma	Basal cell carcinoma
PTEN	10q23.3	Cowden disease	Breast cancer, thyroid cancer, endometrial cancer
rb	13q14	Retinoblastoma	Retinoblastoma, sarcomas, melanoma, and malignant neoplasms of brain and meninges
RET	10q11.2	Multiple endocrine neoplasia type 2	Medullary thyroid cancer, pheochromocytoma, parathyroid hyperplasia
SDHB; SDHC; SDHD	1p363.1-p35; 11q23; 1q21	Hereditary paraganglioma and pheochromocytoma	Paraganglioma, pheochromocytoma
SMAD4/DPC4	18q21.1	Juvenile polyposis coli	Juvenile polyps of the GI tract, GI and colorectal malignancy
STK11	19p13.3	Peutz-Jeghers syndrome	GI tract carcinoma, breast carcinoma, testicular cancer, pancreatic cancer, benign pigmentation of the skin and mucosa
p53	17p13	Li-Fraumeni syndrome	Breast cancer, soft tissue sarcoma, osteosarcoma, brain tumors, adrenocortical carcinoma, Wilms' tumor, phyllodes tumor of the breast, pancreatic cancer, leukemia, neuroblastoma
TSC1; TSC2	9q34; 16p13	Tuberous sclerosis	Multiple hamartomas, renal cell carcinoma, astrocytoma
VHL	3p25	von Hippel-Lindau disease	Renal cell carcinoma, hemangioblastomas of retina and central nervous system, pheochromocytoma
WT	11p13	Wilms' tumor	Wilms' tumor, aniridia, genitourinary abnormalities, mental retardation

Data from Marsh DJ, Zori RT: Genetic insights into familial cancers—update and recent discoveries. *Cancer Lett* 181:125, 2002. Copyright © Elsevier.

15. Certain breast cancer subtypes preferably spread to certain organs. This is an example of
    A. Tumor dormancy
    B. "Seed and soil" theory
    C. Lymphatic spread
    D. In situ carcinoma

Answer: B
One explanation for the tendency of cancer subtypes to spread to certain organs is mechanical and is based on the different circulatory drainage patterns of the tumors. When different tumor types and their preferred metastasis sites were compared, 66% of organ-specific metastases were explained on the basis of blood flow alone. The other explanation for preferential metastasis is

what is referred to as the *'seed and soil' theory*, the dependence of the seed (the cancer cell) on the soil (the secondary organ). According to this theory, once cells have reached a secondary organ, their growth efficiency in that organ is based on the compatibility of the cancer cell's biology with its new microenvironment. (See Schwartz 9th ed., p. 245.)

16. Mutations in the Rb1 gene were first associated with
    A. Breast cancer
    B. Colorectal cancer
    C. Rhabdomyosarcoma
    D. Retinoblastoma

Answer: D

The retinoblastoma gene *rb1* was the first tumor suppressor to be cloned. The *rb1* gene product, the Rb protein, is a regulator of transcription that controls the cell cycle, differentiation, and apoptosis in normal development. Retinoblastoma is a pediatric retinal tumor. Most of these tumors are detected within the first 7 years of life. Bilateral disease usually is diagnosed earlier, at an average age of 12 months. There is a higher incidence of second extraocular primary tumors, especially sarcomas, malignant melanomas, and malignant neoplasms of the brain and meninges in patients with germline mutations. In addition to hereditary retinoblastoma, Rb protein is commonly inactivated directly by mutation in many sporadic tumors. Moreover, other molecules in the Rb pathway, such as p16 and cyclin-dependent kinases 4 and 6 (CDK4 and CDK6), have been identified in a number of sporadic tumors, which suggests that the Rb pathway is critical in malignant transformation. (See Schwartz 9th ed., p. 246.)

17. APC (adenomatosis polyposis coli tumor-suppressor gene) is abnormal in what percentage of sporadic (non-syndromic) colon cancer?
    A. 5%
    B. 15%
    C. 50%
    D. 80%

Answer: D

The product of the adenomatous polyposis coli tumor-suppressor gene (*APC*) is widely expressed in many tissues and plays an important role in cell-cell interactions, cell adhesion, regulation of β-catenin, and maintenance of cytoskeletal microtubules. Alterations in *APC* lead to dysregulation of several physiologic processes that govern colonic epithelial cell homeostasis, including cell-cycle progression, migration, differentiation, and apoptosis. Mutations in the *APC* gene have been identified in FAP and in 80% of sporadic colorectal cancers. Furthermore, *APC* mutations are the earliest known genetic alterations in colorectal cancer progression, which emphasizes its importance in cancer initiation. The germline mutations in *APC* may arise from point mutations, insertions, or deletions that lead to a premature stop codon and a truncated, functionally inactive protein. The risk of developing specific manifestations of FAP is correlated with the position of the FAP mutations, a phenomenon referred to as *genotype-phenotype correlation*. For example, desmoids usually are associated with mutations between codons 1403 and 1578. (See Schwartz 9th ed., p. 248.)

CLINICAL QUESTIONS

1. Which of the following is thought to have contributed to a decrease in the worldwide mortality rate of gastric cancer?
    A. Lower intake of fruits
    B. Better food preservation
    C. Routine laboratory monitoring
    D. More effective therapy after diagnosis

Answer: B

The incidence of stomach cancer varies significantly among different regions of the world. The age-adjusted incidence is highest in Japan (62.1 per 100,000 men, 26.1 per 100,000 women). In comparison, the rates are much lower in North America (7.4 per 100,000 (4.4 to 3.4 per 100,000 men, 2.5 to 3.6 per 100,000 women). The difference in risk by country is presumed to be primarily due to differences in dietary factors. The risk is increased by high consumption of preserved salted foods such as meats and pickles, and decreased by high intake of fruits and vegetables. There also is some international variation in the incidence of infection with *Helicobacter pylori*, which is known to play a major role in gastric cancer development. Fortunately, a steady decline is being observed in the incidence and mortality rates of gastric cancer. This may be related to improvements in preservation and storage of foods as well as due to changes in the prevalence of *H. pylori*. (See Schwartz 9th ed., p. 237.)

2. A patient with breast cancer is considered to be cancer free (no further risk of primary recurrence or metastatic tumor) after
   A. 3 years
   B. 5 years
   C. 10 years
   D. Never

Answer: D

Metastases can sometimes arise several years after the treatment of primary tumors. For example, although most breast cancer recurrences occur within the first 10 years after the initial treatment and recurrences are rare after 20 years, breast cancer recurrences have been reported decades after the original tumor. This phenomenon is referred to as *dormancy*, and it remains one of the biggest challenges in cancer biology. Persistence of solitary cancer cells in a secondary site such as the liver or bone marrow is one possible contributor to dormancy. Another explanation of dormancy is that cells remain viable in a quiescent state and then become reactivated by a physiologically perturbing event. Interestingly, primary tumor removal has been proposed to be a potentially perturbing factor. An alternate explanation is that cells establish preangiogenic metastases in which they continue to proliferate but that the proliferative rate is balanced by the apoptotic rate. Therefore, when these small metastases acquire the ability to become vascularized, substantial tumor growth can be achieved at the metastatic site, leading to clinical detection. (See Schwartz 9th ed., p. 245.)

3. Which of the following is the most common etiology of Li-Fraumeni syndrome?
   A. Exposure to aflatoxin
   B. Exposure to radiation
   C. Mutation in the p53 gene
   D. Mutation in the BRCA1 gene

Answer: C

Li-Fraumeni syndrome (LFS) was first defined on the basis of observed clustering of malignancies, including early-onset breast cancer, soft tissue sarcomas, brain tumors, adrenocortical tumors, and leukemia. Criteria for classic LFS in an individual (the proband) include (a) a bone or soft tissue sarcoma when younger than 45 years, (b) a first-degree relative with cancer before age 45 years, and (c) another first- or second-degree relative with either a sarcoma diagnosed at any age or any cancer diagnosed before age 45 years. Approximately 70% of LFS families have been shown to have germline mutations in the tumor-suppressor gene p53. Breast carcinoma, soft tissue sarcoma, osteosarcoma, brain tumors, adrenocortical carcinoma, Wilms' tumor, and phyllodes tumor of the breast are strongly associated; pancreatic cancer is moderately associated; and leukemia and neuroblastoma are weakly associated with germline p53 mutations. Mutations of p53 have not been detected in approximately 30% of LFS families, and it is hypothesized that genetic alterations in other proteins interacting with p53 function may play a role in these families. (See Schwartz 9th ed., p. 246.)

4. What percentage of breast cancers are hereditary?
   A. <1%
   B. 5-10%
   C. 30%
   D. 50%

Answer: B

It is estimated that 5 to 10% of breast cancers are hereditary. Of women with early-onset breast cancer (aged 40 years or younger), nearly 10% have a germline mutation in one of the breast cancer genes *BRCA1* or *BRCA2*. Mutation carriers are more prevalent among women who have a first- or second-degree relative with premenopausal breast cancer or ovarian cancer at any age. The likelihood of a *BRCA* mutation is higher in patients who belong to a population in which founder mutations may be prevalent, such as in the Ashkenazi Jewish population. (See Schwartz 9th ed., p. 248.)

5. The risk of developing breast cancer by age 70 for a woman with a BRCA1 mutation is approximately
   A. 20%
   B. 40%
   C. 60%
   D. 80%

Answer: D

For a female *BRCA1* mutation carrier, the cumulative risks of developing breast cancer and ovarian cancer by age 70 have been estimated to be 87 and 44%, respectively. The cumulative risks of breast cancer and ovarian cancer by age 70 in families with *BRCA2* mutation have been estimated to be 84 and 27%, respectively. Although male breast cancer can occur with either *BRCA1* or *BRCA2* mutation, the majority of families (76%) with both male and female breast cancer have mutations in *BRCA2*. (See Schwartz 9th ed., p. 248.)

6. BRCA2 mutations are associated with all of the following EXCEPT
   A. Gastric cancer
   B. Lung cancer
   C. Ovarian cancer
   D. Prostate cancer

Answer: B

Besides breast and ovarian cancer, *BRCA1* and *BRCA2* mutations may be associated with increased risks for several other cancers. *BRCA1* mutations confer a fourfold increased risk for colon cancer and threefold increased risk for prostate cancer. *BRCA2* mutations confer a fivefold increased risk for prostate cancer, sevenfold in men younger than 65 years. Furthermore, *BRCA2* mutations confer a fivefold increased risk for gallbladder and bile duct cancers, fourfold increased risk for pancreatic cancer, and threefold increased risk for gastric cancer and malignant melanoma. (See Schwartz 9th ed., p. 248.)

7. A patient with Lynch syndrome 2 is at increased risk for
   A. Carcinoma of the endometrium
   B. Secretory carcinoma of the breast
   C. Osteosarcoma
   D. Melanoma

Answer: A

Hereditary nonpolyposis colorectal cancer (HNPCC), also referred to as *Lynch syndrome*, is an autosomal dominant hereditary cancer syndrome that predisposes to a wide spectrum of cancers, including colorectal cancer without polyposis. Some have proposed that HNPCC consists of at least two syndromes: Lynch syndrome 1, which entails hereditary predisposition for colorectal cancer with early age of onset (approximately age 44 years) and an excess of synchronous and metachronous colonic cancers; and Lynch syndrome 2, featuring a similar colonic phenotype accompanied by a high risk for carcinoma of the endometrium, transitional cell carcinoma of the ureter and renal pelvis, and carcinomas of the stomach, small bowel, ovary, and pancreas. The diagnostic criteria for HNPCC are referred to as the *Amsterdam criteria*, or the *3-2-1-0 rule*. The classic *Amsterdam criteria* were revised to include other HNPCC-related cancers (Table 10-2). (See Schwartz 9th ed., p. 248.)

TABLE 10-2 Revised criteria for hereditary nonpolyposis colon cancer (HNPCC) (Amsterdam criteria II)

Three or more relatives with an HNPCC-associated cancer (colorectal cancer, endometrial cancer, cancer of the small bowel, ureter, or renal pelvis), one of whom is a first-degree relative of the other two
At least two successive generations affected
At least one case diagnosed before age 50 y
Familial adenomatous polyposis excluded
Tumors verified by pathologic examination

Source: Modified with permission from Vasen HF, Watson P, Mecklin JP, et al: New clinical criteria for hereditary nonpolyposis colorectal cancer (HNPCC, Lynch syndrome) proposed by the international Collarbone group on HNPCC. *Gastroenterology* 116:1453, 1999. Copyright © Elsevier.

8. Cowden syndrome is associated with an increased incidence of
   A. Thyroid cancer
   B. Adrenal cancer
   C. Colorectal cancer
   D. Gastric cancer

Answer: A

Somatic deletions or mutations in the tumor-suppressor gene *PTEN* (phosphatase and tensin homologue deleted on chromosome 10) have been observed in a number of glioma and breast, prostate, and renal carcinoma cell lines and several primary tumor specimens. *PTEN* also is referred to as the *gene mutated in multiple advanced cancers 1 (MMAC1)*. *PTEN* was identified as the susceptibility gene for the autosomal dominant syndrome Cowden disease (CD) or multiple hamartoma syndrome. Trichilemmomas, benign tumors of the hair follicle infundibulum, and mucocutaneous papillomatosis are pathognomonic of CD. Other common features include thyroid adenomas and multinodular goiters, breast fibroadenomas, and hamartomatous GI polyps. The diagnosis of CD is made when an individual or family has a combination of pathognomonic major and/or minor criteria proposed by the International Cowden Consortium (Table 10-3). CD is associated with an increased risk of breast and thyroid cancers. Breast cancer develops in 25 to 50% of affected women. (See Schwartz 9th ed., p. 249.)

TABLE 10-3 Cowden disease diagnostic criteria

Pathognomonic criteria
Mucocutaneous lesions
Facial trichilemmomas
Acral keratoses
Papillomatous lesions
Mucosal lesions
Major criteria
Breast cancer
Thyroid cancer, especially follicular thyroid carcinoma type
Macrocephaly (≥97th percentile)
Lhermitte-Duclos disease
Endometrial carcinoma
Minor criteria
Other thyroid lesions (e.g., goiter)
Mental retardation (intelligence quotient ≤75)
GI hamartomas
Fibrocystic disease of the breast
Lipomas
Fibromas
Genitourinary tumors (e.g., uterine fibroids) or malformation
Operational diagnosis in an individual
Mucocutaneous lesions alone if there are:
Six or more facial papules, of which three or more must be trichilemmoma, or
Cutaneous facial papules and oral mucosal papillomatosis, or
Oral mucosal papillomatosis and acral keratoses, or
Palmoplantar keratoses, six or more
Two major criteria, but one must be macrocephaly or Lhermitte-Duclos disease
One major and three minor criteria
Four minor criteria

Source: Modified with permission from Eng C: Will the real Cowden syndrome please stand up: revised diagnostic criteria. *J med Genet* 37:828, 2000. With permission from the BMJ Publishing Group.

9. Patients with hereditary melanoma due to a p16 mutation are also at higher risk for
   A. Thyroid cancer
   B. Pancreatic cancer
   C. Colorectal cancer
   D. Breast cancer

Answer: B

The gene *P16*, also known as INK4A, CDKN1, CDKN2A, and MTS1, is a tumor suppressor that acts by binding CDK4 and CDK6 and that is required for phosphorylation of Rb and subsequent cell-cycle progression. Studies suggest that germline mutations in p16 can be found in 20% of melanoma-prone families. Mutations in p16 that alter its ability to inhibit the catalytic activity of the CDK4-CDK6/cyclin D complex not only increase the risk of melanoma by 75-fold but also increase the risk of pancreatic cancer by 22-fold. (See Schwartz 9th ed., p. 249.)

10. Which of the following chemical carcinogens has been associated with angiosarcoma of the liver?
   A. Benzene
   B. Diethylstilbestrol
   C. Vinyl chloride
   D. Coal tar

Answer: C

(See Schwartz 9th ed., p. 250, and Table 10-4 below.)

TABLE 10-4 Selected IARC group 1 chemical carcinogens[a]

Chemical	Predominant Tumor Type[b]
Aflatoxins	Liver cancer
Arsenic	Skin cancer
Benzene	Leukemia
Benzidine	Bladder cancer
Beryllium	Lung cancer
Cadmium	Lung cancer
Chinese-style salted fish	Nasopharyngeal carcinoma
Chlorambucil	Leukemia
Chromium [VI] compounds	Lung cancer
Coal tar	Skin cancer, scrotal cancer
Cyclophosphamide	Bladder cancer, leukemia
Diethylstilbestrol (DES)	Vaginal and cervical clear cell adenocarcinomas
Ethylene oxide	Leukemia, lymphoma
Estrogen replacement therapy	Endometrial cancer, breast cancer
Nickel	Lung cancer, nasal cancer
Tamoxifen[c]	Endometrial cancer
Vinyl chloride	Angiosarcoma of the liver, hepatocellular carcinoma, brain tumors, lung cancer, malignancies of lymphatic and hematopoietic system
TCDD (2,3,7,8-tetrachlorodibenzo-para-dioxin)	Soft tissue sarcoma
Tobacco products, smokeless	Oral cancer
Tobacco smoke	Lung cancer, oral cancer, pharyngeal cancer, laryngeal cancer, esophageal cancer (squamous cell), pancreatic cancer, bladder cancer, liver cancer, renal cell carcinoma, cervical cancer, leukemia

[a]Based on information in the IARC monographs.
[b]Only tumor types for which causal relationships are established are listed. Other cancer types may be linked to the agents with a lower frequency or with insufficient data to prove causality.
[c]Tamoxifen has been shown to prevent contralateral breast cancer.
IARC = International Agency for Research on Cancer.
Source: Based on data from *http://monographs.iarc.fr/ENG/Classification/index.php:* IARC Monographs on the Evaluation of Carcinogenic Risks to Humans, Complete List of Agents Evaluated and Their Classification, International Agency for Research on Cancer (IARC) [accessed January 16, 2008].

11. Exposure to coal tar is associated with which of the following cancers?
    A. Bladder cancer
    B. Nasopharyngeal cancer
    C. Scrotal cancer
    D. Breast cancer

Answer: C
(See Schwartz 9th ed., p. 250, and Table 10-4.)

12. Epstein Barr virus (EBV) is associated with which of the following cancers?
    A. Nasopharyngeal carcinoma
    B. Non-Hodgkin's lymphoma
    C. Adult T-cell leukemia
    D. Kaposi's sarcoma

Answer: A
(See Schwartz 9th ed., p. 251, and Table 10-5.)

TABLE 10-5 Selected viral carcinogens[a]

Virus	Predominant Tumor Type[b]
Epstein-Barr virus	Burkitt's lymphoma Hodgkin's disease Immunosuppression-related lymphoma Sinonasal angiocentric T-cell lymphoma Nasopharyngeal carcinoma
Hepatitis B virus	Hepatocellular carcinoma
Hepatitis C virus	Hepatocellular carcinoma
HIV type 1	Kaposi's sarcoma Non-Hodgkin's lymphoma
Human papillomavirus 16 and 18	Cervical cancer Anal cancer
Human T-cell lymphotropic viruses	Adult T-cell leukemia/lymphoma

[a]Based on information in the International Agency for Research on Cancer monographs.
[b]Only tumor types for which causal relationships are established are listed. Other cancer types may be linked to the agents with a lower frequency or with insufficient data to prove causality.
Source: Based on data from *http://monographs.iarc.fr/ENG/Classification/crthgr01.php:* IARC Monographs on the Evaluation of Carcinogenic Risks to Humans, Overall Evaluations of Carcinogenicity to Humans: Group 1: Carcinogenic to Humans, International Agency for Research on Cancer (IARC) [accessed January 16, 2008].

13. Which of the following is the most significant risk factor for invasive breast cancer when screening a patient for risk?
    A. >2 first-degree relatives with breast cancer
    B. 2 previous breast biopsies in a patient <50 years of age
    C. Age <12 at menarche
    D. Atypical hyperplasia in a previous breast biopsy

Answer: A
(See Schwartz 9th ed., p. 253, and Table 10-6.)

TABLE 10-6 Assessment of risk for invasive breast cancer

Risk Factor	Relative Risk (%)
Age at menarche (years)	
>14	1.00
12–13	1.10
<12	1.21
Age at first live birth (years)	
Patients with no first-degree relatives with cancer	
<20	1.00
20–24	1.24
25–29 or nulliparous	1.55
≥30	1.93
Patients with one first-degree relative with cancer	
<20	1.00
20–24	2.64
25–29 or nulliparous	2.76
≥30	2.83
Patients with ≥2 first-degree relatives with cancer	
<20	6.80
20–24	5.78
25–29 or nulliparous	4.91
≥30	4.17
Breast biopsies (number)	
Patients aged <50 y at counseling	
0	1.00
1	1.70
≥2	2.88

(*continued*)

TABLE 10-6 (continued)

Risk Factor	Relative Risk (%)
Patients aged ≥50 y at counseling	
0	1.00
1	1.27
≥2	1.62
Atypical hyperplasia	
No biopsies	1.00
At least 1 biopsy, no atypical hyperplasia	0.93
No atypical hyperplasia, hyperplasia status unknown for at least 1 biopsy	1.00
Atypical hyperplasia in at least 1 biopsy	1.82

Source: Modified with permission from Gail MH et al: Projecting individualized probabilities of developing breast cancer for white females who are being examined annually. *J Natl Cancer Inst* 81:1989. By permission of Oxford University Press.

14. For average-risk patients, routine cancer screening is recommended for all but the following disease?
    A. Breast cancer
    B. Colorectal cancer
    C. Cervical cancer
    D. Pancreatic cancer

Answer: D

(See Schwartz 9th ed., p. 254, and Table 10-7.)

TABLE 10-7 American Cancer Society recommendations for early detection of cancer in average-risk, asymptomatic individuals

Cancer Site	Population	Test or Procedure	Frequency
Breast	Women aged ≥20 y	Breast self-examination	Monthly, starting at age 20
		Clinical breast examination	Every 3 y, ages 20–39 Annual, starting at age 40
		Mammography	Annual, starting at age 40
Colorectal	Men and women aged ≥50 y	Fecal occult blood test (FOBT) or fecal immunochemical test (FIT)	Annual, starting at age 50
		or	
		Flexible sigmoidoscopy	Every 5 y, starting at age 50
		or	
		FOBT and flexible sigmoidoscopy	Annual FOBT (or FIT) and flexible sigmoidoscopy every 5 y, starting at age 50
		or	
		Double-contrast barium enema (DCBE)	DCBE every 5 y, starting at age 50
		or	
		Colonoscopy	Colonoscopy every 10 y, starting at age 50
Prostate	Men aged ≥50 y	Digital rectal examination (DRE) and prostate-specific antigen (PSA) test	Offer PSA test and DRE annually, starting at age 50, for men who have life expectancy of at least 10 y
Cervix	Women aged ≥18 y	Pap test	Cervical cancer screening beginning 3 y after first vaginal intercourse, but no later than age 21 y; screening every year with conventional Pap tests or every 2 y using liquid-based Pap tests; at or after age 30 y, women who have had three normal test results in a row may get screened every 2 to 3 y with cervical cytologic analysis alone or every 3 y with a human papillomavirus DNA test plus cervical cytologic analysis.
Endometrial	Women at menopause	—	At the time of menopause, women at average risk should be informed about the risks and symptoms of endometrial cancer and strongly encouraged to report any unexpected bleeding or spotting to their physicians.
Cancer-related checkup	Men and women aged ≥20 y	On the occasion of a periodic health examination, the cancer-related checkup should include examination of the thyroid, testicles, ovaries, lymph nodes, oral cavity, and skin, as well as health counseling about tobacco use, sun exposure, diet and nutrition, risk factors, sexual practices, and environmental and occupational exposures.	

Source: Modified with permission from Smith RA, Cokkinides V, Eyre HJ: American Cancer Society guidelines for the early detection of cancer, 2006. *CA Cancer J Clin* 56:11; quiz 49, 2006.

15. Tumor staging for most epithelial cancers includes all of the following EXCEPT
   A. Tumor size
   B. Tumor mutations
   C. Nodal involvement
   D. Distant spread

Answer: B
Standardization of staging systems is essential to allow comparison of results from different studies from different institutions and worldwide. The staging systems proposed by the American Joint Committee on Cancer (AJCC) and the Union Internationale Contre le Cancer (International Union Against Cancer, or UICC) are among the most widely accepted staging systems. Both the AJCC and the UICC have adopted a shared tumor, node, and metastasis (TNM) staging system that defines the cancer in terms of the anatomic extent of disease and is based on assessment of three components: the size of the primary tumor (T), the presence (or absence) and extent of nodal metastases (N), and the presence (or absence) and extent of distant metastases (M). (See Schwartz 9th ed., p. 254.)

16. Which of the following tumor marker-disease associations is NOT correct?
   A. PSA and prostate cancer
   B. CEA and colon cancer
   C. CA19-9 and pancreatic cancer
   D. AFP and breast cancer

Answer: D
(See Schwartz 9th ed., p. 255, and Table 10-8.)

TABLE 10-8 Sensitivity and specificity of some common tumor markers

Marker	Cancer	Sensitivity (%)	Specificity (%)
Prostate-specific antigen (4 μg/L)	Prostate	57–93	55–68
Carcinoembryonic antigen	Colorectal	40–47	90
	Breast	45	81
	Recurrent disease	84	100
Alpha-fetoprotein	Hepatocellular	98	65
Cancer antigen 19-9	Pancreatic	78–90	95
Cancer antigen 27-29	Breast	62	83
Cancer antigen 15-3	Breast	57	87

Source: Modified with permission from Way BA, Kessler G: Tumor marker overview. *Lab Med Newsl* 4:1, 1996.

17. Which of the following is an alkylating agent?
   A. Cyclophosphamide
   B. Doxorubicin
   C. Pactitaxel
   D. Vincristine

Answer: A
Alkylating agents are cell-cycle–nonspecific agents, that is, they are able to kill cells in any phase of the cell cycle. They act by cross-linking the two strands of the DNA helix or by causing other direct damage to the DNA. The damage to the DNA prevents cell division and, if severe enough, leads to apoptosis. The alkylating agents are composed of three main subgroups: classic alkylators, nitrosoureas, and miscellaneous DNA-binding agents (Table 10-9). (See Schwartz 9th ed., p. 261.)

TABLE 10-9 Classification of chemotherapeutic agents

Alkylating agents
Classic alkylating agents
Busulfan
Chlorambucil
Cyclophosphamide
Ifosfamide
Mechlorethamine (nitrogen mustard)
Melphalan
Mitomycin C
Triethylene thiophosphoramide (thiotepa)
Nitrosoureas
Carmustine (BCNU)
Lomustine (CCNU)
Semustine (MeCCNU)
Streptozocin

(continued)

TABLE 10-9 (continued)

Miscellaneous DNA-binding agents
Carboplatin
Cisplatin
Dacarbazine (DTIC)
Hexamethylmelamine
Procarbazine
Antitumor antibiotics
Bleomycin
Dactinomycin (actinomycin D)
Daunorubicin
Doxorubicin
Idarubicin
Plicamycin (mithramycin)
Antimetabolites
Folate analogues
Methotrexate
Purine analogues
Azathioprine
Mercaptopurine
Thioguanine
Cladribine (2-chlorodeoxyadenosine)
Fludarabine
Pentostatin
Pyrimidine analogues
Capecitabine
Cytarabine
Floxuridine
Gemcitabine
Ribonucleotide reductase inhibitors
Hydroxyurea
Plant alkaloids
Vinca alkaloids
Vinblastine
Vincristine
Vindesine
Vinorelbine
Epipodophyllotoxins
Etoposide
Teniposide
Taxanes
Paclitaxel
Docetaxel
Miscellaneous agents
Asparaginase
Estramustine
Mitotane

18. Which of the following molecularly targeted therapies is directed against the HER2 gene?
    A. Cetuximab
    B. Sunitinib
    C. Trastuzumab
    D. Temsirolimus

Answer: C
(See Schwartz 9th ed., p. 263, and Table 10-10.)

TABLE 10-10 Selected FDA-approved targeted therapies

Generic Name	Trade Name	Company	Target	FDA Approval Date	Initial Indication
Trastuzumab	Herceptin	Genentech	HER2	9/1998	Breast cancer
Imatinib	Gleevec	Novartis	c-kit, bcr-abl, PDGFR	5/2001, 12/2002	CML, GIST
Cetuximab	Erbitux	ImClone Systems	EGFR	2/2004	Colorectal cancer
Bevacizumab	Avastin	Genentech	VEGF	2/2004	Colorectal cancer, lung cancer
Erlotinib	Tarceva	Genentech, OSI Pharmaceuticals	EGFR	11/2004	Non–small cell lung cancer
Sorafenib	Nexavar	Bayer	Raf, PDGF, VEGFR, c-kit	12/2005	RCC
Sunitinib	Sutent	Pfizer	VEGFR PDGFR c-kit, Flt-3, RET	1/2006	GIST, RCC
Dasatinib	Sprycel	Bristol-Myers Squibb	bcr-abl, src family, c-kit, EPHA2, PDGFR-β	6/2006	CML
Lapatinib	Tykerb	GlaxoSmithKline	EGFR and HER2	3/2007	Breast cancer
Temsirolimus	Torisel	Wyeth	mTOR	5/2007	RCC

CML = chronic myelogenous leukemia; EGFR = epidermal growth factor receptor; EPHA2 = ephrin A2; FDA = Food and Drug Administration; Flt-3 = fms-related tyrosine kinase 3; GIST = GI stromal tumor; HER2 = human epidermal growth factor receptor 2; mTOR = mammalian target of rapamycin; PDGF = platelet-derived growth factor; PDGFR = platelet-derived growth factor receptor; RCC = renal cell carcinoma; RET = rearranged during transfection; VEGF = vascular endothelial growth factor; VEGFR = vascular endothelial growth factor receptor.

CHAPTER 11

Transplantation

BASIC SCIENCE QUESTIONS

1. Class I HLA antigens are expressed on the membrane of
   A. All nucleated cells
   B. B lymphocytes
   C. Monocytes
   D. Dendritic cells

Answer: A

The main antigens involved in triggering rejection are coded for by a group of genes known as the *major histocompatibility complex* (MHC). These antigens, and hence genes, define the 'foreign' nature of one individual to another within the same species. In humans, the MHC complex is known as the *human leukocyte antigen* (HLA) system. It comprises a series of genes located on chromosome 6. The HLA antigens are grouped into two classes, which differ in their structure and cellular distribution. Class I molecules (named HLA-A, -B, and -C) are found on the membrane of all nucleated cells. Class II molecules (named HLA-DR, -DP, and -DQ) generally are expressed by antigen-presenting cells (APCs) such as B lymphocytes, monocytes, and dendritic cells. (See Schwartz 9th ed., p 274.)

2. Which of the following immunosuppressive drugs inhibits IL-2 synthesis?
   A. Azathioprine
   B. Mycophenolate mofetil
   C. Tacrolimus
   D. Sirolimus

Answer: C

Azathioprine inhibits DNA and RNA synthesis. Mycophenolate mofetil inhibits the synthesis of purine. Sirolimus inhibits lymphocyte function. (See Schwartz 9th ed., p 275, and Table 11-1.)

TABLE 11-1 Summary of the main immunosuppressive drugs

Drug	Mechanism of Action	Adverse Effects	Clinical Uses	Dosage
Cyclosporine (CSA)	Binds to cyclophilin Inhibits calcineurin and IL-2 synthesis	Nephrotoxicity Tremor Hypertension Hirsutism	Improved bioavailability of microemulsion form Used as mainstay of maintenance protocols	Oral dose is 8–10 mg/kg per day (given in two divided doses)
Tacrolimus (FK506)	Binds to FKBP Inhibits calcineurin and IL-2 synthesis	Nephrotoxicity Hypertension Neurotoxicity GI toxicity (nausea, diarrhea)	Improved patient and graft survival in (liver) primary and rescue therapy Used as mainstay of maintenance, like CSA	IV 0.05–0.1 mg/kg per day PO 0.15–0.3 mg/kg per day (given q12h)
Mycophenolate mofetil	Antimetabolite Inhibits enzyme necessary for de novo purine synthesis	Leukopenia GI toxicity	Effective for primary and rescue therapy (kidney transplants) May replace azathioprine	1 g bid PO (may need 1.5 g in black recipients)

(continued)

TABLE 11-1 (continued)

Drug	Mechanism of Action	Adverse Effects	Clinical Uses	Dosage
Sirolimus	Inhibits lymphocyte effects driven by IL-2 receptor	Thrombocytopenia Increased serum cholesterol/LDL Vasculitis (animal studies)	May allow early withdrawal of steroids and decreased calcineurin doses	2–4 mg/d, adjusted to trough drug levels
Corticosteroids	Multiple actions Anti-inflammatory Inhibits lymphokine production	Cushingoid state Glucose intolerance Osteoporosis	Used in induction, maintenance, and treatment of acute rejection	Varies from mg to several grams/d Maintenance doses, 5–10 mg/d
Azathioprine	Antimetabolite Interferes with DNA and RNA synthesis	Thrombocytopenia Neutropenia Liver dysfunction	Used in maintenance protocols	1–3 mg/kg per day for maintenance

FKBP = FK506-binding protein; IL = interleukin; LDL = low-density lipoprotein.

3. Cyclosporine inhibits T-cell activation by
   A. Directly binding to T-cell surface membrane
   B. Increasing production of IL-2
   C. Decreasing production of IL-10
   D. Inhibiting calcineurin

Answer: D

Cyclosporine binds with its cytoplasmic receptor protein, cyclophilin, which subsequently inhibits the activity of calcineurin. Doing so impairs expression of several critical T-cell activation genes, the most important being for IL-2. As a result, T-cell activation is suppressed. (See Schwartz 9th ed., p 276.)

4. Which of the following is a component of the University of Wisconsin preservation solution?
   A. Glucose
   B. Magnesium
   C. Raffinose
   D. Albumin

Answer: C

The most commonly used fluid worldwide is the University of Wisconsin solution. It contains lactobionate, raffinose, and hydroxyethyl starch. Lactobionate is impermeable and prevents intracellular swelling; it also lowers the concentration of intracellular calcineurin and free iron, which may be beneficial in reducing reperfusion injury. Hydroxyethyl starch, a synthetic colloid, may help decrease hypothermia-induced cell swelling of endothelial cells and reduce interstitial edema. (See Schwartz 9th ed., p 282.)

1. The proportion of patients on the waiting list to patients transplanted is approximately
   A. 1:1 (waiting:transplanted)
   B. 1:3 (waiting:transplanted)
   C. 3:1 (waiting:transplanted)
   D. 8:1 (waiting:transplanted)

Answer: C

In 2005 (see Fig. 11-1), there were approximately 28,000 patients transplanted and 90,000 on the waiting list. (See Schwartz 9th ed., p 272.)

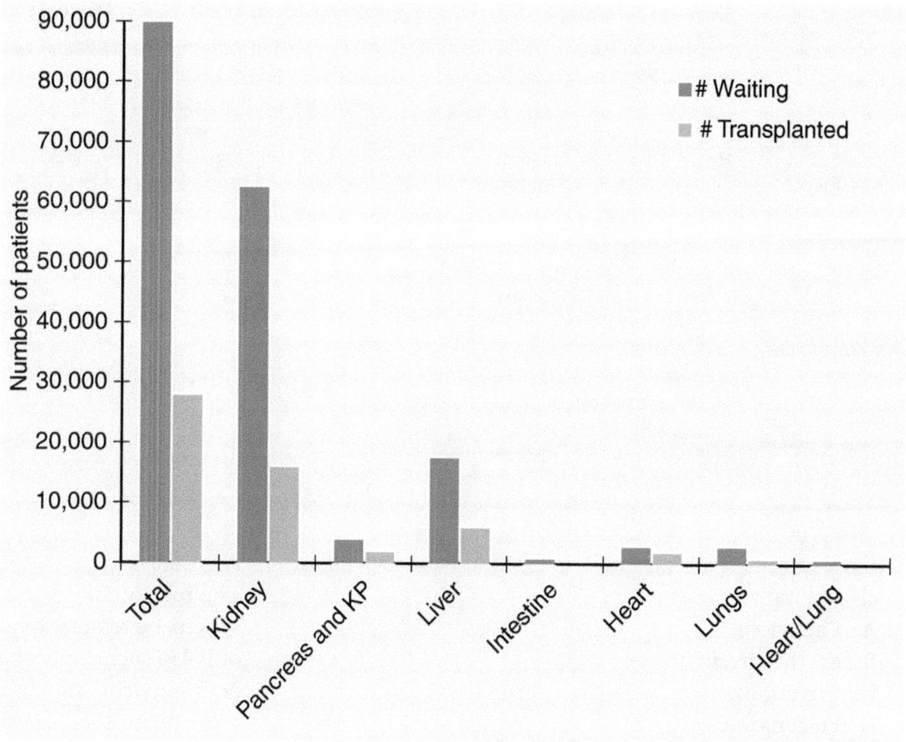

FIG. 11-1. Patients on waiting list and number of organ transplants for 2005. (U.S. data from Organ Procurement and Transplantation Network/Scientific Registry of Transplant Recipients Annual Report, *http://www.ustransplant.org*). KP = kidney and pancreas.

2. Rejection that starts on postoperative day 2 is most likely
   A. Hyperacute rejection
   B. Accelerated acute rejection
   C. Acute rejection
   D. Chronic rejection

Answer: B

[Hyperacute] rejection, which usually occurs within minutes after the transplanted organ is reperfused, is due to the presence of preformed antibodies in the recipient, antibodies that are specific to the donor. These antibodies may be directed against the donor's HLA antigens or they may be anti-ABO blood group antibodies.

[Accelerated acute] rejection, seen within the first few days posttransplant, involves both cellular and antibody-mediated injury. It is more common when a recipient has been sensitized by previous exposure to antigens present in the donor, resulting in an immunologic memory response.

Acute rejection usually is seen within days to a few months posttransplant. It is predominantly a cell-mediated process, with lymphocytes being the main cells involved.

[Chronic] rejection occurs months to years posttransplant. Now that short-term graft survival rates have improved so markedly, chronic rejection is an increasingly common problem. Histologically, the process is characterized by atrophy, fibrosis, and arteriosclerosis. Both immune and nonimmune mechanisms are likely involved. Clinically, graft function slowly deteriorates over months to years posttransplant. (See Schwartz 9th ed., p 274.)

3. The most significant side effect of sirolimus is
   A. Nephrotoxicity
   B. Thrombocytopenia
   C. Glucose intolerance
   D. Leukopenia

Answer: B

The major side effects of sirolimus include neutropenia, thrombocytopenia, and a significant elevation of the serum triglyceride and cholesterol levels. It also has been associated with impaired wound healing, leading to a higher incidence of wound-related complications. (See Schwartz 9th ed., pp 275-277, and Table 11-2.)

TABLE 11-2 Side effects and drug interactions of the main immunosuppressive drugs

	Common Side Effects	Other Medications That Increase Blood Levels	Other Medications That Decrease Blood Levels	Other Medications That Potentiate Toxicity
Cyclosporine (CSA)	Hypertension, nephrotoxicity, hirsutism, neurotoxicity, gingival hyperplasia	Verapamil, clarithromycin, doxycycline, azithromycin, erythromycin, fluconazole, itraconazole, ketoconazole	Isoniazid, carbamazepine, phenobarbital, phenytoin, rifampin	Nephrotoxicity: Acyclovir, ganciclovir, aminoglycosides, NSAIDs
Tacrolimus (FK506)	Hypertension, nephrotoxicity, hyperglycemia, neurotoxicity	Verapamil, clarithromycin, doxycycline, azithromycin, erythromycin, fluconazole, itraconazole, ketoconazole	Isoniazid, carbamazepine, phenobarbital, phenytoin, rifampin	Nephrotoxicity: Acyclovir, ganciclovir, aminoglycosides, NSAIDs
Sirolimus	Thrombocytopenia and nutropenia, elevated cholesterol, extremity edema, impaired wound healing	—	—	—
Mycophenolate mofetil	Leukopenia, thrombocytopenia, GI upset	—	Cholestyramine, antacids	—
Corticosteroids	Hyperglycemia, osteoporosis, cataracts, myopathy, weight gain	—	—	—
Azathioprine	Leukopenia, anemia, thrombocytopenia, GI upset	—	—	Bone marrow suppression: Allopurinol, sulfonamides

4. Cyclosporine levels may be decreased in patients who are also taking
   A. Phenytoin
   B. Erythromycin
   C. Cimetidine
   D. Fluconazole

Answer: A

The metabolism of cyclosporine is via the cytochrome P-450 system, therefore several drug interactions are possible. Inducers of P-450 such as phenytoin decrease blood levels; drugs such as erythromycin, cimetidine, ketoconazole, and fluconazole increase them. (See Schwartz 9th ed., p 276, and Table 11-2.)

5. Bowel removed from a living donor for small bowel transplant is most commonly
   A. Proximal jejunum
   B. Mid to distal jejunum
   C. Proximal ileum
   D. Mid to distal ileum

Answer: D

Living-donor intestinal transplants usually involve removal of about 200 cm of the donor's ileum, with inflow and outflow provided by the ileocolic vessels. (See Schwartz 9th ed., p 282.)

6. Ischemia time of a harvested lung should ideally be less than
   A. 6 hours
   B. 12 hours
   C. 24 hours
   D. 36 hours

Answer: A

With kidneys, cold ischemic times should be kept below 36 to 40 hours; after that, delayed graft function significantly increases. With pancreata, more than 24 hours of ischemia increases problems due to pancreatitis and duodenal leaks. With livers, more than 16 hours of ischemia increases the risk for primary nonfunction and biliary complications. Hearts and lungs tolerate preservation poorly; ideally, ischemia times should be below 6 hours. With marginal donors, all of these times should be adjusted further downward. (See Schwartz 9th ed., p 282.)

7. The most appropriate treatment of a lymphocele following renal transplantation is
   A. Observation until resolution
   B. Percutaneous aspiration
   C. Laparoscopic or open peritoneal window
   D. Open exploration with sclerotherapy

Answer: C

The reported incidence of lymphoceles (fluid collections of lymph that generally result from cut lymphatic vessels in the recipient) is 0.6 to 18%. Lymphoceles usually do not occur until at least 2 weeks posttransplant. Symptoms are generally related to the mass effect and compression of nearby structures (e.g., ureter, iliac vein, allograft renal artery), and patients develop hypertension, unilateral leg swelling on the side of the transplant, and elevated serum creatinine. Ultrasound is used to confirm a fluid collection, although percutaneous aspiration may be necessary to exclude presence of other collections such as urinomas, hematomas, or abscesses. The standard surgical treatment is creation of a peritoneal window to allow for drainage of the lymphatic fluid into the peritoneal cavity, where it can be absorbed. Either a laparoscopic or an open approach may be used. Another option is percutaneous insertion of a drainage catheter, with or without sclerotherapy; however, it is associated with some risk of recurrence or infection. (See Schwartz 9th ed., p 289.)

8. The major cause of death following renal transplantation is
   A. Rejection with acute renal failure
   B. Vascular (myocardial infarction or stroke)
   C. Malignancy
   D. Sepsis

Answer: B

The major cause of death in all kidney recipients is cardiovascular (myocardial infarction or stroke); sepsis accounts for less than 3%, while malignancy accounts for 2%. (See Schwartz 9th ed., p 290.)

9. The leading cause of graft loss following renal transplantation is
   A. Recipient death
   B. Acute rejection
   C. Chronic nephropathy
   D. Pyelonephritis

Answer: A

Currently, the most common cause of graft loss is recipient death (usually from cardiovascular causes) with a functioning graft. The second most common cause is chronic allograft nephropathy. Characterized by a slow, unrelenting deterioration of graft function, it likely has multiple causes (both immunologic and nonimmunologic). The graft failure rate due to surgical technique has remained at about 2%. (See Schwartz 9th ed., p 290.)

10. Back table preparation of a donor pancreas prior to transplantation includes
   A. Removal of the donor duodenum
   B. Removal of the tail of the pancreas with the spleen
   C. Ligation of the proximal splenic vein
   D. Placement of an arterial graft to connect the splenic and superior mesenteric arteries

Answer: D

(See Schwartz 9th ed., p 292, and Fig. 11-2.)

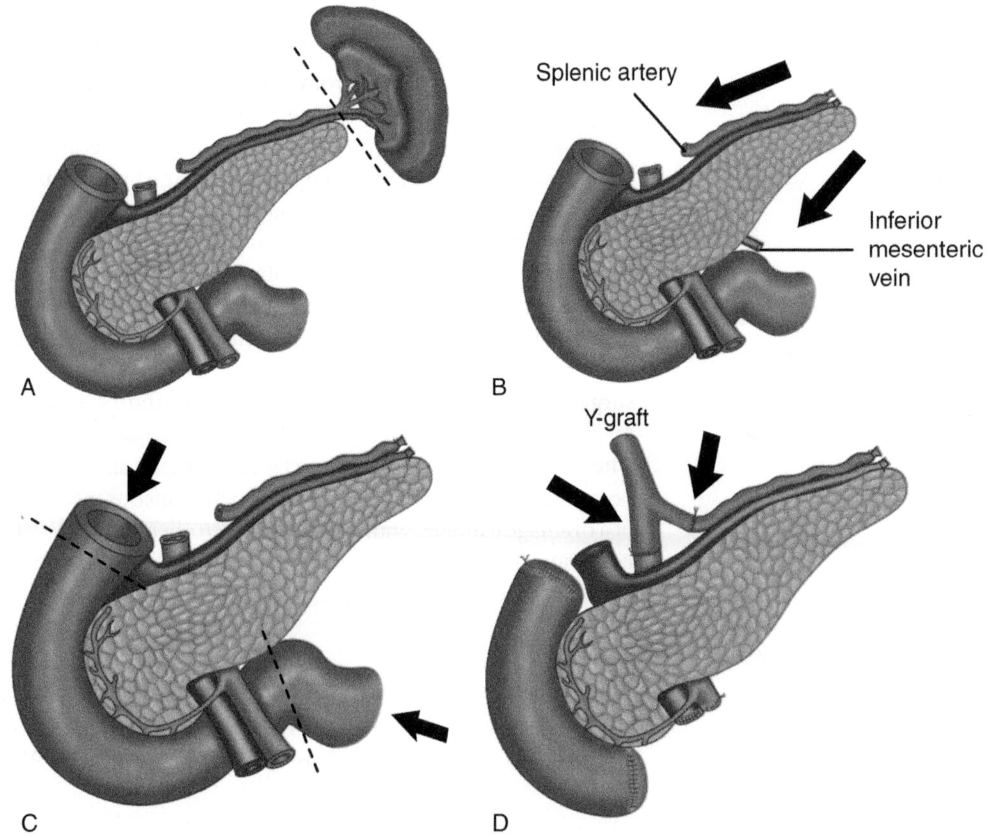

FIG. 11-2. Bench preparation of pancreas graft. Steps include (A) removal of the spleen; (B) removal of tissue along the superior and inferior aspect of the tail of the pancreas; (C) trimming of excess duodenum; and (D) ligation of vessels at the root of the mesentery and placement of arterial Y-graft.

11. The most common etiology of liver failure in patients undergoing liver transplantation is
   A. Alcoholic cirrhosis
   B. Metabolic disease
   C. Chronic hepatitis
   D. Fulminant (acute) liver failure

Answer: C

Chronic liver diseases account for the majority of liver transplants today. The most common cause in North America is chronic hepatitis, usually due to hepatitis C and less commonly to hepatitis B. Chronic alcohol abuse accelerates the process, especially with hepatitis C. Progression from chronic infection to cirrhosis is generally slow, usually occurring over a period of 10 to 20 years. Chronic hepatitis may also result from autoimmune causes, primarily in women. It can present either acutely over months or insidiously over years. Alcohol often plays a role in end-stage liver disease secondary to hepatitis C, but it may also lead to liver failure in the absence of viral infection. In fact, alcohol is the most common cause of end-stage liver disease in the United States. Such patients generally are suitable candidates for a transplant as long as an adequate period of sobriety can be documented. (See Schwartz 9th ed., p 295.)

12. Following biopsy which shows no vascular or lymphatic invasion, which of the following patients with hepatocellular carcinoma would be considered a candidate for liver transplantation?
   A. A single tumor in the left lobe 5.5 cm in diameter
   B. Two tumors, both in the right lobe, 3.5 cm and 2.5 cm in diameter
   C. Three tumors, in the right and left lobes, 2.5 cm, 2.8 cm, and 1.0 cm in diameter
   D. None of the above

Answer: C

Long-term patient survival in early series of OLT for HCC only reached 30 to 40%. It was not until patient selection strategies evolved that OLT became a more effective treatment. In a landmark 1996 study by Mazzaferro and colleagues at the University of Milan, characteristics of patients with HCC that were good candidates for OLT were described. These characteristics, now commonly referred to as the *Milan criteria*, included (a) a single lesion <5 cm or 1 to 3 tumors, each <3 cm; and (b) absence of vascular or lymphatic invasion. Patients meeting these criteria achieved an impressive 85% 4-year overall patient survival, while those patients that exceeded the Milan criteria had only 50% 4-year survival. (See Schwartz 9th ed., p 296.)

13. Which of the following is an indication for liver transplantation in a patient with acute liver failure?
A. INR >6.5
B. Age <40
C. Creatinine >2.0
D. Duration of jaundice >3 days prior to onset of encephalopathy

Answer: A
Acute liver disease, more commonly termed *fulminant hepatic failure*, is defined as the development of hepatic encephalopathy (HE) and profound coagulopathy shortly after the onset of symptoms, such as jaundice, in patients without pre-existing liver disease. The most common causes include acetaminophen overdose, acute hepatitis B infection, various drugs and hepatotoxins, and Wilson's disease; often, however, no cause is identified. Treatment consists of appropriate critical care support, giving patients time for spontaneous recovery. The prognosis for spontaneous recovery depends on the patient's age (those younger than 10 and older than 40 years have a poor prognosis), the underlying cause, and the severity of liver injury (as indicated by degree of HE, coagulopathy, and kidney dysfunction; Table 11-3). (See Schwartz 9th ed., p 296.)

TABLE 11-3 Indications for a liver transplant in patients with acute liver failure

Acetaminophen toxicity
pH <7.30
Prothrombin time >100 s (INR >6.5)
Serum creatinine >300 mmol/L (>3.4 mg/dL)
No acetaminophen toxicity
Prothrombin time >100 s (INR >6.5)
age <10 or >40 y
Non-A, non-B hepatitis
Duration of jaundice before onset of encephalopathy >7 d
Serum creatinine >300 mmol/L (>3.4 mg/dL)

INR = International Normalized Ratio.

14. Which of the following is one of the variables of the MELD score?
A. Creatinine
B. Age
C. Degree of encephalopathy
D. Cause of hepatic failure

Answer: A
Waiting list mortality can be quite accurately predicted in chronic liver failure patients by calculating their MELD (model for end-stage liver disease) score. The formula for calculation of this is:

$$\text{MELD score} = 3.8 \times \log(e)(\text{bilirubin mg/dL}) + 11.2 \times \log(e)(\text{INR}) + 9.6 \log(e)(\text{creatinine mg/dL})$$

A higher MELD score indicates a sicker patient, with a higher risk for mortality. In the United States, this scoring system has proven to be a useful method to determine the allocation of livers, with priority given to the sickest individuals. The calculated score does not take into account special situations such as HCC, which have a definite impact on waiting list mortality, but scoring exceptions are applied to these situations to allow for timely transplants. (See Schwartz 9th ed., p 297.)

15. The most common vascular complication after liver transplantation is
A. Hepatic vein thrombosis
B. Portal vein thrombosis
C. Hepatic artery thrombosis
D. Inferior vena cava thrombosis

Answer: C
The incidence of vascular complications after liver transplants ranges from 8 to 12%. Thrombosis is the most common early event, with stenosis and pseudoaneurysm formation occurring later. Hepatic artery thrombosis (HAT) has a reported incidence of about 3 to 5% in adults and about 5 to 10% in children. The incidence tends to be higher in partial liver transplant recipients. After HAT, liver recipients may be asymptomatic or may develop severe liver failure secondary to extensive necrosis. Doppler ultrasound evaluation is the initial investigative method of choice, with more than 90% sensitivity and specificity. If HAT is suggested by radiologic imaging,

urgent re-exploration is indicated, with thrombectomy and revision of the anastomosis. If hepatic necrosis is extensive, a retransplant is indicated. However, HAT also may present in a less dramatic fashion. Thrombosis may render the common bile duct ischemic, resulting in a localized or diffuse bile leak from the anastomosis or in a more chronic, diffuse biliary stricture. (See Schwartz 9th ed., p 302.)

16. PTLD (posttransplant lymphoproliferative disorder) is caused by
    A. Poorly controlled immunosuppression
    B. Induction of lymphocyte antigens by immunosuppression
    C. Cytomegalovirus infection
    D. Epstein-Barr virus infection

Answer: D
Viral infections generally are not seen until after the first month posttransplant. CMV is the most common pathogen involved. Its presentation ranges from asymptomatic infection to tissue-invasive disease. Epstein-Barr virus (EBV), another member of the herpesvirus family, also may be seen posttransplant. A wide spectrum of clinical presentations is possible, including an asymptomatic rise in antibody titers, a mononucleosis syndrome, hepatitis, and posttransplant lymphoproliferative disorder (PTLD). The most severe form of infection, PTLD can present as a localized tumor of the lymph nodes or GI tract, or rarely as a rapidly progressive, diffuse, often fatal lymphomatous infiltration. (See Schwartz 9th ed., p 304.)

17. The most common indication for pediatric liver transplantation is
    A. Wilson's disease
    B. Alagille's syndrome
    C. Biliary atresia
    D. Tyrosinemia

Answer: C
Biliary atresia is the most common indication for a pediatric liver transplant. The incidence of biliary atresia is about one in 10,000 infant births. Other cholestatic disorders that may eventually require a transplant include sclerosing cholangitis, familial cholestasis syndromes, and paucity of intrahepatic bile ducts (as seen with Alagille syndrome). Metabolic disorders probably account for the next largest group of disorders that may require a liver transplant. Such disorders may directly result in liver failure or may have mainly extrahepatic manifestations. $Alpha_1$-antitrypsin deficiency is the most common metabolic disorder that may require a liver transplant. Such patients may present with jaundice in the neonatal period, but this usually resolves. Subsequently, they may present in late childhood or early adolescence with cirrhosis and portal hypertension. Another metabolic disorder resulting in liver failure is tyrosinemia, a hereditary disorder characterized by deficiency of an enzyme that degrades the metabolic products of tyrosine, resulting in cirrhosis and a greatly increased risk for HCC. Still another is Wilson's disease, an autosomal recessive disorder characterized by copper accumulation in the liver, central nervous system, kidneys, eyes, and other organs, that may present as fulminant, subfulminant, or chronic liver failure. (See Schwartz 9th ed., p 304.)

18. Following transplantation, patients are at increased risk for which of the following malignancies?
    A. Melanoma
    B. Kaposi's sarcoma
    C. Colon cancer
    D. Follicular carcinoma of the thyroid

Answer: B
Transplant recipients are at increased risk for developing certain types of de novo malignancies, including nonmelanomatous skin cancers (three- to sevenfold increased risk), lymphoproliferative disease (two- to threefold increased risk), gynecologic and urologic cancers, and Kaposi's sarcoma. The risk ranges from 1% among renal allograft recipients to approximately 5 to 6% among recipients of small bowel and multivisceral transplants. (See Schwartz 9th ed., p 309.)

CHAPTER 12

Patient Safety

BASIC SCIENCE QUESTIONS

1. Which one of the following high-risk organizations has achieved an exceptionally low accident and error rate?
   A. Navy nuclear submarine program
   B. U.S. Postal Service
   C. Auto manufacturing industry
   D. Food services industry

Answer: A

The nuclear submarine program is an excellent example of an organization that has achieved the distinction of being considered a 'high reliability organization.' High reliability organization theory, which was developed by a group of social scientists at the University of California at Berkeley, recognizes that there are certain high-risk industries and organizations that have achieved very low accident and error rates compared to what would be expected given the inherent risks involved in their daily operations (Fig. 12-1). Other examples of industries or organizations that are regarded as having achieved high reliability status include aircraft carrier flight decks, nuclear power plants, and the Federal Aviation Administration's air traffic control system. In fact, one reason why nuclear power plants have such an excellent reliability record may be that their operators are often former naval submarine officers whose previous experience and training within one highly reliable organization are easily transferable to other organizations. The other three industries listed have all been identified as having a higher error rate (lower quality). (See Schwartz 9th ed., p 314, and Fig. 12-1.)

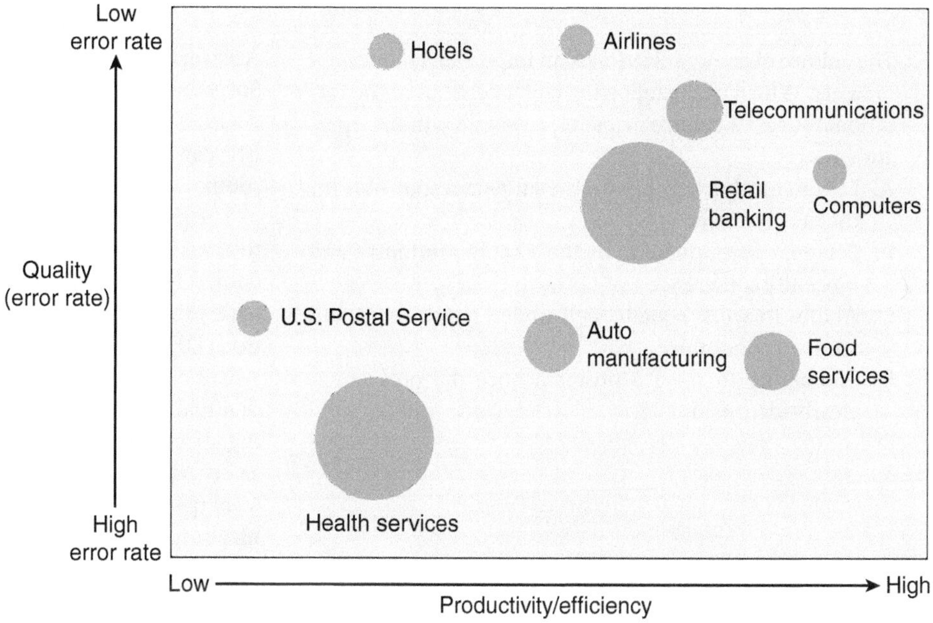

FIG. 12-1. Cross-industry comparison of size, productivity, and efficiency. (Reproduced with permission from the Advisory Board Company, 2005.)

2. A serious medical error is committed by the chief resident. The best way to teach him or her and his or her fellow residents about this situation is
   A. To make the resident personally accountable in a public forum such as morbidity and mortality conference
   B. To make the resident personally accountable in a one-on-one discussion with his or her attending
   C. To have the resident meet with risk management to understand the potential medicolegal implications of the error
   D. To use the error to analyze the system that allowed it to happen, and make suggestions for prevention of the error in the future

Answer: D
One of the assumptions underlying the science of high reliability organizations is the following observation made by Weick in 1987: Humans who operate and manage complex systems are themselves not sufficiently complex to sense and anticipate the problems generated by the system. This introduces another important idea undergirding the science of patient safety: the concept of normal accident theory. Instead of attributing accidents to individual error, this theory states that accidents are intrinsic to high-volume activities and even inevitable in some settings; that is, they are 'normal' and should be expected to occur. Accidents should not be used merely to identify and punish the person at fault. As Reason states, even the 'best people can make the worst errors as a result of latent conditions.' (See Schwartz 9th ed., p 314.)

3. Which of the following characteristics is typically seen in a high-reliability (low error) surgical service?
   A. Personal accountability is stressed in a public forum such as a morbidity and mortality conference on a regular (usually weekly) basis
   B. Hierarchical responsibility is imposed, with final authority resting with the attending surgeon
   C. Friendly open relationships exist between all members of the surgical team including nurses and clerical staff
   D. The culture of the work environment stresses following established protocols.

Answer: C
High reliability organization theory suggests that proper oversight of people, processes, and technology can handle complex and hazardous activities and keep error rates acceptably low. Studies of multiple high reliability organizations have revealed that they share the following common characteristics:

- People are supportive of one another.
- People trust one another.
- People have friendly, open relationships emphasizing credibility and attentiveness.
- The work environment is resilient and emphasizes creativity and goal achievement, providing strong feelings of credibility and personal trust.

Developing these characteristics is an important step toward achieving a low error rate in any organization. (See Schwartz 9th ed., p 314.)

4. The number of medical errors which kill patients in the United States is the equivalent of one jumbo jet crashing every
   A. Day
   B. Week
   C. Month
   D. 3 months

Answer: A
The Institute of Medicine (IOM) report shocked the health care community by concluding that between 44,000 and 98,000 deaths and over 1 million injuries occurred each year in American hospitals due to medical error. In fact, the number of deaths attributed to medical error is the aviation equivalent of one jumbo jet crash per day. (See Schwartz 9th ed., p 315.)

5. The culture of an organization is an important component of safety. Which of the following characteristics of the traditional surgical culture helps improve safety in the operating room?
   A. Hierarchical structure with the surgeon responsible for the final outcome
   B. Personal accountability at the weekly morbidity and mortality conference
   C. Ability to work equally well under nonstressful and stressful conditions
   D. The ability to solve a problem once the problem is clearly identified.

Answer: D
Surgeons have a culture that encourages them to quickly and decisively identify issues and solve problems. This characteristic can easily be applied to improving safety in the operating room.

The hierarchical structure of the operating room, tendency to assess "blame" to a surgeon at a morbidity and mortality conference, and the perception most surgeons have of their ability to work equally well in stressful and nonstressful situations DECREASE safety in the operating room.

Culture is to an organization what personality is to the individual—a hidden, yet unifying theme that provides meaning, direction, and mobilization. Organizations with effective safety cultures share a constant commitment to safety as a top-level priority, a commitment that permeates the entire organization. These organizations frequently share the following characteristics:

- An acknowledgment of the high-risk, error-prone nature of an organization's activities
- A nonpunitive environment where individuals are able to report errors or close calls without fear of punishment or retaliation
- An expectation of collaboration across ranks to seek solutions to vulnerabilities
- A willingness on the part of the organization to direct resources to address safety concerns

Traditional surgical culture stands almost in direct opposition to the values upheld by organizations with effective safety cultures for several reasons. Surgeons are less likely to acknowledge their propensity to make mistakes or to admit these mistakes to others. Surgeons tend to minimize the effects of stress on their ability to make decisions, and often claim that their decision making is equally effective in emergency and normal situations. The surgical culture, especially in the operating room (OR), is traditionally rife with hierarchy. Intimidation of other OR personnel, by surgeons was historically accepted as the norm. This can prevent nurses and other OR staff from pointing out potential errors or mistakes by surgeons. (See Schwartz 9th ed., p 316.)

6. The most common cause of a sentinel event such as wrong-site surgery is
   A. Inadequate training of personnel involved
   B. Poor communication
   C. Inadequate patient assessment prior to the procedure
   D. Critical information unavailable at the time of the procedure

Answer: B

According to the Joint Commission, communication breakdown is the most common root cause of sentinel events such as wrong-site surgery (Fig. 12-2). Poor communication contributed to nearly 70% of sentinel events reported to the Joint Commission on Accreditation of Healthcare Organizations in 2006. Good communication is an essential component of teamwork and should be emphasized in any organization wishing to create a culture of patient safety. It especially is important in the OR, one of the most complex work environments in health care. (See Schwartz 9th ed., p 316.)

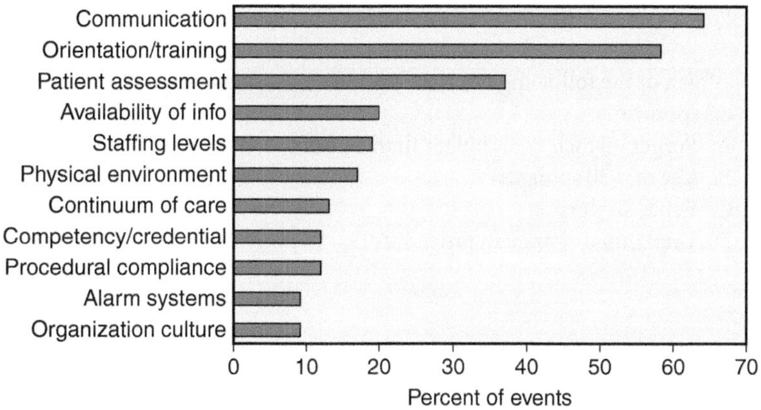

FIG. 12-2. Root causes of sentinel events 1995–2002. (Data from http://www.jointcommission.org/Sentinel Events/Statistics: *Sentinel Event Statistics*. Joint Commission website [accessed February 6, 2008].)

1. A patient with a right popliteal occlusion is scheduled for bypass. The initial incision is made on the left leg. The error is recognized and no further dissection is carried out. The bypass is performed uneventfully on the right (correct) leg. This situation is
   A. An adverse event
   B. Negligence
   C. A sentinel event
   D. All of the above

Answer: D

This constitutes "an injury caused by medical management" (an adverse event), "care falling below the standard of care" (negligence), and "an unexpected occurrence involving death or serious physical or psychological damage" (sentinel event). (See Schwartz 9th ed., p 315, and Table 12-1.)

TABLE 12-1 Types of medical error

Adverse event
- Injury caused by medical management rather than the underlying condition of the patient
- Prolongs hospitalization, produces a disability at discharge, or both
- Classified as preventable or unpreventable

Negligence
- Care that falls below a recognized standard of care
- Standard of care is considered to be care a reasonable physician of similar knowledge, training, and experience would use in similar circumstances

Near miss
- An error that does not result in patient harm
- Analysis of near misses provides the opportunity to identify and remedy system failures before the occurrence of harm

Sentinel event
- An unexpected occurrence involving death or serious physical or psychological injury
- The injury involves loss of limb or function
- This type of event requires immediate investigation and response
- Other examples
  - Hemolytic transfusion reaction involving administration of blood or blood products having major blood group incompatibilities
  - Wrong-site, wrong-procedure, or wrong-patient surgery
  - A medication error or other treatment-related error resulting in death
  - Unintentional retention of a foreign body in a patient after surgery

Reproduced with permission from Woreta TA, Makary MA: Patient safety, in Makary M (ed): *General Surgery Review*. Washington, DC: Ladner-Drysdale, 2008, p 553.

2. Which of the following is a risk factor for a retained surgical sponge?
   A. Surgery which takes longer than 6 hours
   B. Use of >30 sponges
   C. Pelvic surgery
   D. Unplanned change in procedure

Answer: D

An unplanned change in procedure is one of the risk factors for retained surgical sponge. The length of the procedure, unless it involves nurses from more than one shift, is not a risk factor, nor is pelvic surgery. There is no increased risk with an increased number of sponges. (See Schwartz 9th ed., p 325, and Table 12-2.)

TABLE 12-2 Risk factors for retained surgical sponges

- Emergency surgery
- Unplanned changes in procedure
- Patient with higher body-mass index
- Multiple surgeons involved in same operation
- Multiple procedures performed on same patient
- Involvement of multiple operating room nurses/staff members
- Case duration covers multiple nursing "shifts"

3. Which of the following can be used to decrease the risk of a retained sponge?
   A. Limiting the use of sponges by liberal use of suction
   B. Routine radiographs in patients undergoing multiple procedures
   C. Delaying wound closure until the count is completed
   D. Routine radiograph in patients with a BMI >40

Answer: B

The benefit of performing surgical counts to prevent the occurrence of retained surgical items is controversial. The increased risk of a retained surgical item during emergency surgery in the study by Gawande and colleagues appeared to be related to bypassing the surgical count in many of these cases, suggesting that the performance of a surgical count can be useful in reducing the incidence of this sentinel event. However, the 'falsely correct count,' in which a count is performed and declared correct when it is actually incorrect, occurred in 21 to 100% of cases in which a retained surgical item was found. This type of count was the most common circumstance encountered in all retained surgical item cases, which suggests that performing a surgical count in and of itself does not prevent this error from taking place. The counting protocol also imposes significant demands on the nursing staff and distracts them from focusing on other primarily patient-centered tasks.

Although there is no single tool to prevent all errors, the development of multiple lines of defense to prevent retained surgical items and universally standardizing and adhering to OR safety protocols by all members of the surgical team will help reduce the incidence of this never event. Surgeons should take the lead in the prevention of retained surgical items by avoiding the use of small or nonradiologically detectable sponges in large cavities, by performing a thorough wound inspection before closing any surgical incision, and by having a vested interest in the counting procedure performed by nursing staff to keep track of sponges, needles, instruments, and any other potential retained surgical item. The value of routine radiography in the setting of emergency cases or when multiple major procedures involving multiple surgical teams are being performed to prevent a retained surgical item is becoming more apparent. (See Schwartz 9th ed., p 325.)

4. Which of the following increases the risk of wrong-site surgery?
   A. Surgery late in the day
   B. Thin patient (BMI <22)
   C. Surgeon running multiple rooms
   D. Multiple surgeons involved in the same operation

Answer: D

Multiple surgeons involved in the operation has been identified as a risk factor for wrong-site surgery. Morbidly obese patients are at higher risk; thin patients have no increased risk for wrong-site surgery. Although "time pressure" is a risk factor for wrong-site surgery, running multiple rooms in and of itself is not considered a risk factor.

There is a one in four chance that surgeons who work on symmetric anatomic structures will be involved in a wrong-site error sometime during their careers. No surgical specialty is immune.

The risk of performing wrong-site surgery increases when there are multiple surgeons involved in the same operation or multiple procedures are performed on the same patient, especially if the procedures are scheduled or performed on different areas of the body. Time pressure, emergency surgery, abnormal patient anatomy, and morbid obesity are also thought to be risk factors. Communication errors are the root cause in more than 70% of the wrong-site surgeries reported to the Joint Commission. Other risk factors include receiving an incomplete preoperative assessment because documents are either unavailable or not reviewed for other reasons; having inadequate procedures in place to verify the correct surgical site; or having an organizational culture that lacks teamwork or reveres the surgeon as someone whose judgment should never be questioned. (See Schwartz 9th ed., p 326.)

5. Which of the following increases the risk of a complication while placing a central line?
   A. Placing a central line at the request of another surgeon
   B. Placement by a lower level (PGY3) resident
   C. Failure to place the patient in Trendelenburg position
   D. Changing a line when infected, rather than on a protocol set schedule

Answer: A

Failure to ensure that the central line is indicated is a key cause of complications after placing central lines. This most often occurs when the line is placed at the request of another surgeon. Lines should be placed by trained and competent personnel. At a PGY3 level most residents are well trained in this technique. Trendelenburg position is controversial. Lines should only be changed when indicated, not on a routine schedule. (See Schwartz 9th ed., p 327.)

Steps to decrease complications include the following:

- Ensure that central venous access is indicated.
- Experienced (credentialed) personnel should insert the catheter, or should supervise the insertion.
- Use proper positioning and sterile technique. Controversy exists as to whether or not placing the patient in the Trendelenburg position facilitates access.
- Central venous catheters should be exchanged only for specific indications (not as a matter of routine) and should be removed as soon as possible.

6. If air embolism is suspected during placement of a central line, the patient should be placed in which of the following positions?
   A. Supine
   B. Prone
   C. Right lateral decubitus
   D. Left lateral decubitus

Answer: D

Although estimated to occur in only 0.2 to 1% of patients, an air embolism can be dramatic and fatal. Treatment may prove futile if the air bolus is larger than 50 mL. Auscultation over the precordium may reveal a "crunching" noise, but a portable chest xray is required for diagnosis. If an embolus is suspected, the patient should immediately be placed into a left lateral decubitus Trendelenburg position, so the entrapped air can be stabilized within the right ventricle. Aspiration via a central venous line accessing the heart may decrease the volume of gas in the right side of the heart, and minimize the amount traversing into the pulmonary circulation. Subsequent recovery of intracardiac and intrapulmonary air may require open surgical or angiographic techniques. Prevention requires careful attention to technique. (See Schwartz 9th ed., p 328.)

7. During placement of a Swan Ganz catheter, the patient coughs up a significant amount of blood. The initial step to manage this complication is
   A. Nothing
   B. Inflate the balloon on the Swan Ganz catheter
   C. Intubate the patient
   D. Emergent thoracotomy

Answer: B

Flow-directed, pulmonary artery ('Swan-Ganz') catheters can cause pulmonary artery rupture due to excessive advancement of the catheter into the pulmonary circulation. There usually is a sentinel bleed noted when a pulmonary artery catheter balloon is inflated, and then the patient begins to have uncontrolled hemoptysis. Reinflation of the catheter balloon is the initial step in management, followed by immediate airway intubation with mechanical ventilation, an urgent portable chest x-ray, and notification of the OR that an emergent thoracotomy may be required. If there is no further bleeding after the balloon is reinflated, the x-ray shows no significant consolidation of lung fields from ongoing bleeding and the patient is easily ventilated, then a conservative nonoperative approach may be considered. This approach might include observation alone if the patient has no signs of bleeding or hemodynamic compromise; however, more typically a pulmonary angiogram with angioembolization or vascular stenting is required. Hemodynamically unstable patients rarely survive because of the time needed to perform the thoracotomy and identify the branch of the pulmonary artery that has ruptured. (See Schwartz 9th ed., p 328.)

8. 4 days following placement of a tracheostomy tube in the ICU, a significant amount of blood is suctioned from the tracheostomy. The most appropriate next step is
   A. Nothing
   B. Gentle repeat suctioning until clear
   C. Bedside bronchoscopy
   D. Bronchoscopy in the operating room

Answer: D

The most dramatic complication of tracheostomy is tracheoinnominate artery fistula (TIAF). This occurs rarely (~0.3%), but carries a 50 to 80% mortality rate. TIAFs can occur as early as 2 days or as late as 2 months after tracheostomy. The prototypical patient is a thin woman with a long, gracile neck. The patient may have a sentinel bleed, which occurs in 50% of TIAF cases, followed by a most spectacular bleed. Should a TIAF be suspected, the patient should be transported immediately to the OR for fiberoptic evaluation. If needed, remove the tracheostomy, and place a finger through the tracheostomy site to apply direct pressure anteriorly for compression of the innominate artery. (See Schwartz 9th ed., p 329.)

9. Which of the following should be used to prepare a patient with mild renal insufficiency (BUN 38, Creatinine 1.5) for angiography?
   A. Nothing
   B. Oral hydration (3 liters) during the 24 hours before the procedure
   C. Intravenous hydration for 12 hours after the procedure
   D. *N*-acetylcysteine

Answer: D

Renal complications of angiography occur in 1 to 2% of patients. Contrast nephropathy is a temporary and preventable complication of radiologic studies such as CT, angiography, and/or venography. Some studies suggest a benefit of *N*-acetylcysteine for this condition. For the patient with impaired renal function or dehydration before contrast studies, twice-daily dosing 24 hours before and on the day of the radiographic study is suggested. Nonionic contrast also may be of benefit in higher-risk patients. IV hydration before and after the procedure is the most efficient method for preventing contrast nephropathy. (See Schwartz 9th ed., p 329.)

10. Which of the following may help prevent ototoxicity in a patient receiving vancomycin?
   A. *N*-acetylcysteine
   B. Alpha-tocopherol
   C. Ferrous sulfate
   D. Thalidomide

Answer: B

Ototoxicity due to aminoglycoside administration occurs in up to 10% of patients, and is often irreversible. Recent data show that iron chelating agents and alpha-tocopherol may be protective against ototoxicity. Vancomycin-related ototoxicity occurs about 3% of the time when used alone, and as often as 6% when used with other ototoxic agents, but is self limiting. (See Schwartz 9th ed., p 329.)

11. On the third day after a carotid endarterectomy, a 68-year-old patient develops atrial fibrillation with a heart rate of 160 and a blood pressure of 96/58. The initial treatment should be
   A. Digoxin
   B. Cardioversion
   C. A beta blocker
   D. An alpha blocker

Answer: C

Atrial fibrillation is the most common arrhythmia and occurs between postoperative days 3 and 5 in high-risk patients. This is typically when patients begin to mobilize their interstitial fluid into the vascular fluid space. Contemporary evidence suggests that rate control is more important than rhythm control for atrial fibrillation. The first-line treatment includes beta blockade and/or calcium channel blockade. Beta blockade must be used judiciously, because hypotension, as well as withdrawal from beta blockade with rebound hypertension, is possible. Calcium channel blockers are an option if beta blockers are not tolerated by the patient, but caution must be exercised in those with a history of congestive heart failure. Although digoxin is still a faithful standby medication, it has limitations due to the need for optimal dosing levels. Cardioversion may be required if patients become hemodynamically unstable and the rhythm cannot be controlled. (See Schwartz 9th ed., p 332.)

12. Which of the following is the best method to decrease the risk of renal failure in a patient with myoglobinuria?
    A. IV hydration to maintain good urine output
    B. Sodium bicarb to maintain urine pH >8
    C. Mannitol
    D. Lasix

Answer: A
The treatment of renal failure due to myoglobinuria in severe trauma patients has shifted away from the use of sodium bicarbonate for alkalinizing the urine, to merely maintaining brisk urine output of 100 mL/h with crystalloid fluid infusion. Mannitol and furosemide are not recommended as long as the IV fluid achieves the goal rate of urinary output. (See Schwartz 9th ed., p 334.)

13. Ischemic changes to the skin can lead to decubitus ulcers. This ischemia occurs after what period of time in the same position?
    A. 10 minutes
    B. 30 minutes
    C. 1 hour
    D. 2 hours

Answer: D
Decubitus ulcers are preventable complications of prolonged bedrest due to traumatic paralysis, dementia, chemical paralysis, or coma. Ischemic changes in the microcirculation of the skin can be significant after 2 hours of sustained pressure. Routine skin care and turning of the patient helps ensure a reduction in skin ulceration. This can be labor intensive and special mattresses and beds are available to help with this ubiquitous problem. (See Schwartz 9th ed., p 334.)

14. The most common virus transmitted by transfusion is
    A. Hepatitis A
    B. Hepatitis B
    C. Hepatitis C
    D. Human Immunodeficiency Virus (HIV)

Answer: B
Hepatitis B is the most common virus transmitted by blood transfusion, followed by hepatitis C and then HIV. Hepatitis A is transmitted through contaminated food. (See Schwartz 9th ed., p 335, and Table 12-3.)

TABLE 12-3 Rate of viral transmission in blood product transfusions[a]

HIV	1:1.9 million
HBV[b]	1:137,000
HCV	1:1 million

[a]Post–nucleic acid amplification technology (1999). Earlier rates were erroneously reported higher due to lack of contemporary technology.
[b]HBV is reported with pre–nucleic acid amplification technology. Statistical information is unavailable in post–nucleic acid amplification technology at this writing.
Note that bacterial transmission is 50 to 250 times higher than viral transmission per transfusion.
HBV = hepatitis B virus; HCV = hepatitis C virus.

15. Intra-abdominal hypertension is defined by a bladder pressure greater than
    A. 10 mmHg
    B. 15 mmHg
    C. 20 mmHg
    D. 25 mmHg

Answer: C
Measurement of abdominal pressures is easily accomplished by transducing bladder pressures from the urinary catheter after instilling 100 mL of sterile saline into the urinary bladder. A pressure greater than 20 mmHg constitutes intra-abdominal hypertension, but the diagnosis of ACS requires intra-abdominal pressure greater than 25 to 30 mmHg, with at least one of the following: compromised respiratory mechanics and ventilation, oliguria or anuria, or increasing intracranial pressures. (See Schwartz 9th ed., p 335.)

16. Which of the following has been shown to decrease wound infections in a clean contaminated wound (e.g., nonperforated appendicitis)?
    A. Antibiotic impregnated plastic drape placed prior to skin incision
    B. Irrigation of the wound with saline solution prior to closure
    C. Irrigation of the abdomen with antibiotic solution prior to closure
    D. 24 to 28 hours of antibiotics after surgery

Answer: B
There exist no prospective, randomized, double-blind, controlled studies that demonstrate that antibiotics used beyond 24 hours in the perioperative period prevent infections. There is a general trend toward providing a single preoperative dose, as antibiotic prophylaxis may not impart any benefit at all beyond the initial dosing. Irrigation of the operative field and the surgical wound with saline solution has shown benefit in controlling wound inoculum. Irrigation with an antibiotic-based solution has not demonstrated significant benefit in controlling postoperative infection. Antibacterial-impregnated polyvinyl placed over the operative wound area for the duration of

the surgical procedure has not been shown to decrease the rate of wound infection. Although skin preparation with 70% isopropyl alcohol has the best bactericidal effect, it is flammable, and could be hazardous when electrocautery is used. The contemporary formulas of chlorhexidine gluconate with isopropyl alcohol or povidone-iodine and iodophor with alcohol are more advantageous. (See Schwartz 9th ed., p 335.)

17. At the conclusion of an operation for a colostomy closure, the patient is noted to have a HR of 130, temp of 102, and elevated expired pCO_2. The most appropriate treatment is
    A. Irrigation of the abdominal cavity to remove cytokines and lower temperature
    B. Careful exploration to rule out a missed bowel injury
    C. Tylenol per rectum at the end of the procedure and careful observation
    D. Ice packs and intravenous dantrolene

Answer: D

Malignant hyperthermia occurs after exposure to agents such as succinylcholine and some halothane-based inhalational anesthetics. The presentation is dramatic, with rapid onset of increased temperature, rigors, and myoglobinuria related to myonecrosis. Medications must be discontinued immediately and dantrolene administered (2.5 mg/kg every 5 minutes) until symptoms subside. Aggressive cooling methods are also implemented, such as an alcohol bath, or packing in ice. In cases of severe malignant hyperthermia, the mortality rate is nearly 30%. (See Schwartz 9th ed., p 339.)

CHAPTER 13

Physiologic Monitoring of the Surgical Patient

BASIC SCIENCE QUESTIONS

1. Critical oxygen delivery (transition from supply-independent to supply-dependent oxygen delivery) occurs when oxygen delivery falls below
   A. 1.5 mL/kg
   B. 2.0 mL/kg
   C. 4.5 mL/kg
   D. 6.0 mL/kg

Answer: C
Under normal conditions when the supply of O_2 is plentiful, aerobic metabolism is determined by factors other than the availability of O_2. These factors include the hormonal milieu and mechanical workload of contractile tissue. However, in pathologic circumstances when O_2 availability is inadequate, O_2 utilization ($\dot{V}O_2$) becomes dependent upon O_2 delivery ($\dot{D}O_2$). The relationship of $\dot{V}o_2$ to $\dot{D}o_2$ over a broad range of $\dot{D}O_2$ values is commonly represented as two intersecting straight lines. In the region of higher $\dot{D}O_2$ values, the slope of the line is approximately equal to zero, indicating that $\dot{V}O_2$ is largely independent of $\dot{D}O_2$. In contrast, in the region of low $\dot{D}o_2$ values, the slope of the line is nonzero and positive, indicating that $\dot{V}O_2$ is supply dependent. The region where the two lines intersect is called the point of critical O_2 delivery ($\dot{D}O_{2crit}$), and represents the transition from supply-independent to supply-dependent O_2 uptake. Below this critical threshold of O_2 delivery (approximately 4.5 mL/kg per minute), increased O_2 extraction cannot compensate for the delivery deficit; hence, O_2 consumption begins to decrease. (See Schwartz 9th ed., p 344.)

2. Preload is determined by
   A. End systolic volume
   B. End systolic pressure
   C. End diastolic volume
   D. End diastolic pressure

Answer: C
Starlings law of the heart states that the force of muscle contraction depends on the initial length of the cardiac fibers. Using terminology that derives from early experiments using isolated cardiac muscle preparations, preload is the stretch of ventricular myocardial tissue just before the next contraction. Preload is determined by end-diastolic volume (EDV). For the right ventricle, central venous pressure (CVP) approximates right ventricular (RV) end-diastolic pressure (EDP). For the left ventricle, pulmonary artery occlusion pressure (PAOP), which is measured by transiently inflating a balloon at the end of a pressure monitoring catheter positioned in a small branch of the pulmonary artery, approximates left ventricular EDP. The presence of atrioventricular valvular stenosis will alter this relationship. (See Schwartz 9th ed., p 346.)

3. In measuring cardiac output with a Swan-Ganz catheter, a rapid bolus of saline is used. What is the best temperature for that bolus?
   A. 4° centigrade
   B. 15° centigrade
   C. 30° centigrade
   D. Room temperature

Answer: D

Determination of cardiac output by the thermodilution method is generally quite accurate, although it tends to systematically overestimate QT at low values. Changes in blood temperature and QT during the respiratory cycle can influence the measurement. Therefore, results generally should be recorded as the mean of two or three determinations obtained at random points in the respiratory cycle. Using cold injectate widens the difference between TB and TI and thereby increases signal-to-noise ratio. Nevertheless, most authorities recommend using room temperature injectate (normal saline or 5% dextrose in water) to minimize errors resulting from warming of the fluid as it transferred from its reservoir to a syringe for injection. (See Schwartz 9th ed., p 348.)

4. Which of the following will result in a subnormal $S\bar{v}O_2$?
   A. Fluid overload
   B. Increased PaO_2
   C. Anemia
   D. Hypothermia

Answer: C

$S\bar{v}O_2$ is a function of $\dot{V}O_2$ (i.e., metabolic rate), QT, SaO_2, and Hgb. Accordingly, subnormal values of $S\bar{v}O_2$ can be caused by a decrease in Q_T (due, for example, to heart failure or hypovolemia), a decrease in SaO_2 (due, for example, to intrinsic pulmonary disease), a decrease in Hgb (i.e., anemia), or an increase in metabolic rate (due, for example, to seizures or fever). (See Schwartz 9th ed., p 348.)

CLINICAL QUESTIONS

1. In direct measurement of blood pressure, what effect will overdamping have on the mean arterial pressure (MAP)?
   A. The MAP will be artificially high
   B. The MAP will be artificially low
   C. There is no effect on the MAP reading
   D. The MAP cannot be calculated if the system is overdamped

Answer: C

The fidelity of the catheter-tubing-transducer system is determined by numerous factors, including the compliance of the tubing, the surface area of the transducer diaphragm, and the compliance of the diaphragm. If the system is underdamped, then the inertia of the system, which is a function of the mass of the fluid in the tubing and the mass of the diaphragm, causes overshoot of the points of maximum positive and negative displacement of the diaphragm during systole and diastole, respectively. Thus in an underdamped system, systolic pressure will be overestimated and diastolic pressure will be underestimated. In an overdamped system, displacement of the diaphragm fails to track the rapidly changing pressure waveform, and systolic pressure will be underestimated and diastolic pressure will be overestimated. It is important to note that even in an underdamped or overdamped system, mean pressure will be accurately recorded, provided the system has been properly calibrated. For these reasons, when using direct measurement of intra-arterial pressure to monitor patients, clinicians should make clinical decisions based on the measured mean arterial blood pressure. (See Schwartz 9th ed., p 345.)

2. Addition of which of the following leads to continuous EKG monitoring will improve the ability to detect myocardial ischemia?
   A. Left arm
   B. Right arm
   C. V_1
   D. V_4

Answer: D

A standard 3-lead ECG is obtained by placing electrodes that correspond to the left arm (LA), right arm (RA), and left leg (LL). The limb leads are defined as lead I (LA-RA), lead II (LL-RA), and lead III (LL-LA).

Additional information can be obtained from a 12-lead ECG, which is essential for patients with potential myocardial ischemia or to rule out cardiac complications in other acutely ill patients. Continuous monitoring of the 12-lead ECG now is available and is proving to be beneficial in certain patient populations. In a study of 185 vascular surgical patients, continuous 12-lead ECG monitoring was able to detect transient myocardial ischemic episodes in 20.5% of the patients. This study demonstrated that the precordial lead V_4, which is not routinely monitored on a standard 3-lead ECG, is the most sensitive for detecting perioperative ischemia and infarction. To detect 95% of the ischemic episodes, two or more precordial leads were necessary. Thus, continuous 12-lead ECG monitoring may provide greater sensitivity than 3-lead ECG for the detection of perioperative myocardial ischemia, and is likely to become standard for monitoring high-risk surgical patients. (See Schwartz 9th ed., p 346.)

3. The width of a blood pressure cuff should be what percentage of the circumference of the patient's arm?
   A. 30%
   B. 40%
   C. 50%
   D. 60%

Answer: B

Both manual and automated means for the noninvasive determination of blood pressure use an inflatable cuff to increase pressure around an extremity. If the cuff is too narrow (relative to the extremity), the measured pressure will be artifactually elevated. Therefore, the width of the cuff should be approximately 40% of its circumference. (See Schwartz 9th ed., p 344.)

4. In critically ill postoperative patients, monitoring with a pulmonary artery catheter
   A. Decreases mortality
   B. Decreases the rate of postoperative myocardial infarction
   C. Decreases ICU length of stay
   D. None of the above

Answer: D

(See Schwartz 9th ed., p 349, and Table 13-1.)

TABLE 13-1 Summary of randomized, prospective clinical trials comparing pulmonary artery catheter with central venous pressure monitoring

Author	Study Population	Groups	Outcomes
Pearson, et al	"Low-risk" patients undergoing cardiac or vascular surgery	CVP catheter (group 1); PAC (group 2); PAC with continuous $S\bar{v}O_2$, readout (group 3)	No differences among groups for mortality or length of ICU stay; significant differences in costs (group 1 < group 2 < group 3)
Tuman, et al	Cardiac surgical patients	PAC; CVP	No differences between groups for mortality, length of ICU stay, or significant noncardiac complications
Bender, et al	Vascular surgery patients	PAC; CVP	No differences between groups for mortality, length of ICU stay, or length of hospital stay
Valentine, et al	Aortic surgery patients	PAC + hemodynamic optimization in ICU night before surgery; CVP	No difference between groups for mortality or length of ICU stay; significantly higher incidence of postoperative complications in PAC group
Sandham, et al	"High-risk" major surgery	PAC; CVP	No differences between groups for mortality, length of ICU stay; increased incidence of pulmonary embolism in PAC group
Harvey, et al	Medical and surgical ICU patients	PAC vs. no PAC, with option for alternative CO measuring device in non-PAC group	No difference in hospital mortality between the two groups, increased incidence of complications in the PAC group
Binanay, et al	Patients with CHF	PAC vs. no PAC	No difference in hospital mortality between the two groups, increased incidence of adverse events in the PAC group
Wheeler, et al	Patients with ALI	PAC vs. CVC with a fluid and inotropic management protocol	No difference in ICU or hospital mortality, or incidence of organ failure between the two groups; increased incidence of adverse events in the PAC group

ALI = acute lung injury; CHF = congestive heart failure; CO = cardiac output; CVC = central venous catheter; CVP = central venous pressure; ICU = intensive care unit; PAC = pulmonary artery catheter; $S\bar{v}O_2$ = fractional mixed venous (pulmonary artery) hemoglobin saturation.

5. Which of the following is most likely to accurately estimate cardiac output?
   A. Sternal notch ultrasonography
   B. Transesophageal ultrasonography
   C. Impedence cardiography
   D. Partial carbon dioxide rebreathing

Answer: D

Partial carbon dioxide (CO_2) rebreathing uses the Fick principle to estimate Q_T noninvasively. By intermittently altering the dead space within the ventilator circuit via a rebreathing valve, changes in CO_2 production (VCO_2) and end-tidal CO_2 ($ETCO_2$) are used to determine cardiac output using a modified Fick equation ($Q_T = \Delta VCO_2/\Delta ETCO_2$). Commercially available devices use this Fick principle to calculate Q_T using intermittent partial CO_2 rebreathing through a disposable rebreathing loop. These devices consist of a CO_2 sensor based on infrared light absorption, an airflow sensor, and a pulse oximeter. Changes in intrapulmonary shunt and hemodynamic instability impair the accuracy of Q_T estimated by partial CO_2 rebreathing. Continuous in-line pulse oximetry and inspired fraction of inspired O_2 (FiO_2) are used to estimate shunt fraction to correct Q_T.

Two approaches have been developed for using Doppler ultrasonography to estimate Q_T. The first approach uses an ultrasonic transducer, which is manually positioned in the suprasternal notch and focused on the root of the aorta. Aortic cross-sectional area can be estimated using a nomogram, which factors in age, height, and weight, back-calculated if an independent measure of Q_T is available, or by using two-dimensional transthoracic or transesophageal ultrasonography. Although this approach is completely noninvasive, it requires a highly skilled operator to obtain meaningful results, and is labor intensive. Moreover, unless Q_T measured using thermodilution is used to back-calculate aortic diameter, accuracy using the suprasternal notch approach is not acceptable.

The impedance to flow of alternating electrical current in regions of the body is commonly called *bioimpedance*. In the thorax, changes in the volume and velocity of blood in the thoracic aorta lead to detectable changes in bioimpedance. The first derivative of the oscillating component of thoracic bioimpedance (dZ/dt) is linearly related to aortic blood flow. On the basis of this relationship, empirically derived formulas have been developed to estimate SV, and subsequently Q_T, noninvasively. This methodology is called *impedance cardiography*. The approach is attractive because it is noninvasive, provides a continuous readout of Q_T, and does not require extensive training for use. Despite these advantages, studies suggest that measurements of Q_T obtained by impedance cardiography are not sufficiently reliable to be used for clinical decision making and have poor correlation with standard methods such as thermodilution and ventricular angiography. (See Schwartz 9th ed., p 351.)

6. Which of the following does NOT cause a simultaneous increase in peak airway pressure and plateau airway pressure?
   A. Intrinsic PEEP
   B. Endotracheal tube plugging
   C. Bronchospasm
   D. Insufficient expiratory time

Answer: B

If both P_{peak} and $P_{plateau}$ are increased (and tidal volume is not excessive), then the problem is a decrease in the compliance in the lung/chest wall unit. Common causes of this problem include pneumothorax, hemothorax, lobar atelectasis, pulmonary edema, pneumonia, acute respiratory distress syndrome (ARDS), active contraction of the chest wall or diaphragmatic muscles, abdominal distention, and intrinsic PEEP, such as occurs in patients with bronchospasm and insufficient expiratory times. When P_{peak} is increased but $P_{plateau}$ is relatively normal, the primary problem is an increase in airway resistance, such as occurs with bronchospasm, use of a small-caliber endotracheal tube, or kinking or obstruction of the endotracheal tube. (See Schwartz 9th ed., p 354.)

7. A high level of methemoglobin will result in
   A. A falsely high pulse oximetry reading
   B. A falsely low pulse oximetry reading
   C. A pulse oximetry reading of 85%
   D. None of the above—there is no effect on the pulse oximetry reading

Answer: C

Under normal circumstances, the contributions of carboxyhemoglobin and methemoglobin are minimal. However, if carboxyhemoglobin levels are elevated, the pulse oximeter will incorrectly interpret carboxyhemoglobin as oxyhemoglobin and the arterial saturation displayed will be falsely elevated. When the concentration of methemoglobin is markedly increased, the SaO_2 will be displayed as 85%, regardless of the true arterial saturation. The accuracy of pulse oximetry begins to decline at SaO_2 values less than 92%, and tends to be unreliable for values less than 85%. (See Schwartz 9th ed., p 354.)

8. Which of the following is the approximate $PaCO_2$ for a healthy individual with an end-tidal CO_2 ($PETCO_2$) of 25?
   A. 20
   B. 25
   C. 30
   D. None of the above—there is no accurate correlation between $PaCO_2$ and end-tidal CO_2

Answer: C

In healthy subjects, $PETCO_2$ is about 1 to 5 mmHg less than $PaCO_2$. Thus, $PETCO_2$ can be used to estimate $PaCO_2$ without the need for blood gas determination. However, changes in $PETCO_2$ may not correlate with changes in $PaCO_2$ during a number of pathologic conditions. (See Schwartz 9th ed., p 354.)

9. Which of the following is considered confirmatory of the diagnosis of abdominal compartment syndrome?
   A. Bladder pressure >15 mmHg
   B. Bladder pressure >25 mmHg
   C. Bladder pressure >35 mmHg
   D. Bladder pressure >45 mmHg

Answer: B

The triad of oliguria, elevated peak airway pressures, and elevated intra-abdominal pressure is known as the *abdominal compartment syndrome* (ACS). This syndrome, first described in patients after repair of ruptured abdominal aortic aneurysm, is associated with interstitial edema of the abdominal organs, resulting in elevated intra-abdominal pressure. When intra-abdominal pressure exceeds venous or capillary pressures, perfusion of the kidneys and other intra-abdominal viscera is impaired. Oliguria is a cardinal sign. Although the diagnosis of ACS is a clinical one, measuring intra-abdominal pressure is useful to confirm the diagnosis. Ideally, a catheter inserted into the peritoneal cavity could measure intra-abdominal pressure to substantiate the diagnosis. In practice, transurethral bladder pressure measurement reflects intra-abdominal pressure and is most often used to confirm the presence of ACS. After instilling 50 to 100 mL of sterile saline into the bladder via a Foley catheter, the tubing is connected to a transducing system to measure bladder pressure. Most authorities recommend that a bladder pressure greater than 20 to 25 mmHg confirms the diagnosis of ACS. (See Schwartz 9th ed., p 355.)

10. ICP monitoring is indicated for a patient with
    A. An abnormal CT of the brain and a Glasgow Coma Scale score of 10 after traumatic brain injury
    B. A normal CT of the brain after traumatic brain injury, systolic BP <90, and age >40
    C. A normal CT of the brain and hepatic failure with coma
    D. A normal CT of the brain and coma after anoxia

Answer: B

Monitoring of ICP is currently recommended in patients with severe traumatic brain injury (TBI), defined as a Glasgow Coma Scale (GCS) score ≤8 with an abnormal CT scan, and in patients with severe TBI and a normal CT scan if two or more of the following are present: age greater than 40 years, unilateral or bilateral motor posturing, or systolic blood pressure less than 90 mmHg. ICP monitoring also is indicated in patients with acute subarachnoid hemorrhage with coma or neurologic deterioration, intracranial hemorrhage with intraventricular blood, ischemic middle cerebral artery stroke, fulminant hepatic failure with coma and cerebral edema on CT scan, and global cerebral ischemia or anoxia with cerebral edema on CT scan. (See Schwartz 9th ed., p 355.)

11. Titration of sedation in the ICU can be improved by monitoring with
    A. Continuous EEG
    B. Bispectral index (BIS)
    C. Serum levels of the drug(s) being used
    D. Near infrared spectrometry

Answer: B

A recent advance in EEG monitoring is the use of the bispectral index (BIS) to titrate the level of sedative medications. Although sedative drugs usually are titrated to the clinical neurologic examination, the BIS device has been used in the operating room to continuously monitor the depth of anesthesia. The BIS is an empiric measurement statistically derived from a database of more than 5000 EEGs. The BIS is derived from bifrontal EEG recordings and analyzed for burst suppression ratio, relative alpha:beta ratio, and bicoherence. Using a multivariate regression model, a linear numeric index (BIS) is calculated, ranging from 0 (isoelectric EEG) to 100 (fully awake). Its use has been associated with lower consumption of anesthetics during surgery and earlier awakening and faster recovery from anesthesia. The BIS also has been validated as a useful approach for monitoring the level of sedation for ICU patients, using the revised Sedation-Agitation Scale as a gold standard. (See Schwartz 9th ed., p 355.)

CHAPTER 14

Minimally Invasive Surgery, Robotics, and Natural Orifice Transluminal Endoscopic Surgery

BASIC SCIENCE QUESTIONS

1. Pneumoperitoneum results in which of the following?
   A. Decreased plasma rennin
   B. Decreased antidiuretic hormone (ADH)
   C. Decreased glomerular filtration rate
   D. Decreased free water absorption in the distal tubules

Answer: C

Increased intra-abdominal pressure decreases renal blood flow, glomerular filtration rate, and urine output. These effects may be mediated by direct pressure on the kidney and the renal vein. The secondary effect of decreased renal blood flow is to increase plasma renin release, thereby increasing sodium retention. Increased circulating antidiuretic hormone levels also are found during the pneumoperitoneum, increasing free water reabsorption in the distal tubules. (See Schwartz 9th ed., p 362.)

2. When compared to open procedures, laparoscopic procedures
   A. Result in greater immune suppression
   B. Result in greater stress hormone production
   C. Result in higher serum cortisol levels
   D. Result in slower normalization of cytokine levels

Answer: C

Endocrine responses to laparoscopic surgery are not always intuitive. Serum cortisol levels after laparoscopic operations are often higher than after the equivalent operation performed through an open incision. The greatest difference between the endocrine response of open and laparoscopic surgery is the more rapid equilibration of most stress-mediated hormone levels after laparoscopic surgery. Immune suppression also is less after laparoscopy than after open surgery. There is a trend toward more rapid normalization of cytokine levels after a laparoscopic procedure than after the equivalent procedure performed by celiotomy. (See Schwartz 9th ed., p 362.)

3. Which of the following does NOT require an electrical current to coagulate tissue?
   A. Monopolar cautery
   B. Bipolar cautery
   C. Mixed current cautery
   D. Ultrasonic shears device

Answer: D

A third means of using ultrasonic energy is to create rapidly oscillating instruments that are capable of heating tissue with friction; this technology represents a major step forward in energy technology. An example of its application is the laparoscopic coagulation shears device (Harmonic Scalpel), which is capable of coagulating and dividing blood vessels by first occluding them and then providing sufficient heat to weld the blood vessel walls together and to divide the vessel. This nonelectric method of coagulating and dividing tissue with a minimal amount of collateral damage has facilitated the performance of numerous endosurgical procedures. It is especially useful in the control of bleeding from medium-sized vessels that are too big to manage with monopolar electrocautery and require bipolar desiccation followed by cutting. (See Schwartz 9th ed., p 370.)

1. Which of the following statements concerning N_2O pneumoperitoneum is true
   A. N_2O is flammable, therefore, electrosurgery should not be used
   B. Minute ventilation is increased in patients with N_2O pneumoperitoneum when compared to CO_2
   C. N_2O pneumoperitoneum is more analgesic than CO_2 pneumoperitoneum
   D. N_2O is the gas of choice to use for oncologic procedures

Answer: C

N_2O had the advantage of being physiologically inert and rapidly absorbed. It also provided better analgesia for laparoscopy performed under local anesthesia when compared with CO_2 or air. Despite initial concerns that N_2O would not suppress combustion, controlled clinical trials have established its safety within the peritoneal cavity. In addition, N_2O has been shown to reduce the intraoperative end-tidal CO_2 and minute ventilation required to maintain homeostasis when compared to CO_2 pneumoperitoneum. The effect of N_2O on tumor biology and the development of port site metastasis are unknown. As such, caution should be exercised when performing laparoscopic cancer surgery with this agent. Finally, the safety of N_2O pneumoperitoneum in pregnancy has yet to be elucidated. (See Schwartz 9th ed., p 361.)

2. Hypercarbia from a CO_2 pneumoperitoneum can cause
   A. Bradycardia
   B. Increased myocardial oxygen demand
   C. Metabolic acidosis
   D. Hypocalcemia

Answer: B

CO_2 is rapidly absorbed across the peritoneal membrane into the circulation. In the circulation, CO_2 creates a respiratory acidosis by the generation of carbonic acid. Body buffers, the largest reserve of which lies in bone, absorb CO_2 (up to 120 L) and minimize the development of hypercarbia or respiratory acidosis during brief endoscopic procedures. Once the body buffers are saturated, respiratory acidosis develops rapidly, and the respiratory system assumes the burden of keeping up with the absorption of CO_2 and its release from these buffers.

In patients with normal respiratory function, this is not difficult; the anesthesiologist increases the ventilatory rate or vital capacity on the ventilator. If the respiratory rate required exceeds 20 breaths per minute, there may be less efficient gas exchange and increasing hypercarbia. Conversely, if vital capacity is increased substantially, there is a greater opportunity for barotrauma and greater respiratory motion-induced disruption of the upper abdominal operative field. In some situations, it is advisable to evacuate the pneumoperitoneum or reduce the intra-abdominal pressure to allow time for the anesthesiologist to adjust for hypercarbia. Although mild respiratory acidosis probably is an insignificant problem, more severe respiratory acidosis leading to cardiac arrhythmias has been reported. Hypercarbia also causes tachycardia and increased systemic vascular resistance, which elevates blood pressure and increases myocardial oxygen demand. (See Schwartz 9th ed., p 361.)

3. The most common arrhythmia seen with CO_2 pneumoperitoneum is
   A. Ventricular tachycardia
   B. Superventricular tachycardia
   C. Sinus tachycardia
   D. Sinus bradycardia

Answer: D

The pressure effects of the pneumoperitoneum on cardiovascular physiology also have been studied. In the hypovolemic individual, excessive pressure on the inferior vena cava and a reverse Trendelenburg position with loss of lower extremity muscle tone may cause decreased venous return and decreased cardiac output. This is not seen in the normovolemic patient. The most common arrhythmia created by laparoscopy is bradycardia. A rapid stretch of the peritoneal membrane often causes a vagovagal response with bradycardia and, occasionally, hypotension. The appropriate management of this event is desufflation of the abdomen, administration of vagolytic agents (e.g., atropine), and adequate volume replacement. (See Schwartz 9th ed., p 361.)

4. A patient undergoing laparoscopic colon resection is noted to have a decreased urine output during the last hour of the case. A bolus is given at the end of the case. One hour later, there is still very poor urine output. The appropriate treatment is
   A. Repeat the bolus
   B. IV furosemide
   C. Check urine electrolytes
   D. None of the above

Answer: D

Low urine output is a normal physiologic response to increased intra-abdominal pressure for up to 1 hour after surgery. Although the effects of the pneumoperitoneum on renal blood flow are immediately reversible, the hormonally mediated changes such as elevated antidiuretic hormone levels decrease urine output for up to 1 hour after the procedure has ended. Intraoperative oliguria is common during laparoscopy, but the urine output is not a reflection of intravascular volume status; IV fluid administration during an uncomplicated laparoscopic procedure should not be linked to urine output. (See Schwartz 9th ed., p 362.)

5. Laser therapy restores luminal patency in a blood vessel by
   A. Coring out the obstructive lesion
   B. Fracturing the obstructive lesion
   C. Chemically dissolving the obstructive lesion
   D. None of the above

Answer: A

Photodynamic therapy works by coring out the obstructive lesion. (See Schwartz 9th ed., p 372, and Table 14-1.)

TABLE 14-1 Modalities and techniques of restoring luminal patency

Modality	Technique
Core out	Photodynamic therapy Laser Coagulation Endoscopic biopsy forceps Chemical Ultrasound
Fracture	Ultrasound Endoscopic biopsy Balloon
Dilate	Balloon Bougie Angioplasty Endoscope
Bypass	Transvenous intrahepatic portosystemic shunt Surgical (synthetic or autologous conduit)
Stent	Self-expanding metal stent Plastic stent

CHAPTER 15

Molecular Biology

BASIC SCIENCE QUESTIONS

1. Functional genomics is a term used to describe which of the following?
   A. Transcription of DNA
   B. Translation of RNA
   C. Proteomics
   D. All of the above

Answer: D

Functional genomics seeks to assign a biochemical, physiologic, cell biologic, and/or developmental function to each predicted gene. An ever-increasing arsenal of approaches, including transgenic animals, RNA interference (RNAi), and various systematic mutational strategies, will allow dissection of functions associated with newly discovered genes. (See Schwartz 9th ed., p 385, and Fig. 15-1.)

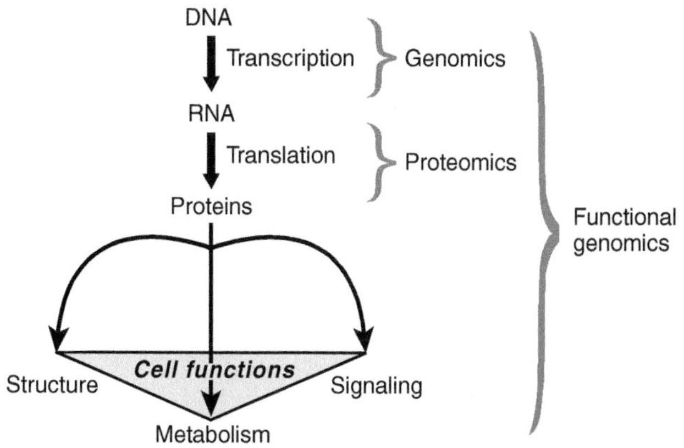

FIG. 15-1. The flow of genetic information from DNA to protein to cell functions. The process of transmission of genetic information from DNA to RNA is called *transcription*, and the process of transmission from RNA to protein is called *translation*. Proteins are the essential controlling components for cell structure, cell signaling, and metabolism. *Genomics* and *proteomics* are the study of the genetic composition of a living organism at the DNA and protein level, respectively. The study of the relationship between genes and their cellular functions is called *functional genomics*.

2. An intron is
   A. A segment of DNA removed prior to transcription
   B. The remaining (functional) segment of DNA after removal of nonfunctional DNA
   C. A segment of mRNA removed prior to translation
   D. The remaining (functional) segment of mRNA after removal of nonfunctional RNA

Answer: A

Living cells have the necessary machinery to enzymatically transcribe DNA into RNA and translate the mRNA into protein. This machinery accomplishes the two major steps required for gene expression in all organisms: transcription and translation. However, gene regulation is far more complex, particularly in eukaryotic organisms. For example, many gene transcripts must be spliced to remove the intervening sequences. The sequences that are spliced off are called *introns*, which appear to be useless, but in fact may carry some regulatory information. The sequences that are joined together, and are eventually translated into protein, are called *exons*. Additional regulation of gene expression includes modification of mRNA, control of mRNA stability, and its nuclear export into cytoplasm (where it is assembled into ribosomes for translation). After mRNA is translated into protein, the levels and functions of the proteins can be further regulated posttranslationally. (See Schwartz 9th ed., p 382.)

3. Translation of mRNA into proteins occurs in the
   A. Mitochondria
   B. Ribosomes
   C. Cytoplasm
   D. Cell membrane

Answer: B

DNA directs the synthesis of RNA; RNA in turn directs the synthesis of proteins. Proteins are variable-length polypeptide polymers composed of various combinations of 20 different amino acids and are the working molecules of the cell. The process of decoding information on mRNA to synthesize proteins is called *translation*. Translation takes place in ribosomes composed of rRNA and ribosomal proteins. (See Schwartz 9th ed., p 383, and Fig. 15-2.)

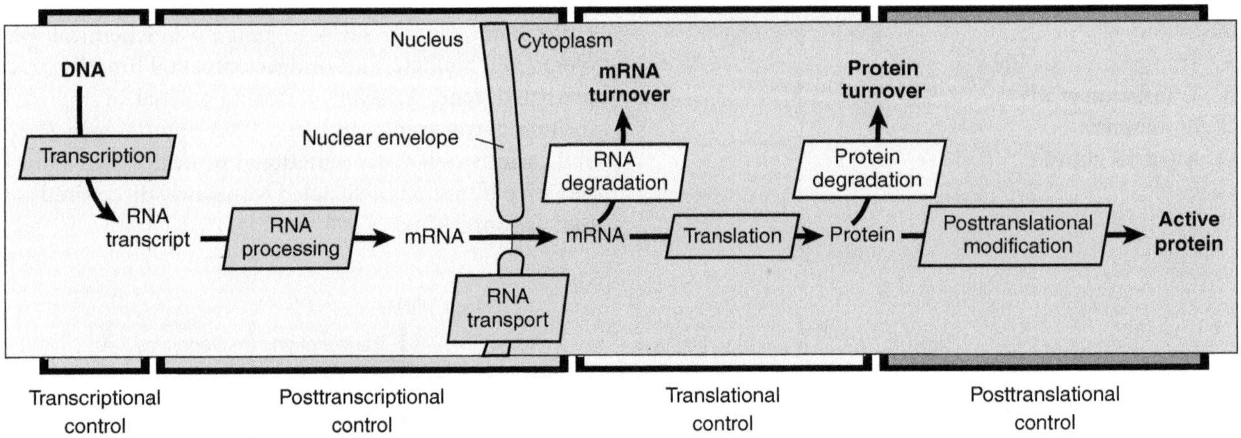

FIG. 15-2. Four major steps in the control of eukaryotic gene expression. Transcriptional and posttranscriptional control determine the level of messenger RNA (mRNA) that is available to make a protein, while translational and posttranslational control determine the final outcome of functional proteins. Note that posttranscriptional and posttranslational controls consist of several steps.

4. Approximately how many genes are present in the human genome?
   A. 25,000
   B. 100,000
   C. 250,000
   D. 750,000

Answer: A

Genome is a collective term for all genes present in one organism. The human genome contains DNA sequences of 3 billion base-pairs, carried by 23 pairs of chromosomes. The human genome has an estimated 25,000 to 30,000 genes, and overall it is 99.9% identical in all people. Approximately 3 million locations where single-base DNA differences exist have been identified and termed *single nucleotide polymorphisms*. Single nucleotide polymorphisms may be critical determinants of human variation in disease susceptibility and responses to environmental factors. (See Schwartz 9th ed., p 385.)

5. DNA replication occurs in which phase of the cell cycle?
   A. G_1
   B. S
   C. G_2
   D. M

Answer: B

Many cells grow, while some cells such as nerve cells and striated muscle cells do not. All growing cells have the ability to duplicate their genomic DNA and pass along identical copies of this genetic information to every daughter cell. Thus, the cell cycle is the fundamental mechanism to maintain tissue homeostasis. A cell cycle comprises four periods: G_1 (first gap phase before DNA synthesis), S (synthesis phase when DNA replication occurs), G_2 (the gap phase before mitosis), and M (mitosis, the phase when two daughter cells with identical

DNA are generated) (Fig. 15-3). After a full cycle, the daughter cells enter G_1 again, and when they receive appropriate signals, undergo another cycle, and so on. The machinery that drives cell cycle progression is made up of a group of enzymes called *cyclin-dependent kinases* (CDK). Cyclin expression fluctuates during the cell cycle, and cyclins are essential for CDK activities and form complexes with CDK. The cyclin A/CDK1 and cyclin B/CDK1 drive the progression for the M phase, while cyclin A/CDK2 is the primary S phase complex. Early G_1 cyclin D/CDK4/6 or late G_1 cyclin E/CDK2 controls the G_1-S transition. There also are negative regulators for CDK termed *CDK inhibitors*, which inhibit the assembly or activity of the cyclin-CDK complex. Expression of cyclins and CDK inhibitors often are regulated by developmental and environmental factors. (See Schwartz 9th ed., pp 385-386.)

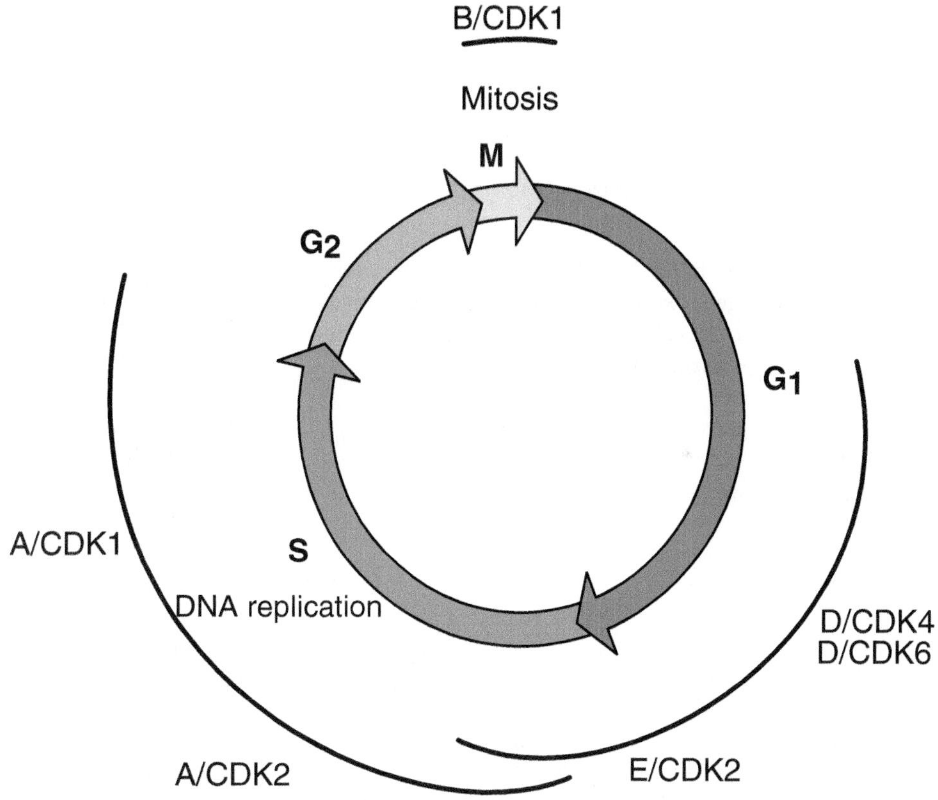

FIG. 15-3. The cell cycle and its control system. M is the mitosis phase, when the nucleus and the cytoplasm divide; S is the phase when DNA is duplicated; G_1 is the gap between M and S; G_2 is the gap between S and M. A complex of cyclin and cyclin-dependent kinase (CDK) controls specific events of each phase. Without cyclin, CDK is inactive. Different cyclin/CDK complexes are shown around the cell cycle. A, B, D, and E stand for cyclin A, cyclin B, cyclin D, and cyclin E, respectively.

6. Apoptosis is accomplished by activation of
   A. Capsases
   B. Metalloproteases
   C. Complement
   D. Heat shock protein

Answer: A

Normal tissues undergo proper apoptosis to remove unwanted cells, those that have completed their jobs or have been damaged or improperly proliferated. Apoptosis can be activated by many physiologic stimuli such as death receptor signals (e.g., Fas or cytokine tumor necrosis factor), growth factor deprivation, DNA damage, and stress signals. Two major pathways control the biochemical mechanisms governing apoptosis: the death receptor and mitochondrial. However, recent advances in apoptosis research suggest an interconnection of the two pathways. What is central to the apoptotic machinery is the activation of a cascade of proteinases called caspases. (See Schwartz 9th ed., pp 385-386, and Fig. 15-4.)

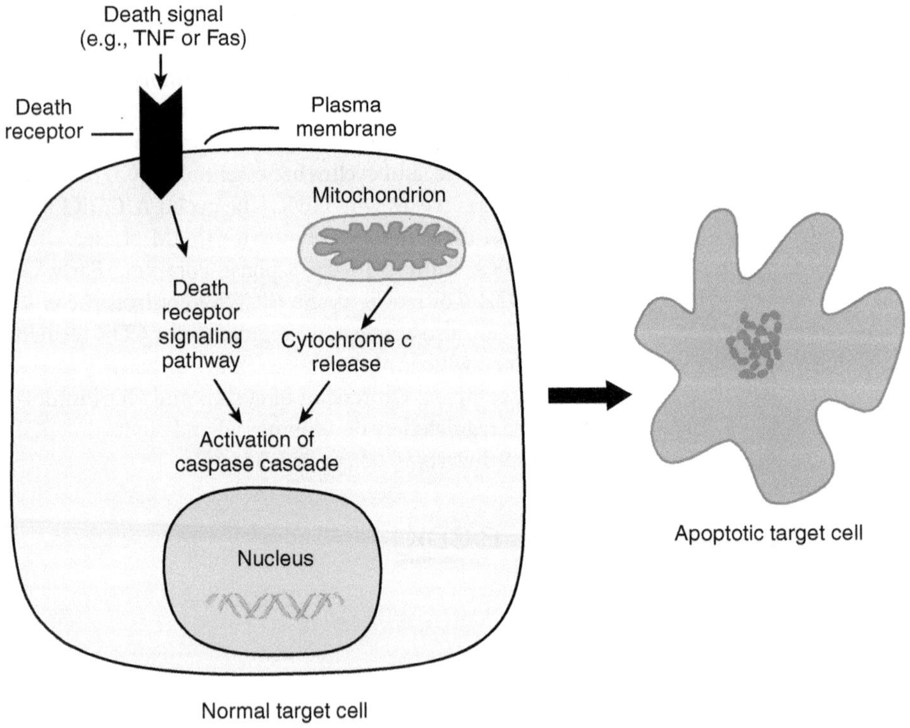

FIG. 15-4. A simplified view of the apoptosis pathways. Extracellular death receptor pathways include the activation of Fas and tumor necrosis factor (TNF) receptors, and consequent activation of the caspase pathway. Intracellular death pathway indicates the release of cytochrome c from mitochondria, which also triggers the activation of the caspase cascade. During apoptosis, cells undergo DNA fragmentation, nuclear and cell membrane breakdown, and are eventually digested by other cells.

7. Cells sense changes in their environment which then subsequently affects gene expression in the cell. These changes are transmitted to the cell by "ligands," substances that interact with receptors on or in the cell. Ligands are
   A. Peptides
   B. Dissolved gases
   C. Retinoids
   D. All of the above

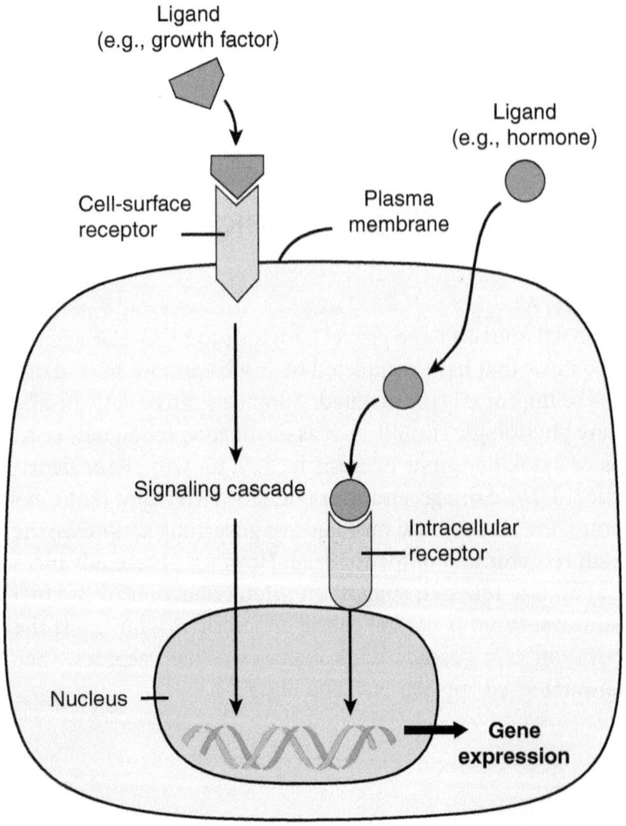

Answer: D

Gene expression in a genome is controlled in a temporal and spatial manner, at least in part by signaling pathways. A signaling pathway generally begins at the cell surface and, after a signaling relay by a cascade of intracellular effectors, ends up in the nucleus (Fig. 15-5). All cells have the ability to sense changes in their external environment. The bioactive substances to which cells can respond are many and include proteins, short peptides, amino acids, nucleotides/nucleosides, steroids, retinoids, fatty acids, and dissolved gases. Some of these substances are lipophilic and thereby can cross the plasma membrane by diffusion to bind to a specific target protein within the cytoplasm (intracellular receptor). Other substances bind directly with a transmembrane protein (cell-surface receptor). Binding of ligand to receptor initiates a series of biochemical reactions (*signal transduction*) typically involving protein-protein interactions and the transfer of high-energy phosphate groups, leading to various cellular end responses. (See Schwartz 9th ed., p 386.)

FIG. 15-5. Cell-surface and intracellular receptor pathways. Extracellular signaling pathway: Most growth factors and other hydrophilic signaling molecules are unable to move across the plasma membrane and directly activate cell-surface receptors such as G-protein coupled receptors and enzyme-linked receptors. The receptor serves as the receiver, and in turn activates the downstream signals in the cell. Intracellular signaling pathway: Hormones or other diffusible molecules enter the cell and bind to the intracellular receptor in the cytoplasm or in the nucleus. Either extracellular or intracellular signals often reach the nucleus to control gene expression.

8. Identification of a specific DNA segment can be accomplished by
   A. Southern blotting
   B. Northern blotting
   C. Western blotting
   D. Eastern blotting

Answer: A

Southern blotting refers to the technique of transferring DNA fragments from an electrophoresis gel to a membrane support, and the subsequent analysis of the fragments by hybridization with a radioactively labeled probe (Fig. 15-6). Southern blotting is named after E. M. Southern, who in 1975 first described the technique of DNA analysis. It enables reliable and efficient analysis of size-fractionated DNA fragments in an immobilized membrane support. (See Schwartz 9th ed., p 392.)

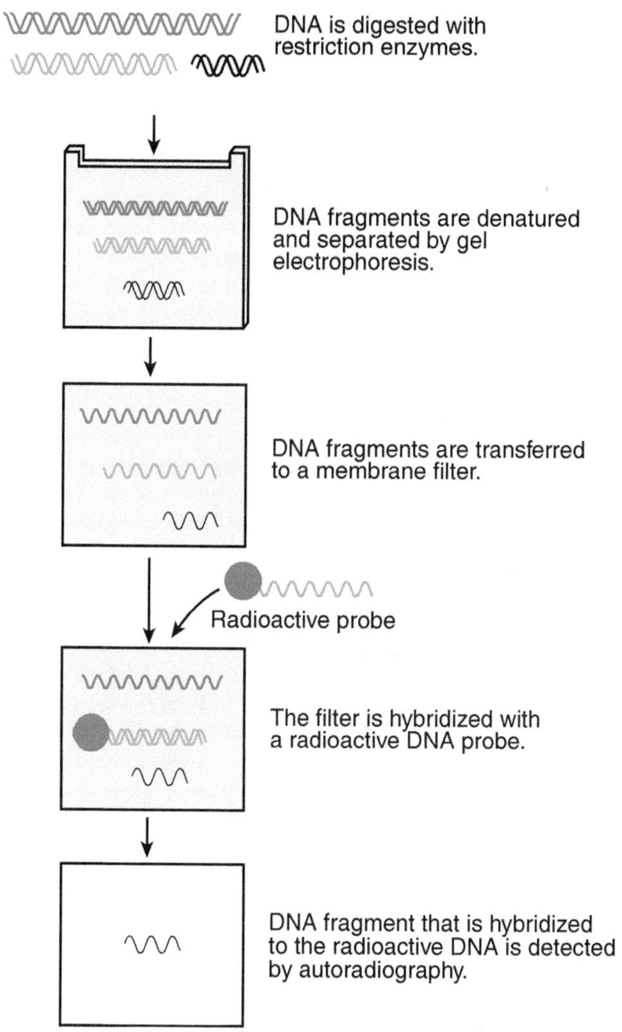

FIG. 15-6. Southern blotting. Restriction enzymatic fragments of DNA are separated by agarose gel electrophoresis, transferred to a membrane filter, and then hybridized to a radioactive probe.

Northern blotting refers to the technique of size fractionation of RNA in a gel and the transferring of an RNA sample to a solid support (membrane) in such a manner that the relative positions of the RNA molecules are maintained. The resulting membrane then is hybridized with a labeled probe complementary to the mRNA of interest. Signals generated from detection of the membrane can be used to determine the size and abundance of the target RNA. In principle, Northern blot hybridization is similar to Southern blot hybridization (and hence its name), with the exception that RNA, not DNA, is on the membrane.

Analyses of proteins are primarily carried out by antibody-directed immunologic techniques. For example, Western blotting, also called *immunoblotting*, is performed to detect protein levels in a population of cells or tissues, whereas immunoprecipitation is used to concentrate proteins from a larger pool.

There is no technique known as Eastern blotting.

9. DNA microarrays allow identification of gene mutations using
   A. Polymerase chain reaction
   B. Hybridization
   C. Western blotting
   D. Molecular cloning

Answer: B

DNA microarray, also called *gene chip*, *DNA chip*, and *gene array*, refers to large sets of probes of known sequences orderly arranged on a small chip, enabling many hybridization reactions to be carried out in parallel in a small device. Like Southern and Northern hybridization, the underlying principle of this technology is the remarkable ability of nucleic acids to form a duplex between two strands with complementary base sequences. DNA microarray provides a medium for matching known and unknown DNA samples based on base-pairing rules, and automating the process of identifying the unknowns. Microarrays require specialized robotics and imaging equipment that spot the samples on a glass or nylon substrate, carry out the hybridization, and analyze the data generated. DNA microarrays containing different sets of genes from a variety of organisms are now commercially available, allowing biologists to simply purchase the chips and perform hybridization and data collection.

Polymerase chain reaction (PCR) is an in vitro method for the polymerase-directed amplification of specific DNA sequences using two oligonucleotide primers that hybridize to opposite strands and flank the region of interest in the target DNA.

Western blotting, also called *immunoblotting*, is performed to detect protein levels in a population of cells.

Molecular cloning refers to the process of cloning a DNA fragment of interest into a DNA vector that ultimately is delivered into bacterial or mammalian cells or tissues. (See Schwartz 9th ed., p 394.)

1. Trastuzumab is a monoclonal antibody which targets which of the following cell receptors in susceptible patients with breast cancer?
   A. BRCA-1
   B. BRCA-2
   C. HER2
   D. CAD-1

Answer: C

One of the most exciting applications of immunotherapy has come from the identification of certain tumor targets called *antigens* and the aiming of an antibody at these targets. This was first used as a means of localizing tumors in the body for diagnosis, and was more recently used to attack cancer cells. Trastuzumab (Herceptin) is an example of such a drug. Trastuzumab is a monoclonal antibody that neutralizes the mitogenic activity of cell-surface growth factor receptor HER2. Approximately 25% of breast cancers overexpress HER2. These tumors tend to grow faster and generally are more likely to recur than tumors that do not overproduce HER2. Trastuzumab is designed to attack cancer cells that overexpress HER2. Trastuzumab slows or stops the growth of these cells and increases the survival of HER2-positive breast cancer patients. (See Schwartz 9th ed., p 390.)

2. STI157, also known as Gleevec, is a molecularly targeted therapy for
   A. Acute lymphocytic leukemia
   B. Acute myeloid leukemia
   C. Chronic lymphocytic leukemia
   D. Chronic myeloid leukemia

Answer: D

The primary function of anticancer chemicals is to block different steps involved in cell growth and replication. These chemicals often block a critical chemical reaction in a signal transduction pathway or during DNA replication or gene expression. For example, STI571, also known as *Gleevec*, is one of the first molecularly targeted drugs based on the changes that cancer causes in cells. STI571 offers promise for the treatment of chronic myeloid leukemia (CML) and may soon surpass interferon-γ as the standard treatment for the disease. In CML, STI571 is targeted at the Bcr-Abl kinase, an activated oncogene product in CML (Fig. 15-7). Bcr-Abl is an overly activated protein kinase resulting from a specific genetic abnormality generated by chromosomal translocation that is found in the cells of patients with CML. STI571-mediated inhibition of Bcr-Abl-kinase activity not only prevents cell growth of Bcr-Abl–transformed leukemic cells, but also induces apoptosis. Clinically, the drug quickly corrects the blood cell abnormalities caused by the leukemia in a majority of patients, achieving a complete disappearance of the leukemic blood cells and the return of normal blood cells. (See Schwartz 9th ed., p 390.)

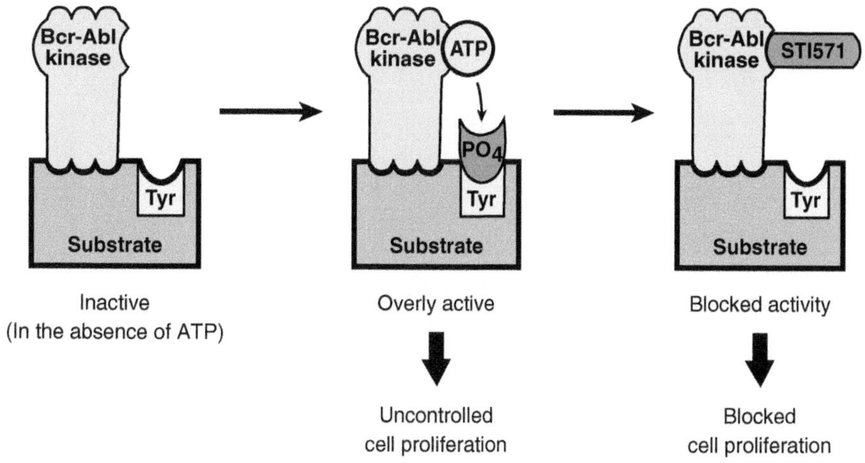

FIG. 15-7. Mechanism of STI571 as a molecular drug. Bcr-Abl is an overly activated oncogene product resulting from a specific genetic abnormality generated by chromosomal translocation that is found in cells of patients with chronic myeloid leukemia. Bcr-Abl is an activated protein kinase and thus requires adenosine triphosphate (ATP) to phosphorylate substrates, which in turn promote cell proliferation. STI571 is a small molecule that competes with the ATP-binding site and thus blocks the transfer of phosphoryl group to substrate. PO_4 = phosphate; Tyr = tyrosine.

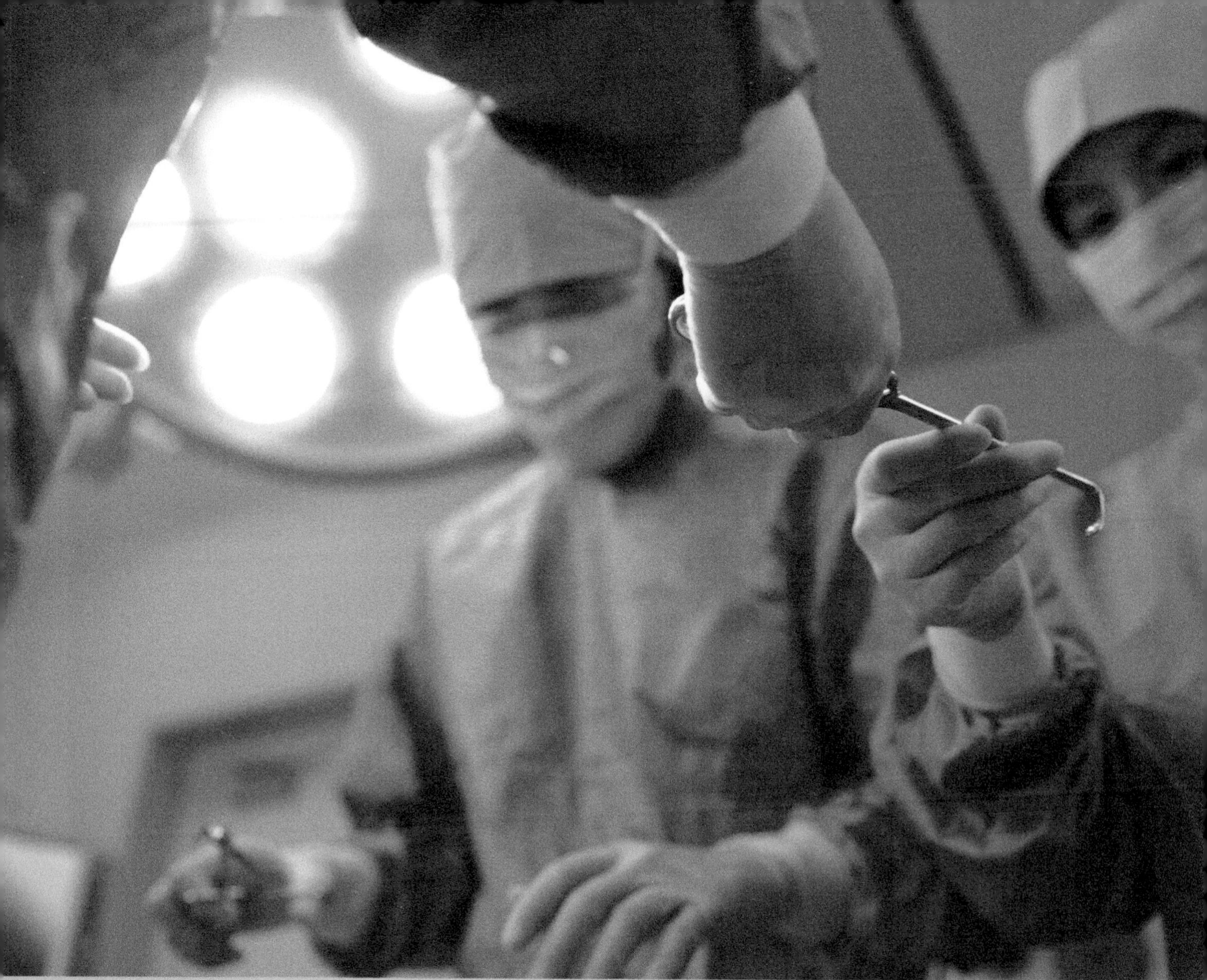

PART II
Specific Considerations

CHAPTER 16

The Skin and Subcutaneous Tissue

BASIC SCIENCE QUESTIONS

1. Approximately how long does it take from migration of a keratinocyte from the base layer to the time it is shed from the epidermis?
   A. 10 days
   B. 30 days
   C. 50 days
   D. 70 days

Answer: C

Composed primarily of keratinocytes, the epidermis is a dynamic, multilayered composite of maturing cells. From internal to external most layer, the epidermis is composed of the (a) stratum germinatum (b) stratum spinosum, (c) stratum granulosum, (d) stratum lucidum, and finally, (e) stratum corneum. Basal cells are a mitotically active, single-cell layer of the least-differentiated keratinocytes at the base of epidermal structure. As basal cells multiply, they leave the basal lamina to begin their differentiation and upward migration. In the spinous layer, keratinocytes are linked together by tonofibrils and produce keratin. As these cells drift upward, they lose their mitotic ability. With entry into the granular layer, cells accumulate keratohyalin granules. In the horny layer, keratinocytes age, lose their intercellular connections, and shed. From basal layer exit to shedding, keratinocyte transit time approximates 40 to 56 days. (See Schwartz 9th ed., p 406.)

2. What is the embryologic origin of melanocytes?
   A. Ectoderm
   B. Mesoderm
   C. Endoderm
   D. Neural crest

Answer: D

Melanocytes and other cellular components within the skin deter absorption of harmful radiation. Initially derived from precursor cells of the neural crest, melanocytes extend dendritic processes upward into epidermal tissues from their position beneath the basal cell layer. They number approximately one for every 35 keratinocytes, and produce melanin from tyrosine and cysteine. Once the pigment is packaged into melanosomes within the melanocyte cell body, these pigment molecules are transported into the epidermis via dendritic processes. As dendritic processes (apocopation) are sheared off, melanin is transferred to keratinocytes via phagocytosis. Despite differences in skin tone, the density of melanocytes is constant among individuals. It is the rate of melanin production, transfer to keratinocytes, and melanosome degradation that determine the degree of skin pigmentation. (See Schwartz 9th ed., p 406.)

3. Which of the following is the primary type of collagen present in fetal skin?
   A. Type I collagen
   B. Type II collagen
   C. Type III collagen
   D. Type IV collagen

Answer: C
Collagen, the main functional protein within the dermis, constitutes 70% of dermal dry weight and is responsible for its remarkable tensile strength. Tropocollagen, a collagen precursor, consists of three polypeptide chains (hydroxyproline, hydroxylysine, and glycine) wrapped in a helix. These long molecules are then cross-linked to one another to form collagen fibers. Of the seven structurally distinct collagens, the skin primarily contains type I. Fetal dermis contains mostly type III (reticulin fibers) collagen, but this only remains in the basement membrane zone and perivascular regions during postnatal development. (See Schwartz 9th ed., p 407.)

4. Which of the following is NOT a component of a mechanoreceptor in the skin (i.e., used to transmit information about mechanical forces on the skin to the central nervous system)?
   A. Meissner's corpuscles
   B. Ruffini's corpuscles
   C. Pacini's corpuscles
   D. Glomus bodies

Answer: D
Cutaneous sensation is achieved via activation of a complicated plexus of dermal autonomic fibers synapsed to sweat glands, erector pili, and vasculature control points. These fibers also connect to corpuscular receptors that relay information from the skin back to the central nervous system. Meissner's, Ruffini's, and Pacini's corpuscles transmit information on local pressure, vibration, and touch. In addition, 'unspecialized' free nerve endings report temperature, touch, pain, and itch sensations.

Glomus bodies are tortuous arteriovenous shunts that allow a substantial increase in superficial blood flow when stimulated to open. (See Schwartz 9th ed., p 407.)

5. A pressure of 60 mmHg can result in pressure necrosis of the skin and underlying soft tissue after
   A. 20 minutes
   B. 1 hour
   C. 4 hours
   D. 12 hours

ANSWER: B
As little as 1 hour of 60 mmHg pressure produces histologically identifiable venous thrombosis, muscle degeneration, and tissue necrosis. Although normal arteriole, capillary, and venule pressures are 32, 20, and 12 mmHg, respectively, sitting can produce pressures as high as 300 mmHg at the ischial tuberosities. Healthy individuals regularly shift their body weight, even while asleep. However, sacral pressure can build to 150 mmHg when lying on a standard hospital mattress. Patients unable to sense pain or shift their body weight, such as paraplegics or bedridden individuals, may develop prolonged elevated tissue pressures and local necrosis. Because muscle tissue is more sensitive to ischemia than skin, necrosis usually extends to a deeper area than that apparent on superficial inspection. (See Schwartz 9th ed., p 409.)

6. Which of the following radiation wavelengths is primarily responsible for the development of skin cancer after exposure to the sun?
   A. UVA (400-315 nm)
   B. UVB (315-290 nm)
   C. UVC (290-200 nm)
   D. FUV (200-122 nm)

Answer: B
Solar or UV radiation is the most common form of radiation exposure. The UV spectrum is divided into UVA (400 to 315 nm), UVB (315 to 290 nm), and UVC (290 to 200 nm). With regard to skin damage and development of skin cancers, significant wavelengths are in the UV spectrum. The ozone layer absorbs UVC wavelengths below 290 nm, allowing only UVA and UVB to reach the earth. UVB is responsible for the acute sunburns and for the chronic skin damage leading to malignant degeneration, although it makes up less than 5% of the solar UV radiation that hits the earth. FUV (far ultraviolet) is also absorbed by the ozone layer. (See Schwartz 9th ed., p 409.)

CLINICAL QUESTIONS

1. Which of the following is the best initial treatment of a burn with hydrofluoric acid?
   A. Copious irrigation with water
   B. Copious irrigation with a dilute solution of sodium bicarbonate
   C. Application of a topical quaternary ammonium compound
   D. Application of topical calcium carbonate gel

Answer: A

The effect of acid exposure on the skin is determined by the concentration, duration of contact, amount, and penetrability. Deep tissue *coagulative* injury may result, damaging nerves, blood vessels, tendons, and bone. The initial treatment should include copious skin irrigation for at least 30 minutes with either saline or water. This dilutes active acid solution and helps return the skin to normal pH. Injuries associated with hydrofluoric acid present an additional treatment challenge. Fluoride ions continue to injure underlying tissue until they are neutralized with calcium, and absorb the body's calcium supply, which may prompt cardiac arrythmia. Topical quaternary ammonium compounds are widely used, and topical calcium carbonate gel also effectively detoxifies fluoride ions. (See Schwartz 9th ed., p 407.)

2. What is the causative agent of the lesion shown in Fig. 16-1?
   A. *Staphyloccocus epidermidis*
   B. *Actinomyces israelii*
   C. *Nocardia brasiliensis*
   D. Papillomavirus Type 2

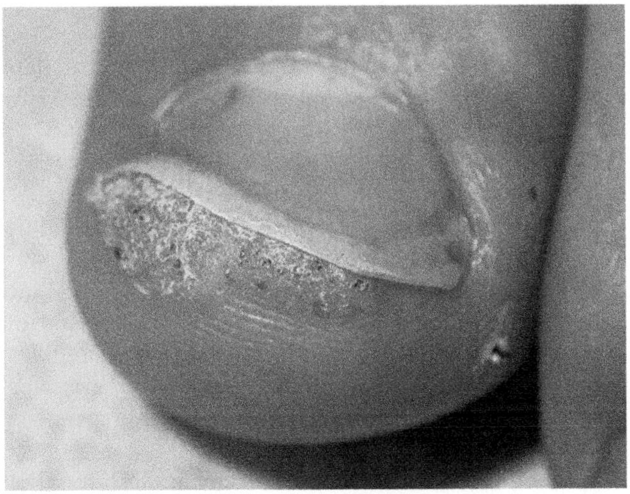

FIG. 16-1.

Answer: D

Warts are epidermal growths resulting from human papillomavirus (HPV) infection. Different morphologic types have a tendency to occur at different areas of the body. The common wart (verruca vulgaris) is found on the fingers and toes and is rough and bulbous (Fig. 16-1). Plantar warts (verruca plantaris) occur on the soles and palms, and may resemble a common callus. Flat warts (verruca plana) are slightly raised and flat. This particular subtype tends to appear on the face, legs, and hands. Venereal warts (condylomata acuminata) grow in the moist areas around the vulva, anus, and scrotum.

Actinomycosis is a granulomatous suppurative bacterial disease caused by *Actinomyces*. In addition to *Nocardia*, *Actinomadura*, and *Streptomyces*, *Actinomyces* infections may produce deep cutaneous infections that present as nodules and spread to form draining tracts within surrounding soft tissue. Forty to 60% of the actinomycotic infections occur within the face or head. Actinomycotic infection usually results following tooth extraction, odontogenic infection, or facial trauma. Accurate diagnosis depends on careful histologic analysis, and the presence of sulfur granules within purulent specimen is pathognomonic. Penicillin and sulfonamides are typically effective against these infections. However, areas of deep-seated infection, abscess, or chronic scarring may require surgical therapy. (See Schwartz 9th ed., p 410.)

3. Which of the following is associated with pyoderma gangrenosum?
   A. Monoclonal immunoglobulin A gammopathy
   B. Degenerative arthritis
   C. Adenocarcinoma of the colon
   D. Glioblastoma

Answer: A

Pyoderma gangrenosum is a relatively uncommon destructive cutaneous lesion. Clinically, a rapidly enlarging, necrotic lesion with undermined border and surrounding erythema characterize this disease. Linked to underlying systemic disease in 50% of cases, these lesions are commonly associated with inflammatory bowel disease, rheumatoid arthritis, hematologic malignancy, and monoclonal immunoglobulin A gammopathy. Recognition of the underlying disease is of paramount importance. Management of pyoderma gangrenosum ulcerations without correction of underlying systemic disorders is fraught with complication. A majority of patients receive systemic steroids or cyclosporine. Although medical management alone may slowly result in wound healing many physicians advocate chemotherapy with aggressive wound care and skin graft coverage. (See Schwartz 9th ed., p 410.)

4. Staphylococcal scalded skin syndrome (see Fig. 16-2) is most likely to be associated with which of the following?
   A. Phenytoin
   B. Barbiturates
   C. Tetracycline
   D. Otitis media

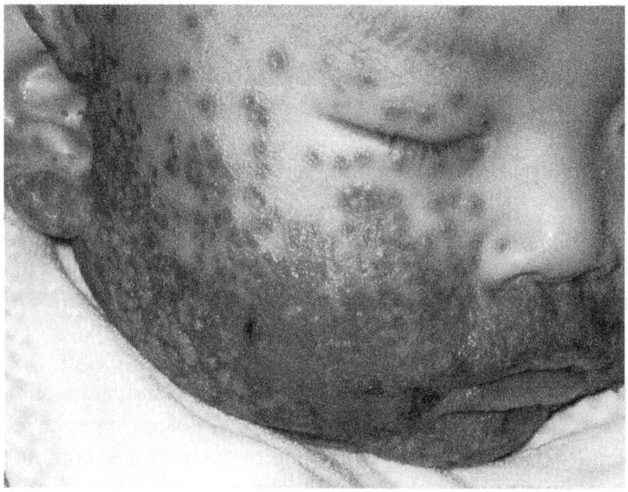

FIG. 16-2.

Answer: D

Staphylococcal scalded skin syndrome (SSSS) is caused by an exotoxin produced during staphylococcal infection of the nasopharynx or middle ear. Toxic epidermal necrolysis (TEN) is an immune response to certain drugs such as sulfonamides, phenytoin, barbiturates, and tetracycline. Diagnosis is made via skin biopsy. Histologic analysis of SSSS reveals a cleavage plane in the granular layer of the epidermis. In contrast, TEN results in structural defects at the dermoepidermal junction and is similar to a second-degree burn. Treatment involves fluid and electrolyte replacement, as well as wound care similar to burn therapy. Whereas those with more than 30% of total body surface area involvement are classified as TEN, patients with less than 10% of epidermal detachment are categorized as Stevens-Johnson syndrome. In Stevens-Johnson syndrome, respiratory and alimentary tract epithelial sloughing may result in intestinal malabsorption and pulmonary failure. Patients with significant soft-tissue loss should be treated in burn units with specially trained staff and critical equipment. Although corticosteroid therapy has not been efficacious, temporary coverage via cadaveric, porcine skin, or semisynthetic biologic dressings (Biobrane) allows the underlying epidermis to regenerate spontaneously. (See Schwartz 9th ed., p 411.)

5. A "sebaceous" cyst is removed from the scalp of a 48-year-old woman. Which of the following would be expected on histologic examination?
   A. Presence of sebum
   B. Presence of a granular layer
   C. Presence of eccrine glands
   D. The presence of epidermis covered by an external basal layer

Answer: D

Cutaneous cysts are categorized as either epidermal, dermoid, or trichilemmal. Although surgeons often refer to cutaneous cysts as sebaceous cysts because they appear to contain sebum, this is a misnomer and the substance is actually keratin. Epidermal cysts are the most common type of cutaneous cyst, and may present as a single, firm nodule anywhere on the body. Dermoid cysts are congenital lesions that result when epithelium is trapped during fetal midline closure. Although the eyebrow is the most frequent site of presentation, dermoid cysts are common anywhere from the nasal tip to the forehead. Trichilemmal (pilar) cysts, the second most common cutaneous cyst, occur more often on the scalp of females.

Histologic examination reveals several key features. Cyst walls consist of an epidermal layer oriented with the basal layer superficial, and the more mature layers deep (i.e., with the epidermis growing into the center of the cyst). The desquamated cells (keratin) collect in the center to form the cyst. Epidermal cysts have a mature epidermis complete with granular layer. Dermoid cysts demonstrate squamous epithelium, eccrine glands, and ilosebaceous units. In addition, these particular cysts may develop bone, tooth, or nerve tissue on occasion. Trichilemmal cyst walls do not contain a granular layer; however, these cysts contain a distinctive outer layer resembling the root sheath of a hair follicle (trichilemmoma). (See Schwartz 9th ed., p 411.)

6. Which of the following is indicated in the patient shown in Fig. 16-3?
   A. CT of the brain
   B. MRI of the sinuses
   C. Ultrasound of the spleen
   D. Doppler ultrasound of the femoral vessels

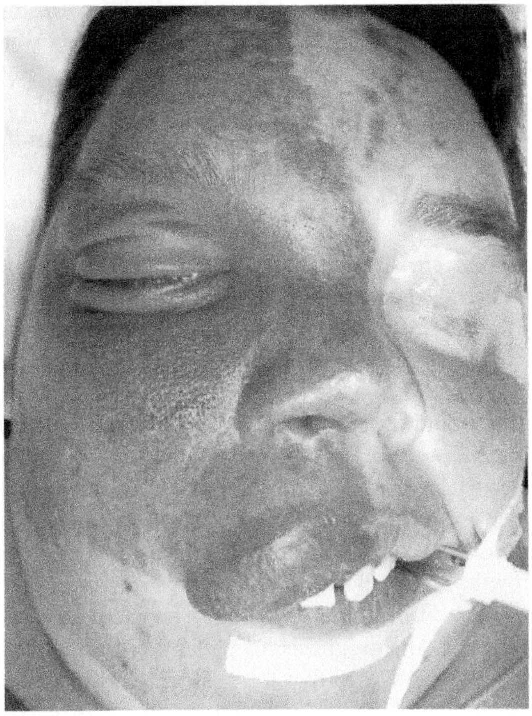

FIG. 16-3.

Answer: A

A capillary hemangioma (also known as a *port-wine stain*) present upon the midface may signify Churg-Strauss syndrome, and computed tomography of the brain is appropriate to rule out intracranial berry aneurysms. (See Schwartz 9th ed., p 412.)

7. Which of the following is the most common form of basal cell carcinoma?
   A. Morpheaform
   B. Superficial spreading
   C. Pigmented
   D. Nodular

Answer: D

Arising from the basal layer of the epidermis, BCC is the most common type of skin cancer. Based on gross and histologic morphology, BCC has been divided into several subtypes: nodular, superficial spreading, micronodular, infiltrative, pigmented, and morpheaform. Nodulocystic or noduloulcerative type accounts for 70% of BCC tumors. Waxy and frequently cream colored, these lesions present with rolled, pearly borders surrounding a central ulcer. Although superficial basal cell tumors commonly occur on the trunk and form a red, scaling lesion, pigmented BCC lesions are tan to black in color. Morpheaform BCC often appears as a flat, plaque-like lesion. This particular variant is considered relatively aggressive and should prompt early excision. A rare form of BCC is the basosquamous type, which contains elements of both basal cell and squamous cell cancer. These lesions may metastasize similar to squamous cell carcinoma SCC, and should be treated aggressively. (See Schwartz 9th ed., p 413.)

8. A Marjolin's ulcer arises in areas exposed to
   A. External beam radiation
   B. Thermal injury
   C. Pressure
   D. Lymphedema

Answer: B

Marjolin's ulcers arise in burn scars. Squamous cell carcinoma (SCC) may arise in Marjolin's ulcers. Along with SCCs associated with osteomyelitis and areas of previous injury, these lesions tend to be more aggressive and metastasize earlier than other SCCs. (See Schwartz 9th ed., p 414.)

9. Angiosarcoma associated with Stewart-Treves syndrome arises in areas exposed to
   A. External beam radiation
   B. Thermal injury
   C. Pressure
   D. Lymphedema

Answer: D

Angiosarcomas may arise spontaneously, mostly on the scalp, face, and neck. They usually appear as a bruise that spontaneously bleeds or enlarges without trauma. Tumors also may arise in areas of prior radiation therapy or in the setting of chronic lymphedema of the arm, such as after mastectomy (Stewart-Treves syndrome). The angiosarcomas that arise in these areas of chronic change occur decades later. The tumors consist of anaplastic endothelial cells surrounding vascular channels. Although total excision of early lesions can provide occasional cure, the prognosis usually is poor, with 5-year survival rates of less than 20%. Chemotherapy and radiation therapy are used for palliation. (See Schwartz 9th ed., p 418.)

10. Which type of melanoma has the best overall prognosis?
    A. Superficial spreading
    B. Nodular
    C. Lentigo maligna
    D. Acral lentiginous

Answer: C

In order of decreasing frequency, the four types of melanoma are superficial spreading, nodular, lentigo maligna, and acral lentiginous. The most common type, superficial spreading, accounts for up to 70% of melanomas. These lesions occur anywhere on the skin except the hands and feet. They are typically flat and measure 1 to 2 cm in diameter at diagnosis. Before vertical extension, a prolonged radial growth phase is characteristic of these lesions. Typically of darker coloration and often raised, the nodular type accounts for 15 to 30% of melanomas. These lesions are noted for their lack of radial growth; hence, all nodular melanomas are in the vertical growth phase at diagnosis. Although considered a more aggressive lesion, the prognosis for patients with nodular-type melanomas is similar to that for a patient with a superficial spreading lesion of the same depth. Lentigo maligna accounts for 4 to 15% of melanomas, and occurs most frequently on the neck, face, and hands of the elderly. Although they tend to be quite large at diagnosis, these lesions have the best prognosis because invasive growth occurs late. Less than 5% of lentigo maligna are estimated to evolve into melanoma. Acral lentiginous melanoma is the least common subtype, and constitutes only 2 to 8% of melanomas in white populations. Although acral lentiginous melanoma among dark-skinned people is relatively rare, this type accounts for 29 to 72% of all melanomas in dark-skinned people (African Americans, Asians, and Hispanics). Acral lentiginous melanoma most frequently is encountered on the palms, soles, and subungual regions. Most common on the great toe or thumb, subungual lesions appear as blue-black discolorations of the posterior nail fold. The additional presence of pigmentation in the proximal or lateral nail folds (Hutchinson's sign) is diagnostic of subungual melanoma. (See Schwartz 9th ed., p 415.)

11. A patient presents with a biopsy proven melanoma of the thigh which is 3 mm thick on histologic examination. At the time of excision, how wide should the margins be?
    A. 1 cm
    B. 2 cm
    C. 3 cm
    D. 4 cm

Answer: B

Regardless of tumor depth or extension, surgical excision is the management of choice. Lesions 1 mm or less in thickness can be treated with a 1-cm margin. For lesions 1 mm to 4 mm thick, a 2-cm margin is recommended. Lesions of greater than 4 mm may be treated with 3-cm margins. The surrounding tissue should be removed down to the fascia to remove all lymphatic channels. If the deep fascia is not involved by the tumor, removing it does not affect recurrence or survival rates, so the fascia is left intact. (See Schwartz 9th ed., pp 415-416, and Fig. 16-4.)

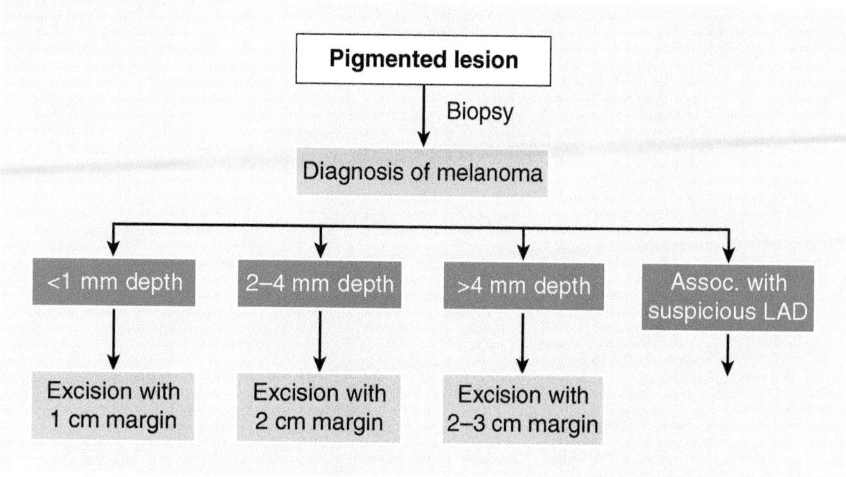

FIG. 16-4. The diagnosis of melanoma should be made via excisional biopsy. Based on tumor depth, appropriate margins may be planned. Indications for lymph node evaluation continue to advance as our understanding of tumor behavior improves and outcome data become available. LAD = lymphadenopathy.

12. A patient presents with a biopsy proven Merkel cell carcinoma 2 mm in diameter. At the time of excision, how wide should the margins be?
    A. 1 cm
    B. 2 cm
    C. 3 cm
    D. 4 cm

Answer: C

Once thought to be a variant of squamous cell carcinoma (SCC), Merkel cell carcinomas are actually of neuroepithelial differentiation. These tumors are associated with a synchronous or metasynchronous SCC 25% of the time. Due to their aggressive nature, wide local resection with 3-cm margins is recommended. Local recurrence rates are high, and distant metastases occur in one third of patients. Prophylactic regional LN dissection and adjuvant radiation therapy are recommended. Overall, the prognosis is worse than for malignant melanoma. (See Schwartz 9th ed., p 417.)

13. Which of the following chemotherapeutic agents is used in the treatment of some patients with dermatofibrosarcoma protuberans (DFSP)?
    A. Imatinib
    B. Carboplatin
    C. Methotrexate
    D. None of the above—DFSP is not chemosensitive

Answer: A

Continued study of chemotherapy efficacy on dermatofibrosarcoma protuberans (DFSP) also has produced optimistic results. Imatinib, a selective inhibitor of platelet-derived growth factor (PDGF) β-chain alpha and PDGF receptor beta protein-tyrosine kinase activity, alters the biologic effects of deregulated PDGF receptor signaling. Clinical trials have shown activity against localized and metastatic DFSP containing the t(17:22) translocation, suggesting that targeting the PDGF receptors may become a new therapeutic option for DFSP. Phase II clinical trials are under way. (See Schwartz 9th ed., p 418.)

14. Nevus sebaceous of Jadassohn is most commonly associated with
    A. Melanoma
    B. Squamous cell carcinoma
    C. Basal cell carcinoma
    D. Neurofibroma

Answer: C

Nevus sebaceous of Jadassohn is a lesion containing several cutaneous tissue elements that develops during childhood. This lesion is associated with a variety of neoplasms of the epidermis, but most commonly basal cell carcinoma (BCC). (See Schwartz 9th ed., p 418.)

CHAPTER 17

The Breast

BASIC SCIENCE QUESTIONS

1. How many lactiferous ducts drain into the nipple of the mature female breast?
   A. 5-10
   B. 15-20
   C. 25-30
   D. 35-40

Answer: B

The breast is composed of 15 to 20 lobes, which are each composed of several lobules.

Each lobe of the breast terminates in a major (lactiferous) duct (2 to 4 mm in diameter), which opens through a constricted orifice (0.4 to 0.7 mm in diameter) into the ampulla of the nipple. (See Schwartz 9th ed., p 426.)

2. During pregnancy, alveolar epithelium develops in the breast which is responsible after delivery for the production of milk. Which portion of the alveolar epithelial cell is responsible for production of the fat present in human milk?
   A. Endoplasmic reticulum
   B. Mitochondria
   C. Cell membrane
   D. Cytoplasm

Answer: D

With pregnancy, the breast undergoes proliferative and developmental maturation. As the breast enlarges in response to hormonal stimulation, lymphocytes, plasma cells, and eosinophils accumulate within the connective tissues. The minor ducts branch and alveoli develop. Development of the alveoli is asymmetric, and variations in the degree of development may occur within a single lobule. With parturition, enlargement of the breasts occurs via hypertrophy of alveolar epithelium and accumulation of secretory products in the lumina of the minor ducts.

Two distinct substances are produced by the alveolar epithelium: (a) the protein component of milk, which is synthesized in the endoplasmic reticulum (merocrine secretion); and (b) the lipid component of milk (apocrine secretion), which forms as free lipid droplets in the cytoplasm. (See Schwartz 9th ed., p 427.)

3. The medial mammary artery is a tributary of the
   A. 2nd, 3rd, and 4th intercostal arteries
   B. Lateral thoracic artery
   C. Thoracoacromial artery
   D. Posterior intercostal arteries

Answer: A

The breast receives its principal blood supply from (a) perforating branches of the internal mammary artery; (b) lateral branches of the posterior intercostal arteries; and (c) branches from the axillary artery, including the highest thoracic, lateral thoracic, and pectoral branches of the thoracoacromial artery. The second, third, and fourth anterior intercostal perforators and branches of the internal mammary artery arborize in the breast as the medial mammary arteries. The lateral thoracic artery gives off branches to the serratus anterior, pectoralis major and pectoralis minor, and subscapularis muscles. It also gives rise to lateral mammary branches. (See Schwartz 9th ed., p 428.)

4. Which of the following hormones is primarily responsible for differentiation of the breast ductal epithelium?
   A. Estrogen
   B. Testosterone
   C. Progesterone
   D. Prolactin

Answer: C
Estrogen initiates ductal development, whereas progesterone is responsible for differentiation of epithelium and for lobular development. Prolactin is the primary hormonal stimulus for lactogenesis in late pregnancy and the postpartum period. It upregulates hormone receptors and stimulates epithelial development. (See Schwartz 9th ed., p 429.)

CLINICAL QUESTIONS

1. Absence of the breast (amastia) is associated with
   A. Turner's syndrome
   B. Kleinfelter's syndrome
   C. Poland syndrome
   D. Fleischer's syndrome

Answer: C
Absence of the breast (*amastia*) is rare and results from an arrest in mammary ridge development that occurs during the sixth fetal week. Poland's syndrome consists of hypoplasia or complete absence of the breast, costal cartilage and rib defects, hypoplasia of the subcutaneous tissues of the chest wall, and brachysyndactyly. (See Schwartz 9th ed., p 426.)

Turner's syndrome (ovarian agenesis and dysgenesis) and Fleischer's syndrome (displacement of the nipples and bilateral renal hypoplasia) may have polymastia as a component.

Klinefelter's syndrome (XXY) is manifested by gynecomastia, hypergonadotropic hypogonadism, and azoospermia. This is an increased risk of breast cancer in men with Klinefelter's syndrome. (See Schwartz 9th ed., p 431.)

2. The treatment of choice for Zuska's disease is
   A. Observation and nonsteroidal anti-inflammatory drugs (NSAIDs)
   B. Antibiotics, incision, and drainage
   C. Wide resection of the affected area
   D. Mastectomy

Answer: B
Zuska's disease, also called *recurrent periductal mastitis*, is a condition of recurrent retroareolar infections and abscesses. This syndrome is managed symptomatically, by antibiotics coupled with incision and drainage as necessary. Attempts to obtain durable long-term control by wide débridement of chronically infected tissue and/or terminal duct resection are frequently frustrated by postoperative infections. Smoking has been implicated as a risk factor for this condition. (See Schwartz 9th ed., p 433.)

3. A clinically positive subclavicular lymph node is a
   A. Level I node
   B. Level II node
   C. Level III node
   D. Level IV node

Answer: C
The lymph node groups are assigned levels according to their anatomic relationship to the pectoralis minor muscle. Lymph nodes located lateral to or below the lower border of the pectoralis minor muscle are referred to as *level I lymph nodes*, which include the axillary vein, external mammary, and scapular groups. Lymph nodes located superficial or deep to the pectoralis minor muscle are referred to as *level II lymph nodes*, which include the central and interpectoral groups. Lymph nodes located medial to or above the upper border of the pectoralis minor muscle are referred to as *level III lymph nodes*, which consist of the subclavicular group. (See Schwartz 9th ed., p 429, and Fig. 17-1.)

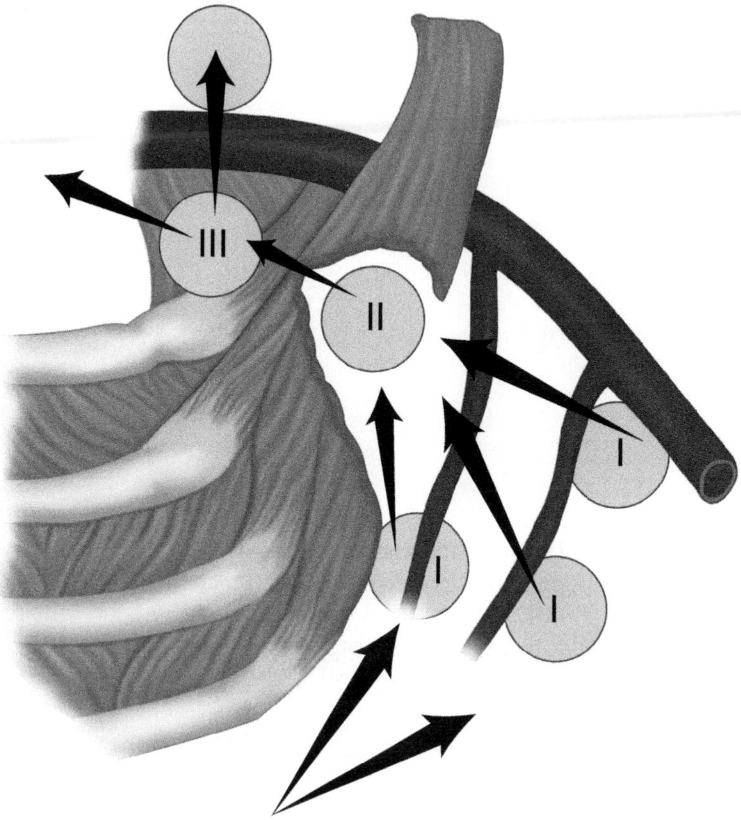

FIG. 17-1. Axillary lymph node groups. Level I includes lymph nodes located lateral to the pectoralis minor muscle (PM); level II includes lymph nodes located deep to the PM; and level III includes lymph nodes located medial to the PM. *Arrows* indicate the direction of lymph flow. The axillary vein with its major tributaries and the supraclavicular lymph node group are also illustrated. (Reproduced with permission from Romrell LJ, Bland KI: Anatomy of the breast, axilla, chest wall, and related metastatic sites, in Bland KI, Copeland EM III (eds): *The Breast: Comprehensive Management of Benign and Malignant Diseases*. Philadelphia: W.B. Saunders, 1998, p 32. Copyright © Elsevier.)

4. Which of the following conditions leads to gynecomastia due to an increased production of estrogen?
   A. Klinefelter's syndrome
   B. Hepatocellular carcinoma
   C. Aging (senescence)
   D. Renal failure

Answer: B

Estrogen excess results from an increase in the secretion of estradiol by the testicles or by nontesticular tumors, nutritional alterations such as protein and fat deprivation, endocrine disorders (hyperthyroidism, hypothyroidism), and hepatic disease (nonalcoholic and alcoholic cirrhosis). (See Schwartz 9th ed., p 431, and Table 17-1.)

Klinefelter's syndrome, aging, and renal failure all cause gynecomastia by a decrease in testosterone production.

TABLE 17-1 Pathophysiologic mechanisms of gynecomastia

- I. Estrogen excess states
  - A. Gonadal origin
    - 1. True hermaphroditism
    - 2. Gonadal stromal (nongerminal) neoplasms of the testis
      - a. Leydig cell (interstitial)
      - b. Sertoli cell
      - c. Granulosa-theca cell
    - 3. Germ cell tumors
      - a. Choriocarcinoma
      - b. Seminoma, teratoma
      - c. Embryonal carcinoma
  - B. Nontesticular tumors
    - 1. Adrenal cortical neoplasms
    - 2. Lung carcinoma
    - 3. Hepatocellular carcinoma
  - C. Endocrine disorders
  - D. Diseases of the liver—nonalcoholic and alcoholic cirrhosis
  - E. Nutrition alteration states
- II. Androgen deficiency states
  - A. Senescence
  - B. Hypoandrogenic states (hypogonadism)

(*continued*)

TABLE 17-1 (continued)

1. Primary testicular failure
a. Klinefelter's syndrome (XXY)
b. Reifenstein's syndrome
c. Rosewater-Gwinup-Hamwi familial gynecomastia
d. Kallmann syndrome
e. Kennedy's disease with associated gynecomastia
f. Eunuchoidal state (congenital anorchia)
g. Hereditary defects of androgen biosynthesis
h. Adrenocorticotropic hormone deficiency
2. Secondary testicular failure
a. Trauma
b. Orchitis
c. Cryptorchidism
d. Irradiation
C. Renal failure
III. Drug effects
IV. Systemic diseases with idiopathic mechanisms

5. The treatment of choice for Mondor's disease is
   A. Observation and nonsteroidal anti-inflammatory drugs (NSAIDs)
   B. Antibiotics, incision, and drainage
   C. Wide resection of the affected area
   D. Mastectomy

Answer: A

Mondor's disease is a variant of thrombophlebitis that involves the superficial veins of the anterior chest wall and breast. In 1939, Mondor described the condition as "string phlebitis," a thrombosed vein presenting as a tender, cord-like structure. Frequently involved veins include the lateral thoracic vein, the thoracoepigastric vein, and, less commonly, the superficial epigastric vein. Typically, a woman presents with acute pain in the lateral aspect of the breast or the anterior chest wall. A tender, firm cord is found to follow the distribution of one of the major superficial veins. Rarely, the presentation is bilateral, and most women have no evidence of thrombophlebitis in other anatomic sites. This benign, self-limited disorder is not indicative of a cancer. When the diagnosis is uncertain, or when a mass is present near the tender cord, biopsy is indicated. Therapy for Mondor's disease includes the liberal use of anti-inflammatory medications and application of warm compresses along the symptomatic vein. Restriction of motion of the ipsilateral extremity and shoulder as well as brassiere support of the breast are important. The process usually resolves within 4 to 6 weeks. When symptoms persist or are refractory to therapy, excision of the involved vein segment is appropriate. (See Schwartz 9th ed., p 433.)

6. The appropriate therapy for Paget's disease of the nipple is
   A. Topical steroid cream
   B. Topical antifungal medication
   C. Intralesional steroid injection
   D. Resection

Answer: D

Paget's disease of the nipple was described in 1874. It frequently presents as a chronic, eczematous eruption of the nipple, which may be subtle but may progress to an ulcerated, weeping lesion. Paget's disease usually is associated with extensive DCIS and may be associated with an invasive cancer. A palpable mass may or may not be present. A nipple biopsy specimen will show a population of cells that are identical to the underlying DCIS cells (pagetoid features or pagetoid change). Pathognomonic of this cancer is the presence of large, pale, vacuolated cells (Paget cells) in the rete pegs of the epithelium. Paget's disease may be confused with superficial spreading melanoma. Differentiation from pagetoid intraepithelial melanoma is based on the presence of S-100 antigen immunostaining in melanoma and carcinoembryonic antigen immunostaining in Paget's disease. Surgical therapy for Paget's disease may involve lumpectomy, mastectomy, or modified radical mastectomy, depending on the extent of involvement and the presence of invasive cancer. (See Schwartz 9th ed., pp 444-445.)

7. In the ANDI (aberrations of normal development and involution) classification, a 2-cm fibroadenoma is considered
   A. Normal
   B. A disorder
   C. A disease
   D. A premalignant disease

Answer: B

The basic principles underlying the aberrations of normal development and involution (ANDI) classification of benign breast conditions are the following: (a) benign breast disorders and diseases are related to the normal processes of reproductive life and to involution; (b) there is a spectrum of breast conditions that ranges from normal to disorder to disease; and (c) the ANDI classification encompasses all aspects of the breast condition, including pathogenesis and the degree of abnormality. The horizontal component of Table 17-2 defines ANDI along a spectrum from normal, to mild abnormality (disorder), to severe abnormality (disease). The vertical component indicates the period during which the condition develops. (See Schwartz 9th ed., p 433.)

Fibroadenomas are seen predominantly in younger women aged 15 to 25 years. Fibroadenomas usually grow to 1 or 2 cm in diameter and then are stable but may grow to a larger size. Small fibroadenomas (≤1 cm in size) are considered normal, whereas larger fibroadenomas (≤3 cm) are disorders and giant fibroadenomas (>3 cm) are disease. Similarly, multiple fibroadenomas (more than five lesions in one breast) are very uncommon and are considered disease. (See Schwartz 9th ed., p 434.)

TABLE 17-2 ANDI classification of benign breast disorders

	Normal	Disorder	Disease
Early reproductive years (age 15–25 y)	Lobular development Stromal development Nipple eversion	Fibroadenoma Adolescent hypertrophy Nipple inversion	Giant fibroadenoma Gigantomastia Subareolar abscess Mammary duct fistula
Later reproductive years (age 25–40 y)	Cyclical changes of menstruation Epithelial hyperplasia of pregnancy	Cyclical mastalgia Nodularity Bloody nipple discharge	Incapacitating mastalgia
Involution (age 35–55 y)	Lobular involution	Macrocysts Sclerosing lesions	—
	Duct involution Dilatation Sclerosis Epithelial turnover	 Duct ectasia Nipple retraction Epithelial hyperplasia	 Periductal mastitis — Epithelial hyperplasia with atypia

ANDI = aberrations of normal development and involution.

Source: Modified with permission from Hughes LE: Aberrations of normal development and involution (ANDI): A concept of benign breast disorders based on pathogenesis, in Hughes LE, et al (eds): *Benign Disorders and Diseases of the Breast: Concepts and Clinical Management*. London: WB Saunders, 2000, p 23. Copyright © Elsevier.

8. Which of the following conditions increases a woman's risk of breast cancer?
   A. Sclerosing adenosis
   B. Fibroadenoma
   C. Atypical lobular hyperplasia
   D. Intraductal papilloma

Answer: C

Atypical proliferative diseases include ductal and lobular hyperplasia, both of which display some features of carcinoma in situ. Women with atypical ductal or lobular hyperplasia have a four-fold increase in breast cancer risk. (See Schwartz 9th ed., p 434, and Table 17-3.)

TABLE 17-3	Cancer risk associated with benign breast disorders and in situ carcinoma of the breast
Abnormality	**Relative Risk**
Nonproliferative lesions of the breast	No increased risk
Sclerosing adenosis	No increased risk
Intraductal papilloma	No increased risk
Florid hyperplasia	1.5 to 2-fold
Atypical lobular hyperplasia	4-fold
Atypical ductal hyperplasia	4-fold
Ductal involvement by cells of atypical ductal hyperplasia	7-fold
Lobular carcinoma in situ	10-fold
Ductal carcinoma in situ	10-fold

Data from Dupont WD, et al: Risk factors for breast cancer in women with proliferative breast disease. *N Engl J Med* 312:146, 1985.

9. A 35-year-old woman with a BRCA1 gene mutation seeks your advice about her known increased risk of breast cancer. You should recommend
   A. Mammograms and physical examination every 6 months until she is 50, then bilateral prophylactic mastectomy
   B. Mammograms and physical examination every 6 months + tamoxifen
   C. Prophylactic bilateral mastectomy and, if she has completed childbearing, prophylactic bilateral oophorectomy
   D. None of the above

Answer: C

Present screening recommendations for *BRCA* mutation carriers who do not undergo prophylactic mastectomy include clinical breast examination every 6 months and mammography every 12 months beginning at age 25 years, because the risk of breast cancer in *BRCA* mutation carriers increases after age 30 years.

Despite a 49% reduction in the incidence of breast cancer in high-risk women taking tamoxifen, it is too early to recommend the use of tamoxifen uniformly for *BRCA* mutation carriers. Cancers arising in *BRCA1* mutation carriers are usually high grade and are most often hormone receptor negative. Approximately 66% of *BRCA1*-associated DCIS lesions are estrogen receptor negative, which suggests early acquisition of the hormone-independent phenotype. Tamoxifen appears to be more effective at preventing estrogen receptor–positive breast cancers.

The risk of ovarian cancer in *BRCA1* and *BRCA2* mutation carriers ranges from 20 to 40%, which is 10 times higher than that in the general population. Prophylactic oophorectomy is a reasonable prevention option in mutation carriers. The American College of Obstetrics and Gynecology recommends that women with a documented *BRCA1* or *BRCA2* mutation consider prophylactic oophorectomy at the completion of childbearing or at the time of menopause. Hormone replacement therapy is discussed with the patient at the time of oophorectomy. (See Schwartz 9th ed., pp 439-440.)

10. Which of the following statements about lobular carcinoma in situ (LCIS) is true?
    A. In general, LCIS occurs at an older age than ductal carcinoma in situ (DCIS)
    B. The majority of women with LCIS are premenopausal
    C. LCIS is bilateral in 10 to 20% of women
    D. Invasive ductal carcinoma can be expected to occur an average of 5 to 10 years later in approximately 75% of women with LCIS

Answer: B

LCIS tends to occur at a younger age than DCIS and the majority (approximately two thirds) of women with LCIS are premenopausal. LCIS is bilateral in 50 to 70% of women. Approximately 25 to 35% of women with LCIS can be expected to develop invasive ductal carcinoma an average of 15 to 20 years after diagnosis. (See Schwartz 9th ed., p 444, and Table 17-4.)

TABLE 17-4 Salient characteristics of in situ ductal (DCIS) and lobular (LCIS) carcinoma of the breast

	LCIS	**DCIS**
Age (years)	44–47	54–58
Incidence[a]	2–5%	5–10%
Clinical signs	None	Mass, pain, nipple discharge
Mammographic signs	None	Microcalcifications
Premenopausal	2/3	1/3

(continued)

TABLE 17-4 (continued)		
	LCIS	DCIS
Incidence of synchronous invasive carcinoma	5%	2–46%
Multicentricity	60–90%	40–80%
Bilaterality	50–70%	10–20%
Axillary metastasis	1%	1–2%
Subsequent carcinomas:		
Incidence	25–35%	25–70%
Laterality	Bilateral	Ipsilateral
Interval to diagnosis	15–20 y	5–10 y
Histologic type	Ductal	Ductal

[a]In biopsy specimens of mammographically detected breast lesions.
Source: Reproduced with permission from Frykberg ER, et al: Current concepts on the biology and management of in situ (Tis, stage 0) breast carcinoma, in Bland KI, et al (eds): *The Breast: Comprehensive Management of Benign and Malignant Diseases.* Philadelphia: WB Saunders, 1998, p 1020. Copyright © Elsevier.

11. Moderate ductal hyperplasia of the breast is characterized by the microscopic finding of
    A. 3 to 4 cell layers above the basement membrane
    B. 5 or more cell layers above the basement membrane
    C. Obstruction of >50% of the ductal lumen by hyperplastic cells
    D. Obstruction of >70% of the ductal lumen by hyperplastic cells

Answer: B

Mild ductal hyperplasia is characterized by the presence of three or four cell layers above the basement membrane. Moderate ductal hyperplasia is characterized by the presence of five or more cell layers above the basement membrane. Florid ductal epithelial hyperplasia occupies at least 70% of a minor duct lumen. It is found in >20% of breast tissue specimens, is either solid or papillary, and is associated with an increased cancer risk. (See Schwartz 9th ed., p 435, and Table 17-5.)

TABLE 17-5 Cancer risk associated with benign breast disorders and in situ carcinoma of the breast

Abnormality	Relative Risk
Nonproliferative lesions of the breast	No increased risk
Sclerosing adenosis	No increased risk
Intraductal papilloma	No increased risk
Florid hyperplasia	1.5 to 2-fold
Atypical lobular hyperplasia	4-fold
Atypical ductal hyperplasia	4-fold
Ductal involvement by cells of atypical ductal hyperplasia	7-fold
Lobular carcinoma in situ	10-fold
Ductal carcinoma in situ	10-fold

Data from Dupont WD, et al: Risk factors for breast cancer in women with proliferative breast disease. *N Engl J Med* 312:146, 1985.

12. Which of the following is appropriate treatment for a 3-cm fibroadenoma?
    A. Resection
    B. Cryoablation
    C. Observation
    D. All of the above

Answer: D

Removal of all fibroadenomas has been advocated irrespective of patient age or other considerations, and solitary fibroadenomas in young women are frequently removed to alleviate patient concern. Yet most fibroadenomas are self-limiting and many go undiagnosed, so a more conservative approach is reasonable. Careful ultrasound examination with core-needle biopsy will provide for an accurate diagnosis. Ultrasonography may reveal specific features that are pathognomonic for fibroadenoma. In this situation a core-needle biopsy may not be necessary. Subsequently, the patient is counseled concerning the ultrasound and biopsy results, and excision of the fibroadenoma may be avoided. Cryoablation is an approved treatment for fibroadenomas of the breast. With short-term follow-up a significant percentage of fibroadenomas will decrease in size and will no longer be palpable. However, many will remain palpable, especially those larger than 2 cm. Therefore, women should be counseled that the options for treatment include surgical removal, cryoablation, or observation. (See Schwartz 9th ed., p 436.)

13. Which of the following women with recurrent subareolar infection should undergo a total duct excision (rather than a fistulotomy)?
    A. 55-year-old with nipple inversion
    B. 55-year-old without nipple inversion
    C. 35-year-old with nipple inversion
    D. 35-year-old without nipple inversion

Answer: A
In general, the criteria for performing a total duct excision in a woman with recurrent subareolar abscess are: older age, large or diffuse infection, and nipple inversion. (See Schwartz 9th ed., p 436, and Table 17-6.)

TABLE 17-6 Treatment of recurrent subareolar sepsis

Suitable for Fistulectomy	Suitable for Total Duct Excision
Small abscess localized to one segment	Large abscess affecting >50% of the areolar circumference
Recurrence involving the same segment	Recurrence involving a different segment
Mild or no nipple inversion	Marked nipple inversion
Patient unconcerned about nipple inversion	Patient requests correction of nipple inversion
Younger patient	Older patient
No discharge from other ducts	Purulent discharge from other ducts
No prior fistulectomy	Recurrence after fistulectomy

Source: Modified with permission from Hughes LE: The duct ectasia/periductal mastitis complex, in Hughes LE, et al (eds): *Benign Disorders and Diseases of the Breast: Concepts and Clinical Management*. London: WB Saunders, 2000, p 162. Copyright © Elsevier.

14. The average lifetime risk for a woman to develop breast cancer is approximately
    A. 7%
    B. 12%
    C. 17%
    D. 22%

Answer: B
The average lifetime risk of breast cancer for newborn U.S. females is 12%. The longer a woman lives without cancer, the lower her risk of developing breast cancer. Thus, a woman aged 50 years has an 11% lifetime risk of developing breast cancer, and a woman aged 70 years has a 7% lifetime risk of developing breast cancer. (See Schwartz 9th ed., p 437.)

15. Routine mammography in women over 50 years of age decreases mortality from breast cancer by approximately
    A. 10%
    B. 25%
    C. 33%
    D. 45%

Answer: C
Routine use of screening mammography in women ≥50 years of age reduces mortality from breast cancer by 33%. This reduction comes without substantial risks and at an acceptable economic cost. However, the use of screening mammography in women <50 years of age is more controversial for several reasons: (a) breast density is greater and screening mammography is less likely to detect early breast cancer; (b) screening mammography results in more false-positive test findings, which results in unnecessary biopsies; and (c) younger women are less likely to have breast cancer, so fewer young women will benefit from screening. On a population basis, however, the benefits of screening mammography in women between the ages of 40 and 49 years still appear to outweigh the risks.

Current recommendations are that women undergo baseline mammography at age 35 and then have annual mammographic screening beginning at age 40. (See Schwartz 9th ed., pp 437-438.)

16. The most common genetic cause of breast cancer is a mutation in
    A. PTEN (Cowden syndrome)
    B. BRCA2
    C. P53 (Li-Fraumeni syndrome)
    D. MSH2 (Muir-Torre syndrome)

Answer: B

Mutations in *BRCA1* and *BRCA2* are the most common mutations associated with breast cancer (see Table 17-7).

Both *BRCA1* and *BRCA2* function as tumor-suppressor genes, and for each gene, loss of both alleles is required for the initiation of cancer.

The breast cancer risk for *BRCA2* mutation carriers is close to 85%, and the lifetime ovarian cancer risk, while lower than for *BRCA1*, is still estimated to be close to 20%.... Unlike male carriers of *BRCA1* mutations, men with germline mutations in *BRCA2* have an estimated breast cancer risk of 6%, which represents a 100-fold increase over the risk in the general male population.

Other hereditary syndromes associated with an increased risk of breast cancer include Cowden disease (*PTEN* mutations, in which cancers of the thyroid, GI tract, and benign skin and subcutaneous nodules are also seen), Li-Fraumeni syndrome (p53 mutations, also associated with sarcomas, lymphomas, and adrenocortical tumors), and syndromes of breast and melanoma. (See Schwartz 9th ed., p 438.)

TABLE 17-7 Incidence of sporadic, familial, and hereditary breast cancer

Sporadic breast cancer	65–75%
Familial breast cancer	20–30%
Hereditary breast cancer	5–10%
BRCA1[a]	45%
BRCA2	35%
p53[a] (Li-Fraumeni syndrome)	1%
STK11/LKB1[a] (Peutz-Jeghers syndrome)	<1%
PTEN[a] (Cowden disease)	<1%
MSH2/MLH1[a] (Muir-Torre syndrome)	<1%
ATM[a] (Ataxia-telangiectasia)	<1%
Unknown	20%

[a]Affected gene.
Data from Martin AM, Weber BL: Genetic and hormonal risk factors in breast cancer. *J Natl Cancer Inst* 92:1126, 2000.

CHAPTER 18

Disorders of the Head and Neck

BASIC SCIENCE QUESTIONS

1. The relative risk of developing a squamous cell carcinoma of the head and neck for a patient who abuses both cigarettes and alcohol is
   A. 4-fold increased risk
   B. 10-fold increased risk
   C. 22-fold increased risk
   D. 35-fold increased risk

Answer: D

It should come as no surprise that abuse of tobacco and alcohol are the most common preventable risk factors associated with the development of head and neck cancers. This relationship is synergistic rather than additive. Smoking confers a 1.9-fold increased risk to males and a threefold increased risk to females for developing a head and neck carcinoma, when compared to nonsmokers. The risk increases as the number of years smoking and number of cigarettes smoked per day increases. Alcohol alone confers a 1.7-fold increased risk to males drinking one to two drinks per day, when compared to nondrinkers. This increased risk rises to greater than threefold for heavy drinkers. Individuals who both smoke (two packs per day) and drink (four units of alcohol per day) had an odds ratio of 35 for the development of a carcinoma when compared to controls. Users of smokeless tobacco have a four times increased risk of oral cavity carcinoma when compared to nonusers. (See Schwartz 9th ed., p 489.)

2. The primary lymphatic drainage of the midline of the upper lip is
   A. Submandibular nodes
   B. Submental nodes
   C. Intraparotid nodes
   D. Preauricular nodes

Answer: D

The midline of the upper lip drains initially to the preauricular nodes (Fig. 18-1). (See Schwartz 9th ed., p 491.)

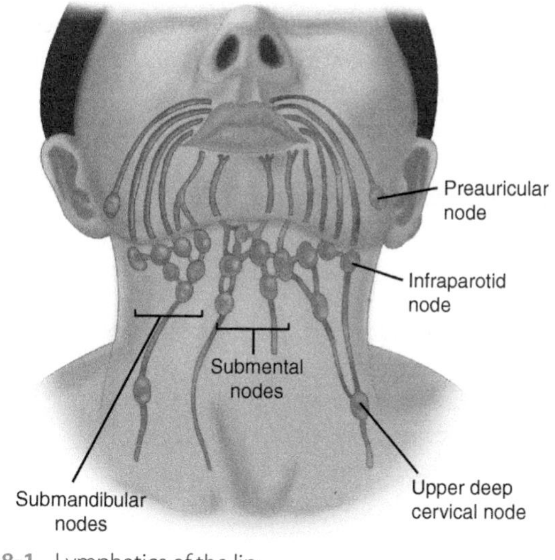

FIG. 18-1. Lymphatics of the lip.

3. Lymphatic drainage from the supraglottic larynx is primarily to
   A. The prelaryngeal (Delphian) node
   B. Paratracheal nodes
   C. Deep cervical nodes
   D. Superior jugular nodes

Answer: D

Lymphatic drainage of the larynx is distinct for each subsite. Two major groups of laryngeal lymphatic pathways exist: those that drain areas superior to the ventricle, and those that drain areas inferior to it. Supraglottic drainage routes pierce the thyrohyoid membrane with the superior laryngeal artery, vein, and nerve, and drain mainly to the subdigastric and superior jugular nodes. Those from the glottic and subglottic areas exit via the cricothyroid ligament and end in the prelaryngeal node (the Delphian node), the paratracheal nodes, and the deep cervical nodes along the inferior thyroid artery. Limited glottic cancers typically do not spread to regional lymphatics (1 to 4%). However, there is a high incidence of lymphatic spread from supraglottic (30 to 50%) and subglottic cancers (40%). (See Schwartz 9th ed., p 498, and Fig. 18-2.)

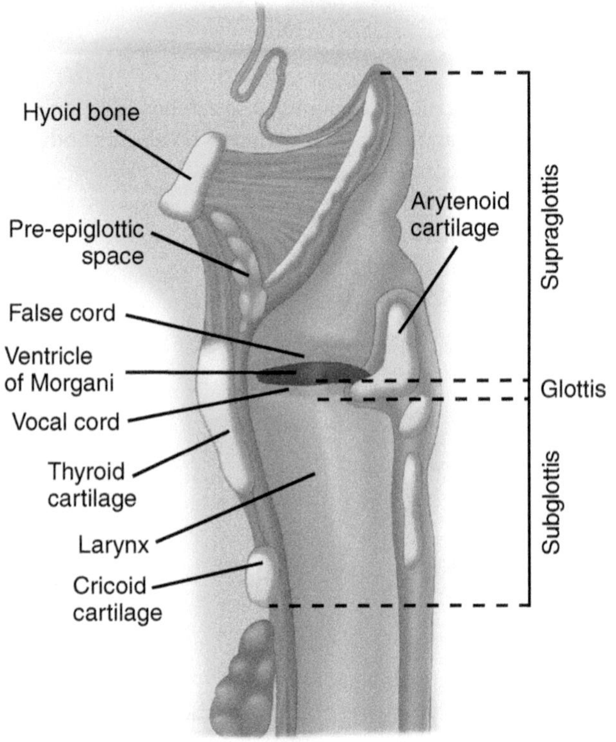

FIG. 18-2. Sagittal view of the larynx with the divisions of the supraglottis, glottis, and subglottis demonstrated.

4. Which of the following infections have been correlated with nasopharyngeal carcinoma?
   A. Herpes simplex virus (HSV)
   B. Epstein Barr virus (EBV)
   C. Cytomegalovirus (CMV)
   D. Human immunodeficiency virus (HIV)

Answer: B

Risk factors for nasopharyngeal carcinoma include area of habitation, ethnicity, and tobacco use. There is an increased incidence of nasopharyngeal cancer in southern China, Africa, Alaska, and in Greenland Eskimos. A strong correlation exists between nasopharyngeal cancer and the presence of EBV infection, such that EBV titers may be used as a means to follow a patient's response to treatment. (See Schwartz 9th ed., p 502.)

5. Level V lymph nodes in the neck are located
   A. In the submental area
   B. In the anterior triangle
   C. In the posterior triangle
   D. In the inferior jugular chain

Answer: C

The regional lymphatic drainage of the neck is divided into seven levels. These levels allow for a standardized format for radiologists, surgeons, pathologists, and radiation oncologists to communicate concerning specific sites within the neck (Fig. 18-3). (See Schwartz 9th ed., p 503.) The levels are defined as the following:

Level I—the submental and submandibular nodes

Level Ia—the submental nodes; medial to the anterior belly of the digastric muscle bilaterally, symphysis of mandible superiorly, and hyoid inferiorly

Level Ib—the submandibular nodes and gland; posterior to the anterior belly of digastric, anterior to the posterior belly of digastric, and inferior to the body of the mandible

Level II—upper jugular chain nodes

Level IIa—jugulodigastric nodes; deep to sternocleidomastoid (SCM) muscle, anterior to the posterior border of the muscle, posterior to the posterior aspect of the posterior belly of digastric, superior to the level of the hyoid, inferior to spinal accessory nerve (CN XI)

Level IIb—submuscular recess; superior to spinal accessory nerve to the level of the skull base

Level III—middle jugular chain nodes; inferior to the hyoid, superior to the level of the cricoid, deep to SCM muscle from posterior border of the muscle to the strap muscles medially

Level IV—lower jugular chain nodes; inferior to the level of the cricoid, superior to the clavicle, deep to SCM muscle from posterior border of the muscle to the strap muscles medially

Level V—posterior triangle nodes

Level Va—lateral to the posterior aspect of the SCM muscle, inferior and medial to splenius capitis and trapezius, superior to the spinal accessory nerve

Level Vb—lateral to the posterior aspect of SCM muscle, medial to trapezius, inferior to the spinal accessory nerve, superior to the clavicle

Level VI—anterior compartment nodes; inferior to the hyoid, superior to suprasternal notch, medial to the lateral extent of the strap muscles bilaterally

Level VII—paratracheal nodes; inferior to the suprasternal notch in the upper mediastinum

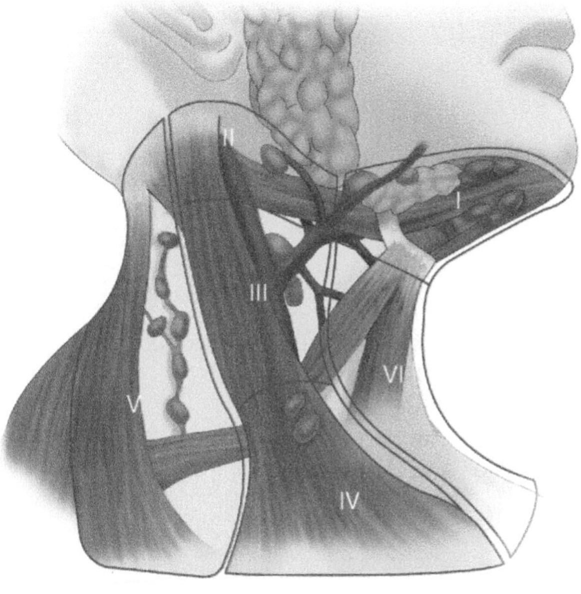

FIG. 18-3. Levels of the neck denoting lymph node bearing regions.

1. The most common causative organism in otitis externa is
   A. Staphylococcus aureus
   B. Pseudomonas aeruginosa
   C. Streptococcus pneumonia
   D. Herpes simplex type 1

Answer: B

Acute otitis externa is commonly known as *swimmer's ear*, because moisture that persists within the canal after swimming often initiates the process and leads to skin maceration and itching. Typically, the patient subsequently traumatizes the canal skin by scratching (i.e., with a cotton swab or fingernail), thus eroding the normally protective skin/cerumen barrier. Because the environment within the external ear canal is already dark, warm, and humid, it then becomes susceptible to rapid microbial proliferation and tissue cellulitis. The most common organism responsible is *Pseudomonas aeruginosa*, although other bacteria and fungi may also be implicated. Table 18-1 summarizes the microbiology of common otolaryngologic conditions. (See Schwartz 9th ed., p 476.)

Diabetic, elderly, and immunodeficient patients are susceptible to a condition called *malignant otitis externa*, a fulminant necrotizing infection of the otologic soft tissues combined with osteomyelitis of the temporal bone. In addition to the above findings, cranial neuropathies may be observed. The classic physical finding is granulation tissue along the floor of the EAC. Symptoms include persistent otalgia for longer than 1 month and purulent otorrhea for several weeks. These patients require aggressive medical therapy, including IV antibiotics covering *Pseudomonas*. (See Schwartz 9th ed., p 476.)

TABLE 18-1 Microbiology of common otolaryngologic infections

Condition	Microbiology
Otitis externa and malignant otitis externa	*Pseudomonas aeruginosa*, fungi (*Aspergillus* most common)
Acute otitis media	*Streptococcus pneumoniae*, *Haemophilus influenzae*, *Moraxella catarrhalis*
Chronic otitis media	Above bacteria, staphylococci, other streptococci; may be polymicrobial; exact role of bacteria unclear
Acute sinusitis	Viral upper respiratory infection, *S. pneumoniae*, *H. influenzae*, *M. catarrhalis*
Chronic sinusitis	Above bacteria, staphylococci, other streptococci; may be polymicrobial; exact role of bacteria unclear; may represent immune response to fungi
Pharyngitis	Viral, streptococci (usually pyogenes)

2. Bell's palsy is most commonly associated with
   A. Injury to the temporal bone
   B. Acute sinusitis
   C. Infection with Herpes simplex
   D. Infection with Herpes zoster

Answer: C

Bell's palsy, or idiopathic facial paralysis, may be considered within the spectrum of otologic disease given the facial nerve's course through the temporal bone. This entity is the most common etiology of facial nerve paralysis and is clinically distinct from that occurring as a complication of otitis media in that the otologic exam is normal. Historically, Bell's palsy was synonymous with 'idiopathic' facial paralysis. It is now accepted, however, that the majority of these cases represent a viral neuropathy caused by herpes simplex. Treatment includes oral steroids plus antiviral therapy (i.e., acyclovir). Complete recovery is the norm, but does not occur universally, and selected cases may benefit from surgical decompression of the nerve within its bony canal. Electrophysiologic testing has been used to identify those patients in whom surgery might be indicated. The procedure involves decompression of the nerve via exposure in the middle cranial fossa. Varicella zoster virus may also cause facial nerve paralysis when the virus reactivates from dormancy in the nerve. This condition, known as *Ramsay Hunt syndrome*, is characterized by severe otalgia followed by the eruption of vesicles of the external ear. Treatment is similar to Bell's palsy, but full recovery is only seen in approximately two thirds of cases. (See Schwartz 9th ed., p 478.)

3. Which of the following meet the diagnostic criteria for acute sinusitis?
   A. Symptoms of facial pressure, headache, cough
   B. Symptoms of nasal discharge and ear pain
   C. Opacification of sinus on plain radiograph
   D. Opacification of sinus on CT scan

Answer: A

Sinusitis is a clinical diagnosis based on patient signs and symptoms. The Task Force on Rhinosinusitis (sponsored by the American Academy of Otolaryngology–Head and Neck Surgery) has established criteria to define 'a history consistent with sinusitis' (Table 18-2). To qualify for the diagnosis, the patient must exhibit at least two major factors or one major and two minor factors. The classification of sinusitis as acute vs. subacute or chronic is primarily based on the time course over which those criteria have been met. If signs and symptoms are present for at least 7 to 10 days, but for less than 4 weeks, the process is designated acute sinusitis. Subacute sinusitis is present for 4 to 12 weeks and chronic sinusitis is diagnosed when the patient has had signs and symptoms for at least 12 weeks. In addition, the diagnosis of chronic sinusitis requires some objective demonstration of mucosal inflammatory disease. This may be accomplished by endoscopic examination or radiologically (i.e., CT scan). (See Schwartz 9th ed., p 478.)

TABLE 18-2 Factors associated with a history of rhinosinusitis[a]

Major Factors	Minor Factors
Facial congestion/fullness	Headache
Facial pain/pressure	Maxillary dental pain
Nasal drainage/discharge	Cough
Postnasal drip	Halitosis (bad breath)
Nasal obstruction/blockage	Fatigue
Hyposmia/anosmia (decreased or absent sense of smell)	Ear pain, pressure, or fullness
Fever (acute sinusitis only)	Fever
Purulence on nasal endoscopy (diagnostic by itself)	

[a]Either two major factors or one major and two minor factors are required. Purulence on nasal endoscopy is diagnostic. Fever is a major factor only in the acute stage.

4. Initial treatment of a patient with allergic rhinitis and chronic sinusitis includes
   A. Oral antibiotics for 3-6 weeks alone
   B. Oral antibiotics for 3-6 weeks + tapering oral steroids
   C. Antihistamines and nasal steroid spray alone
   D. Endoscopic debridement + oral antibiotics for 3-6 weeks

Answer: B

Medical management of chronic sinusitis includes a prolonged course of oral antibiotics for 3 to 6 weeks, nasal and/or oral steroids, and nasal irrigations with saline or antibiotic solutions. Underlying allergic disease may be managed with antihistamines and possible allergy immunotherapy. Although the role of these treatments in resolving chronic sinusitis remains questionable, they may be considered in patients with comorbid allergic rhinitis or as part of empiric management before consideration of surgery. (See Schwartz 9th ed., p 479, and Fig. 18-4.)

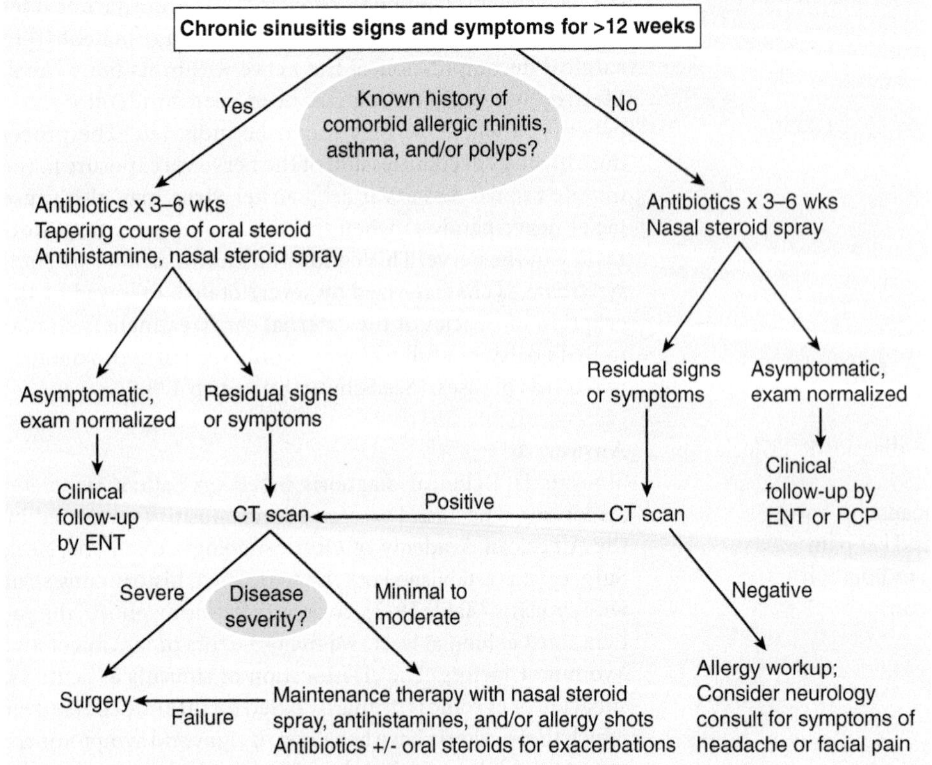

FIG. 18-4. Algorithm of chronic sinusitis signs and symptoms for 12 weeks. CT = computed tomography; ENT = ear, nose, and throat; PCP = primary care physician.

5. Timely antibiotic therapy is most likely to prevent which of the following complications of Streptococcal pharyngitis?
   A. Endocarditis
   B. Glomerulonephritis
   C. Scarlet fever
   D. Rheumatic fever

Answer: D

It is particularly important to identify group A beta-hemolytic streptococci in pediatric patients to initiate timely antibiotic therapy, given the risk of rheumatic fever, which may occur in up to 3% of cases if antibiotics are not used.

Complications of *S. pyogenes* pharyngitis may be systemic, including rheumatic fever, poststreptococcal glomerulonephritis, and scarlet fever. The incidence of glomerulonephritis is not influenced by antibiotic therapy. Scarlet fever results from production of erythrogenic toxins by streptococci. This causes a punctate rash, first appearing on the trunk and then spreading distally, sparing the palms and soles. The so-called *strawberry tongue* also is seen. (See Schwartz 9th ed., p 481.)

6. Which of the following is an indication for tonsillectomy in children?
   A. >5 infections
   B. >3 infections with strong family history
   C. >3 infections in one year
   D. >1 week missed from school in a year due to tonsillar infections

Answer: C

Tonsillectomy and adenoidectomy are indicated for chronic or recurrent acute infection and for obstructive hypertrophy. The American Academy of Otolaryngology–Head and Neck Surgery Clinical Indicators Compendium suggests tonsillectomy after three or more infections per year despite adequate medical therapy. Some feel that tonsillectomy is indicated in children who miss 2 or more weeks of school annually secondary to tonsil infections. (See Schwartz 9th ed., p 482.)

7. Which of the following is the most common therapy used in the treatment of recurrent respiratory papillomatosis?
   A. Laryngoscopy with excision and/or ablation of lesions
   B. Oral acyclovir
   C. Intralesional cidofovir injection
   D. Intralesional steroid injection

Answer: A

Recurrent respiratory papillomatosis (RRP) reflects involvement of human papillomavirus (HPV) within the mucosal epithelium of the upper aerodigestive tract. The larynx is the most frequently involved site, and subtypes 6 and 11 are the most often implicated. The disorder typically presents in early childhood, secondary to viral acquisition during vaginal delivery. Many cases resolve after puberty, but the disorder may progress into adulthood. Adult-onset RRP typically occurs in the third or fourth decade of life, is usually less severe, and is more likely to involve extralaryngeal sites of the upper aerodigestive tract. With laryngeal involvement, RRP is most likely to present with hoarseness, although airway compromise may be observed. The diagnosis can be established with office endoscopy. Currently, there is no 'cure' for RRP. Treatment involves operative microlaryngoscopy with excision or laser ablation, and the natural history is eventual recurrence. Therefore, surgery has an ongoing role for palliation of the disease. Multiple procedures are typically required over the patient's lifetime. Several medical therapies, including intralesional cidofovir injection and oral indole-3-carbinol, are being investigated to determine their abilities to retard recurrence. Additionally, the advent of HPV vaccines has suggested a role for this therapy in prevention of RRP. (See Schwartz 9th ed., p 482.)

8. What is the most likely diagnosis for the lesion seen in the photo below? (See Fig. 18-5.):

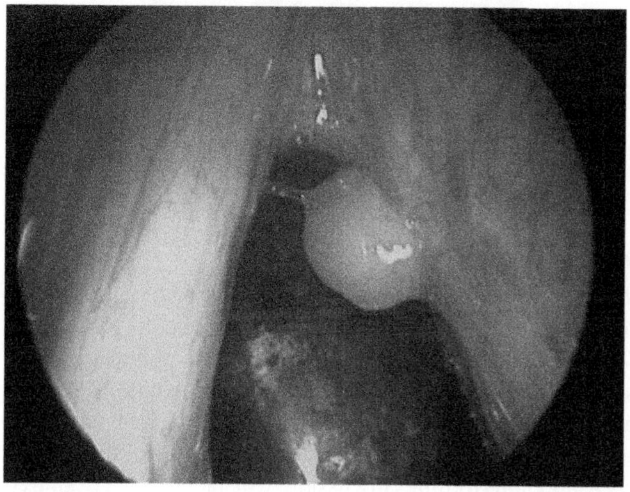

FIG. 18-5.

A. Laryngeal granuloma
B. Polypoid laryngitis
C. Vocal cord cyst
D. Leukoplakia of the vocal cord

Answer: A

Laryngeal granulomas typically occur in the posterior larynx on the arytenoid mucosa.

Edema in the superficial lamina propria of the vocal cord is known as *polypoid corditis, polypoid laryngitis, polypoid degeneration of the vocal cord*, or *Reinke's edema.*

Vocal cord cysts may occur under the laryngeal mucosa, particularly in regions containing mucous-secreting glands, such as the supraglottic larynx.

Leukoplakia of the vocal fold represents a white patch (which cannot be wiped off) on the mucosal surface, usually on the superior surface of the true vocal cord. (See Schwartz 9th ed., p 484.)

9. A classic Le Fort Type I fracture involves the
A. Forehead
B. Nose
C. Maxilla
D. Mandible

Answer: C

Le Fort I fractures occur transversely across the alveolus, above the level of the teeth apices. In a pure Le Fort I fracture, the palatal vault is mobile while the nasal pyramid and orbital rims are stable. The Le Fort II fracture extends through the nasofrontal buttress, medial wall of the orbit, across the infraorbital rim, and through the gomaticomaxillary articulation. The nasal dorsum, palate, and medial part of the infraorbital rim are mobile. The Le Fort III fracture is also known as *craniofacial disjunction*. The frontozygomaticomaxillary, frontomaxillary, and frontonasal suture lines are disrupted. The entire face is mobile from the cranium. It is convenient to conceptualize complex midface fractures according to these patterns (Fig. 18-6); however, in reality, fractures reflect a combination of these three types. Also, the fracture pattern may vary between the left and right sides of the midface. (See Schwartz 9th ed., p 487.)

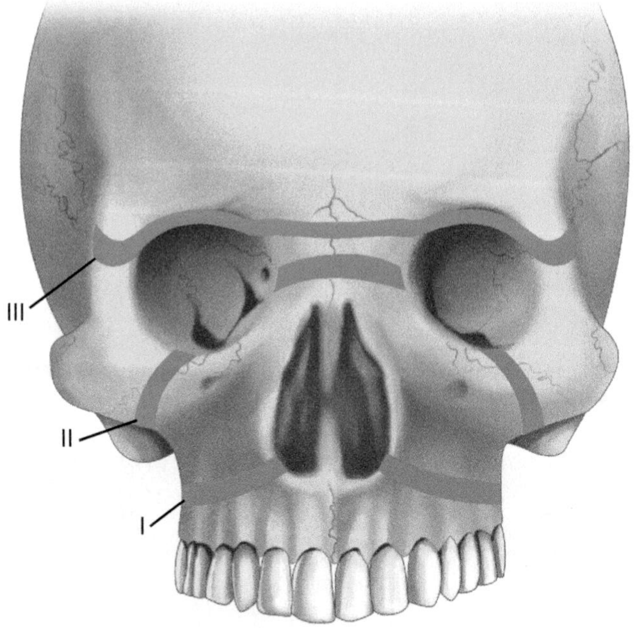

FIG. 18-6. Classic Le Fort fracture patterns.

10. Which of the following temporal bone fractures is most likely to have an associated facial nerve injury?
    A. Transverse
    B. Longitudinal
    C. Oblique
    D. Open

Answer: A

Temporal bone fractures are divided into two patterns (Fig. 18-7), longitudinal and transverse, based on the clinical picture and CT imaging. In practice, most fractures are oblique. By classical descriptions, longitudinal fractures constitute 80% and are associated with lateral skull trauma. Signs and symptoms include conductive hearing loss, ossicular injury, bloody otorrhea, and labyrinthine concussion. The facial nerve is injured in approximately 20% of cases. In contrast, the transverse pattern constitutes only 20% of temporal bone fractures and occurs secondary to fronto-occipital trauma. The facial nerve is injured in 50% of cases. These injuries frequently involve the otic capsule to cause sensorineural hearing loss and loss of vestibular function. Hemotympanum may be observed. A cerebrospinal fluid (CSF) leak must be suspected in temporal bone trauma. This resolves with conservative measures in most cases. The most significant consideration in the management of temporal bone injuries is the status of the facial nerve. Delayed or partial paralysis will almost always resolve with conservative management. However, immediate paralysis that does not recover within 1 week should be considered for nerve decompression. (See Schwartz 9th ed., p 488.)

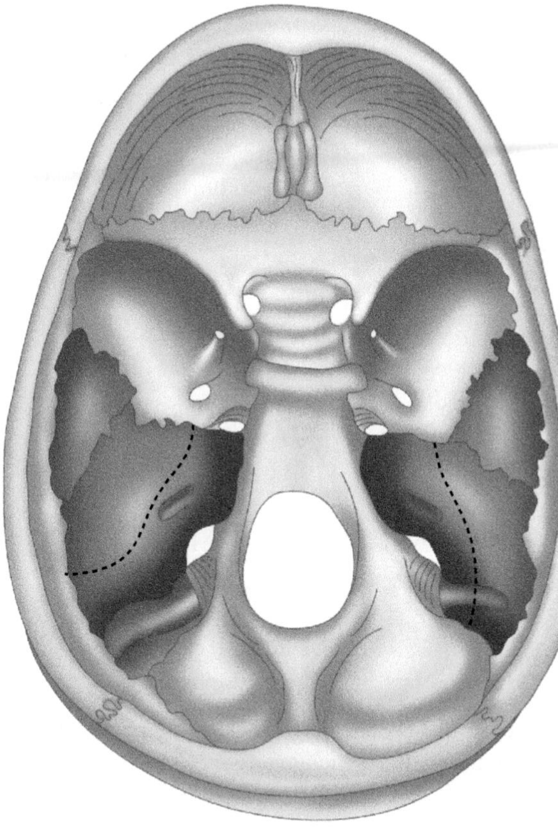

FIG. 18-7. View of cranial surface of skull base. Longitudinal (*left*) and transverse (*right*) temporal bone fractures.

11. The treatment of choice for a small squamous carcinoma of the lip is
    A. Surgical excision alone
    B. Radiotherapy alone
    C. Surgical excision + adjuvant chemotherapy
    D. Radiotherapy + adjuvant chemotherapy

Answer: A

The treatment for lip cancer is determined by the overall health of the patient, size of the primary lesion, and the presence of regional metastases. Small primary lesions may be treated with surgery or radiation with equal success and acceptable cosmetic results. However, surgical excision with histologic confirmation of tumor-free margins is the preferred treatment modality. Lymph node metastasis occurs in fewer than 10% of patients with lip cancer. The primary echelon of nodes at risk is in the submandibular and submental regions. In the presence of clinically evident neck metastasis, neck dissection is indicated. The overall 5-year cure rate of lip cancer approximates 90% and drops to 50% in the presence of neck metastases. Postoperative radiation is administered to the primary site and neck for patients with close or positive margins, lymph node metastases, or perineural invasion. (See Schwartz 9th ed., p 491.)

12. Primary repair is possible after excision of what percentage of the lip?
    A. <10%
    B. <25%
    C. <33%
    D. <50%

Answer: C

Resection with primary closure is possible with a defect of up to one third of the lip. When the resection includes one third to one half of the lip, rectangular excisions can be closed using Burow's triangles in combination with advancement flaps and releasing incisions in the mental crease. Borrowing tissue from the upper lip can repair other medium-size defects. For larger defects of up to 75%, the Karapandzic flap uses a sensate, neuromuscular flap that includes the remaining orbicularis oris muscle, conserving its blood supply from branches of the labial artery (Fig. 18-8). The lip-switch (Abbe-Estlander) flap or a stairstep advancement technique can be used to repair defects of either the upper or lower lip. (See Schwartz 9th ed., p 492.)

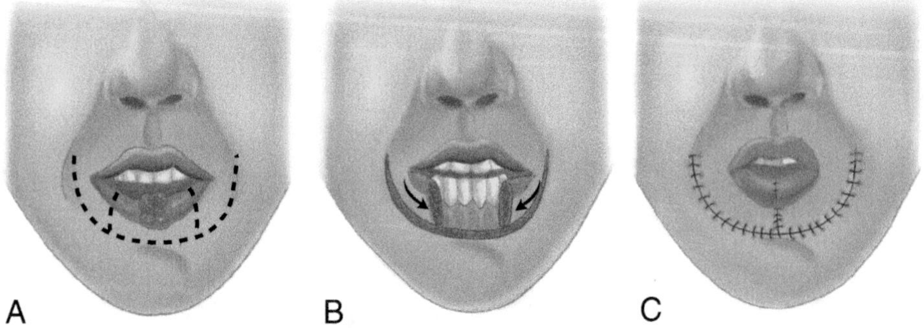

FIG. 18-8. A through C. Karapandzic labioplasty for lower lip carcinoma.

13. The most common location for Kaposi's sarcoma of the oropharynx is
    A. Tongue
    B. Palate
    C. Floor of the mouth
    D. Tonsil

Answer: B
Squamous cell carcinoma and minor salivary gland tumors are the most common malignancies of the palate. The latter include adenoid cystic carcinoma, mucoepidermoid carcinoma, adenocarcinoma, and polymorphous low-grade adenocarcinoma. Mucosal melanoma may occur on the palate and presents as a nonulcerated, pigmented plaque. Kaposi's sarcoma of the palate is the most common intraoral site for this tumor. (See Schwartz 9th ed., p 495.)

14. What is the probability that a neck mass measuring 2.5 cm in an adult is malignant?
    A. 20%
    B. 40%
    C. 60%
    D. 80%

Answer: D
In the adult population, a neck mass greater than 2 cm in diameter has a greater than 80% probability of being malignant. (See Schwartz 9th ed., p 503.)

15. Which of the following is removed in a modified radical neck dissection?
    A. Level I-V lymph nodes
    B. Internal jugular vein
    C. Sternocleidomastoid muscle
    D. All of the above

Answer: A
Traditionally, the gold standard for control of cervical metastasis has been the radical neck dissection (RND) first described by Crile. The classic RND removes levels I to V of the cervical lymphatics in addition to the SCM, internal jugular vein, and the spinal accessory nerve (CN XI). Any modification of the RND that preserves nonlymphatic structures (i.e., CN XI, SCM muscle, or internal jugular vein) is defined as a *modified radical neck dissection* (MRND). A neck dissection that preserves lymphatic compartments normally removed as part of a classic RND is termed a *selective neck dissection* (SND). (See Schwartz 9th ed., p 504.)

16. Which of the following is also removed when resecting a thyroglossal duct cyst?
    A. Anterior jugular vein
    B. External jugular vein
    C. Hyoid bone
    D. Superior laryngeal cartilage

Answer: C
Thyroglossal duct cysts represent the vestigial remainder of the tract of the descending thyroid gland from the foramen cecum, at the tongue base, into the lower anterior neck during fetal development. They present as a midline or paramedian cystic mass adjacent to the hyoid bone. After an upper respiratory infection, the cyst may enlarge or become infected. Surgical management of a thyroglossal duct cyst requires removal of the cyst, the tract, and the central portion of the hyoid bone (Sistrunk procedure), as well as a portion of the tongue base up to the foramen cecum. Before excision of a thyroglossal duct cyst, an imaging study such as ultrasound is performed to identify if normal thyroid tissue exists in the lower neck, and lab assay is performed to assess if the patient is euthyroid. (See Schwartz 9th ed., p 506.)

17. Branchial cleft anomalies involving the pyriform sinus arise from the
    A. 1st branchial cleft
    B. 2nd branchial cleft
    C. 3rd branchial cleft
    D. 4th branchial cleft

Answer: C

First branchial cleft cysts and sinuses are associated intimately with the EAC and the parotid gland. Second and third branchial cleft cysts are found along the anterior border of the SCM muscle and can produce drainage via a sinus tract to the neck skin. Secondary infections can occur, producing enlargement, cellulitis, and neck abscess that requires operative drainage. The removal of branchial cleft cysts and fistula requires removal of the fistula tract to the point of origin to decrease the risk of recurrence. The second branchial cleft remnant tract courses between the internal and external carotid arteries and proceeds into the tonsillar fossa. The third branchial cleft remnant courses posterior to the common carotid artery, ending in the pyriform sinus region. (See Schwartz 9th ed., p 506.)

18. The most common parotid tumor is
    A. Warthin's tumor
    B. Pleomorphic adenoma
    C. Mucoepidermoid carcinoma
    D. Adenoid cystic carcinoma

Answer: B

Eighty-five percent of salivary gland neoplasms arise within the parotid gland. The majority of these neoplasms are benign, with the most common histology being pleomorphic adenoma (benign mixed tumor). In contrast, approximately 50% of tumors arising in the submandibular and sublingual glands are malignant. Tumors arising from minor salivary gland tissue carry an even higher risk for malignancy (75%).

Benign and malignant tumors of the salivary glands are divided into epithelial, nonepithelial, and metastatic neoplasms. Benign epithelial tumors include pleomorphic adenoma (80%), monomorphic adenoma, Warthin's tumor, oncocytoma, or sebaceous neoplasm. Nonepithelial benign lesions include hemangioma, neural sheath tumor, and lipoma.

The most common malignant epithelial neoplasm of the salivary glands is mucoepidermoid carcinoma. The low-grade mucoepidermoid carcinoma is composed of largely mucin-secreting cells, whereas in high-grade tumors, the epidermoid cells predominate. High-grade mucoepidermoid carcinomas resemble nonkeratinizing squamous cell carcinoma in their histologic features and clinical behavior. Adenoid cystic carcinoma, which has a propensity for neural invasion, is the second most common malignancy in adults. Skip lesions along nerves are common and can lead to treatment failures because of the difficulty in treating the full extent of invasion. Adenoid cystic carcinomas have a high incidence of distant metastasis but display indolent growth. It is not uncommon for patients to experience lengthy survival despite the presence of disseminated disease. The most common malignancies in the pediatric population are mucoepidermoid carcinoma and acinic cell carcinoma. For minor salivary glands, the most common malignancies are adenoid cystic carcinoma, mucoepidermoid carcinoma, and low-grade polymorphous adenocarcinoma. Carcinoma expleomorphic adenoma is an aggressive malignancy that arises from a pre-existing benign mixed tumor. (See Schwartz 9th ed., p 507.)

CHAPTER 19

Chest Wall, Lung, Mediastinum, and Pleura

BASIC SCIENCE QUESTIONS

1. What is the approximate length of the trachea distal to the subglottic space?
   A. 7-8 cm
   B. 10-13 cm
   C. 14-16 cm
   D. 20-24 cm

Answer: B

The trachea is composed of cartilaginous and membranous portions, beginning with the cricoid cartilage, the first complete cartilaginous ring of the airway. The cricoid cartilage consists of an anterior arch and a posterior broad-based plate. Articulating with the posterior cricoid plate are the arytenoid cartilages. The vocal cords originate from the arytenoid cartilages and then attach to the thyroid cartilage. The subglottic space, the narrowest part of the trachea with an internal diameter of approximately 2 cm, begins at the inferior surface of the vocal cords and extends to the first tracheal ring. The remainder of the distal trachea is 10.0 to 13.0 cm long, consists of 18 to 22 rings, and has an internal diameter of 2.3 cm. (See Schwartz 9th ed., p 514.)

2. The lymphatic drainage from the pulmonary (N1) nodes of the lung terminates in the lymphatic sump of Borrie which, on the right side, is located
   A. Around the bronchus intermedius
   B. In the intralobar fissure
   C. In the posterior mediastinum
   D. At the level of the carina

Answer: A

Lymph nodes that drain the lungs are divided into two groups according to the tumor, node, and metastasis (TNM) staging system for lung cancer: the pulmonary lymph nodes, N1; and the mediastinal nodes, N2 (Fig. 19-1).

The N1 lymph nodes consist of the following: (a) intrapulmonary or segmental nodes that lie at points of division of segmental bronchi or in the bifurcations of the pulmonary artery; (b) lobar nodes that lie along the upper, middle, and lower lobe bronchi; (c) interlobar nodes that are located in the angles formed by the bifurcation of the main bronchi into the lobar bronchi; and (d) hilar nodes that are located along the main bronchi. The interlobar lymph nodes lie in the depths of the interlobar fissure on each side and constitute a lymphatic sump for each lung, referred to as the *lymphatic sump of Borrie*; all of the pulmonary lobes of the corresponding lung drain into this group of nodes (Fig. 19-2). On the right side, the nodes of the lymphatic sump lie around the bronchus intermedius (bounded above by the right upper lobe bronchus and below by the middle lobe and superior segmental bronchi). On the left side, the lymphatic sump is confined to the interlobar fissure, with the lymph nodes in the angle between the lingular and lower lobe bronchi and in apposition to the pulmonary artery branches. (See Schwartz 9th ed., p 520.)

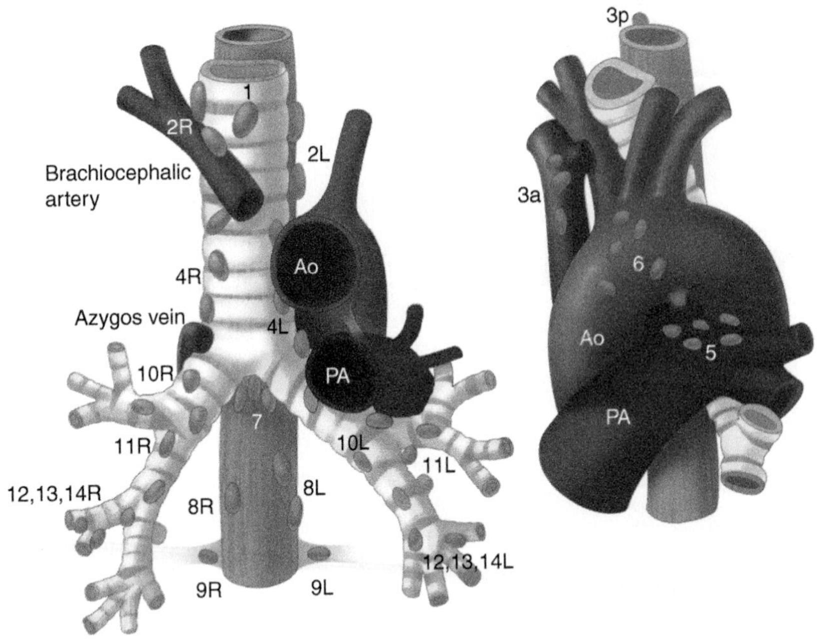

FIG. 19-1. The location of regional lymph node stations for lung cancer staging. Station, Description: 1, highest mediastinal lymph nodes; 2, upper paratracheal nodes; 3, prevascular, precarinal, and retrotracheal nodes; 4, lower paratracheal nodes; 5, aorto-pulmonary nodes; 6, pre-aortic nodes; 7, subcarnal nodes; 8, paraesophageal nodes; 9, pulmonary ligament nodes; 10, tracheobronchial nodes; 11, interlobular nodes; 12, lobar bronchial nodes; 13, segmental nodes; 14, subsegmental nodes. Note: Stations 12, 13, and 14 are not shown in their entirety. (Reproduced with permission from Ferguson, MK: *Thoracic Surgery Atlas*. W.B. Saunders, Inc., Philadelphia, PA, 2007. Copyright © Elsevier.)

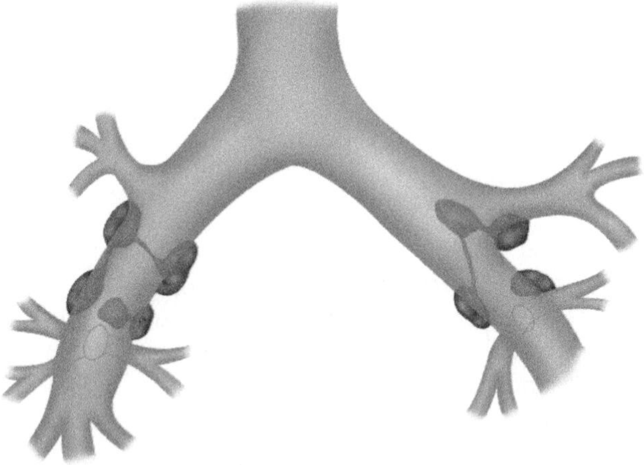

FIG. 19-2. The lymphatic sump of Borrie includes the groups of lymph nodes that receive lymphatic drainage from all pulmonary lobes of the corresponding lung.

3. Which of the following genes is associated with desmoid tumors of the chest wall?
   A. p53
   B. BRAC-2
   C. Adenomatous polyposis coli (APC)
   D. HER2

Answer: C
Desmoid tumors have recently been shown to possess alterations in the adenomatous polyposis coli/β-catenin pathway, and cyclin D1 dysregulation is thought to play a significant role in their pathogenesis. Associations with other diseases and conditions are well documented, especially those with similar alterations in the adenomatous polyposis coli pathway, such as familial adenomatous polyposis (Gardner's syndrome). (See Schwartz 9th ed., p 565.)

4. How many segments are in the left lung?
   A. 7
   B. 8
   C. 9
   D. 10

Answer: C
There are 9 segments in the left lung and 10 segments in the right lung. (See Schwartz 9th ed., p 520, and Fig. 19-3).

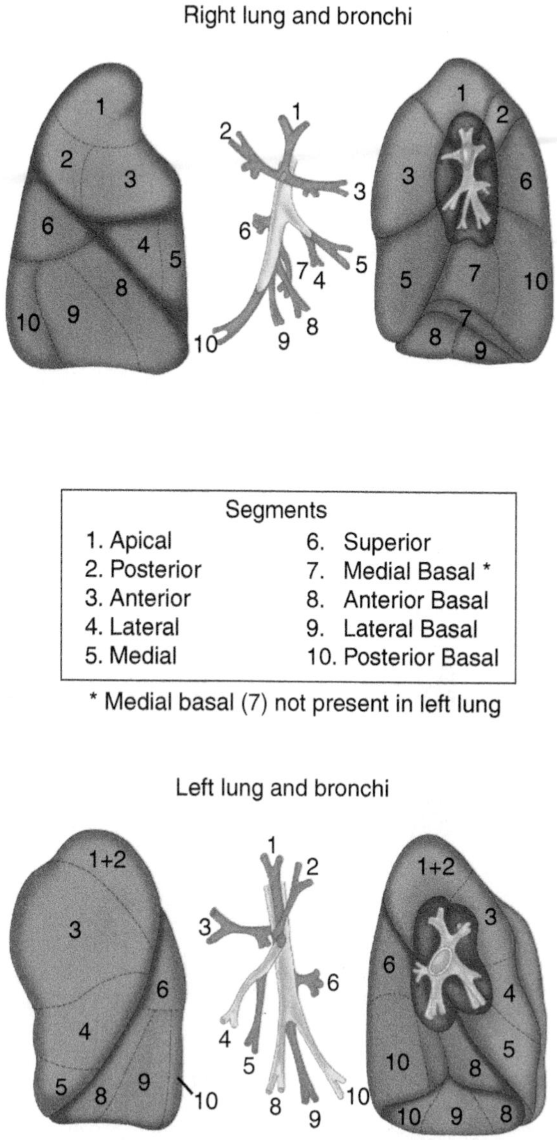
Right lung and bronchi
Segments
1. Apical
2. Posterior
3. Anterior
4. Lateral
5. Medial
6. Superior
7. Medial Basal *
8. Anterior Basal
9. Lateral Basal
10. Posterior Basal
* Medial basal (7) not present in left lung
Left lung and bronchi

FIG. 19-3. Segmental anatomy of the lungs and bronchi.

CLINICAL QUESTIONS

1. The most appropriate treatment for clinically significant tracheal stenosis is
   A. Endoscopic balloon dilation
   B. Endoscopic placement of a wire stent
   C. Laser ablation
   D. Resection and primary anastomosis

Answer: D

The treatment of tracheal stenosis is resection and primary anastomosis. In nearly all postintubation injuries the injury is transmural, and significant portions of the cartilaginous structural support are destroyed (Fig. 19-4). Measures such as laser ablation are temporizing. In the early phase of evaluating patients, dilation using a rigid bronchoscope is useful to gain immediate relief of dyspnea and to allow full assessment of the lesion. It is important to carefully document the length and position of the stenosis as well as the location in relation to the vocal cords. Rarely, if ever, is a tracheostomy necessary. For patients who are not operative candidates due to associated comorbidities, internal stents, typically silicone T tubes, are useful. Wire mesh stents should not be used, given their known propensity to erode through the wall of the airway. The use of balloon dilation and tracheoplasty also has been described, although their efficacy is marginal. Efforts focused on tissue engineering may provide suitable material for tracheal replacement in long-segment tracheal stenosis in the future.

Most intubation injuries are located in the upper third of the trachea, so tracheal resection usually is done through a collar incision. Resection typically involves 2 to 4 cm of trachea for benign stenosis. However, a primary anastomosis can still be performed without undue tension, even if up to one half of the trachea needs to be resected. When resection for a postintubation injury is performed, it is critical to fully resect all inflamed and scarred tissue. Tracheostomies and stents are not required postoperatively, and the patient often is extubated in the operating room or shortly thereafter. (See Schwartz 9th ed., pp 516-517.)

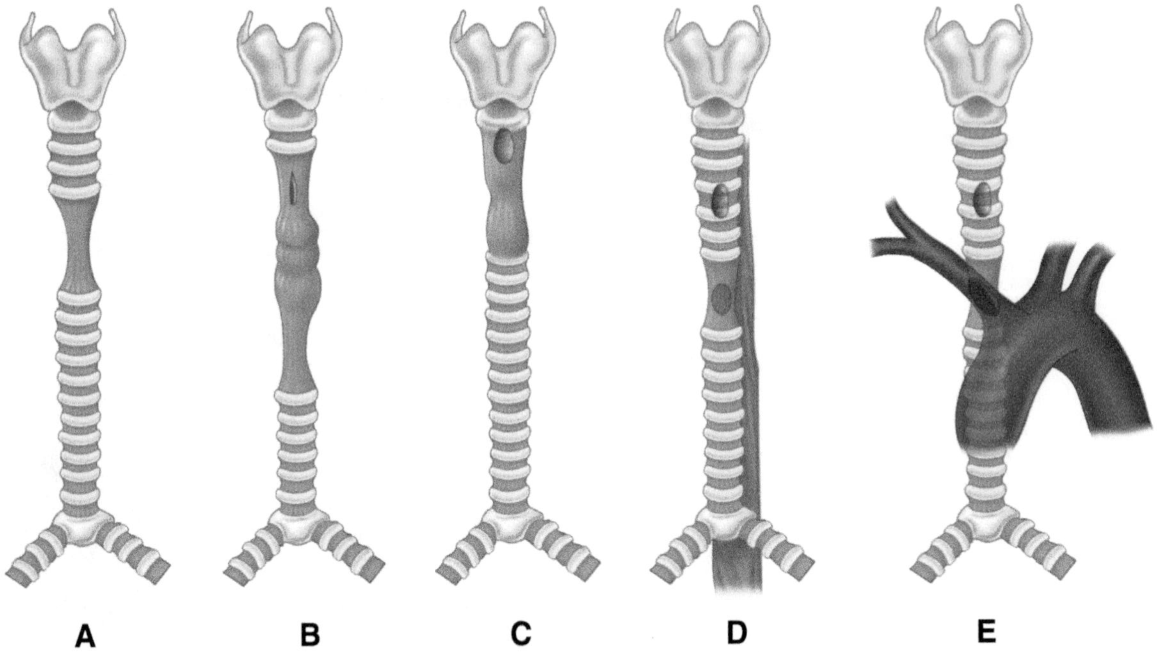

FIG. 19-4. Diagram of the principal postintubation lesions. A. A circumferential lesion at the cuff site after the use of an endotracheal tube. B. Potential lesions after the use of tracheostomy tubes. Anterolateral stenosis can be seen at the stomal level. Circumferential stenosis can be seen at the cuff level (lower than with an endotracheal tube). The segment in between is often inflamed and malacotic. C. Damage to the subglottic larynx. D. Tracheoesophageal fistula occurring at the level of the tracheostomy cuff. Circumferential damage is usual at this level. E. Tracheoinnominate artery fistula. (Adapted with permission from Grillo HC: Surgical treatment of postintubation tracheal injuries. *J Thorac Cardiovasc Surg* 8:860, 1979.)

2. Which of the following is an indication for drainage of a peri-pneumonic effusion?
   A. pH <7.20
   B. Glucose <60 mg/dL
   C. LDH <100 units/L
   D. WBC >10,000/dl

Answer: A

The finding of grossly purulent, foul-smelling pleural fluid makes the diagnosis of empyema obvious on visual examination at the bedside. In the early stage, small to moderate turbid pleural effusions in the setting of a pneumonic process may require further pleural fluid analysis. Close clinical follow-up also is imperative to determine if progression to empyema is occurring. A deteriorating clinical course or a pleural pH of <7.20 and a glucose level of <40 mg/dL indicates the need to drain the fluid.

As organisms enter the pleural space, an influx of polymorphonuclear cells occurs, with a subsequent release of inflammatory mediators and toxic oxygen radicals. In attempting to control the invading organisms, these mechanisms lead to variable degrees of endothelial injury and capillary instability. An influx of fluid into the pleural space then occurs, followed by a process that overwhelms the normal exit avenues of the pleural lymphatic network. This early effusion is watery and free flowing in the pleural cavity. Thoracentesis at this stage yields fluid with a pH typically >7.3, a glucose level of >60 mg/dL, and a low LDH level (<500 units/L). If relatively thin, purulent pleural fluid is found early in the setting of a pneumonic process, the fluid often can be completely drained with simple large-bore thoracentesis. If complete lung expansion is obtained and the pneumonic process is responding to antibiotics, no further drainage may be necessary. A finding of pleural fluid with a pH <7.2 and with a low glucose level means that a more aggressive approach to drainage should be pursued. (See Schwartz 9th ed., pp 579-580.)

3. A 55-year-old nonsmoker is noted to have a solitary pulmonary nodule on plain radiograph. Based on the CT finding in Fig. 19-5, what is the most likely diagnosis for this patient?

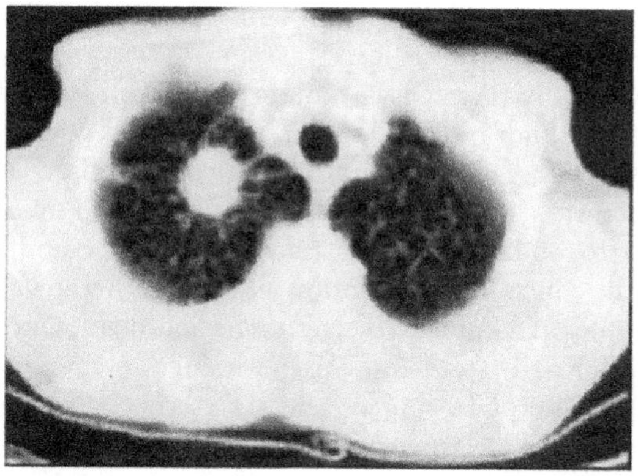

FIG. 19-5.

A. Benign neoplasm
B. Malignant neoplasm
C. Granulomatous nodule
D. Hamartoma

Answer: B

This CT shows a solitary pulmonary nodule with a corona radiata sign. Irregular, lobulated, or speculated edges strongly suggest malignancy. The corona radiata sign (consisting of fine linear strands extending 4 to 5 mm outward and appearing spiculated on radiographs) is highly cancer specific. (See Schwartz 9th ed., p 527.)

4. Lung cancer in a patient who has never smoked is most likely to be
A. Large cell carcinoma
B. Adenocarcinoma
C. Squamous cell carcinoma
D. Bronchoalveolar carcinoma

Answer: B

Approximately 25% of all lung cancers worldwide and 53% of cancers in women are not related to smoking, and the majority of these (62%) are adenocarcinomas. (See Schwartz 9th ed., p 529.)

5. A patient with a primary tracheal tumor is found on bronchoscopy to have a sessile tumor with extensive submucosal infiltration. The most likely diagnosis is
A. Adenocarcinoma
B. Squamous cell carcinoma
C. Adenoid cystic carcinoma
D. Small cell carcinoma

Answer: C

Squamous cell carcinomas of the trachea often present with regional lymph node metastases and are frequently not resectable at the time of presentation. Their biologic behavior is similar to that of squamous cell carcinomas of the lung. Adenoid cystic carcinomas, which are a type of salivary gland tumor, are generally slow growing, spread submucosally, and tend to infiltrate along nerve sheaths and within the tracheal wall. Spread to regional lymph nodes can occur. Although indolent in nature, adenoid cystic carcinomas are malignant and can spread to the lungs and bones. Squamous cell carcinomas and adenoid cystic carcinomas represent approximately 65% of all tracheal neoplasms.

The remaining 35% is composed of small cell carcinomas, mucoepidermoid carcinomas, adenocarcinomas, lymphomas, and others. (See Schwartz 9th ed., p 519.)

6. The treatment of choice for a patient with a Pancoast tumor, no metastases, and good pulmonary function is
   A. Surgical resection followed by radiation therapy
   B. Surgical resection followed by chemotherapy and radiotherapy
   C. Induction chemotherapy followed by surgical resection
   D. Induction chemotherapy and radiotherapy followed by surgical resection

Answer: D

Carcinoma arising in the extreme apex of the chest with associated arm and shoulder pain, atrophy of the muscles of the hand, and Horner syndrome was first described by Henry Pancoast in 1932. Any tumor of the superior sulcus, including tumors without evidence of involvement of the neurovascular bundle, is now commonly known as *Pancoast's tumor*. The designation should be reserved for those tumors involving the parietal pleura or deeper structures overlying the first rib. Chest wall involvement at or below the second rib should not be considered Pancoast's tumor. Treatment involves a multidisciplinary approach. Goals of operative treatment obviously include curative resection; however, due to the location of the tumor and involvement of the neurovascular bundle that supplies the ipsilateral extremity, preserving postoperative function of the extremity also is critical.

Historically, Pancoast's tumors have been difficult to treat, with high rates of local recurrence and poor 5-year survival with radiation and/or surgical resection. Tumor invasion into surrounding structures prompted investigations into modalities such as induction radiation and, more recently, concomitant radiation and chemotherapy, to improve rates of complete resection. The Southwest Oncology Group formally studied the use of induction chemoradiotherapy followed by surgery, and long-term results are now available. The treatment regimen was well tolerated, with 95% of patients completing induction treatment. Complete resection was achieved in 76%. Five-year survival was 44% overall and 54% when complete resection was achieved. Disease progression with this regimen was predominantly at distant sites, with the brain being the most common. A treatment algorithm for Pancoast's tumors is presented in Fig. 19-6. (See Schwartz 9th ed., pp 544-545.)

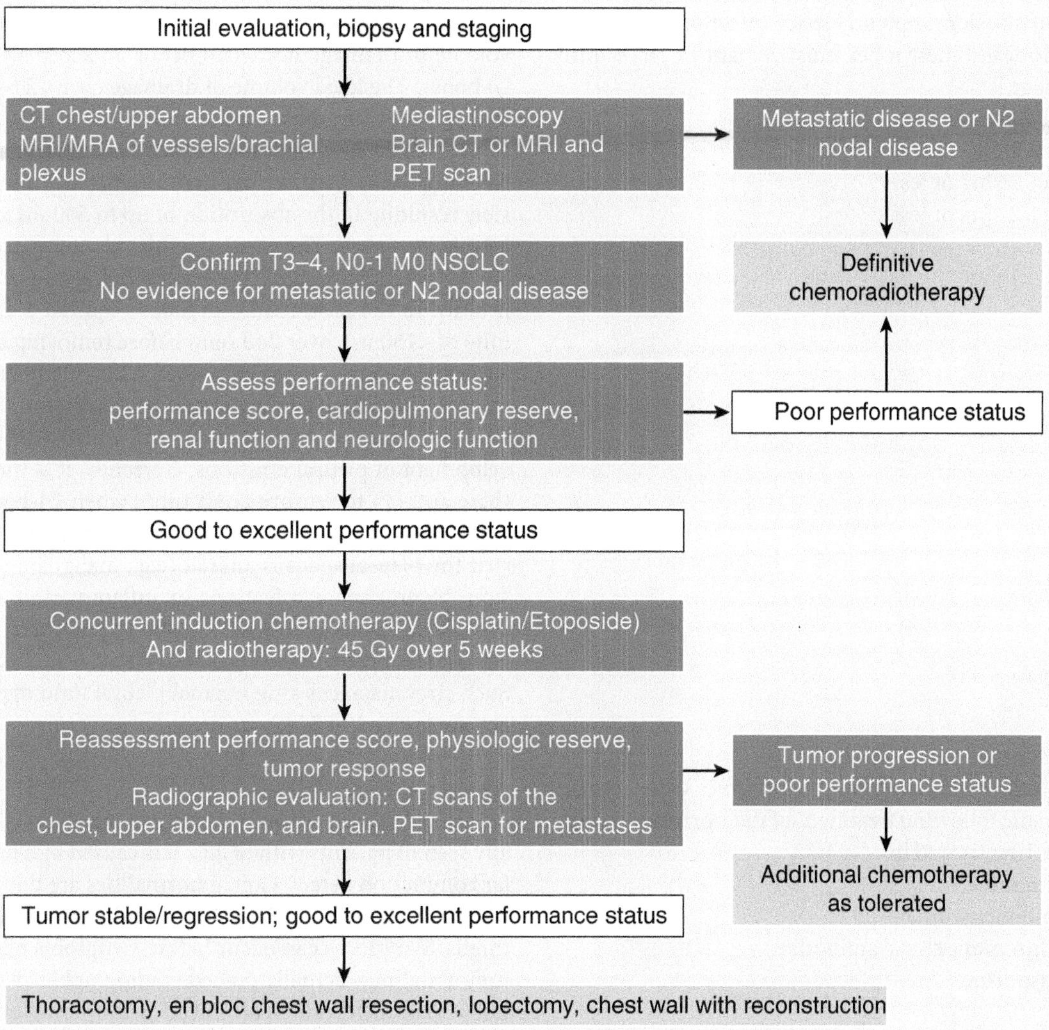

FIG. 19-6. Treatment algorithm for Pancoast's tumors. CT = computed tomography; MRA = magnetic resonance angiography; MRI = magnetic resonance imaging; NSCLC = non–small cell lung cancer; PET = positron emission tomography.

7. When compared to open thoracotomy, VATS (video-assisted thoracic surgery) has been shown to result in
   A. Reduced mortality
   B. Slower recovery of respiratory function
   C. Faster return to work
   D. Decreased ability to tolerate chemotherapy

Answer: C

Thoracic surgical approaches have changed over recent years with advancements in minimally invasive approaches. A surgeon trained in advanced minimally invasive techniques can now perform sympathectomy, segmental lung resections, lobectomies, and mediastinal resections through multiple thoracoscopic ports and small access incisions without the need for a substantial, rib-spreading incision. Although there has not been a documented change in mortality using these approaches, subjective measures of quality of life after video-assisted thoracic surgery (VATS), such as pain level and perceived functional recovery, consistently and reproducibly favor VATS over thoracotomy. Objective measures such as functional status as measured by 6-minute walk, return to work, and ability to tolerate chemotherapy also favor VATS over thoracotomy. Finally, recovery of respiratory function occurs earlier in patients undergoing VATS. These findings are pronounced in patients with chronic obstructive pulmonary disease (COPD) and in the elderly, populations whose quality of life can be dramatically impacted by changes in their respiratory symptoms and function, thoracic pain, and physical performance. (See Schwartz 9th ed., p 522.)

8. If the pleural space is altered by disease processes such as malignant effusion or pleural space infections or following pleurodesis, chest tubes must remain in place until the drainage is
   A. 50 ml/24 hrs or less
   B. 150 ml/24 hrs or less
   C. 400 ml/24 hrs or less
   D. 750 ml/24 hrs or less

Answer: B

The tube is removed when the air leak is resolved and when the volume of drainage decreases below an acceptable level over 24 hours. The ideal volume of drainage over a 24-hour period that predicts safe chest tube removal is unknown. The ability of the pleural lymphatics to absorb fluid is substantial. It can be as high as 0.40 mL/kg per hour in a healthy individual, possibly resulting in the absorption of up to 500 mL of fluid over a 24-hour period. The capacity of the pleural space to manage and absorb fluid is high if the pleural lining and lymphatics are healthy. In the past, many surgeons required a drainage volume of <150 mL over 24 hours before removing a chest tube. Recently, however, it has been shown that pleural tubes can be removed after VATS lobectomy or thoracotomy with 24-hour drainage volumes as high as 400 mL without subsequent development of pleural effusions. Currently, it is the practice of these authors to remove chest tubes when 24-hour output is ≤400 mL after lobectomy or lesser pulmonary resections.

If the pleural space is altered (e.g., malignant pleural effusion, pleural space infections or inflammation, or pleurodesis), strict adherence to a volume requirement before tube removal is appropriate (typically 100 to 150 mL over 24 hours). Such circumstances alter normal pleural fluid dynamics. (See Schwartz 9th ed., p 524.)

9. Patients with Lambert-Eaton syndrome who remain symptomatic following treatment of their primary malignancy are best treated by
   A. Neostigmine
   B. Guanidine hydrochloride
   C. Anti IgA monoclonal antibodies
   D. Cyclosporine

Answer: B

Lambert-Eaton syndrome is a myasthenia-like syndrome usually seen in patients with SCLC. It is caused by a neuromuscular conduction defect. Gait abnormalities are due to proximal muscle weakness and fatigability, and particularly affect the thighs. Symptoms can occur before symptoms of the primary tumor and may actually precede radiographic evidence of the tumor. The syndrome is produced by immunoglobulin G antibodies targeting voltage-gated calcium channels, which function in the release of acetylcholine from presynaptic sites at the motor end plate. Therapy is directed at the primary tumor with resection, radiation, and/or chemotherapy. Many patients have dramatic improvement after resection or successful medical therapy. For patients with refractory symptoms, treatment consists of administration of guanidine hydrochloride, immunosuppressive agents such as prednisone and azathioprine, and occasionally plasma exchange. Unlike in myasthenia gravis patients, neostigmine is usually ineffective. (See Schwartz 9th ed., p 536.)

10. Which of the following chest wall sarcomas is most likely to respond to preoperative chemotherapy?
    A. Fibrosarcoma
    B. Malignant fibrous histiocytoma
    C. Synovial sarcoma
    D. Primitive neuroectodermal tumor

Answer: D

Sarcomas can be divided into two broad groups according to potential responsiveness to chemotherapy (Table 19-1). Preoperative (neoadjuvant) chemotherapy offers the ability to (a) assess tumor chemosensitivity by the degree of tumor size reduction and microscopic necrosis, (b) determine to which chemotherapeutic agents the tumor is sensitive, and (c) lessen the extent of surgical resection by reducing tumor size. Patients whose tumors are responsive to preoperative chemotherapy (as judged by the reduction in the size of the primary tumor and/or by the degree of necrosis seen histologically after resection) have a much better prognosis than those whose tumors show a poor response. (See Schwartz 9th ed., p 565.)

TABLE 19-1 Classification of sarcomas by therapeutic response

Tumor Type	Chemotherapy Sensitivity
Osteosarcoma	+
Rhabdomyosarcoma	+
Primitive neuroectodermal tumor	+
Ewing's sarcoma	+
Malignant fibrous histiocytoma	±
Fibrosarcoma	±
Liposarcoma	±
Synovial sarcoma	±

11. What percent of the trachea can be safely resected?
    A. 20%
    B. 30%
    C. 40%
    D. 50%

Answer: D

The length limit of tracheal resection is roughly 50% of the trachea. To prevent tension on the anastomosis postoperatively, specialized maneuvers are necessary, such as anterolateral tracheal mobilization, suturing of the chin to the sternum with the head flexed forward for 7 days, laryngeal release, and right hilar release. For most tracheal resections (which involve much less than 50% of the airway), anterolateral tracheal mobilization and suturing of the chin to the sternum for 7 days are done routinely. Use of laryngeal and hilar release is determined at the time of surgery, based on the surgeon's judgment of the degree of tension present. (See Schwartz 9th ed., p 519.)

12. Which of the following mediastinal masses is most likely to be found in the anterior mediastinum?
    A. Pleuropericardial cyst
    B. Ganglioneuroma
    C. Pheochromocytoma
    D. Germ cell tumor

Answer: D

(See Schwartz 9th ed., p 570, and Table 19-2.)

TABLE 19-2 Usual location of the common primary tumors and cysts of the mediastinum

Anterior Compartment	Visceral Compartment	Paravertebral Sulci
Thymoma	Enterogenous cyst	Neurilemoma-schwannoma
Germ cell tumor	Lymphoma	Neurofibroma
Lymphoma	Pleuropericardial cyst	Malignant schwannoma
Lymphangioma	Mediastinal granuloma	Ganglioneuroma
Hemangioma	Lymphoid hamartoma	Ganglioneuroblastoma
Lipoma	Mesothelial cyst	Neuroblastoma
Fibroma	Neuroenteric cyst	Paraganglioma
Fibrosarcoma	Paraganglioma	Pheochromocytoma
Thymic cyst	Pheochromocytoma	Fibrosarcoma
Parathyroid adenoma	Thoracic duct cyst	Lymphoma

Source: Reproduced with permission from Shields TW: The mediastinum and its compartments, in Shields TW (ed): *Mediastinal Surgery*. Philadelphia: Lea & Febiger, 1991, p 5.

13. The primary treatment for oat cell carcinoma of the lung is
    A. Surgery followed by chemotherapy
    B. Chemotherapy alone
    C. Chemotherapy and radiation therapy
    D. Immunotherapy

Answer: C

Small cell lung carcinoma (SCLC) accounts for approximately 20% of primary lung cancers and generally is not treated surgically. These aggressive neoplasms have early, widespread metastases. Histologically, they can be difficult to distinguish from lymphoproliferative lesions and atypical carcinoid tumors. Therefore, a definitive diagnosis must be established with adequate tissue samples. Three groups of SCLC are recognized: pure small cell carcinoma (sometimes referred to as *oat cell carcinoma*), small cell carcinoma with a large cell component, and combined (mixed) tumors. Unlike with NSCLC, the clinical stage of SCLC is defined broadly by the presence of either local "limited" or distant "disseminated" disease. SCLC presenting with bulky locoregional disease but no evidence for distant metastatic disease is termed *limited* SCLC. Most often, the primary tumor is large and associated with bulky mediastinal adenopathy, which may lead to obstruction of the superior vena cava. SCLC falling into the other clinical stage, termed *disseminated*, usually presents with metastatic disease throughout the patient's body. Regardless of the stage of presentation, treatment is primarily chemotherapy and radiation. Surgery is appropriate for the rare patient with an incidentally discovered peripheral nodule that is found to be SCLC. If a stage I SCLC is identified after resection, postoperative chemotherapy usually is given. (See Schwartz 9th ed., pp 548-549.)

14. A 65-year-old who has smoked 2 packs a day for 45 years is found to have a 2-cm solitary pulmonary nodule 1 cm from the surface of the superior segment of the right lower lobe. The best initial diagnostic procedure is
    A. Observation with biopsy if this increases in size over 3-6 months
    B. Bronchoscopy
    C. Fine-needle aspiration
    D. Open thoracotomy for excisional biopsy

Answer: C

The surgeon must have an evidence-based algorithm for approaching the diagnosis and treatment of a pulmonary nodule. Guidelines have been developed based on a systematic literature review and consensus of clinical experts in the field (Fig. 19-7). Only through biopsy can a pulmonary nodule be definitively diagnosed. Bronchoscopy has a 20 to 80% sensitivity for detecting a neoplastic process within a solitary pulmonary nodule, depending on the nodule size, its proximity to the bronchial tree, and the prevalence of cancer in the population being sampled. Transthoracic fine-needle aspiration (FNA) biopsy can accurately identify the status of peripheral pulmonary lesions in up to 95% of patients; the false-negative rate ranges from 3 to 29%. Complications may occur at a relatively high rate (e.g., a 30% rate of pneumothorax). VATS often is used for excising and diagnosing indeterminate pulmonary nodules. Lesions most suitable for VATS are those that are located in the outer one third of the lung and those that are <3 cm in diameter. Certain principles must be followed when excising potentially malignant lesions via VATS. The nodule must not be directly manipulated with instruments, the visceral pleura overlying the nodule must not be violated, and the excised nodule must be extracted from the chest within a bag to prevent seeding of the chest wall. Some groups advocate proceeding directly to VATS in the workup of a solitary pulmonary nodule in appropriate clinical circumstances, citing superior diagnostic accuracy and low surgical risks. (See Schwartz 9th ed., pp 527-528.)

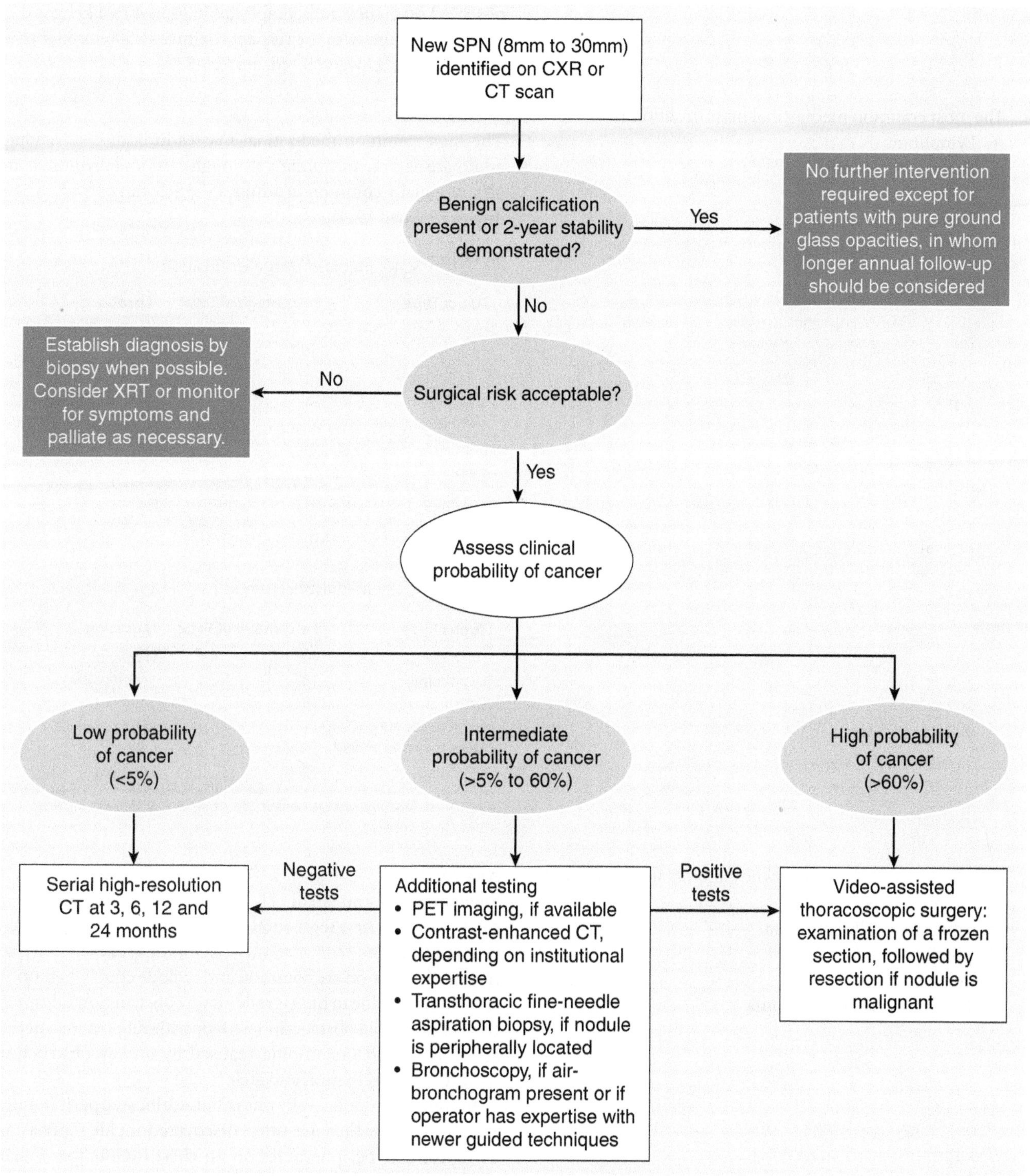

FIG. 19-7. Recommended management algorithm for patients with solitary pulmonary nodules (SPNs) measuring 8 mm to 30 mm in diameter. CT = computed tomography; CXR = chest radiograph; PET = positron emission tomography; XRT = radiotherapy. (Adapted from Ost D, Fein AM, Feinsilver SH. Clinical practice: the solitary pulmonary nodule. *N Engl J Med* 2003; 348:2535–2542.)

15. What is the probability that a solitary pulmonary nodule is malignant in a patient whose smoke exposure is unknown?
    A. 0-20%
    B. 20-40%
    C. 40-60%
    D. >60%

Answer: B

The differential diagnosis of a solitary pulmonary nodule can be distilled down to a differentiation between malignancy and other numerous benign conditions. Ideally, diagnostic approaches would provide a clear distinction between the two, so that definitive surgical resection could be reserved for the malignant nodule and resection avoided when the nodule is benign. In unselected patient populations, a new solitary pulmonary nodule observed on a chest radiograph has a 20 to 40% likelihood of being malignant, with the risk approximately 50% or higher in smokers. (See Schwartz 9th ed., pp 526-527.)

16. The most common mediastinal mass in children is
    A. Lymphoma
    B. Neurogenic tumor
    C. Congenital cyst
    D. Germ cell tumor

Answer: B

The most common mediastinal masses in both children and adults are neurogenic tumors, although cysts and thymomas are almost equally common in adults. (See Schwartz 9th ed., p 570, Tables 19-3 and 19-4).

TABLE 19-3 Mediastinal tumors in adults

Tumor Type	Percentage of Total	Location
Neurogenic tumors	21	Posterior
Cysts	20	All
Thymomas	19	Anterior
Lymphomas	13	Anterior/middle
Germ cell tumors	11	Anterior
Mesenchymal tumors	7	All
Endocrine tumors	6	Anterior/middle

Source: Reproduced from Shields TW: Primary lesions of the mediastinum and their investigation and treatment, in Shields TW (ed): *General Thoracic Surgery*, 4th ed. Baltimore: Lippincott Williams & Wilkins, 1994, p 1731.

TABLE 19-4 Mediastinal tumors in children

Tumor Type	Percentage of Total	Location
Neurogenic tumors	40	Posterior
Lymphomas	18	Anterior/middle
Cysts	18	All
Germ cell tumors	11	Anterior
Mesenchymal tumors	9	All
Thymomas	Rare	Anterior

Source: Reproduced with permission from Silverman NA, et al: Mediastinal masses. *Surg Clin North Am* 60:760, 1980.

17. A patient with lung cancer who presents with chest wall pain is most likely to have
    A. Squamous cell carcinoma
    B. Small cell carcinoma
    C. Adenocarcinoma
    D. Bronchoalveolar carcinoma

Answer: C

Squamous cell and small cell carcinomas frequently arise in main, lobar, or first segmental bronchi, which are collectively referred to as the *central airways*. Symptoms of airway irritation or obstruction are common and include cough, hemoptysis, wheezing (due to high-grade airway obstruction), dyspnea (due to bronchial obstruction with or without postobstructive atelectasis), and pneumonia (caused by airway obstruction with secretion retention and atelectasis).

In contrast, adenocarcinomas often are located peripherally. For this reason, they are often discovered incidentally as an asymptomatic peripheral lesion on chest radiograph. When symptoms occur, they are due to pleural or chest wall invasion (pleuritic or chest wall pain) or pleural seeding with malignant pleural effusion.

BAC (a variant of adenocarcinoma) may present as a solitary nodule, as multifocal nodules, or as a diffuse infiltrate mimicking an infectious pneumonia (pneumonic form). In the pneumonic form, severe dyspnea and hypoxia may occur, sometimes with expectoration of large volumes (over 1 L/d) of light tan fluid, with resultant dehydration and electrolyte imbalance. Because BAC tends to fill the alveolar spaces as it grows (as opposed to the typical invasion, destruction, and compression of lung architecture seen with other cell types), air bronchograms may be seen radiographically within the tumor. (See Schwartz 9th ed., p 533.)

Peripherally located tumors (often adenocarcinomas) extending through the visceral pleura lead to irritation or growth into the parietal pleura and potentially to continued growth into the chest wall structures. Three types of symptoms are possible, depending on the extent of chest wall involvement: (a) pleuritic pain, from noninvasive contact of the parietal pleura with inflammatory irritation and from direct parietal pleural invasion; (b) localized chest wall pain, with deeper invasion and involvement of the rib and/or intercostal muscles; and (c) radicular pain, from involvement of the intercostal nerve(s). Radicular pain may be mistaken for renal colic in the case of lower lobe tumors that invade the posterior chest wall. (See Schwartz 9th ed., p 534.)

18. What percent of patients with myasthenia gravis and a thymoma will experience improvement or resolution of muscle weakness after resection of the thymoma?
    A. 25%
    B. 50%
    C. 75%
    D. 95%

Answer: A

Thymoma is the most frequently encountered neoplasm of the anterior mediastinum in adults (seen most frequently between 40 and 60 years of age). They are rare in children. Most patients with thymomas are asymptomatic, but depending on the institutional referral patterns, between 10 and 50% have symptoms suggestive of myasthenia gravis or have circulating antibodies to acetylcholine receptor. However, <10% of patients with myasthenia gravis are found to have a thymoma on CT. Thymectomy leads to improvement or resolution of symptoms of myasthenia gravis in only approximately 25% of patients with thymomas. In contrast, in patients with myasthenia gravis and no thymoma, thymectomy results are superior: up to 50% of patients have a complete remission and 90% improve. In 5% of patients with thymomas, other paraneoplastic syndromes, including red cell aplasia, hypogammaglobulinemia, systemic lupus erythematosus, Cushing's syndrome, or syndrome of inappropriate secretion of antidiuretic hormone may be present. Large thymic tumors may present with symptoms related to a mass effect, which may include cough, chest pain, dyspnea, or superior vena caval syndrome. (See Schwartz 9th ed., p 573.)

19. Hypertrophic pulmonary osteoarthropathy
    A. Occurs most commonly in patients with bronchoalveolar carcinoma
    B. May develop months before patients become symptomatic from a primary malignancy
    C. Is best treated by normalizing serum calcium
    D. Is most commonly seen in the vertebrae of patients with lung cancer

Answer: B

One of the more common paraneoplastic syndromes in patients with small cell lung cancer (SCLC) is hypertrophic pulmonary osteoarthropathy (HPO). Clinically, the syndrome is characterized by tenderness and swelling of the ankles, feet, forearms, and hands. It is due to periostitis of the fibula, tibia, radius, metacarpals, and metatarsals. Symptoms may be severe and debilitating. Clubbing of the digits occurs with or independently of HPO in up to 30% of patients with SCLC. Symptoms of HPO may antedate the diagnosis of cancer by months. Radiographically, plain films of the affected areas show periosteal inflammation and elevation. A bone scan demonstrates intense but symmetric uptake of radiotracer in the long bones. Relief is afforded by treatment with aspirin or NSAIDs and by successful surgical or medical eradication of the tumor. (See Schwartz 9th ed., p 535.)

20. Surgical intervention in a patient with a lung abscess should be considered
    A. If the abscess is >3 cm in diameter
    B. If there is no decrease in size after 2 weeks of antibiotic therapy
    C. If the abscess is under tension
    D. If there are bilateral abscesses

Answer: C

Surgical drainage of lung abscesses is uncommon, because drainage usually occurs spontaneously via the tracheobronchial tree. Indications for intervention are listed in Table 19-5.

External drainage may be accomplished with tube thoracostomy, percutaneous drainage, or surgical cavernostomy. The choice between thoracostomy placement and radiologic placement of a drainage catheter depends on the treating physician's preference and the availability of interventional radiology. Surgical resection is required in <10% of lung abscess patients. Lobectomy is the preferred intervention for bleeding from a lung abscess or pyopneumothorax. An important intraoperative consideration is to protect the contralateral lung with a double-lumen tube, bronchial blocker, or contralateral main stem intubation. Surgical treatment has a 90% success rate, with an associated mortality of 1 to 13%. (See Schwartz 9th ed., p 551.)

The duration of antimicrobial therapy is variable: 1 to 2 weeks for simple aspiration pneumonia and 3 to 12 weeks for necrotizing pneumonia and lung abscess. It is probably best to treat until the cavity is resolved or until serial radiographs show significant improvement. (See Schwartz 9th ed., p 550.)

TABLE 19-5	Indications for surgical drainage procedures for lung abscesses
1. Failure of medical therapy	
2. Abscess under tension	
3. Abscess increasing in size during appropriate treatment	
4. Contralateral lung contamination	
5. Abscess >4–6 cm in diameter	
6. Necrotizing infection with multiple abscesses, hemoptysis, abscess rupture, or pyopneumothorax	
7. Inability to exclude a cavitating carcinoma	

21. Which of the following infections is a significant cause of bronchiectasis?
    A. Pneumococcus
    B. Nontuberculous mycobacterial infection
    C. Rhinovirus
    D. Aspergillus

Answer: B

Development of bronchiectasis can be attributed to either congenital or acquired causes. The principal congenital diseases that lead to bronchiectasis include cystic fibrosis, primary ciliary dyskinesia, and immunoglobulin deficiencies (e.g., selective immunoglobulin A deficiency). Congenital causes tend to produce a diffuse pattern of bronchial involvement.

Acquired causes are categorized broadly as infectious and inflammatory. Adenoviruses and influenza viruses are the predominant childhood viral infections associated with the development of bronchiectasis. Chronic infection with tuberculosis remains an important worldwide cause of bronchiectasis.

More significant in the United States are nontuberculous mycobacterial (NTM) infections that cause bronchiectasis, particularly infection by *Mycobacterium avium-intracellulare* complex. Recently, several studies have suggested an association between chronic gastroesophageal reflux disease, acid suppression, and NTM infection with bronchiectasis. This interaction is thought to be related to chronic aspiration of colonized gastric secretions in the setting of acid suppression. Although a causative relationship has not been proven, these findings suggest a role for gastroesophageal reflux disease in the pathogenesis of this disease process. (See Schwartz 9th ed., pp 551-552.)

22. A mediastinal germ cell tumor with normal alpha-fetoprotein levels and minimally elevated beta-hCG levels is most likely a
    A. Teratoma
    B. Seminoma
    C. Choriocarcinoma
    D. Embryonal cell carcinoma

Answer: B

About one third of all primary mediastinal germ cell tumors are seminomatous. Two thirds are nonseminomatous tumors or teratomas. Treatment and prognosis vary considerably within these two groups. Mature teratomas are benign and can generally be diagnosed by the characteristic CT findings of a multilocular cystic tumor encapsulated with combinations of fluid, soft tissue, calcium, and/or fat attenuation in the anterior compartment. FNA biopsy alone may be diagnostic for seminomas, and usually levels of serum markers, including hCG and AFP, are normal. In 10% of seminomas, hCG levels are slightly elevated. FNA findings, along with high hCG and AFP levels, can accurately diagnose nonseminomatous tumors.

Nonseminomatous germ cell tumors include embryonal cell carcinomas, choriocarcinomas, endodermal sinus tumors, and mixed types. They are often bulky, irregular tumors of the anterior mediastinum with areas of low attenuation on CT scan because of necrosis, hemorrhage, or cyst formation. Frequently, adjacent structures have become involved, with metastases to regional lymph nodes, pleura, and lungs. Lactate-dehydrogenase (LDH), AFP, and hCG levels are frequently elevated. (See Schwartz 9th ed., pp 575-576.)

The use of serum markers to evaluate a mediastinal mass can be invaluable in some patients. For example, seminomatous and nonseminomatous germ cell tumors can frequently be diagnosed and often distinguished from one another by the levels of alpha-fetoprotein (AFP) and human chorionic gonadotropin (hCG). In over 90% of nonseminomatous germ cell tumors, either the AFP or the hCG level will be elevated. Results are close to 100% specific if the level of either AFP or hCG is >500 ng/mL. (See Schwartz 9th ed., p 571.)

23. How much protein will be lost per day in a patient with a chylothorax whose chest tube drains 1000 ml/day?
    A. 10-15 g
    B. 25-50 g
    C. 70-85 g
    D. 100-120 g

Answer: B

The usual composition of chyle is 2.2 to 5.9 g of protein/100 ml (22-60 g/1000 ml). Therefore, B is the most appropriate answer. (See Schwartz 9th ed., p 582, and Table 19-6.)

TABLE 19-6 Composition of chyle

Component	Amount (per 100 mL)
Total fat	0.4–5 g
Total cholesterol	65–220 mg
Total protein	2.21–5.9 g
Albumin	1.1–4.1 g
Globulin	1.1–3.1 g
Fibrinogen	16–24 g
Sugars	48–200 g
Electrolytes	Similar to levels in plasma
Cellular elements	
Lymphocytes	400–6800/mm³
Erythrocytes	50–600/mm³
Antithrombin globulin	>25% of plasma concentration
Prothrombin	>25% of plasma concentration
Fibrinogen	>25% of plasma concentration

Source: Reproduced with permission from Miller JI Jr.: Diagnosis and management of chylothorax. *Chest Surg Clin N Am* 6:139, 1996. 180.

24. A patient with a chronic draining sinus with yellow granules in the pus most likely has an infection with
    A. *Aspergillus flavus*
    B. *Nocardia asteroides*
    C. *Actinomyces israelii*
    D. *Cryptococcus neoformans*

Answer: C

Actinomycosis is a chronic disease usually caused by *Actinomyces israelii.* It is characterized by chronic suppuration, sinus formation, and discharge of purulent material containing yellow-brown sulfur granules. Approximately 15% of infections involve the thorax; organisms enter the lungs via the oral cavity (where they normally reside). Because the disease is uncommon, making the correct diagnosis can be challenging, and the clinician must first suspect the disease and then perform appropriate culture analysis under anaerobic conditions. Lung involvement can present with progressive pulmonary fibrosis in the periphery. Pleural and chest wall involvement (periostitis of the ribs) is an associated finding. Treatment consists of prolonged high-dose penicillin, which is very effective. Because of the intense fibrotic reaction surrounding affected parenchyma, surgery is seldom possible.

Aspergillosis can manifest as one of three clinical syndromes: *Aspergillus* hypersensitivity lung disease, aspergilloma, or invasive pulmonary aspergillosis. Overlap occurs between these syndromes, depending on the patient's immune status. Hypersensitivity results in productive cough, fever, wheezing, pulmonary infiltrates, eosinophilia, and elevated levels of immunoglobulin E antibodies to *Aspergillus.*

Nocardia asteroides is an aerobic, acid-fast, grampositive organism that usually causes nocardiosis, a disease similar to actinomycosis with additional CNS involvement. In addition, hematogenous dissemination from a pulmonary focus may lead to generalized systemic infection. The disease process ranges from benign, self-limited suppuration of skin and subcutaneous tissues to pulmonary (extensive parenchymal necrosis and abscesses) and systemic (e.g., CNS) manifestations. In immunosuppressed patients, pulmonary cavitation or hematogenous dissemination may be accelerated. Prolonged treatment (2 to 3 months) with sulfadiazine, minocycline, or trimethoprim-sulfamethoxazole is typically required. Surgery to drain abscesses and empyema is indicated.

Cryptococcosis is a subacute or chronic infection caused by *Cryptococcus neoformans*, a round, budding yeast (5 to 20 μm in diameter) that is sometimes surrounded by a characteristic wide gelatinous capsule. (See Schwartz 9th ed., pp 555-556.)

25. Initial treatment of a patient with massive hemoptysis with airway compromise is
    A. Angiography with embolization of the bleeding bronchial artery
    B. Rigid bronchoscopy with ice water lavage
    C. Rigid bronchoscopy and laser ablation of the bleeding site
    D. Thoracotomy with external control of the site of hemorrhage

Answer: B

Massive hemoptysis generally is defined as expectoration of >600 mL of blood within a 24-hour period. It is a medical emergency associated with a mortality rate of 30 to 50%. (See Schwartz 9th ed., p 559.)

Life-threatening bleeding requires emergency airway control and preparation for potential surgery. Such patients are best cared for in an operating room equipped with rigid bronchoscopy equipment. Immediate orotracheal intubation may be necessary to gain control of ventilation and suctioning. However, rapid transport to the operating room and rigid bronchoscopy should be facilitated. Rigid bronchoscopy allows adequate suctioning of bleeding with visualization of the bleeding site; the nonbleeding side can be cannulated with the rigid scope and the patient ventilated. After stabilization, ice-saline lavage of the bleeding site can then be performed (up to 1 L in 50-mL aliquots); bleeding stops in up to 90% of patients.

Alternatively, blockade of the main stem bronchus of the affected side can be accomplished with a double-lumen endotracheal tube, with a bronchial blocker, or by intubation of the nonaffected side using an uncut standard endotracheal tube. Placement of a double-lumen endotracheal tube is challenging in these circumstances, given the bleeding and secretions. Proper placement and suctioning may be difficult, and attempts could compromise the patient's ventilation. The best option is to place a bronchial blocker in the affected bronchus with inflation. The blocker is left in place for 24 hours and the area is then re-examined bronchoscopically. After this 24-hour period, bronchial artery embolization can be performed. (See Schwartz 9th ed., p 561.)

26. A 2-cm isolated osteochondroma of the rib should be treated by
    A. Shave biopsy
    B. Local excision
    C. Segmental resection of the rib with grossly clear margins
    D. Segmental resection of the rib with 2-cm margins

Answer: B

Osteochondromas are the most common benign bone tumor. Many are detected as incidental radiographic findings. Most are solitary. If a patient has multiple osteochondromas, the surgeon must have a high index of suspicion for malignancy, because the incidence of chondrosarcoma is significantly higher in this population.

Osteochondromas occur in the first 2 decades of life, and they arise at or near the growth plate of bones. The lesions are benign during youth or adolescence. Osteochondromas that enlarge after completion of skeletal growth have the potential to develop into chondrosarcomas.

Osteochondromas in the thorax arise from the rib cortex. They are one of several components of the autosomal dominant syndrome known as *hereditary multiple exostoses*. When part of this syndrome, osteochondromas have a high rate of degeneration into chondrosarcomas. Any patient with hereditary multiple exostoses syndrome who develops new pain at the site of an osteochondroma or who notes gradual growth in the mass over time should be carefully evaluated for osteosarcoma. Local excision of a benign osteochondroma is sufficient treatment. If malignancy is determined, wide excision is performed, with a 4-cm margin. (See Schwartz 9th ed., p 564.)

27. Which of the following preoperative functional assessments is associated with poor outcome after lobectomy or pneumonectomy for resectable lung neoplasm?
    A. Predicted postoperative DLCO <70%
    B. FEV_1 <2 L
    C. VO_2 max <10 mL/kg
    D. Unable to walk up 4 flights of stairs

Answer: C

See Fig. 19-8. When obtaining the patient's history, specific questions should be routinely asked that help determine the amount of lung that the patient will likely tolerate having resected. Can the patient walk on a flat surface indefinitely, without oxygen and without having to stop and rest secondary to dyspnea? If so, the patient will be very likely to tolerate thoracotomy and lobectomy. Can the patient walk up two flights of stairs (up two standard levels), without having to stop and rest secondary to dyspnea? If so, the patient will likely tolerate pneumonectomy. Finally, nearly all patients, except those who show carbon dioxide retention on arterial blood gas analysis, will be able to tolerate periods of single-lung ventilation and wedge resection. (See Schwartz 9th ed., p 539.)

General guidelines for the use of FEV_1 in assessing the patient's ability to tolerate pulmonary resection are as follows: patients with an FEV_1 of >2.0 L can tolerate pneumonectomy, and those with an FEV_1 of >1.5 L can tolerate lobectomy. It must be emphasized that these are guidelines only. It is also

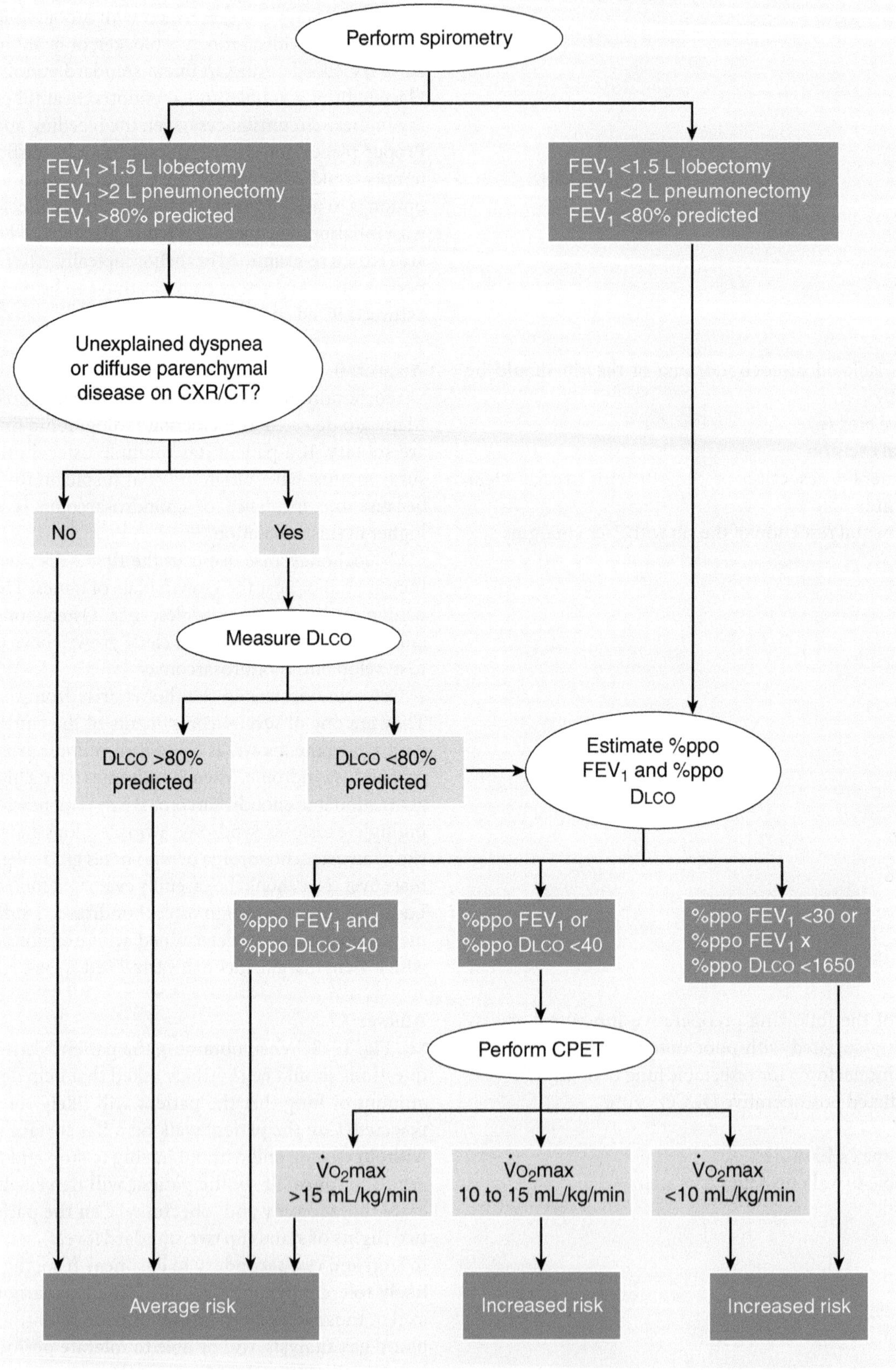

FIG. 19-8. Algorithm for preoperative evaluation of pulmonary function and reserve before resectional lung surgery. CPET = cardiopulmonary exercise test; CT = computed tomographic scan; CXR = chest radiograph; DLCO = carbon monoxide diffusion capacity; FEV_1 = forced expiratory volume in 1 second; %ppo = percent predicted postoperative lung function; VO_2max = maximum oxygen consumption. (Reproduced with permission from Colice GL, Shafazand S, Griffin JP, et al: Physiologic evaluation of the patient with lung cancer being considered for resectional surgery: ACCP evidence-based clinical practice guidelines (2nd edition). *Chest* 132(3 Suppl):161S, 2007.)

important to note that the raw value is often imprecise, because normal values are reported as 'percent predicted' based on corrections made for age, height, and gender.

The percent predicted value for both FEV_1 and DLCO correlates with the risk of development of complications postoperatively, particularly pulmonary complications. Complication rates are significantly higher among patients with percent predicted values of <50%, with the risk of complications increasing in a stepwise fashion for each 10% decline. Figure 19-9 shows the relationship between predicted postoperative DLCO and estimated operative mortality. (See Schwartz 9th ed., p 540.)

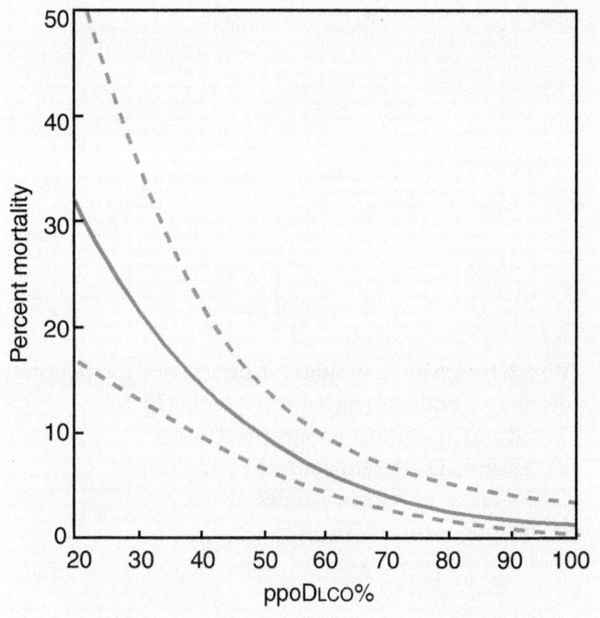

FIG. 19-9. Operative mortality after major pulmonary resection for non–small cell lung cancer (334 patients) as a function of the percent predicted postoperative carbon monoxide diffusion capacity (ppoDLCO%). *Solid line* is the logistic regression model; *dashed lines* represent the 95% confidence limits. (Adapted with permission from Wang J, et al: Diffusing capacity predicts operative mortality but not long-term survival after resection for lung cancer. *J Thorac Cardiovasc Surg* 117:582, 1999. Copyright © Elsevier.)

Exercise testing that yields maximum oxygen consumption (VO_2max) has emerged as a valuable decision-making technique to help in evaluation of patients with abnormal FEV_1 and DLCO. Table 19-7 provides a summary of the existing data regarding the relationship between VO_2max and postoperative mortality risk. It is not uncommon to encounter patients with significant reductions in percent predicted FEV_1 and DLCO whose history shows a functional status that is inconsistent with the pulmonary function test results. In these circumstances, and in other situations in which decision making is difficult, the VO_2max should be measured. Values of <10 mL/kg per minute generally prohibit any major pulmonary resection, because the mortality associated with this level is 26%, compared with only 8.3% for VO_2max levels of ≥10 mL/kg per minute; VO_2max levels >15 mL/kg per minute generally indicate the patient's ability to tolerate pneumonectomy. (See Schwartz 9th ed., pp 541-542.)

TABLE 19-7 Relation between maximum oxygen consumption ($\dot{V}o_2max$) as determined by preoperative exercise testing and perioperative mortality

Study	Deaths/Total
$\dot{V}o_2max$ 10–15 mL/kg per minute	
Smith et al	1/6 (33%)
Bechard and Wetstein	0/15 (0%)
Olsen et al	1/14 (7.1%)
Walsh et al	1/5 (20%)
Bolliger et al	2/17 (11.7%)
Markos et al	1/11 (9.1%)
Wang et al	0/12 (0%)
Win et al	2/16 (12.5%)
Total	8/96 (8.3%)
$\dot{V}o_2max$ <10 mL/kg per minute	
Bechard and Wetstein	2/7 (29%)
Olsen et al	3/11 (27%)
Holden et al	2/4 (50%)
Markos et al	0/5 (0%)
Total	7/27 (26%)

Source: Reproduced with permission from Colice GL, Shafazand S, Griffin JP, et al: Physiologic evaluation of the patient with lung cancer being considered for resectional surgery: ACCP evidence-based clinical practice guidelines (2nd edition). *Chest* 132(3 Suppl):161S, 2007.

28. Which lymph node stations can be assessed for metastatic disease via endoesophageal ultrasound (EUS)?
    A. 2R and 2L—upper paratracheal nodes
    B. 4R and 4L—lower paratracheal nodes
    C. 5—aorto-pulmonary nodes
    D. 6—pre-aortic nodes

Answer: B

Endoesophageal ultrasound (EUS) has recently emerged as a method of staging in NSCLC. EUS can accurately visualize mediastinal paratracheal lymph nodes (stations 4R, 7, and 4L) and other lymph node stations (stations 8 and 9). It is able to visualize primary lung lesions contiguous with or near the esophagus (see Fig. 19-1). Using FNA techniques and, more recently, core-needle biopsy, samples of lymph nodes or primary lesions can be obtained. Diagnostic yield is improved with intraoperative cytologic evaluation, which can be performed with the cytopathologist in the operating room. Limitations of EUS include the inability to visualize the anterior (pretracheal) mediastinum, and thus it does not replace mediastinoscopy for complete mediastinal nodal staging. However, it may not be necessary to perform mediastinoscopy if findings on EUS are positive for N2 nodal disease, particularly if more than one station is found to harbor metastases. (See Schwartz 9th ed., p 538, and Fig. 19-1.)

29. Surgical intervention is required in most patients infected with
    A. *Actinomyces israelii*
    B. *Mycobacterium tuberculosis*
    C. *Mycobacterium kansasii*
    D. *M. avium-intracellulare* complex

Answer: D

Rifampin and isoniazid augmented with one or more second-line drugs are most commonly used to treat NTM infections. Generally, therapy lasts approximately 18 months. The overall response is satisfactory in 70 to 80% of patients with *M. kansasii* infection. Surgical intervention rarely is required in those 20 to 30% who do not respond to medical therapy. In contrast, pulmonary MAC [*M. avium-intracellulare* complex] infections respond poorly, even to combinations of four or more drugs, and most patients eventually require surgical intervention. (See Schwartz 9th ed., p 554.)

Actinomycosis is a chronic disease usually caused by *Actinomyces israelii*. It is characterized by chronic suppuration, sinus formation, and discharge of purulent material containing yellow-brown sulfur granules. Approximately 15% of infections involve the thorax; organisms enter the lungs via the oral cavity (where they normally reside). Because the disease is uncommon, making the correct diagnosis can be challenging, and the clinician must first suspect the disease and then perform appropriate culture analysis under anaerobic conditions. Lung involvement can present with progressive pulmonary fibrosis in the periphery. Pleural and chest wall involvement (periostitis of the ribs) is an associated finding. Treatment consists of prolonged high-dose penicillin, which is very effective. Because of the intense fibrotic reaction surrounding affected parenchyma, surgery is seldom possible. (See Schwartz 9th ed., p 555.)

30. Which of the following is a primary indication for the use of indwelling pleural catheters to treat malignant pleural effusion?
   A. Poor expansion of the lung
   B. Purulent, foul-smelling pleural fluid
   C. Long life expectancy
   D. Positive results of D-dimer blood test

Answer: A

Before the pleural cavity is sclerosed, whether by chest tube or VATS, the lung should be nearly fully expanded. Poor expansion of the lung (because of entrapment by tumor or adhesions) generally predicts a poor result with pleurodesis and is the primary indication for placement of indwelling pleural catheters. These catheters have dramatically changed the management of end-stage cancer treatment because they substantially shorten the amount of time patients spend in the hospital during their final weeks of life. The choices for sclerosing agent include talc, bleomycin, and doxycycline. Success rates for controlling the effusion range from 60 to 90%, depending on the exact scope of the clinical study, the degree of lung expansion after the pleural fluid is drained, and the care with which the outcomes were reported. Figure 19-10 presents a decision algorithm for the management of malignant pleural effusion. (See Schwartz 9th ed., p 579.)

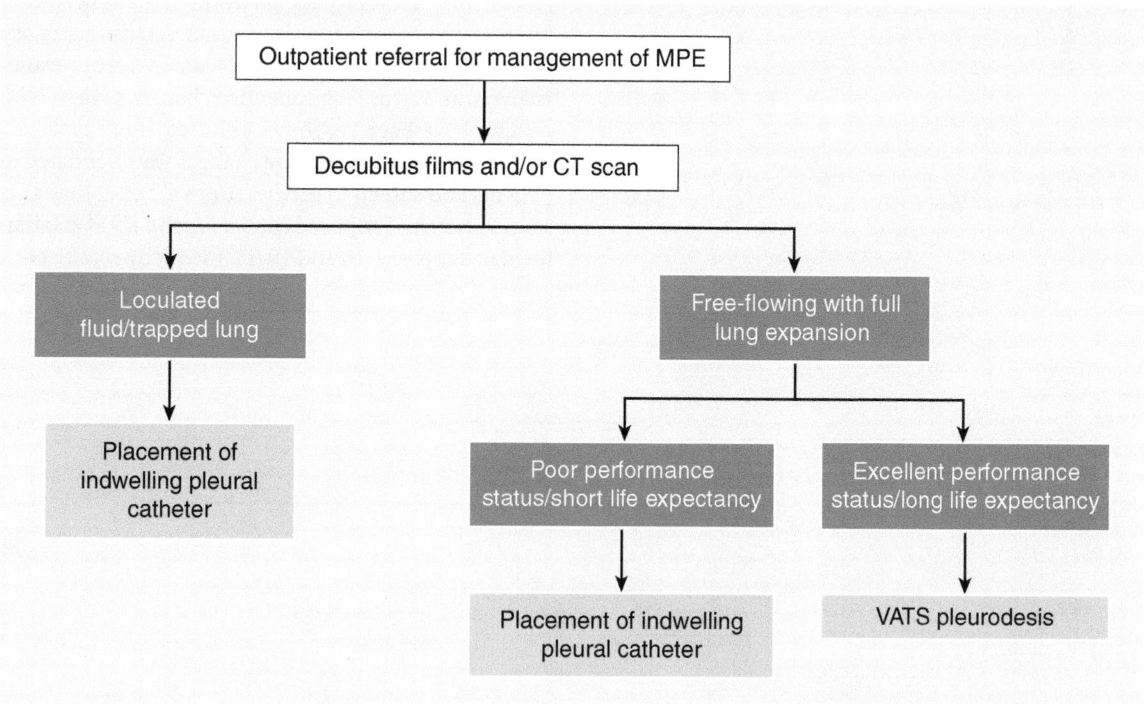

FIG. 19-10. Treatment decision algorithm for the management of malignant pleural effusion (MPE). CT = computed tomography; VATS = video-assisted thoracic surgery.

31. When treating trauma victims, which thoracic surgical approach is typically used?
 A. Median sternotomy
 B. Video-assisted thoracoscopic surgery
 C. Posterolateral thoracotomy
 D. Anterolateral thoracotomy

Answer: D
The anterolateral thoracotomy has traditionally been used in trauma victims. This approach allows quick entry into the chest with the patient supine. (See Schwartz 9th ed., p 523.)

32. Using the proposed changes to the lung cancer staging system, which of the following is the appropriate TNM stage for a patient with a 2-cm squamous cell cancer in the right upper lobe with positive left level 4 mediastinal lymph nodes and a right malignant pleural effusion?
 A. T1a N1 M0, Stage IIa
 B. T1b N2 M1a, Stage IV
 C. T2a N1 M0, Stage IIa
 D. T1b N2 M0, Stage IIIa

Answer: B
In 1986, an international staging system for lung cancer was developed by Mountain and applied to a database of >3000 patients from the M. D. Anderson Hospital in Houston, Texas, and the Lung Cancer Study Group. In 1997, Mountain reviewed the survival data from an additional 1524 patients beyond the original database. Taking into account the combined total of 5319 patients, he revised the staging system. These changes were subsequently adopted by the American Joint Committee on Cancer. The 1997 version of the international staging system, which is still in use, is shown in Table 19-8.

Significant variation in survival is seen within stage groupings, however (Table 19-9), which has prompted a critical evaluation of the variables that predict poor long-term survival. For example, a tumor that is ≤1.0 cm in diameter has a significantly better prognosis than tumors 2.0 to 3.0 cm in diameter. The wide range of postoperative 5-year survival rates (5 to 25%) after surgical resection of patients with N2 nodal involvement demonstrates the effect of the number and location of involved nodal stations and of the presence of extracapsular nodal extension.

To address the wide variability in survival within stages, the International Association for the Study of Lung Cancer Staging Committee was created in 1999. A database encompassing over 100,000 patients worldwide has been created and intensively examined for important determinants of survival by tumor, node, and metastasis staging. The results of this analysis, as well as recommended changes to the TNM staging system, have been recently published after vigorous analysis of multinational data. These changes were validated in 23,583 patients and shown to predict survival better than the current staging system. Proposed changes to the TNM staging are outlined in Tables 19-10 and 19-11. (See Schwartz 9th ed., p 542.)

TABLE 19-8 American Joint Committee on Cancer staging system for lung cancer

Stage	TNM
IA	T1 N0 M0
IB	T2 N0 M0
IIA	T1 N1 M0
IIB	T2 N1 M0
	T3 N0 M0
IIIA	T3 N1 M0
	T1–3 N2 M0
IIIB	T4 Any N M0
	Any T N3 M0
IV	Any T Any N M1

TNM definitions

T	**TX**	Positive malignant cell, but primary tumor not visualized by imaging or bronchoscopy
	T0	No evidence of primary tumor
	Tis	Carcinoma in situ
	T1	Tumor ≤3 cm, surrounded by lung or visceral pleura, without bronchoscopic evidence of invasion more proximal than the lobar bronchus
	T2	Tumor with any of the following features of size or extent: • >3 cm in greatest dimension • Involves main bronchus, ≥2 cm distal to the carina • Invades the visceral pleura • Associated with atelectasis or obstructive pneumonitis that extends to the hilar region but does not involve the entire lung
	T3	Tumor of any size that directly invades any of the following: chest wall (including superior sulcus tumors), diaphragm, mediastinal pleura, parietal pericardium; or tumor in the main bronchus <2 cm distal to the carina, but without involvement of the carina; or associated atelectasis or obstructive pneumonitis of the entire lung
	T4	Tumor of any size that invades any of the following: mediastinum, heart, great vessels, trachea, esophagus, vertebral body, carina; or tumor with a malignant pleural or pericardial effusion, or with satellite tumor nodule(s) within the ipsilateral primary-tumor lobe of the lung
N	**NX**	Regional lymph nodes cannot be assessed
	N0	No regional lymph node metastasis
	N1	Metastasis to ipsilateral peribronchial and/or ipsilateral hilar lymph nodes, and intrapulmonary nodes involved by direct extension of the primary tumor
	N2	Metastasis to ipsilateral mediastinal and/or subcarinal lymph node(s)
	N3	Metastasis to contralateral mediastinal, contralateral hilar, ipsilateral or contralateral scalene, or supraclavicular lymph node(s)
M	**MX**	Presence of distant metastasis cannot be assessed
	M0	No distant metastasis
	M1	Distant metastasis present [including metastatic tumor nodule(s) in the ipsilateral nonprimary tumor lobe(s) of the lung]

Summary of staging definitions

Occult stage	Microscopically identified cancer cells in lung secretions on multiple occasions (or multiple daily collections); no discernible primary cancer in the lung
Stage 0	Carcinoma in situ
Stage IA	Tumor surrounded by lung or visceral pleura ≤3 cm arising more than 2 cm distal to the carina (T1 N0)
Stage IB	Tumor surrounded by lung >3 cm, or tumor of any size with visceral pleura involved arising more than 2 cm distal to the carina (T2 N0)
Stage IIA	Tumor ≤3 cm not extended to adjacent organs, with ipsilateral peribronchial and hilar lymph node involvement (T1 N1)
Stage IIB	Tumor >3 cm not extended to adjacent organs, with ipsilateral peribronchial and hilar lymph node involvement (T2 N1)
	Tumor invading chest wall, pleura, or pericardium but not involving carina, nodes negative (T3 N0)
Stage IIIA	Tumor invading chest wall, pleura, or pericardium and nodes in hilum or ipsilateral mediastinum (T3, N1–2) or tumor of any size invading ipsilateral mediastinal or subcarinal nodes (T1–3, N2)
Stage IIIB	Direct extension to adjacent organs (esophagus, aorta, heart, cava, diaphragm, or spine); satellite nodule same lobe, or any tumor associated with contralateral mediastinal or supraclavicular lymph node involvement (T4 or N3)
Stage IV	Separate nodule in different lobes or any tumor with distant metastases (M1)

TABLE 19-9 Cumulative percentage of survival by stage after treatment for lung cancer

	Time after Treatment	
Pathologic Stage	**24 mo (%)**	**60 mo (%)**
pT1 N0 M0 ($n = 511$)	86	67
pT2 N0 M0 ($n = 549$)	76	57
pT1 N1 M0 ($n = 76$)	70	55
pT2 N1 M0 ($n = 288$)	56	39
pT3 N0 M0 ($n = 87$)	55	38

Data from Mountain CF: Revisions in the International System for Staging Lung Cancer. *Chest* 111:1710, 1997.

TABLE 19-10 Summary of proposed lung cancer staging revisions

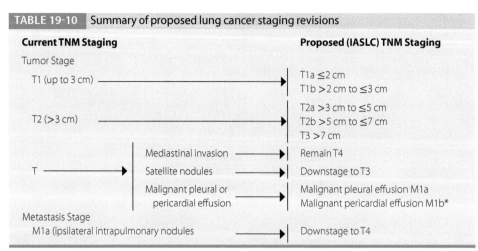

Current TNM Staging		Proposed (IASLC) TNM Staging
Tumor Stage		
T1 (up to 3 cm) →		T1a ≤2 cm T1b >2 cm to ≤3 cm
T2 (>3 cm) →		T2a >3 cm to ≤5 cm T2b >5 cm to ≤7 cm T3 >7 cm
T →	Mediastinal invasion →	Remain T4
	Satellite nodules →	Downstage to T3
	Malignant pleural or pericardial effusion →	Malignant pleural effusion M1a Malignant pericardial effusion M1b*
Metastasis Stage		
M1a (ipsilateral intrapulmonary nodules	→	Downstage to T4

*Additional recommendation after further validation that was not in the proposal for changes to the TNM system by Goldstraw et al.
IASLC = International Association for the Study of Lung Cancer; TNM = tumor, nodes, and metastasis.

TABLE 19-11 International Association for the Study of Lung Cancer proposed changes to the tumor, nodes, and metastasis (TNM) staging system for 2009

Sixth Edition T/M Descriptor	Proposed T/M	N0	N1	N2	N3
T1 (≤2 cm)	T1a	IA	IIA	IIIA	IIIB
T1 (>2 to 3 cm)	T1b	IA	IIA	IIIA	IIIB
T2 (≤5 cm)	T2a	IB	**IIA**	IIIA	IIIB
T2 (>5 to 7 cm)	T2b	**IIA**	IIB	IIIA	IIIB
T2 (>7 cm)	T3	**IIB**	**IIIA**	IIIA	IIIB
T3 invasion	—	IIB	IIIA	IIIA	IIIB
T4 (same-lobe nodules)	—	**IIB**	**IIIA**	**IIIA**	IIIB
T4 (extension)	T4	**IIIA**	**IIIA**	IIIB	IIIB
M1 (ipsilateral lung)	—	**IIIA**	**IIIA**	**IIIB**	**IIIB**
T4 (pleural effusion)	M1a	**IV**	**IV**	**IV**	**IV**
M1 (contralateral lung)	—	IV	IV	IV	IV
M1 (distant)	M1b	IV	IV	IV	IV

Cells in bold represent a change from the sixth edition for a particular TNM category.
Source: Reproduced with permission from Goldstraw P, Crowley J, Chansky K, et al: The IASLC Lung Cancer Staging Project: Proposals for the revision of the TNM stage groupings in the forthcoming (seventh) edition of the TNM classification of malignant tumours. *J Thorac Oncol* 2:706, 2007.

CHAPTER 20

Congenital Heart Disease

BASIC SCIENCE QUESTIONS

1. The ductus arteriosus is derived from
   A. The 2nd aortic arch
   B. The 3rd aortic arch
   C. The 4th aortic arch
   D. The 6th aortic arch

Answer: D

The ductus arteriosus is derived from the sixth aortic arch and normally extends from the main or left PA to the upper descending thoracic aorta, distal to the left subclavian artery. In the normal fetal cardiovascular system, ductal flow is considerable (approximately 60% of the combined ventricular output), and is directed exclusively from the PA to the aorta. (See Schwartz 9th ed., p 597.)

2. The primary stimulus for closure of the ductus arteriosus after birth is
   A. Loss of PGE_2 made in the placenta
   B. Increased PGI_2 levels
   C. Increased oxygen tension in the newborn's blood
   D. Decreased bradykinin

Answer: C

Locally produced and circulating prostaglandin E_2 (PGE_2) and PGI_2 induce active relaxation of the ductal musculature, maintaining maximal patency during the fetal period. At birth, increased pulmonary blood flow metabolizes these prostaglandin products, and absence of the placenta removes an important source of them, resulting in a marked decrease in these ductal-relaxing substances. In addition, release of histamines, catecholamines, bradykinin, and acetylcholine all promote ductal contraction. Despite all of these complex interactions, the rising oxygen tension in the fetal blood is the main stimulus causing smooth muscle contraction and ductal closure within 10 to 15 hours postnatally. Anatomic closure by fibrosis produces the ligamentum arteriosum connecting the PA to the aorta. (See Schwartz 9th ed., p 598.)

3. Truncus arteriosus is often seen in patients with DiGeorge syndrome. This association suggests a common embryologic defect involving early development of
   A. Ectoderm
   B. Mesoderm
   C. Endoderm
   D. Neural crest

Answer: D

During embryonic life, the truncus arteriosus normally begins to separate and spiral into a distinguishable anterior PA and posterior aorta. Persistent truncus, therefore, represents an arrest in embryologic development at this stage. Other implicated events include twisting of the dividing truncus because of ventricular looping, subinfundibular atresia, and abnormal location of the semilunar valve anlages.

The neural crest may also play a crucial role in the normal formation of the great vessels, as experimental studies in chick embryos have shown that ablation of the neural crest results in persistent truncus arteriosus. The neural crest also develops into the pharyngeal pouches that give rise to the thymus and parathyroids, which likely explains the prevalent association of truncus arteriosus and DiGeorge syndrome. (See Schwartz 9th ed., p 602.)

CLINICAL QUESTIONS

1. Which of the following best describes the therapeutic approach to a child with hypoplastic left heart syndrome (HLHS)?
   A. Palliation is the only option, repair is not possible
   B. Reasonable palliation is not possible, repair must be attempted
   C. Either palliation or repair is possible in the newborn period and the decision is made based on the physiology of the child
   D. Palliation is possible in the newborn period with definitive repair later in childhood

Answer: B

Hypoplastic left heart syndrome (HLHS) includes a spectrum of conditions in which there is underdevelopment of the left-sided heart structures. The left heart is therefore inadequate to support the systemic circulation. The traditional strategy of initial palliation followed by definitive correction at a later age, which had pervaded the thinking of most surgeons, began to evolve to one emphasizing early repair, even in the tiniest patients. Furthermore, some of the defects that were virtually uniformly fatal [such as hypoplastic left heart syndrome (HLHS)] now can be successfully treated with aggressive forms of palliation using cardiopulmonary bypass (CPB), resulting in outstanding survival for many of these children.

Because the goal in most cases of CHD is now early repair, as opposed to subdividing lesions into cyanotic or noncyanotic lesions, a more appropriate classification scheme divides particular defects into three categories based on the feasibility of achieving this goal: (a) defects that have no reasonable palliation and for which repair is the only option; (b) defects for which repair is not possible and for which palliation is the only option; and (c) defects that can either be repaired or palliated in infancy. It bears mentioning that all defects in the second category are those in which the appropriate anatomic components either are not present, as in HLHS, or cannot be created from existing structures. (See Schwartz 9th ed., p 592.)

2. The most common type of atrial septal defect (ASD) is
   A. Sinus venosus defect
   B. Ostium primum defect
   C. Ostium secundum defect
   D. Atrioventricular defect

Answer: C

ASDs can be classified into three different types: (a) sinus venosus defects, comprising approximately 5 to 10% of all ASDs; (b) ostium primum defects, which are more correctly described as partial AV canal defects; and (c) ostium secundum defects, which are the most prevalent subtype, comprising 80% of all ASDs. Ostium secundum defects are due to defects of the septum primum and those situated within the fossa ovalis. The secundum defects therefore included patent foramen ovales. (See Schwartz 9th ed., p 592.)

3. The most common type of ventricular septal defect (VSD) is
   A. Supracristal
   B. Muscular
   C. Perimembranous
   D. AV canal

Answer: C

VSD refers to a hole between the [left and right ventricles]. These defects are common, comprising 20 to 30% of all cases of CHD, and may occur as an isolated lesion or as part of a more complex malformation. VSDs vary in size from 3 to 4 mm to more than 3 cm, and are classified into four types based on their location in the ventricular septum: perimembranous, AV canal, outlet or supracristal, and muscular. Perimembranous VSDs are the most common type requiring surgical intervention, constituting approximately 80% of cases. These defects involve the membranous septum and include the malalignment defects seen in TOF. (See Schwartz 9th ed., p 619.)

4. The standard treatment for a small ASD is
   A. Elective closure in infancy
   B. Elective closure at age 4-5
   C. Surgery or placement of an occlusion device only for symptomatic patients
   D. Surgery or placement of an occlusion device for patients with a fixed PVR >12 U/ml

Answer: B

In general, ASDs are closed when patients are between 4 and 5 years of age. Children of this size can usually be operated on without the use of blood transfusion and generally have excellent outcomes. Patients who are symptomatic may require repair earlier, even in infancy. Some surgeons, however, advocate routine repair in infants .and children, as even smaller defects are associated with the risk of paradoxical embolism, particularly during pregnancy. (See Schwartz 9th ed., p 594.)

The advent of two-dimensional echocardiography with color flow Doppler has largely obviated the need for cardiac catheterization because the exact nature of the ASD can be precisely defined by echo alone. However, in cases where the patient is older than age 40 years, catheterization can quantify the degree of pulmonary hypertension present, because those with a fixed PVR greater than 12 U/mL are considered inoperable. (See Schwartz 9th ed., p 593.)

First performed in 1976, transcatheter closure of ASDs with the use of various occlusion devices is gaining widespread acceptance. Certain types of ASDs, including patent foramen ovale (PFO), secundum defects, and some fenestrated secundum defects, are amenable to device closure, as long as particular anatomic criteria (e.g., an adequate superior and inferior rim for device seating and distance from the [atrioventricular] valve) are met. Since the introduction of percutaneous closure, there has been a dramatic rise in device closure prevalence to the point where device closure has supplanted surgical therapy as the dominant treatment modality for secundum ASD. (See Schwartz 9th ed., p 594.)

5. Infants with critical aortic stenosis and good left ventricular function are initially treated with
   A. Aortic valve replacement
   B. Surgical aortic valvotomy
   C. Balloon (catheter) valvotomy
   D. Observation, with surgery planned when they achieve 10 kg weight

Answer: C

Patients who have a [left ventricle] capable of providing systemic output are candidates for intervention to relieve [aortic stenosis], generally through balloon valvotomy. Very rarely, if catheter-based therapy is not an option, relief of valvular AS in infants and children can be accomplished with surgical valvotomy using standard techniques of CPB and direct exposure to the aortic valve. Considerable debate exists, however, in the most accurate method to delineate patients in a morphologic grey zone, whereupon the decision between a single ventricle or biventricular strategy is unclear. The decision is critical as balloon valvotomy in a neonate without an adequate left ventricle can be disastrous. (See Schwartz 9th ed., p 595.)

Considerable debate exists, however, regarding the most accurate method to delineate patients in a morphologic gray zone, whereupon the decision between a single ventricle or biventricular strategy is unclear. The decision is critical as balloon valvotomy in a neonate without an adequate left ventricle can be disastrous.

6. The most common cause of death in patients with patent ductus arteriosus (PDA) is
   A. Respiratory failure
   B. Congestive heart failure
   C. Respiratory infection
   D. Endocarditis

Answer: B

PDA is not a benign entity, although prolonged survival has been reported. The estimated death rate for infants with isolated, untreated PDA is approximately 30%. The leading cause of death is [congestive heart failure], with respiratory infection as a secondary cause. Endocarditis is more likely to occur with a small ductus and is rarely fatal if aggressive antibiotic therapy is initiated early. (See Schwartz 9th ed., p 598.)

7. Which of the following is the most common presenting manifestation in patients with supravalvular aortic stenosis?
   A. Angina
   B. Syncope
   C. Poor exercise tolerance
   D. Asymptomatic murmur

Answer: D

The signs and symptoms of supravalvular AS are similar to other forms of [left ventricular outflow tract obstruction]. An asymptomatic murmur is the presenting manifestation in approximately one half of these patients. Syncope, poor exercise tolerance, and angina may all occur with nearly equal frequency. (See Schwartz 9th ed., p 597.)

8. The treatment of choice for an infant with coarctation of the aorta is
   A. Catheterization with balloon dilation
   B. Catheterization with placement of an aortic stent
   C. Surgical aortoplasty
   D. Resection with primary anastomosis

Answer: D

The routine management of hemodynamically significant COA [coarctation] in all age groups has traditionally been surgical. Transcatheter repairs are used with increasing frequency in older patients and those with recoarctation following surgical repair. Balloon dilatation of native coarctation in neonates has been used with poor results. The most common surgical techniques in current use are resection with end-to-end anastomosis or extended end-to-end anastomosis, taking care to remove all residual ductal tissue. Extended end-to-end anastomosis may also allow the surgeon to treat transverse arch hypoplasia which is commonly encountered in infants with aortic coarctation. The subclavian flap aortoplasty is another repair, although it is used less frequently in the modern era because of the risk of late aneurysm formation and possible underdevelopment of the left upper extremity or ischemia.

Although operative repair is still the gold standard, treatment of COA by catheter-based intervention has become more widespread. Both balloon dilatation and primary stent implantation have been used successfully. The most extensive study of the results of balloon angioplasty reported on 970 procedures: 422 native and 548 recurrent COAs. Mean gradient reduction was 74 ± 24% for native and 70 ± 31% for recurrent COA. This demonstrated that catheter- based therapy could produce equally effective results both in recurrent and in primary COA, a finding with far-reaching implications in the new paradigm of multidisciplinary treatment algorithms for CHD.

In summary, children younger than age 6 months with native COA should be treated with surgical repair, while those requiring intervention at later ages may be ideal candidates for balloon dilatation or primary stent implantation. Additionally, catheter-based therapy should be used for those cases of restenosis following either surgical or primary endovascular management. (See Schwartz 9th ed., p 601.)

9. Cor triatriatum results from division of which of the following chambers into two chambers?
   A. Left atrium
   B. Right atrium
   C. Left ventricle
   D. Right ventricle

Answer: A

Cor triatriatum is a rare CHD characterized by the presence of a fibromuscular diaphragm that partitions the left atrium into two chambers: a superior chamber that receives drainage from the pulmonary veins, and an inferior chamber that communicates with the mitral valve and the [left ventricle] . An ASD frequently exists between the superior chamber and the right atrium, or, more rarely, between the right atrium and the inferior chamber. (See Schwartz 9th ed., p 605.)

10. Which of the following is the most common associated anomaly in patients with coarctation of the aorta?
    A. Rib notching
    B. Bicuspid aortic valve
    C. Ventricular septal defect (VSD)
    D. Patent ductus arteriosus (PDA)

Answer: B

Other associated anomalies, such as VSD, PDA, and ASD, may be seen with COA, but the most common is that of a bicuspid aortic valve, which can be demonstrated in 25 to 42% of cases.

Rib notching is a result of coarctation, not an associated anomaly. Extensive collateral circulation develops, predominantly involving the intercostals and mammary arteries as a direct result of aortic flow obstruction. This translates into the well-known finding of 'rib-notching' on chest radiograph, as well as a prominent pulsation underneath the ribs. (See Schwartz 9th ed., p 601.)

11. Which of the following is the appropriate treatment of a newborn with TAPVC (total anomalous pulmonary venous connection)?
    A. Pharmacologic treatment to maintain a patent ductus arteriosus
    B. Surgical closure of any associated patent ductus arteriosus
    C. Palliation with pulmonary artery banding
    D. Definitive repair in the newborn period

Answer: D

Unique to this lesion is the absence of a definitive form of palliation. Thus, TAPVC with concomitant obstruction represents one of the only true surgical emergencies across the entire spectrum of congenital heart surgery.

Operative correction of TAPVC requires anastomosis of the common pulmonary venous channel to the left atrium, obliteration of the anomalous venous connection, and closure of the atrial septal defect (ASD). (See Schwartz 9th ed., p 604.)

12. Which of the following lesions is exclusively treated with a palliative operation rather than definitive repair as the first stage of treatment?
    A. Tricuspid atresia
    B. Coarctation of the aorta
    C. Tetralogy of Fallot
    D. Truncus arteriosus

Answer: A

Tricuspid atresia and hypoplastic left heart syndrome represent two forms of single ventricle physiology, and are therefore universally treated with palliation as a first stage of repair. Tricuspid atresia, however, is a more favorable morphologic subtype, as the right ventricle is underdeveloped rather than the left ventricle. The left ventricle, therefore, becomes the systemic ventricle.

The treatment for tricuspid atresia in the earlier era of palliation was aimed at correcting the defect in the pulmonary circulation. That is, patients with too much pulmonary flow received a pulmonary band, and those with insufficient flow received a systemic-to-PA [pulmonary artery] (PA) shunt. Systemic-to-PA shunts, or Blalock-Taussig (B-T) shunts, were first applied to patients with tricuspid atresia in the 1940s and 1950s. Likewise, PA banding was applied to patients with tricuspid atresia and congestive failure in 1957. However, despite the initial relief of either cyanosis or CHF, long-term mortality was high, as the single ventricle was left unprotected from either volume or pressure overload.

Recognizing the inadequacies of the initial repairs, Glenn described the first successful cavopulmonary anastomosis, an end-to-side SVC-to-RPA shunt in 1958, and later modified this to allow flow to both pulmonary arteries. This end-to-side SVC-to-RPA anastomosis was known as the *bidirectional Glenn*, and is the first stage to final Fontan repair in widespread use today. (See Schwartz 9th ed., p 608.)

13. Which valve is primarily affected in Ebstein's anomaly?
    A. Aortic
    B. Mitral
    C. Pulmonary
    D. Tricuspid

Answer: D

Ebstein's anomaly is a rare defect, occurring in less than 1% of CHD patients. The predominant maldevelopment in this lesion is the inferior displacement of the tricuspid valve into the [right ventricle], although Bove and others have emphasized that Ebstein's anomaly is primarily a defect in right ventricular morphology rather than an isolated defect in the tricuspid valve. (See Schwartz 9th ed., p 613.)

14. Which of the following is almost universally present in a patient with TAPVC (total anomalous pulmonary vein connection)?
    A. Atrial septal defect
    B. Ventricular septal defect (VSD)
    C. Patent ductus arteriosus (PDA)
    D. Pulmonary valve stenosis

Answer: A

Total anomalous pulmonary venous connection (TAPVC) occurs in 1 to 2% of all cardiac malformations and is characterized by abnormal drainage of the pulmonary veins into the right heart, whether through connections into the right atrium or into its tributaries. Accordingly, the only mechanism by which oxygenated blood can return to the left heart is through an ASD, which is almost uniformly present with TAPVC. (See Schwartz 9th ed., p 603.)

15. The Norwood procedure is used in the treatment of
    A. Coarctation of the aorta
    B. Aortic stenosis
    C. Hypoplastic left heart syndrome
    D. Tetralogy of Fallot

Answer: C

In 1983, Norwood and colleagues described a two-stage palliative surgical procedure for relief of hypoplastic left heart syndrome that was later modified to the currently used three-stage method of palliation. Stage 1 palliation, also known as the *modified Norwood procedure*, bypasses the LV by creating a single outflow vessel, the neoaorta, which arises from the RV. (See Schwartz 9th ed., p 611.)

16. Which valve is most often congenitally abnormal?
    A. Mitral
    B. Tricuspid
    C. Aortic
    D. Pulmonary

Answer: C

The spectrum of aortic valve abnormality represents the most common form of CHD, with the great majority of patients being asymptomatic until midlife. (See Schwartz 9th ed., p 594.)

17. Which of the following can be seen in an infant with severe aortic stenosis?
    A. Crying during feeding
    B. Upper body cyanosis
    C. Hyperactive precordium
    D. Machinery murmur

Answer: A

Neonates and infants with severe valvular AS may have a relatively nonspecific history of irritability and failure to thrive. Angina, if present, is usually manifested by episodic, inconsolable crying that coincides with feeding. As discussed previously, evidence of poor peripheral perfusion, such as extreme pallor, indicates severe left ventricular outflow tract obstruction (LVOTO). Differential cyanosis is an uncommon finding, but is present when enough antegrade flow occurs only to maintain normal upper body perfusion, while a large PDA produces blue discoloration of the abdomen and legs.

Hyperactive precordium and machinery murmur are typical findings in a patient with a patent ductus arteriosus. (See Schwartz 9th ed., p 595.)

18. The Fontan procedure is used to treat
    A. Hypoplastic left heart syndrome
    B. Tetralogy of Fallot
    C. Total anomalous pulmonary venous connection (TAPVC)
    D. Mitral stenosis

Answer: A

Although surgical palliation with the Norwood procedure is still the mainstay of therapy for infants with HLHS, a combined surgical and percutaneous option (hybrid procedure), which consists of bilateral PA banding and placement of a ductal stent, has emerged as a promising alternative that obviates the need for CPB in the fragile neonatal period. The hybrid procedure can also be used as a bridge to heart transplantation in those infants with severe AV valve regurgitation or otherwise unsuitable single-ventricle anatomy.

Following stage 1 palliation, the second surgical procedure is the creation of a bidirectional cavopulmonary shunt or hemi-Fontan, generally at 3 to 6 months of life when the [pulmonary vascular resistance] has decreased to normal levels. This is the first step in separating the pulmonary and systemic circulations, and it decreases the volume load on the single ventricle. The existing innominate artery-to-pulmonary shunt (or RV-to-pulmonary artery shunt) is eliminated during the same operation.

The third stage of surgical palliation, known as the *Fontan procedure*, completes the separation of the systemic and pulmonary circulations and is performed between 18 months and 3 years of age, or when the patient experiences increased cyanosis (i.e., has outgrown the capacity to perfuse the systemic circulation with adequately oxygenated blood) from inadequate flow through their superior cavopulmonary anastomosis. (See Schwartz 9th ed., pp 611-612.)

19. The best initial treatment of D-transposition of the great arteries (D-TGA) in a 6-month-old child is
    A. Atrial septectomy
    B. Atrial septectomy and PA banding
    C. Senning procedure (atrial repair)
    D. Arterial switch

Answer: B

Complete transposition is characterized by connection of the atria to their appropriate ventricles with inappropriate ventriculoarterial connections. Thus, the aorta arises anteriorly from the RV, while the PA arises posteriorly from the LV. Van Praagh and coworkers introduced the term *D-transposition of the great arteries* (D-TGA) to describe this defect, while L-TGA describes a form of corrected transposition where there is concomitant [atrioventricular] discordance.

Blalock and Hanlon introduced the first operative intervention for D-TGA with the creation of an atrial septectomy to enhance intracardiac mixing. Later, Rashkind and Cuaso developed a catheter-based balloon septostomy, which largely obviated the need for open septectomy. These early palliative maneuvers, however, met with limited success, and it was not until the late 1950s, when Senning and Mustard developed the first "atrial repair," that outcomes improved. The Senning operation consisted of rerouting venous flow at the atrial level by incising and realigning the atrial septum over the pulmonary veins and using the right atrial free wall to create a pulmonary venous baffle (Fig. 20-1). Although the Mustard repair was similar, it made use of either autologous pericardium or synthetic material to create an intraatrial baffle. (See Schwartz 9th ed., pp 614-615.)

Despite the improved early survival rates, long-term problems, such as [systemic venous or pulmonary venous obstruction], baffle leak, arrhythmias, tricuspid valve regurgitation, and right ventricular failure, prompted the development of the arterial switch procedure by Jatene in 1975. The arterial switch procedure involves the division of the aorta and the PA, posterior translocation of the aorta (Lecompte maneuver), mobilization of the coronary arteries, placement of a pantaloon shaped pericardial patch, and proper alignment of the coronary arteries on the neoaorta. [The arterial switch operation is now the standard of care for neonates with transposition and coronary artery morphology amenable to transfer].

The most important consideration is the timing of surgical repair, because the arterial switch should be performed within 2 weeks after birth, before the LV loses its ability to pump against systemic afterload. In patients presenting later than 2 weeks, the LV can be retrained with preliminary PA banding and aortopulmonary shunt followed by definitive repair. (See Schwartz 9th ed., p 615.)

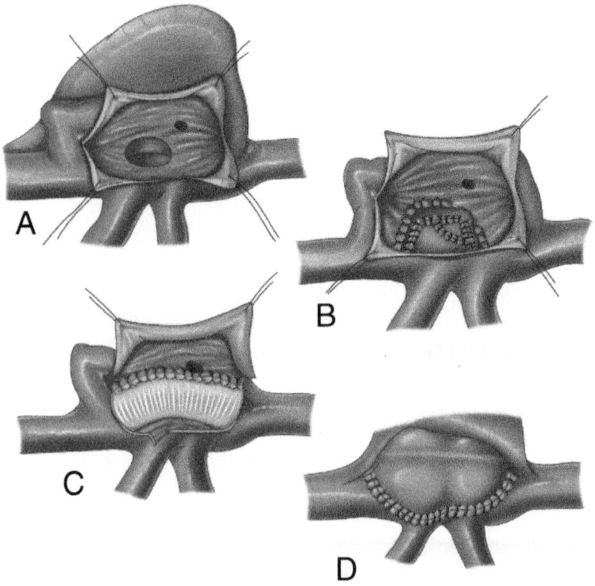

FIG. 20-1. The Senning operation. A. The atrial septum is cut near the tricuspid valve, creating a flap attached posteriorly between the caval veins. B. The flap of atrial septum is sutured to the anterior lip of the orifices of the left pulmonary veins, effectively separating the pulmonary and systemic venous channels. C. The posterior edge of the right atrial incision is sutured to the remnant of the atrial septum, diverting the systemic venous channel to the mitral valve. D. The anterior edge of the right atrial incision (lengthened by short incisions at each corner) is sutured around the cava above and below to the lateral edge of the LA incision, completing the pulmonary channel and diversion of pulmonary venous blood to the tricuspid valve area. (Reproduced with permission from D-Transposition of the great arteries, in Mavroudis C, Backer CL (eds): *Pediatric Cardiac Surgery*, 2nd ed. St. Louis: Mosby, 1994, p 345.)

20. Which of the following is NOT one of the four anomalies found in the Tetralogy of Fallot?
    A. Atrial septal defect (ASD)
    B. Overriding aorta
    C. Right ventricular outflow obstruction
    D. Right ventricular hypertrophy

Answer: A

The original description of TOF by Ettienne Louis Fallot, as the name implies, included four abnormalities: a large perimembranous VSD adjacent to the tricuspid valve; an overriding aorta; a variable degree of RVOT obstruction, which might include hypoplasia and dysplasia of the pulmonary valve as well as obstruction at the subvalvular and PA level; and right ventricular hypertrophy. More recently, Van Praagh and colleagues pointed out that TOF could be more correctly termed *monology of Fallot*, because the four components are explained by the malposition of the infundibular septum. When the infundibular septum is displaced anteriorly and leftward, the RVOT is narrowed and its anterior displacement results in failure of fusion of the ventricular septum between the arms of the trabecula-septomarginalis. (See Schwartz 9th ed., pp 617-618.)

21. The most significant late complication in patients who have had repair of a Tetralogy of Fallot is
    A. Arrhythmias
    B. Myocardial ischemia or infarction
    C. Ventricular aneurysm
    D. Brain abscess

Answer: A

Arrhythmias are potentially the most serious late complication following TOF repair. In a multicenter cohort of 793 patients studied by Gatzoulis and colleagues, a steady increase was documented in the prevalence of ventricular and atrial tachyarrhythmia and sudden cardiac death in the first 5 to 10 years following intracardiac repair. Clinical events were reported in 12% of patients at 35 years after repair. Prevalence of atrial arrhythmias from other studies, however, ranges from 1 to 11%, which is a reflection of the strong time dependence of arrhythmia onset.

Underlying causes of arrhythmia following repair are complex and multifactorial, resulting in poorly defined optimum screening and treatment algorithms. Older repair age has been associated with an increased frequency of both atrial and ventricular arrhythmias. Impaired ventricular function secondary to a protracted period of cyanosis before repair might contribute to the propensity for arrhythmia in older patients. (See Schwartz 9th ed., p 619.)

22. What is the probability of spontaneous closure for a VSD diagnosed in the 1st week of life?
    A. 10%
    B. 32%
    C. 65%
    D. 80%

Answer: D

VSDs may close or narrow spontaneously, and the probability of closure is inversely related to the age at which the defect is observed. Thus, infants at 1 month of age have an 80% incidence of spontaneous closure, whereas a child at 12 months of age has only a 25% chance of closure. This has an important impact on operative decision making, because a small or moderate-size VSD may be observed for a period of time in the absence of symptoms. Large defects and those in severely symptomatic neonates should be repaired during infancy to relieve symptoms and because irreversible changes in PVR may develop during the first year of life. (See Schwartz 9th ed., p 621.)

23. The Ross procedure is used to treat
    A. Mitral insufficiency
    B. Aortic stenosis
    C. Coarctation of the aorta
    D. Patent ductus arteriosus

Answer: B

The use of allografts and the advent of the Ross procedure have made early definitive correction of critical [aortic stenosis] a viable option. Donald Ross first described transposition of the pulmonary valve into the aortic position with allograft reconstruction of the pulmonary outflow tract in 1967. The result of this operation is a normal trileaflet semilunar valve made of a patient's native tissue with the potential for growth to adult size in the aortic position in place of the damaged aortic valve. The Ross procedure has become a useful option for aortic valve replacement in children, because it has improved durability and can be performed with acceptable morbidity and mortality rates. The placement of a pulmonary conduit, which does not grow and becomes calcified and [either insufficient or] stenotic over time, does obligate the patient to reoperation to replace the right-ventricle to [pulmonary artery] conduit. [However, the advent of percutaneously placed pulmonary valves may obviate the need for surgical intervention]. (See Schwartz 9th ed., p 596.)

CHAPTER 21

Acquired Heart Disease

BASIC SCIENCE QUESTIONS

1. Which of the following is the primary physiologic change in patients with heart failure?
   A. Elevated left atrial (LA) end-diastolic pressure
   B. Elevated LA end-systolic pressure
   C. Elevated left ventricular (LV) end-diastolic pressure
   D. Elevated LV end-systolic pressure

Answer: C

The physiologic change in most patients with heart failure is a rise in LV end-diastolic pressure, followed by cardiac enlargement. While Starling's law describes the compensatory mechanism of the heart of increased work in response to increased diastolic fiber length, symptoms develop as this compensatory mechanism fails, resulting in a progressive rise in LV end-diastolic pressure. (See Schwartz 9th ed., p 628.)

2. The arterioventricular (AV) node is supplied by the right coronary artery in what percentage of patients?
   A. 5%
   B. 20%
   C. 45%
   D. 80%

Answer: D

The left coronary system supplies the major portion of the left ventricular (LV) myocardium through the left main, left anterior descending, and circumflex coronary arteries. The right coronary artery supplies the right ventricle, and the posterior descending artery supplies the inferior wall of the left ventricle. The AV nodal artery arises from the right coronary artery in 80 to 85% of patients, termed *right dominant circulation*. In 15 to 20% of cases, the circumflex branch of the left coronary system supplies the posterior descending branch and the AV nodal artery, termed *left dominant*, while 5% are codominant. (See Schwartz 9th ed., p 631.)

CLINICAL QUESTIONS

1. Classic angina occurs in what percentage of patients with coronary artery disease?
   A. 40%
   B. 56%
   C. 75%
   D. 90%

Answer: C

Classic angina is precordial pain described as squeezing, heavy, or burning in nature, lasting from 2 to 10 minutes. The pain is usually substernal, radiating into the left shoulder and arm, but occasionally occurs in the midepigastrium, jaw, right arm, or midscapular region. Angina usually is provoked by exercise, emotion, sexual activity, or eating, and is relieved by rest or nitroglycerin. Angina is present in its classic form in 75% of patients with coronary disease, while atypical symptoms occur in 25% of patients and more frequently in women. (See Schwartz 9th ed., p 628.)

2. Dyspnea is an early symptom in which of the following conditions?
   A. Mitral stenosis
   B. Mitral insufficiency
   C. Aortic stenosis
   D. Aortic insufficiency

Answer: A

Dyspnea may appear as an early sign in patients with mitral stenosis due to restriction of flow from the left atrium into the left ventricle. However, with other forms of heart disease, dyspnea is a late sign, as it develops only after the left ventricle has failed and the end-diastolic pressure rises significantly.

Dyspnea associated with mitral insufficiency, aortic valve disease, or coronary disease represents relatively advanced pathophysiology. (See Schwartz 9th ed., p 628.)

The main symptoms of mitral stenosis are exertional dyspnea and decreased exercise capacity. Dyspnea occurs when the left atrial pressure becomes elevated due to the stenotic valve, resulting in pulmonary congestion. Orthopnea and paroxysmal nocturnal dyspnea may also occur, or in advanced cases, hemoptysis. (See Schwartz 9th ed., p 641.)

3. The most common cause of aortic stenosis is
   A. Congenital
   B. Acquired calcific disease
   C. Bicuspid aortic valve
   D. Rheumatic disease

Answer: B

In the adult North American population, the primary causes of aortic stenosis include acquired calcific disease, bicuspid aortic valve, and rheumatic disease. Acquired calcific aortic stenosis typically occurs in the seventh or eighth decade of life, and is the most frequent etiology, accounting for over half of the cases. Acquired calcific stenosis, also termed *degenerative aortic stenosis* or *senile aortic stenosis*, appears to be related to the aging process, with progressive degeneration leading to valve damage and calcification, although a causative role of lipids has been demonstrated recently. Lipid-lowering drugs seem to slow the progression of acquired calcific stenosis. Bicuspid aortic valve accounts for approximately one third of the cases of aortic stenosis in adults, typically presenting in the fourth or fifth decade of life, after years of turbulent flow through the bicuspid valve result in damage and calcification.

The third major cause of aortic stenosis, rheumatic heart disease, accounts for approximately 10 to 15% of patients in North America, but is more common in underdeveloped countries. With rheumatic disease, the degree of stenosis progresses with time. Concomitant MV disease almost always is present, although not always clinically significant. (See Schwartz 9th ed., p 647.)

4. Which of the following statements about thallium stress tests is FALSE?
   A. A reversible defect on a thallium scan indicates a well-healed area of previous infarction
   B. Initial uptake of thallium is dependent on myocardial perfusion
   C. Delayed uptake of thallium is dependent on myocardial viability
   D. The dipyridamole thallium study should be used in patients who cannot exercise

Answer: A

Currently the most widely used myocardial perfusion screening study is the thallium scan, which uses the nuclide thallium-201. Initial uptake of thallium-201 into myocardial cells is dependent upon myocardial perfusion, while delayed uptake depends on myocardial viability. Thus, reversible defects occur in underperfused, ischemic, but viable zones, while fixed defects occur in areas of infarction. Fixed defects on the thallium scan suggest nonviable myocardium and may be of prognostic value. The exercise thallium test is widely used to identify inducible areas of ischemia and is 95% sensitive in detecting multivessel coronary disease. This is the best overall test to detect myocardial ischemia, but requires the patient to exercise on the treadmill. The study also gives excellent, specific information about the patient's cardiac functional status. The dipyridamole thallium study is a provocative study using IV dipyridamole, which induces vasodilation and consequently unmasks myocardial ischemia in response to stress. This is the most widely used provocative study for risk stratification for patients who cannot exercise. In patients undergoing noncardiac surgery, the predictive value of a positive dipyridamole thallium study is 5 to 20% for MI or death, while a negative study is 99 to 100% predictive that a cardiac event will not occur. It is, therefore, a very effective screening study for moderate- to high-risk patients who require a general surgery procedure. (See Schwartz 9th ed., p 630.)

5. Which of the following is commonly seen in patients with chronic pericarditis?
   A. Dyspnea at rest
   B. Ascites
   C. Chest pain
   D. Cough

Answer: B

The pathophysiology of this disease remains the limitation of diastolic filling of the ventricles. This results in a decrease in cardiac output from a decrease in stroke volume. The right ventricular diastolic pressure is increased, with a corresponding increase in right atrial and central venous pressure ranging from 10 to 30 mmHg. This venous hypertension may produce hepatomegaly, ascites, peripheral edema, and a generalized increase in blood volume. The disease is slowly progressive with increasing ascites and edema. Fatigability and dyspnea on exertion are common, but dyspnea at rest is unusual. The ascites often is severe, and the diagnosis is easily confused with cirrhosis. Hepatomegaly and ascites often are the most prominent physical abnormalities. Peripheral edema is moderate in some patients, but severe in others. These findings are manifestations of advanced congestive failure from any form of heart disease. With constrictive pericarditis, however, the usual cardiac findings are a heart of normal size without murmurs or abnormal sounds. Atrial fibrillation is present in about one third of the patients, and a pleural effusion is common in more severe cases. A paradoxical pulse is found in a small proportion of patients. (See Schwartz 9th ed., pp 659-660.)

6. A patient who develops angina after walking one city block has
   A. Canadian Cardiovascular Society Class I angina
   B. Canadian Cardiovascular Society Class II angina
   C. Canadian Cardiovascular Society Class III angina
   D. Canadian Cardiovascular Society Class IV angina

Answer: C

(See Schwartz 9th ed., p 629, and Table 21-1.)

TABLE 21-1	Canadian Cardiovascular Society angina classification
Class I: Ordinary physical activity, such as walking or climbing stairs, does not cause angina. Angina may occur with strenuous or rapid or prolonged exertion at work or recreation.	
Class II: There is slight limitation of ordinary activity. Angina may occur with walking or climbing stairs rapidly, walking uphill, walking or stair climbing after meals or in the cold, in the wind, or under emotional stress, or walking more than two blocks on the level, or climbing more than one flight of stairs under normal conditions at a normal pace.	
Class III: There is marked limitation of ordinary physical activity. Angina may occur after walking one or more blocks on the level or climbing one flight of stairs under normal conditions at a normal pace.	
Class IV: There is inability to carry on any physical activity without discomfort; angina may be present at rest.	

7. Which of the following is the most common primary cardiac tumor?
   A. Myxoma
   B. Angiosarcoma
   C. Fibroma
   D. Fibrosarcoma

Answer: A

Primary cardiac neoplasms are rare, reported to occur with incidences ranging from 0.001 to 0.3% in autopsy series. Benign tumors account for 75% of primary neoplasms and malignant tumors account for 25%. The most frequent primary cardiac neoplasm is myxoma, comprising 30 to 50%. Other benign neoplasms, in decreasing order of occurrence, include lipoma, papillary fibroelastoma, rhabdomyoma, fibroma, hemangioma, teratoma, lymphangioma, and others. Most primary malignant neoplasms are sarcomas (angiosarcoma, rhabdomyosarcoma, fibrosarcoma, leiomyosarcoma, and liposarcoma), with malignant lymphomas accounting for 1 to 2%. (See Schwartz 9th ed., p 660.)

8. The differential diagnosis of syncope includes all of the following EXCEPT
   A. Aortic stenosis
   B. Hypertrophic cardiomyopathy
   C. Tricuspid insufficiency
   D. Vasovagal reaction

Answer: C
Syncope, or sudden loss of consciousness, is usually a result of sudden decreased perfusion of the brain. The differential diagnosis includes: (a) third-degree heart block with bradycardia or asystole, (b) malignant ventricular tachyarrhythmias or ventricular fibrillation, (c) aortic stenosis, (d) hypertrophic cardiomyopathy, (e) carotid artery disease, (f) seizure disorders, and (g) vasovagal reaction. Any episode of syncope must be evaluated thoroughly, as many of these conditions can result in sudden death. (See Schwartz 9th ed., p 629.)

9. Which of the following symptoms is a LATE symptom of chronic, untreated mitral insufficiency?
   A. Atrial flutter
   B. Pulmonary edema
   C. Decreased LV ejection fraction
   D. Decreased LA stroke volume

Answer: C
The basic physiologic abnormality in patients with mitral insufficiency is regurgitation of a portion of the LV stroke volume into the left atrium. This results in decreased forward blood flow and an elevated left atrial pressure, producing pulmonary congestion and volume overload of the left ventricle. As mitral insufficiency progresses, there is a corresponding increase in the size of the left atrium, and eventually, atrial fibrillation results. Concurrently, the left ventricle dilates. Initially the LV stroke volume increases by Starling's law, but eventually, this compensatory mechanism fails, and the ejection fraction decreases. However, decreased systolic function of the heart is a relatively late finding, because the ventricle is "unloaded" as a result of the valvular insufficiency. Once LV dysfunction and heart failure develop, the left ventricle usually has been significantly and often irreversibly injured. (See Schwartz 9th ed., p 642.)

10. Indications for aortic valve replacement in a patient with aortic stenosis include
   A. Any LV dysfunction
   B. Progressive pulmonary hypertension
   C. Right ventricular dysfunction during exercise
   D. All of the above

Answer: D
Aortic valve replacement is indicated for virtually all symptomatic patients with aortic stenosis. Even in patients with NYHA class IV symptoms and poor ventricular function, surgery has been found to improve both functional status and survival. In asymptomatic patients with moderate to severe stenosis, periodic echocardiographic studies are performed to assess the transvalvular gradient, valve area, LV size, and LV function. Surgery is indicated with the first sign of LV systolic dysfunction, manifest on echocardiography as either a rise in the LV end-systolic size or a drop in the LVEF. Surgery also may be recommended for asymptomatic patients with aortic stenosis who have a progressive increase in the transvalvular gradient on serial echocardiographic studies, a rapid rise in diastolic dimensions, a valve area $<0.80\ cm^2$, progressive pulmonary hypertension, or right ventricular dysfunction during exercise testing. (See Schwartz 9th ed., p 648.)

11. Which of the following is NOT a risk factor for coronary artery disease?
   A. Elevated serum homocysteine
   B. Female gender
   C. Elevated lipoprotein (a)
   D. Sedentary lifestyle

Answer: B
The etiology of CAD is primarily atherosclerosis. The disease is multifactorial, with the primary risk factors being hyperlipidemia, smoking, diabetes, hypertension, obesity, sedentary lifestyle, and male gender. Newly identified risk factors include elevated levels of C-reactive protein, lipoprotein (a), and homocysteine. (See Schwartz 9th ed., p 633.)

12. The most common cause of mitral valve stenosis is
   A. Coronary artery disease
   B. Congenital stenosis
   C. Bacterial endocarditis
   D. Rheumatic heart disease

Answer: D
MV stenosis or mixed mitral stenosis and insufficiency almost always are caused by rheumatic heart disease, although a definite clinical history can be obtained in only 50% of patients. (See Schwartz 9th ed., p 640.)

13. In the Ross procedure, the aortic valve is replaced with
    A. A bileaflet mechanical valve
    B. A stented porcine tissue valve
    C. An unstented bovine tissue valve
    D. The patient's pulmonary valve

Answer: D
The Ross procedure involves replacement of the aortic valve with an autograft from the patient's native pulmonary valve. The resected pulmonary valve is then replaced with a pulmonary homograft. (See Schwartz 9th ed., p 652.)

14. A patient with cardiac disease who is comfortable at rest but experiences angina if he walks 2 to 3 city blocks has
    A. New York Heart Association Class 1 disease
    B. New York Heart Association Class 2 disease
    C. New York Heart Association Class 3 disease
    D. New York Heart Association Class 4 disease

Answer: B
See Table 21-2. An important part of the history is the assessment of the patient's overall cardiac functional disability, which is a good approximation of the severity of the patient's underlying disease. The New York Heart Association (NYHA) has developed a classification of patients with heart disease based on symptoms and functional disability (Table 21-2). The NYHA classification has been extremely useful in evaluating a patient's severity of disability, in comparing treatment regimens, and in predicting operative risk. (See Schwartz 9th ed., p 629.)

TABLE 21-2 New York Heart Association functional classification
Class I: Patients with cardiac disease but without resulting limitation of physical activity. Ordinary physical activity does not cause undue fatigue, palpitation, dyspnea, or angina pain.
Class II: Patients with cardiac disease resulting in slight limitation of physical activity. They are comfortable at rest. Ordinary physical activity results in fatigue, palpitation, dyspnea, or angina pain.
Class III: Patients with cardiac disease resulting in marked limitation of physical activity. They are comfortable at rest. Less than ordinary physical activity causes fatigue, palpitation, dyspnea, or angina pain.
Class IV: Patients with cardiac disease resulting in an inability to carry on any physical activity without discomfort. Symptoms of cardiac insufficiency or of the anginal syndrome may be present even at rest. If any physical activity is undertaken, discomfort is increased.

15. Which of the following patients is most likely to benefit from coronary artery bypass?
    A. Patients with CCS class I angina and double-vessel disease
    B. Patients with single-vessel proximal right coronary artery disease and congestive heart failure
    C. Patients with CCS class I angina and diabetes
    D. Patients with CCS class II angina with hypertension

Answer: C
In some patients with chronic angina, CABG is associated with improved survival and improved complication-free survival when compared to medical management. In general, patients with more severe angina (CCS class III or IV symptoms) are most likely to benefit from bypass. For patients with less severe angina (CCS class I or II), other factors, such as the anatomic distribution of disease (left main coronary disease or triple-vessel) and the degree of LV dysfunction, are used to determine which patients will most benefit from surgical revascularization.

To summarize, although medical therapy may be appropriate for many patients with chronic stable angina, bypass surgery is indicated for most patients with multivessel disease and CCS class III or IV symptoms. In patients with milder (CCS class I or II) symptoms, surgery results in improved survival in those with left main stenosis and those with triple-vessel disease and depressed LV function or diabetes. (See Schwartz 9th ed., p 634.)

16. Which of the following is an indication for surgical repair or replacement of the mitral valve in a patient with mitral insufficiency?
    A. Abnormal exercise testing
    B. Recent onset of atrial fibrillation
    C. Any symptom, even if LV function is normal
    D. All of the above

Answer: D
According to the American College of Cardiology/American Heart Association guidelines, MV repair or replacement is recommended in any symptomatic patient with mitral insufficiency, even with normal LV function (defined as ejection fraction >60% and end-systolic dimension <45 mm). Surgery also is currently recommended in asymptomatic patients with severe mitral

insufficiency if there are signs of LV systolic dysfunction (increased end-systolic dimension or decreased ejection fraction). Recent onset of atrial fibrillation, pulmonary hypertension, or an abnormal response to exercise testing are considered relative indications for surgery. (See Schwartz 9th ed., p 643.)

17. Cardiac myxomas are most commonly found in the
    A. Right atrium
    B. Right ventricle
    C. Left atrium
    D. Left ventricle

Answer: C
Sixty to 75% of cardiac myxomas develop in the left atrium, almost always from the atrial septum near the fossa ovalis. Most other myxomas develop in the right atrium; <20 have been reported in the right or left ventricle. (See Schwartz 9th ed., p 660.)

18. Which of the following is NOT a clinical marker of increased risk for a patient undergoing a general surgical procedure?
    A. Prior stroke
    B. Advanced age
    C. Hypertension (controlled on medication)
    D. Atrial fibrillation

Answer: C
Cardiac risk stratification for patients undergoing noncardiac surgery is a critical part of the preoperative evaluation of the general surgery patient. The joint American College of Cardiology/American Heart Association task force, chaired by Eagle, recently reported guidelines and recommendations, which are summarized in this section. In general, the preoperative cardiovascular evaluation involves an assessment of clinical markers, the patient's underlying functional capacity, and various surgery-specific risk factors.

The *clinical markers* that predict an increased risk of a cardiac event during noncardiac surgery are divided into three grades. *Major* predictors include unstable coronary syndromes, including acute or recent MI and unstable angina (CCS class III or IV), decompensated heart failure (NYHA class IV), and significant arrhythmias and severe valvular disease. *Intermediate* predictors are mild angina (CCS class I or II), old MI, compensated heart failure (NYHA class II and III), diabetes, and renal insufficiency. *Mild* predictors are advanced age, uncontrolled systemic hypertension, irregular rhythm, prior stroke, abnormal electrocardiogram (ECG), and mild functional disability. (See Schwartz 9th ed., p 629.)

19. When compared to percutaneous coronary intervention, coronary artery bypass
    A. Is less expensive
    B. Provides a more complete relief of angina
    C. Has a higher mortality rate
    D. Has a lower morbidity rate

Answer: B
When comparing CABG to PCI for the treatment of patients with CAD, results demonstrate that with appropriate patient selection both procedures are safe and effective, with little difference in mortality. PCI is associated with less short-term morbidity, decreased cost, and shorter hospital stay, but requires more late reinterventions. CABG provides more complete relief of angina, requires fewer reinterventions, and is more durable. Additionally, CABG appears to offer a survival advantage in diabetic patients with multivessel disease. (See Schwartz 9th ed., p 634.)

20. Which of the following does NOT increase operative risk for patients undergoing coronary artery bypass?
    A. Female gender
    B. NYHA class II functional status
    C. Hypertension
    D. Large body surface area

Answer: B
Variables that have been identified as influencing operative risk according to STS risk modeling include: female gender, age, race, body surface area, NYHA class IV status, low ejection fraction, hypertension, PVD, prior stroke, diabetes, renal failure, chronic obstructive pulmonary disease, immunosuppressive therapy, prior cardiac surgery, recent MI, urgent or emergent presentation, cardiogenic shock, left main coronary disease, and concomitant valvular disease. (See Schwartz 9th ed., p 636.)

CHAPTER 22

Thoracic Aneurysms and Aortic Dissection

BASIC SCIENCE QUESTIONS

1. A mutation in the fibrillin gene is associated with which of the following?
   A. Ehlers-Danlos syndrome
   B. Marfan syndrome
   C. Loeys-Dietz syndrome
   D. Congenital bicuspid aortic valve

Answer: B

Marfan syndrome is an autosomal dominant genetic disorder characterized by a specific connective tissue defect that leads to aneurysm formation. The phenotype of patients with Marfan syndrome typically includes a tall stature, high palate, joint hypermobility, eye lens dislocation, mitral valve prolapse, and aortic aneurysms. The aortic wall is weakened by fragmentation of elastic fibers and deposition of extensive amounts of mucopolysaccharides (a process previously called *cystic medial degeneration*). Patients with Marfan syndrome have a mutation in the fibrillin gene located on the long arm of chromosome 15.

Vascular type Ehlers-Danlos syndrome is characterized by an autosomal dominant defect in type III collagen synthesis.

Recently described, Loeys-Dietz syndrome is phenotypically distinct from Marfan syndrome. It is characterized as an aneurysmal syndrome with widespread systemic involvement. Loeys-Dietz syndrome is an aggressive, autosomal dominant condition that is distinguished by the triad of arterial tortuosity and aneurysms, hypertelorism (widely spaced eyes), and bifid uvula or cleft palate. It is caused by heterozygous mutations in the genes encoding TGF-β receptors, rather than fibrillin 1.

Bicuspid aortic valve is the most common congenital malformation of the heart or great vessels, affecting up to 2% of Americans. Compared to patients with normal, trileaflet aortic valves, patients with bicuspid aortic valves have an increased incidence of ascending aortic aneurysm formation and, often, a more rapid rate of aortic enlargement. The exact mechanism responsible for aneurysm formation in patients with bicuspid aortic valves remains controversial. The two most popular theories posit that the dilatation is caused by (a) a congenital defect involving the aortic wall matrix that results in progressive degeneration, or (b) ongoing hemodynamic stress caused by turbulent flow through the diseased valve. It is likely that both proposed mechanisms are involved: patients with bicuspid aortic valves may have a congenital connective tissue abnormality that predisposes the aorta to aneurysm formation, especially in the presence of chronic turbulent flow through a deformed valve. (See Schwartz 9th ed., pp 667-668.)

2. Elastin levels are highest in the wall of the
   A. Ascending thoracic aorta
   B. Aortic arch
   C. Descending thoracic aorta
   D. Abdominal aorta

Answer: A
The normal aorta derives its elasticity from the medial layer, which contains approximately 45 to 55 lamellae of elastin, collagen, smooth muscle cells, and ground substance. Elastin content is highest within the ascending aorta, as would be expected because of its compliant nature, and decreases distally into the descending and abdominal aorta. Maintenance of the aortic matrix involves complex interactions among smooth muscle cells, macrophages, proteases, and protease inhibitors. Any alteration in this delicate balance can lead to aortic disease. (See Schwartz 9th ed., p 667.)

CLINICAL QUESTIONS

1. Which of the following is a common cause of mycotic thoracic aortic aneurysms?
   A. *Candida glabrata*
   B. *Staphylococcus aureus*
   C. *Aspergillus clavatus*
   D. *Stenotrophomonas maltophilia*

Answer: B
Primary infection of the aortic wall resulting in aneurysm formation is rare. Although these lesions are termed *mycotic aneurysms*, the responsible pathogens usually are bacteria rather than fungi. Bacterial invasion of the aortic wall may result from bacterial endocarditis, endothelial trauma caused by an aortic jet lesion, or extension from an infected laminar clot within a pre-existing aneurysm. The most common causative organisms are *Staphylococcus aureus*, *Staphylococcus epidermidis*, *Salmonella*, and *Streptococcus*. Unlike most other causes of thoracic aortic aneurysms, which generally produce fusiform aneurysms, infection often produces saccular aneurysms located in areas of aortic tissue destroyed by the infectious process. (See Schwartz 9th ed., p 668.)

2. Which of the following is NOT a cause of thoracic aortic aneurysms?
   A. Marfan syndrome
   B. Osteogenesis imperfecta
   C. Ehlers-Danlos syndrome
   D. Takayasu's arteritis

Answer: B
See Table 22-1. Osteogenesis imperfecta is not associated with an increased risk of aortic aneurysm. (See Schwartz 9th ed., p 667.)

TABLE 22-1 Causes of thoracic aortic aneurysms
Nonspecific medial degeneration
Aortic dissection
Genetic disorders
Marfan syndrome
Loeys-Dietz syndrome
Ehlers-Danlos syndrome
Familial aortic aneurysms
Congenital bicuspid aortic valve
Poststenotic dilatation
Infection
Aortitis
Takayasu's arteritis
Giant cell arteritis
Rheumatoid aortitis
Trauma

3. Patients with which of the following should undergo elective surgical repair of their condition?
   A. 5-cm ascending aortic aneurysm
   B. 5-cm descending aortic aneurysm
   C. 5-cm ascending aortic aneurysm in a patient with Marfan syndrome
   D. Any aneurysm that has grown 0.5 cm in diameter in 1 year

Answer: C
Thoracic aortic aneurysms are repaired to prevent fatal rupture. Therefore, on the basis of the natural history studies discussed earlier, elective operation is recommended when the diameter of an ascending aortic aneurysm is >5.5 cm, when the diameter of a descending thoracic aortic aneurysm is >6.5 cm, or when the rate of dilatation is >1 cm/y. In patients with connective tissue disorders, such as Marfan and Loeys-Dietz syndromes, the threshold for operation is lower with regard to both absolute size (5.0 cm for the ascending aorta and

6.0 cm for the descending thoracic aorta) and rate of growth. Smaller ascending aortic aneurysms (4.0 to 5.5 cm) also are considered for repair when they are associated with significant aortic valve regurgitation. (See Schwartz 9th ed., p 671.)

4. Which of the following is NOT used to protect perfusion to the spinal cord during open repair of descending thoracic and thoracoabdominal aortic aneurysms?
   A. Permissive mild hypothermia (32–34°C)
   B. Left heart bypass
   C. Reattachment of intercostal arteries
   D. Perfusion of intercostal or lumbar arteries with 4°C cystalloid solution

Answer: D

Clamping the descending thoracic aorta causes ischemia of the spinal cord and abdominal viscera. Clinically significant manifestations of hepatic, pancreatic, and bowel ischemia are relatively uncommon. However, both acute renal failure and spinal cord injury resulting in paraplegia or paraparesis remain major causes of morbidity and mortality after these operations. Therefore, several aspects of the operation are devoted to minimizing spinal and renal ischemia (Table 22-2). Our multimodal approach to spinal cord protection includes expeditious repair to minimize aortic clamping time, moderate systemic heparinization (1.0 mg/kg) to prevent small-vessel thrombosis, mild permissive hypothermia [32° to 34°C (89.6° to 93.2°F)] nasopharyngeal temperature], and reattachment of segmental intercostal and lumbar arteries. (See Schwartz 9th ed., p 678.)

Left heart bypass, which provides perfusion of the distal aorta and its branches during the clamping period, is also used during extensive thoracoabdominal aortic repairs. Because left heart bypass unloads the heart, it is also useful in patients with poor cardiac reserve. Balloon perfusion cannulas connected to the left heart bypass circuit can be used to deliver blood directly to the celiac axis and superior mesenteric artery during their reattachment. The potential benefits of reducing hepatic and bowel ischemia include reduced risks of postoperative coagulopathy and bacterial translocation, respectively. Whenever possible, renal protection is achieved by perfusing the kidneys with cold [4°C (39.2°F)] crystalloid. In a randomized clinical trial, reduced kidney temperature was found to be associated with renal protection, and the use of cold crystalloid independently predicted preserved renal function. (See Schwartz 9th ed., p 679.)

TABLE 22-2	Current strategy for spinal cord and visceral protection during repair of distal thoracic aortic aneurysms

All extents
- Permissive mild hypothermia [32–34°C (89.6–93.2°F), nasopharyngeal]
- Moderate heparinization (1 mg/kg)
- Aggressive reattachment of segmental arteries, especially between T8 and L1
- Sequential aortic clamping when possible
- Perfusion of renal arteries with 4°C (39.2°F) crystalloid solution when possible

Crawford extent I and II thoracoabdominal repairs
- Cerebrospinal fluid drainage
- Left heart bypass during proximal anastomosis
- Selective perfusion of celiac axis and superior mesenteric artery during intercostal and visceral anastomoses

5. The most common symptom in a patient with an acute aortic dissection is
   A. Shortness of breath
   B. Pain
   C. Palpitations
   D. Syncope

Answer: B

The European Society of Cardiology Task Force on Aortic Dissection stated, 'The main challenge in managing acute aortic dissection is to suspect and thus diagnose the disease as early as possible.' A high index of suspicion is critical, particularly in younger, atypical patients, who may have connective tissue disorders or other, less common risk factors. Most patients with acute aortic dissection (80 to 90%) experience severe pain in the chest, back, or abdomen. The pain usually occurs suddenly, has a sharp or tearing quality, and often migrates distally as the dissection progresses along the aorta. For classification purposes (acute vs. subacute vs. chronic), the onset of pain is generally considered to represent the beginning of the dissection process. Most of the other common symptoms either are nonspecific or are caused by the secondary manifestations of dissection. (See Schwartz 9th ed., p 688.)

6. The acute phase of aortic dissection lasts for
   A. 48 hours
   B. 7 days
   C. 14 days
   D. 3 months

Answer: C

Aortic dissection also is categorized according to the time elapsed since the initial tear. Dissection is considered acute within the first 14 days after the initial tear; after 14 days, the dissection is considered chronic. Although arbitrary, the distinction between acute and chronic dissections has important implications not only for decision making about perioperative management strategies and operative techniques, but also for evaluating surgical results. In light of the importance of acuity, Borst and associates have proposed a third phase—termed *subacute*—to describe the transition between the acute and chronic phases. The subacute period encompasses days 15 through 60 after the initial tear. Although this is past the traditional 14-day acute phase, patients with subacute dissection continue to have extremely fragile aortic tissue, which may complicate operative treatment and increase the risks associated with surgery. (See Schwartz 9th ed., p 686.)

For classification purposes (acute vs. subacute vs. chronic), the onset of pain is generally considered to represent the beginning of the dissection process. (See Schwartz 9th ed., p 688.)

7. A patient with a thoracoabdominal aneurysm that involves the entire descending thoracic aorta and extends to the iliac arteries (involving the entire abdominal aorta) is a
   A. Crawford Extent I aneurysm
   B. Crawford Extent II aneurysm
   C. Crawford Extent III aneurysm
   D. Crawford Extent IV aneurysm

Answer: B

Thoracoabdominal aneurysms can involve the entire thoracoabdominal aorta, from the origin of the left subclavian artery to the aortic bifurcation, and are categorized according to the Crawford classification scheme (Fig. 22-1). Extent I thoracoabdominal aortic aneurysms involve most of the descending thoracic aorta, usually beginning near the left subclavian artery, and extend down to encompass the aorta at the origins of the celiac axis and superior mesenteric arteries. The renal arteries also may be involved. Extent II aneurysms also arise near the left subclavian artery but extend distally into the infrarenal abdominal aorta, and they often reach the aortic bifurcation. Extent III aneurysms originate in the lower descending thoracic aorta (below the sixth rib) and extend into the abdomen. Extent IV aneurysms begin within the diaphragmatic hiatus and often involve the entire abdominal aorta. (See Schwartz 9th ed., p 678.)

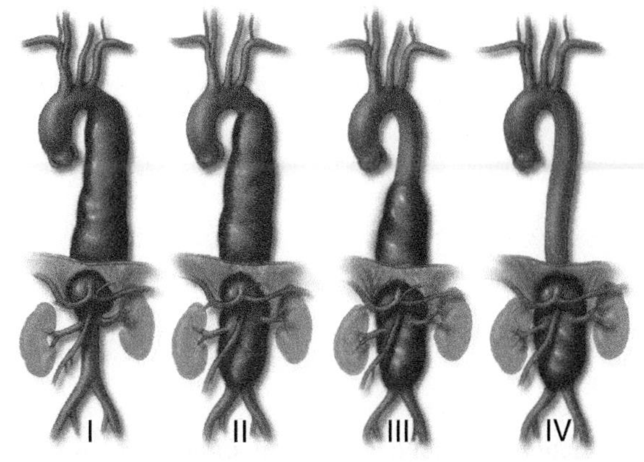

FIG. 22-1. Illustration of the Crawford classification of thoracoabdominal aortic aneurysms based on the extent of aortic involvement. (Reproduced with permission from Coselli JS, LeMaire SA: Descending and Thoracoabdominal Aortic Aneurysms, in Cohn LH (ed): *Cardiac Surgery in the Adult*, 3rd ed. New York: McGraw-Hill, Inc., 2008, Chap. 54, Fig. 54-5.)

8. The "critical diameter" (i.e., associated with a marked increase in risk of complications) for aneurysms of the descending thoracic aorta is
   A. 5 cm
   B. 6 cm
   C. 7 cm
   D. 8 cm

Answer: C

Treatment decisions in cases of thoracic aortic aneurysm are guided by our current understanding of the natural history of these aneurysms, which classically is characterized as progressive aortic dilatation and eventual dissection, rupture, or both. An analysis by Elefteriades of data from 1600 patients with thoracic aortic disease has helped quantify these well-recognized risks. Average expansion rates were 0.07 cm/y in ascending aortic aneurysms and 0.19 cm/y in descending thoracic aortic aneurysms. As expected, aortic diameter was a strong predictor of rupture, dissection, and mortality. For thoracic aortic aneurysms >6 cm in diameter, annual rates of catastrophic complications were 3.6% for rupture, 3.7% for dissection, and 10.8% for death. Critical diameters, at which the incidence of expected complications significantly increased, were 6.0 cm for aneurysms of the ascending aorta and 7.0 cm for aneurysms of the descending thoracic aorta; the corresponding risks of rupture after reaching these diameters were 31 and 43%, respectively. (See Schwartz 9th ed., p 669.)

9. Which of the following is used to protect the spinal cord during endovascular repair of descending thoracic aortic aneurysms?
   A. Heparinization (ACT >300 seconds)
   B. Hypothermia
   C. Spinal fluid drainage
   D. Trendelenburg position

Answer: C

To protect patients against spinal cord ischemia during these endovascular repairs, many surgeons use cerebrospinal fluid drainage. Fluid is drained to maintain a cerebrospinal fluid pressure of approximately 12 to 14 mmHg. (See Schwartz 9th ed., p 679.)

10. Which of the following is the most sensitive test for the diagnosis of an acute aortic dissection?
    A. EKG
    B. Chest x-ray
    C. Cardiac enzymes
    D. D-dimer

Answer: D

Several reports have demonstrated that D-dimer is an extremely sensitive indicator of acute aortic dissection; elevated levels are found in approximately 97% of affected patients. Tests that are commonly used to detect acute coronary events—including ECG and tests for serum markers of myocardial injury—deserve special consideration and need to be interpreted carefully. Normal ECGs and serum marker levels in patients with acute chest pain should raise suspicion about the possibility of aortic dissection. It is important to remember that ECG changes and elevated serum marker levels associated with myocardial infarction do not exclude the diagnosis of aortic dissection, because dissection can cause coronary malperfusion. Ultimately, although the issue has not been well studied, ECGs seem to have little utility for detecting or ruling out dissection. Similarly, although chest x-rays (CXRs) may show a widened mediastinum or abnormal aortic contour, up to 16% of patients with dissection have a normal appearing CXR. The value of the CXR for detecting aortic dissection is limited, with a sensitivity of 67% and a specificity of 86%. (See Schwartz 9th ed., pp 688-689.)

11. Which of the following in an indication for delayed (rather than emergent) repair of an acute ascending thoracic dissection?
    A. Recent (<3 weeks) cardiac surgery
    B. Evidence of acute myocardial infarction
    C. Mesenteric ischemia
    D. Marfan syndrome

Answer: C

In most patients with acute ascending aortic dissection, the risk of a fatal complication, such as aortic rupture, during medical management outweighs the risk associated with early operation. Therefore, acute ascending aortic dissection has traditionally been considered an absolute indication for emergency surgical repair. However, specific patient groups may benefit from nonoperative management or delayed operation. Delayed repair should be considered for patients who (a) present with acute stroke or mesenteric ischemia, (b) are elderly and have substantial comorbidity, (c) are in stable condition and may benefit from transfer to specialized centers, or (d) have undergone a cardiac operation in the remote past. Regarding the last group, it is important that the previous operation not be too recent; dissections that occur during the first 3 weeks after cardiac surgery pose a high risk of rupture and tamponade, and such dissections warrant early operation. (See Schwartz 9th ed., p 690.)

12. Which of the following is the imaging modality of choice for the diagnosis of thoracic aortic aneurysms?
    A. Plain radiograph of the chest
    B. Ultrasound
    C. CT scan
    D. Aortography

Answer: C

Computed tomographic (CT) scanning is widely available and provides visualization of the entire thoracic and abdominal aorta. Consequently, CT is the most common—and arguably the most useful—imaging modality for evaluating thoracic aortic aneurysm. Systems capable of constructing multiplanar images and performing three- dimensional aortic reconstructions are widely available. In addition to establishing the diagnosis, CT provides information about an aneurysm's location, extent, anatomic anomalies, and relationship to major branch vessels. CT is particularly useful in determining the absolute diameter of the aorta, especially in the presence of laminated clot. Contrast-enhanced CT provides information about the aortic lumen and can detect mural thrombus, aortic dissection, inflammatory periaortic fibrosis, and mediastinal or retroperitoneal hematoma due to contained aortic rupture.

Chest radiographs (CXRs) often appear normal in patients with thoracic aortic disease and thus cannot exclude the diagnosis of aortic aneurysm.

Although useful in evaluating infrarenal abdominal aortic aneurysms, standard transabdominal ultrasonography does not allow visualization of the thoracic aorta.

Although diagnostic aortography was, until recently, considered the gold standard for evaluating thoracic aortic disease, CT and MRA have largely replaced this modality. Technologic improvements have enabled CT and MRA to provide excellent aortic imaging while causing less morbidity than catheter-based studies do, so CT and MRA should now be considered the gold standard. Therefore, the role of diagnostic angiography in patients with thoracic aortic disease is currently limited. In selected cases, aortography is used to gain important information when other types of studies are contraindicated or have not provided satisfactory results. For example, information about obstructive lesions of the brachiocephalic, visceral, renal, or iliac arteries is useful when surgical treatment is being planned; if other imaging studies have not provided adequate detail, aortograms can be obtained in patients with suspected branch vessel occlusive disease. (See Schwartz 9th ed., pp 669-671.)

13. Which of the following is NOT a typical complication of an acute ascending aortic dissection?
    A. Myocardial infarction
    B. Pleural effusion
    C. Aortic valve regurgitation
    D. Pericardial effusion

Answer: B

Ascending aortic dissection can directly injure the aortic valve, causing regurgitation. The severity of the regurgitation varies with the degree of commissural disruption, which ranges from partial separation of only one commissure, producing mild valvular regurgitation, to full separation of all three commissures and complete prolapse of the valve into the left ventricle, producing severe acute heart failure.

Ascending dissections also can extend into the coronary arteries or shear the coronary ostia off of the true lumen, causing acute coronary occlusion; when this occurs, it most often involves the right coronary artery. The sudden disruption of coronary blood flow can cause a myocardial infarction.

The thin and inflamed outer wall of a dissected ascending aorta often produces a serosanguineous pericardial effusion that can accumulate and cause tamponade. Suggestive signs include jugular venous distention, muffled heart tones, pulsus paradoxus, and low voltage electrocardiogram (ECG) tracings. Free rupture into the pericardial space produces rapid tamponade and is generally fatal.

As the dissection progresses, any branch vessel from the aorta can become involved, which results in compromised blood flow and ischemic complications (i.e., *malperfusion*). Therefore, depending on which arteries are involved, the dissection can produce acute stroke, paraplegia, hepatic failure, bowel infarction, renal failure, or a threatened ischemic limb. (See Schwartz 9th ed., p 688, and Table 22-3.)

TABLE 22-3 Anatomic complications of aortic dissection and their associated symptoms and signs

Anatomic Manifestation	Symptoms and Signs
Aortic valve insufficiency	Dyspnea Murmur Pulmonary rales Shock
Coronary malperfusion	Chest pain with characteristics of angina Nausea, vomiting Shock Ischemic changes on electrocardiogram Elevated levels of cardiac enzymes
Pericardial tamponade	Dyspnea Jugular venous distention Pulsus paradoxus Muffled cardiac tones Shock Low-voltage electrocardiogram

(*continued*)

TABLE 22-3 (continued)

Anatomic Manifestation	Symptoms and Signs
Subclavian or iliofemoral artery malperfusion	Cold, painful extremity Extremity sensory and motor deficits Peripheral pulse deficit
Carotid artery malperfusion	Syncope Focal neurologic deficit (transient or persistent) Carotid pulse deficit Coma
Spinal malperfusion	Paraplegia Incontinence
Mesenteric malperfusion	Nausea, vomiting Abdominal pain
Renal malperfusion	Oliguria or anuria Hematuria

14. Which of the following is indicated in the initial treatment of a patient with an acute aortic dissection?
    A. Nitroprusside
    B. Labetalol
    C. Emergency catheterization and stenting of the aorta
    D. Emergency surgery to repair the aorta

Answer: B

The initial management strategy, commonly described as *antihypertensive therapy* or *blood pressure control*, focuses on reducing aortic wall stress, the force of left ventricular ejection, chronotropy, and the rate of change in blood pressure (dP/dT). Reductions in dP/dT are achieved by lowering both cardiac contractility and blood pressure. The drugs initially used to accomplish these goals include IV beta-adrenergic blockers, direct vasodilators, calcium channel blockers, and angiotensin-converting enzyme inhibitors. These agents are used to achieve a heart rate between 60 and 80 bpm, a systolic blood pressure between 100 and 110 mmHg, and a mean arterial blood pressure between 60 and 75 mmHg. These hemodynamic targets are maintained as long as urine output remains adequate and neurologic function is not impaired. Achieving adequate pain control with IV opiates, such as morphine and fentanyl, is important for maintaining acceptable blood pressure control.

Beta antagonists are administered to all patients with acute aortic dissections unless there are strong contraindications, such as severe heart failure, bradyarrhythmia, high-grade atrioventricular conduction block, or bronchospastic disease. Esmolol can be useful in patients with bronchospastic disease because it is a cardioselective, ultra-fast-acting agent with a short half-life. Labetalol, which causes both nonselective beta blockade and postsynaptic alpha$_1$-blockade, reduces systemic vascular resistance without impairing cardiac output. Doses of beta antagonists are titrated to achieve a heart rate of 60 to 80 bpm. In patients who cannot receive beta antagonists, calcium channel blockers such as diltiazem are an effective alternative. Nitroprusside, a direct vasodilator, can be administered once beta blockade is adequate. When used alone, however, nitroprusside can cause reflex increases in heart rate and contractility, elevated dP/dT, and progression of aortic dissection. Enalapril and other angiotensin-converting enzyme inhibitors are useful in patients with renal malperfusion. These drugs inhibit renin release, which may improve renal blood flow. (See Schwartz 9th ed., p 690.)

15. The imaging study of choice in a hemodynamically stable patient with a suspected acute thoracic aortic dissection is
    A. Transesophageal echocardiography
    B. CT scan
    C. Chest x-ray
    D. Aortography

Answer: B

Contrast-enhanced CT has a sensitivity of 98% and a specificity of 87% for diagnosis of aortic dissection. Although MRA is now considered the gold standard, with both a sensitivity and a specificity of 98%, CT scanning is the preferred imaging modality in the emergency department, mainly because of its swift image acquisition. In appropriate hands, TEE has a demonstrated sensitivity and specificity as high as 98 and 95%, respectively. Furthermore, TEE offers important information about ventricular function and aortic valve competency. Finally, TEE is the diagnostic modality of choice for hemodynamically unstable patients in whom the diagnosis of ascending dissection is suspected; ideally, these patients should be taken to the operating room, where the TEE can be performed and, if the TEE is confirmatory, surgery can be started immediately. (See Schwartz 9th ed., p 689.)

16. An aortic dissection that extends from the left subclavian artery to the aortic bifurcation is a
    A. DeBakey Type I dissection
    B. DeBakey Type II dissection
    C. DeBakey Type IIIa dissection
    D. DeBakey Type IIIb dissection

Answer: D

Dissections are categorized according to their anatomic location and extent to guide treatment. The two traditional classification schemes that remain in common use are the DeBakey and the Stanford classification systems (Fig. 22-2). In their current forms, both of these schemes describe the segments of aorta that are involved in the dissection, rather than the site of the initial intimal tear. The main drawback of the Stanford classification system is that it does not distinguish between patients with isolated ascending aortic dissection and patients with dissection involving the entire aorta. (See Schwartz 9th ed., pp 684, 686.)

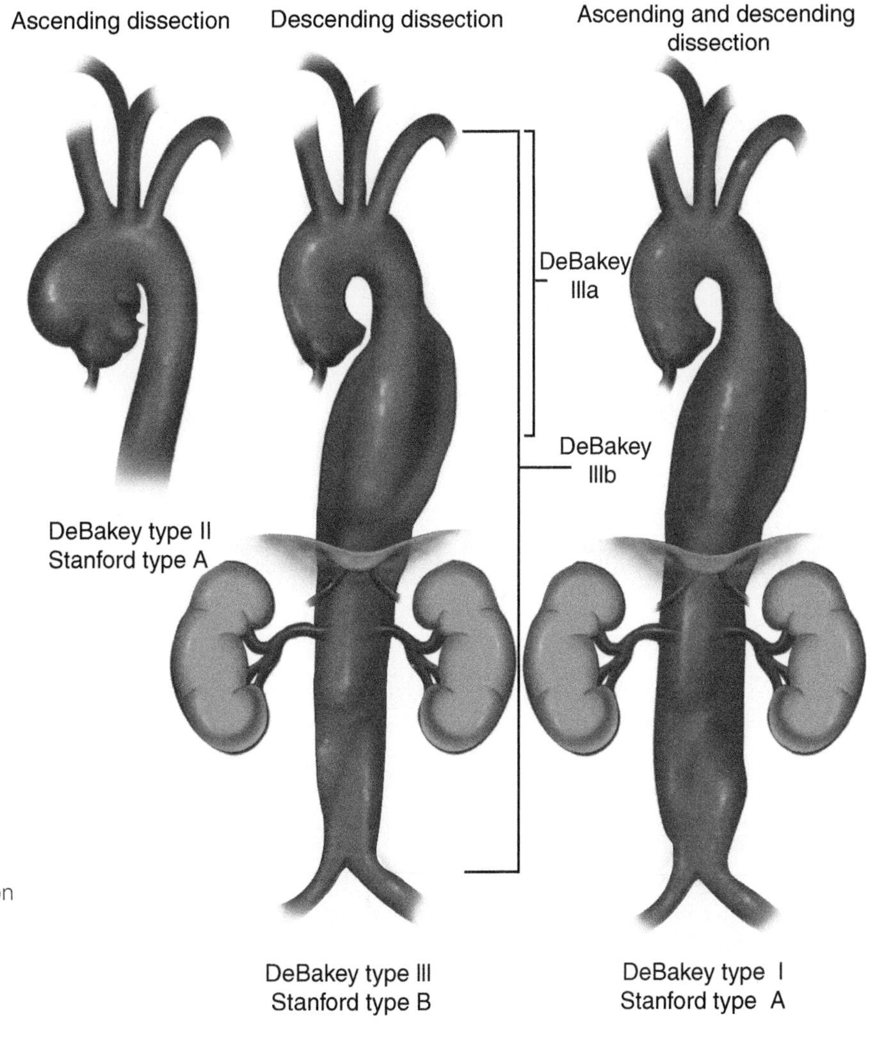
Ascending dissection
Descending dissection
Ascending and descending dissection
DeBakey IIIa
DeBakey IIIb
DeBakey type II
Stanford type A
DeBakey type III
Stanford type B
DeBakey type I
Stanford type A

FIG. 22-2. Illustration of the classification schemes for aortic dissection based on which portions of the aorta are involved. Dissection can be confined to the ascending aorta *(left)* or descending aorta *(middle)*, or it can involve the entire aorta *(right)*. (Reproduced with permission from Creager MA, Dzau VS, Loscalzo J (eds): *Vascular Medicine*. Philadelphia: WB Saunders, 2006. Copyright © Saunders/Elsevier, 2006, Fig. 35-2.)

17. The best treatment for a patient with an uncomplicated descending thoracic dissection is
   A. Nonoperative management
   B. Catheterization with placement of an aortic stent
   C. Replacement of the involved aorta with a graft (single stage repair)
   D. Elephant trunk procedure (staged repair)

Answer: A

Nonoperative, pharmacologic management of acute descending aortic dissection results in lower morbidity and mortality rates than surgical treatment does. The most common causes of death during nonoperative treatment are aortic rupture and end-organ malperfusion. Therefore, patients are continually reassessed for new complications. At least two serial CT scans—usually obtained on day 2 or 3 and on day 8 or 9 of treatment—are compared with the initial scan to rule out significant aortic expansion. (See Schwartz 9th ed., p 690-692.)

Many patients can be discharged after their blood pressure is well controlled with oral agents and after serial CT scans confirm the absence of aortic expansion. Surgery is typically reserved for patients who experience complications. In general terms, surgical intervention for acute descending aortic dissection is intended to prevent or repair ruptures and relieve ischemic manifestations.

During the acute phase of a dissection, the specific indications for operative intervention include aortic rupture, increasing periaortic or pleural fluid volume, rapidly expanding aortic diameter, uncontrolled hypertension, and persistent pain despite adequate medical therapy. Acute dissection superimposed on a pre-existing aneurysm is considered a life-threatening condition and is therefore another indication for operation. Finally, patients who have a history of noncompliance with medical therapy may ultimately benefit more from surgical treatment if they are otherwise reasonable operative candidates. (See Schwartz 9th ed., p 692.)

CHAPTER 23

Arterial Disease

BASIC SCIENCE QUESTIONS

1. The normal ratio between the blood pressure in the brachial artery and the distal arteries of the leg is
   A. <0.8
   B. 0.8
   C. 1.0
   D. >1.0

Answer: D

The ABI is determined in the following ways. Blood pressure (BP) is measured in both upper extremities using the highest systolic BP as the denominator for the ABI. The ankle pressure is determined by placing a BP cuff above the ankle and measuring the return to flow of the posterior tibial and dorsalis pedis arteries using a pencil Doppler probe over each artery. The ratio of the systolic pressure in each vessel divided by the highest arm systolic pressure can be used to express the ABI in both the posterior tibial and dorsalis pedis arteries (Fig. 23-1). Normal is more than 1. (See Schwartz 9th ed., p 704.)

Right ABI = ratio of

Higher of the right ankle systolic pressures (posterior tibial or dorsalis pedis)

Higher arm systolic pressure (left or right arm)

Left ABI = ratio of

Higher of the left ankle systolic pressures (posterior tibial or dorsalis pedis)

Higher arm systolic pressure (left or right arm)

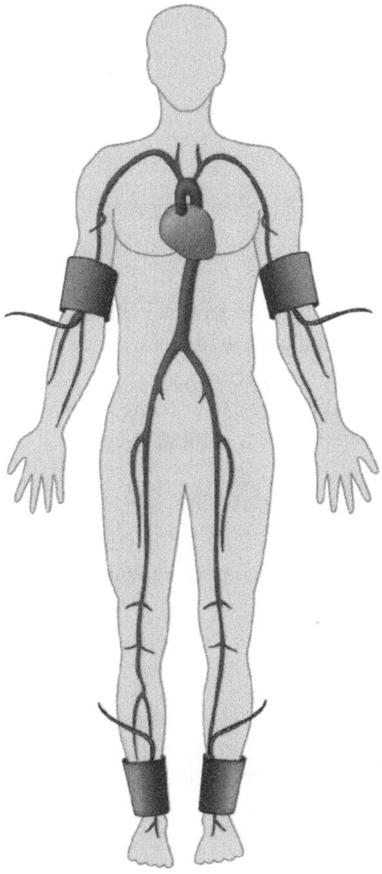

FIG. 23-1. Calculating the ankle-brachial index.

2. Collateral flow between the celiac artery and superior mesenteric artery is primarily through the
   A. Arc of Riolan
   B. Meandering mesenteric arteries
   C. Pancreaticoduodenal arteries
   D. Marginal artery of Drummond

Answer: C

Collateral networks between the celiac artery (CA) and the superior mesenteric artery (SMA) exist primarily through the superior and inferior pancreaticoduodenal arteries. The inferior mesenteric artery (IMA) may provide collateral arterial flow to the SMA through the marginal artery of Drummond, the arc of Riolan, and other unnamed retroperitoneal collateral vessels termed *meandering mesenteric arteries*. (See Schwartz 9th ed., p 731.)

3. Mutations in the ATP-binding cassette subfamily C member 6 (ABCC6) gene are found in patients with
   A. Ehlers-Danlos syndrome
   B. Pseudoxanthoma elasticum
   C. Takayasu's arteritis
   D. Marfan syndrome

Answer: B

Pseudoxanthoma elasticum is a rare inherited disorder of connective tissue that is characterized by an unbalanced elastic fiber metabolism and synthesis, resulting in fragmentation and calcification of the fibers. Clinical manifestations occur in the skin, ocular, GI, and cardiovascular systems. Characteristic skin lesions are seen in the axilla, antecubital and popliteal fossae, and groin. The yellow, xanthoma-like papules occur in redundant folds of skin and are said to resemble plucked chicken skin. The inheritance pattern includes both autosomal dominant and recessive types and has a prevalence of one in 160,000 individuals. The ATP-binding cassette subfamily C member 6 (ABCC6) gene has been demonstrated to be responsible, and 43 mutations have been identified, all of which lead to calcification of the internal elastic laminae of medium-sized vessel walls.

Ehlers-Danlos syndrome is a disorder of fibrillar collagen metabolism with identifiable, specific defects that have been found in the collagen biosynthetic pathway that produce clinically distinct forms of this disease.

Takayasu's arteritis is a rare but well-recognized chronic inflammatory arteritis affecting large vessels, predominantly the aorta and its main branches.

Marfan syndrome is characterized by abnormal musculoskeletal, ocular, and cardiovascular features first described by Antoine Marfan in 1896. The inborn error of metabolism in this syndrome has been localized to the long arm of chromosome 15 (15q21.3). Defects occur in fibrillin, a basic protein in the microfibrillar apparatus that serves as a backbone for elastin, which is one of the main extracellular structural proteins in blood vessels. (See Schwartz 9th ed., p 767.)

4. The superficial peroneal nerve is located in the
   A. Anterior compartment
   B. Lateral compartment
   C. Superficial posterior compartment
   D. Deep posterior compartment

Answer: B

The superficial peroneal nerve is located in the lateral compartment. The deep peroneal nerve is located in the anterior compartment. (See Schwartz 9th ed., p 757, and Table 23-1.)

TABLE 23-1 Fascial compartments of the lower leg

	Anterior Compartment	Lateral Compartment	Superficial Posterior Compartment	Deep Posterior Compartment
Muscles	Tibialis anterior Extensor digitorum longus Peroneus tertius Extensor hallucis longus Extensor digitorum brevis Extensor hallucis brevis	Peroneus longus Peroneus brevis	Gastrocnemius Plantaris Soleus	Tibialis posterior Flexor digitorum longus Flexor hallucis longus
Artery	Anterior tibial artery	Anterior and posterior tibial branches of the popliteal artery	—	Posterior tibial artery Peroneal artery
Nerve	Deep peroneal nerve	Superficial peroneal nerve	—	Tibial nerve

5. The origin of the carotid body is
   A. Ectoderm
   B. Mesoderm
   C. Endoderm
   D. Neural crest cells

Answer: D

The carotid body originates from the third branchial arch and from neuroectodermal-derived neural crest lineage. The normal carotid body is located in the adventitia or periadventitial tissue at the bifurcation of the CCA. The gland is innervated by the glossopharyngeal nerve. Its blood supply is derived predominantly from the external carotid artery, but also can come from the vertebral artery. Carotid body tumor is a rare lesion of the neuroendocrine system. Other glands of neural crest origin are seen in the neck, parapharyngeal spaces, mediastinum, retroperitoneum, and adrenal medulla. Tumors involving these structures have been referred to as *paraganglioma, glomus tumor,* or *chemodectoma*. (See Schwartz 9th ed., p 721.)

CLINICAL QUESTIONS

1. Approximately what percentage of vascular patients are diabetic?
   A. 5%
   B. 15%
   C. 30%
   D. 50%

Answer: C

Appropriate history should be focused on the presenting symptoms related to the vascular system (Table 23-2). Of particular importance in the previous medical history is noting prior vascular interventions (endovascular or open surgical), and all vascular patients should have inquiry made about their prior cardiac history and current cardiac symptoms. Approximately 30% of vascular patients will be diabetic. A history of prior and current smoking status should be noted. (See Schwartz 9th ed., p 703.)

TABLE 23-2 Pertinent elements in vascular history

- History of stroke or transient ischemic attack
- History of coronary artery disease, including previous myocardial infarction and angina
- History of peripheral arterial disease
- History of diabetes
- History of hypertension
- History of tobacco use
- History of hyperlipidemia

2. The most common type of fibromuscular dysplasia of the carotid artery is
   A. Intimal fibroplasia
   B. Medial fibroplasia
   C. Premedial dysplasia
   D. Medial hyperplasia

Answer: B

Four histological types of fibromuscular dysplasia (FMD) have been described in the literature. The most common type is medial fibroplasia, which may present as a focal stenosis or multiple lesions with intervening aneurysmal outpouchings. The disease involves the media with the smooth muscle being replaced by fibrous connective tissue. Commonly, mural dilations and microaneurysms can be seen with this type of FMD. Medial hyperplasia is a rare type of FMD, with the media demonstrating excessive amounts of smooth muscle. Intimal fibroplasia accounts for 5% of all cases and occurs equally in both sexes. The media and adventitia remain normal, and there is accumulation of subendothelial mesenchymal cells with a loose matrix of connective tissue causing a focal stenosis in adults. Finally, premedial dysplasia represents a type of FMD with elastic tissue accumulating between the media and adventitia. (See Schwartz 9th ed., p 720.)

3. Which of the following types of stents would be the best choice for a long segment stenosis of the internal carotid artery?
   A. Self-expanding stent
   B. Stent graft
   C. Balloon-expandable stent
   D. Drug-eluting stent

Answer: A
Self-expanding stents generally come in longer lengths than balloon-expandable stents and are therefore used to treat long and tortuous lesions. Their ability to continually expand after delivery allows them to accommodate adjacent vessels of different size. This makes these stents ideal for placement in the internal carotid artery (ICA). (See Schwartz 9th ed., p 711.)

4. The conduit of choice for infrainguinal bypass grafting is
   A. Autogenous vein
   B. Human umbilical vein
   C. PTFE
   D. Dacron

Answer: A
Autogenous vein is superior to prosthetic conduits for all infrainguinal bypasses, even in the above-knee (AK) position. This preference is applicable not only for the initial bypass but also for reoperative cases. For long bypasses, ipsilateral great saphenous vein (GSV), contralateral GSV, small saphenous vein, arm vein, and spliced vein are used, in decreasing order of preference. (See Schwartz 9th ed., p 765.)

5. Which of the following is NOT one of the characteristics evaluated to determine if a patient is a candidate for endovascular repair of an abdominal aortic aneurysm?
   A. Neck length
   B. Neck mural calcification
   C. Common iliac artery length
   D. Common iliac artery calcification

Answer: D
Anatomic eligibility for endovascular repair is mainly based on three areas: the proximal aortic neck, common iliac arteries (CIAs), and the external iliac and common femoral arteries, which relate to the proximal and distal landing zones or fixation sites and the access vessels, respectively. See Table 23-3 for specific characteristics used to establish anatomic eligibility for endovascular repair. (See Schwartz 9th ed., p 727.)

TABLE 23-3 Ideal characteristics of an aneurysm for endovascular abdominal aortic aneurysm repair

Neck length (mm)	>15
Neck diameter (mm)	>18, <32
Aortic neck angle (°)	<60
Neck mural calcification (% circumference)	<50
Neck luminal thrombus (% circumference)	<50
Common iliac artery diameter (mm)	between 8–20
Common iliac artery length (mm)	>20
External iliac artery diameter (mm)	>7

6. The risk of stroke is markedly increased in patients who have a decrease in internal carotid artery (ICA) luminal diameter of
   A. 40%
   B. 50%
   C. 60%
   D. 70%

Answer: D
With increasing degree of stenosis in the ICA, flow becomes more turbulent, and the risk of atheroembolization escalates. The severity of stenosis is commonly divided into three categories according to the luminal diameter reduction: mild (less than 50%), moderate (50 to 69%), and severe (70 to 99%). Severe carotid stenosis is a strong predictor for stroke. (See Schwartz 9th ed., p 712.)

7. Which of the following patients should be offered revascularization (endoluminal or by endarterectomy) of their carotid stenosis?
   A. Symptomatic patient with 35% unilateral stenosis
   B. Symptomatic patient with 35% bilateral stenosis
   C. Asymptomatic patient with 80% unilateral stenosis
   D. None of the above

Answer: C
In patients with symptomatic carotid stenosis, the degree of stenosis appears to be the most important predictor in determining risk for an ipsilateral stroke. The risk of a recurrent ipsilateral stroke in patients with severe carotid stenosis approaches 40%.

It is generally agreed that asymptomatic patients with severe carotid stenosis (80 to 99%) are at significantly increased risk for stroke and stand to benefit from either surgical or endovascular revascularization. However, revascularization for asymptomatic patients with a less severe degree of stenosis (60 to 79%) remains controversial. (See Schwartz 9th ed., p 715.)

8. Which of the following is NOT a cause of intermittent claudication?
   A. Popliteal cyst
   B. Takayasu's disease
   C. Popliteal entrapment
   D. Acute radiation injury

Answer: D

See Table 23-4 for additional non-atherosclerotic causes of intermittent claudication. (See Schwartz 9th ed., p 754.)

TABLE 23-4	Non-atherosclerotic causes of intermittent claudication

- Aortic coarctation
- Arterial fibrodysplasia
- Iliac syndrome of the cyclist
- Peripheral emboli
- Persistent sciatic artery
- Popliteal aneurysm
- Popliteal cyst
- Popliteal entrapment
- Primary vascular tumors
- Pseudoxanthoma elasticum
- Remote trauma or radiation injury
- Takayasu's disease
- Thromboangiitis obliterans

9. When performing a four-compartment fasciotomy for compartment syndrome, medial and lateral incisions are created. Which of the following compartments is opened through the medial incision?
   A. Anterior compartment
   B. Deep posterior compartment
   C. Peroneal compartment
   D. None of the above

Answer: B

Compartment pressures are relieved in the leg by medial and lateral incisions. Through the medial incision, long openings are then made in the fascia of the superficial and deep posterior compartments. Through the lateral incision, the anterior and peroneal compartments are opened. (See Schwartz 9th ed., p 757, and Fig. 23-2.)

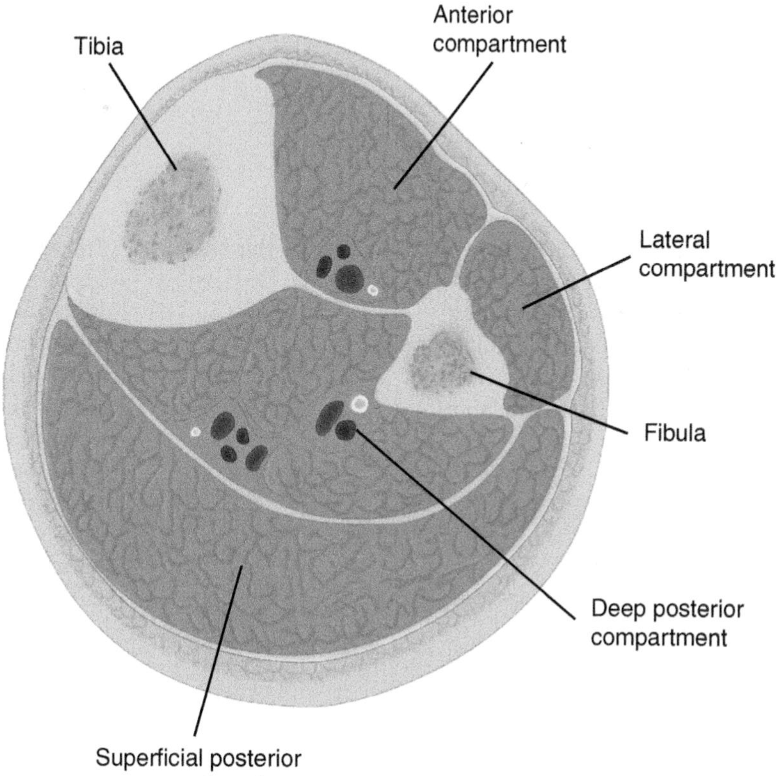

FIG. 23-2. Schematic illustration of fascial compartments of the lower extremity.

10. Amaurosis fugax is a symptom of occlusion of the
   A. Posterior cerebral artery
   B. Circle of Willis
   C. Internal carotid artery
   D. External carotid artery

Answer: C

The common ocular symptoms associated with extracranial carotid artery occlusive disease include amaurosis fugax and presence of Hollenhorst plaques. Amaurosis fugax, commonly referred to as *transient monocular blindness*, is a temporary loss of vision in one eye that patients typically describe as a window shutter coming down or gray shedding of the vision. This partial blindness usually lasts for a few minutes and then resolves. Most of these phenomena (>90%) are due to embolic occlusion of the main artery or the upper or lower divisions. Monocular blindness progressing over a 20-minute period suggests a migrainous etiology. Occasionally, the patient will recall no visual symptoms while the optician notes a yellowish plaque within the retinal vessels, which is also known as the *Hollenhorst plaque*. These are frequently derived from cholesterol embolization. (See Schwartz 9th ed., p 713.)

11. The average annual growth of abdominal aortic aneurysms is approximately
   A. 1 mm
   B. 3 mm
   C. 1 cm
   D. 3 cm

Answer: B

The natural history of an abdominal aortic aneurysm (AAA) is to expand and rupture. AAA exhibits a 'staccato' pattern of growth, where periods of relative quiescence may alternate with expansion. Therefore, although an individual pattern of growth cannot be predicted, average aggregate growth is approximately 3 to 4 mm/y. There is some evidence to suggest that larger aneurysms may expand faster than smaller aneurysms, but there is significant overlap between the ranges of growth rates at each strata of size. (See Schwartz 9th ed., p 723.)

12. What is the approximate 90-day risk of a stroke in a patient with a transient ischemic attack?
   A. <2%
   B. 10-15%
   C. 25-30%
   D. 40-50%

Answer: B

Conventionally, patients with carotid bifurcation occlusive disease are divided into two broad categories: patients without prior history of ipsilateral stroke or transient ischemic attack (TIA) (asymptomatic) and those with prior or current ipsilateral neurologic symptoms (symptomatic). It is estimated that 15% of all strokes are preceded by a TIA. The 90-day risk of a stroke in a patient presenting with a TIA is 3 to 17%. (See Schwartz 9th ed., p 715.)

13. Which of the following is the "gold standard" for the diagnosis of renal artery hypertension?
   A. Captopril renal scanning
   B. Renal artery duplex ultrasonography
   C. Selective angiography
   D. MRA with IV gadolinium

Answer: C

Digital subtraction angiography (DSA) remains the gold standard to assess renal artery occlusive disease. A flush aortogram is performed first so that any accessory renal arteries can be detected and the origins of all the renal arteries are adequately displayed. The presence of collateral vessels circumventing a renal artery stenosis strongly supports the hemodynamic importance of the stenosis. A pressure gradient of 10 mmHg or greater is necessary for collateral vessel development, which also is associated with activation of the renin-angiotensin cascade.

Captopril renal scanning is a functional study that assesses renal perfusion before and after administration of the ACE inhibitor captopril. Captopril inhibits the secretion of angiotensin II. Through this mechanism it reduces the efferent arteriole vasoconstriction and, as a result, the glomerular filtration rate (GFR). The test consists of a baseline renal scan, and a second renal scan after captopril administration. Positive result indicates that captopril administration (a) increases the time to peak activity to more than 11 minutes or (b) increases the GFR ratio between sides to greater than 1.5:1 compared to a normal baseline scan.

Renal artery duplex ultrasonography is a noninvasive test of assessing renal artery stenosis both by visualization of the vessel and measurement of the effect of stenosis on blood flow velocity and waveforms. The presence of a severe renal artery stenosis correlates with peak systolic velocities of >180 cm/s and the ratio of these velocities to those in the aorta of >3.5.

Magnetic resonance angiography (MRA) with IV gadolinium contrast enhancement has been increasingly used for renal artery imaging because of its ability to provide high-resolution images (Figs. 23-3 and 23-4) while using a minimally nephrotoxic agent. Flow void may be inaccurately interpreted as occlusion or stenosis in MRA. Therefore, unless the quality of the image analysis software is superior, MRA should be interpreted with caution and used in conjunction with other modalities before making plans for operative or endovascular treatment. (See Schwartz 9th ed., p 738.)

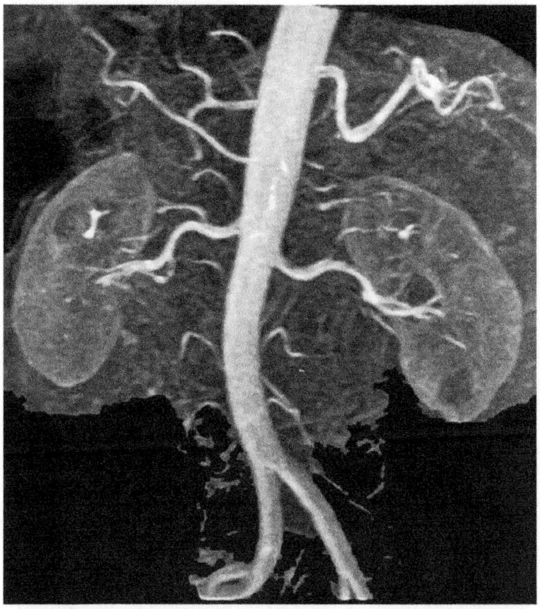

FIG. 23-3. Magnetic resonance angiography of the abdominal aorta revealed bilateral normal renal arteries.

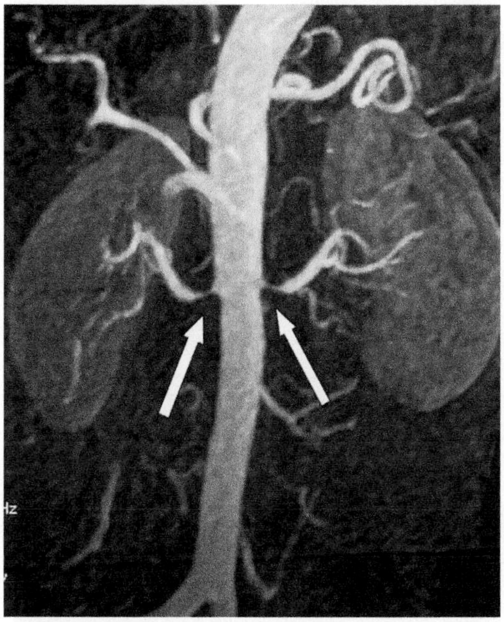

FIG. 23-4. Magnetic resonance angiography of the abdominal aorta revealed bilateral ostial renal artery stenosis (*arrows*).

14. Which of the following is NOT a complication of temporal arteritis?
    A. Aortic dissection
    B. Blindness
    C. Jaw claudication
    D. Temporal aneurysm

Answer: D

The clinical syndrome of temporal arteritis (giant cell arteritis) begins with a prodromal phase of constitutional symptoms, including headache, fever, malaise, and myalgia. As a result of vascular narrowing and end-organ ischemia, complications may occur such as visual alterations, including blindness and mural weakness, resulting in acute aortic dissection that may be devastating. Ischemic optic neuritis resulting in partial or complete blindness occurs in up to 40% of patients and is considered a medical emergency. Cerebral symptoms occur when the disease process extends to the carotid arteries. Jaw claudication and temporal artery tenderness may be experienced. Aortic lesions usually are asymptomatic until later stages and consist of thoracic aneurysms and aortic dissections. (See Schwartz 9th ed., p 767.)

15. Which of the following is a contraindication to carotid artery stenting?
    A. 1.5-cm segment of stenosis
    B. >80% occlusion of the luminal diameter
    C. Extensive calcification
    D. Occluded middle cerebral artery

Answer: C

There are anatomical conditions based on angiographic evaluation in which carotid artery stenting should be avoided due to increased procedural-related risks (Table 23-5). (See Schwartz 9th ed., p 719.)

TABLE 23-5	Unfavorable carotid angiographic appearance in which carotid stenting should be avoided
	• Extensive carotid calcification • Polypoid or globular carotid lesions • Severe tortuosity of the common carotid artery • Long segment stenoses (>2 cm in length) • Carotid artery occlusion • Severe intraluminal thrombus (angiographic defects) • Extensive middle cerebral artery atherosclerosis

16. When compared to open repair of an abdominal aortic aneurysm, endovascular repair
    A. Requires lifelong follow-up imaging
    B. Results in an increased transfusion requirement
    C. Costs about the same
    D. Results in longer ICU stays

Answer: A

Lifelong follow-up is essential to the long-term success after endovascular AAA repair. Indeed, one may go so far as to say that absence of appropriate follow-up is tantamount to not having had a repair at all. A triple-phase (noncontrast, contrast, delayed) spiral CT scan and a four-view (anteroposterior, lateral, and two obliques) abdominal x-ray should be obtained within the first month. Subsequent imaging can be obtained at 6-month intervals in the first 1 to 2 years and yearly thereafter.

The primary success rate after endovascular repair of AAA has been reported to be as high as 95%. The less invasive nature of this procedure is appealing to many physicians and patients. In addition, virtually all reports indicate decreased blood loss, transfusion requirements, and length of ICU and hospital stay for endovascular repair of AAAs when compared to the standard surgical approach. With the advent of bifurcated grafts and improved delivery systems in the future, the only real limitation will be cost. (See Schwartz 9th ed., p 728.)

The in-hospital costs for both endovascular and open repair include graft cost, OR fees, radiology, pharmacy, ancillary care, ICU charges, and floor charges. Despite the improved morbidity and mortality rates, several early studies have reported no cost benefit with the application of endovascular repair. The limiting factor appears to be the cost of the device. Despite commercialization of endovascular repair, the device costs are still in the range of $5000 to $6000 with no signs of abating. A recent report by Angle and associates further corroborates previous studies. In their review, despite decreased hospital and ICU stays and use of pharmacy and respiratory services, cost of endovascular repair was 1.74 times greater than the standard surgical approach. (See Schwartz 9th ed., p 729.)

17. Type 1 aortoiliac disease is associated with
    A. Diabetes
    B. Hypertension
    C. Hyperlipidemia
    D. Elevated levels of homocysteine

Answer: C

Type I aortoiliac disease, which occurs in 5 to 10% of patients, is confined to the distal abdominal aorta and common iliac vessels. This type of aortoiliac occlusive disease occurs in a relatively younger group of patients (aged in their mid-50s), compared with patients who have more femoropopliteal disease. Patients with a type I disease pattern have a lower incidence of hypertension and diabetes, but a significant frequency of abnormal blood lipid levels, particularly type IV hyperlipoproteinemia.

Type II aortoiliac disease represents a more diffuse atherosclerotic progression that involves predominately the abdominal aorta with disease extension into the CIA.

Type III aortoiliac occlusive disease, which affects approximately 65% of patients with aortoiliac occlusive disease, is widespread disease that is seen above and below the inguinal ligament. (See Schwartz 9th ed., p 744, and Fig. 23-5.)

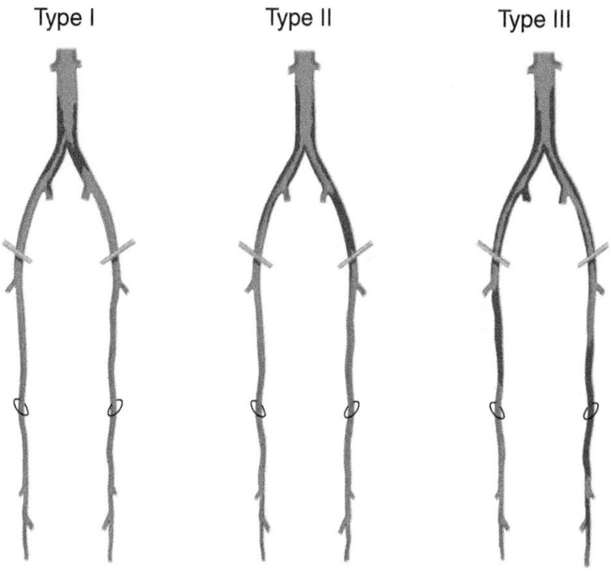

FIG. 23-5. Aortoiliac disease can be classified into three types. Type I represents focal disease affecting the distal aorta and proximal common iliac artery. Type II represents diffuse aortoiliac disease above the inguinal ligament. Type III represents multisegment occlusive disease involving aortoiliac and infrainguinal arterial vessels.

18. Which of the following patients should undergo elective repair of an asymptomatic abdominal aortic aneurysm?
    A. A man with a 4.5-cm aneurysm
    B. A woman with a 5.0-cm aneurysm
    C. A man with an aneurysm that has grown 0.5 cm in the last year
    D. A woman with an aneurysm that has grown 0.5 cm in the last year

Answer: B

Based on best available evidence, the annualized risk of rupture is given in Table 23-6. The rupture risk is quite low for aneurysms <5.5 cm and begins to rise exponentially thereafter. This size can serve as an appropriate threshold for recommending elective repair provided one's surgical mortality is below 5%. For each size strata, however, women appear to be at higher risk for rupture than men, and a lower threshold of 4.5 to 5.0 cm may be reasonable in good-risk patients. Although data are less compelling, a pattern of rapid expansion of >0.5 cm within 6 months can be considered a relative indication for elective repair. (See Schwartz 9th ed., p 723.)

TABLE 23-6 Annualized risk of rupture of abdominal aortic aneurysm (AAA) based on size

Description	Diameter of Aorta (cm)	Estimated Annual Risk of Rupture (%)	Estimated 5-y Risk of Rupture (%)[a]
Normal aorta	2–3	0	0 (unless AAA develops)
Small AAA	4–5	1	5–10
Moderate AAA	5–6	2–5	30–40
Large AAA	6–7	3–10	>50
Very large AAA	>7	>10	Approaching 100

[a]The estimated 5-y risk is more than five times the estimated annual risk because over that 5 y, the AAA, if left untreated, will continue to grow in size.

19. Carotid artery stenting is indicated for patients who are at "high risk" for endarterectomy. Which of the following is NOT one of the criteria for a high-risk patient?
    A. Age >70 years
    B. Previous neck irradiation
    C. Severe chronic obstructive pulmonary disease
    D. End stage renal disease on dialysis

Answer: A

Since carotid artery stenting was approved by the FDA in 2004 for clinical application, this percutaneous procedure has become a treatment alternative in patients who are deemed 'high-risk' for endarterectomy (Table 23-7). Patients older than 80 years of age are considered high risk. (See Schwartz 9th ed., p 716.)

TABLE 23-7 Conditions qualifying patients as "high surgical risk" for carotid endarterectomy

Anatomical Factors	Physiological Factors
• High carotid bifurcation (above C2 vertebral body) • Low common carotid artery (below clavicle) • Contralateral carotid occlusion • Restenosis of ipsilateral prior carotid endarterectomy • Previous neck irradiation • Prior radical neck dissection • Contralateral laryngeal nerve palsy • Presence of tracheostomy	• Age ≥80 y • Left ventricular ejection fraction ≤30% • New York Heart Association Class III/IV congestive heart failure • Unstable angina: Canadian Cardiovascular Society Class III/IV angina pectoris • Recent myocardial infarction • Clinically significant cardiac disease (congestive heart failure, abnormal stress test, or need for coronary revascularization) • Severe chronic obstructive pulmonary disease • End-stage renal disease on dialysis

20. Approximately what percent of carotid body tumors are familial in origin?
    A. <2%
    B. 10%
    C. 35%
    D. 50%

Answer: C

Approximately 5 to 7% of carotid body tumors are malignant. Although chronic hypoxemia has been invoked as a stimulus for hyperplasia of carotid body, approximately 35% of carotid body tumors are hereditary. The risk of malignancy is greatest in young patients with familial tumors. (See Schwartz 9th ed., p 722, and Fig. 23-6.)

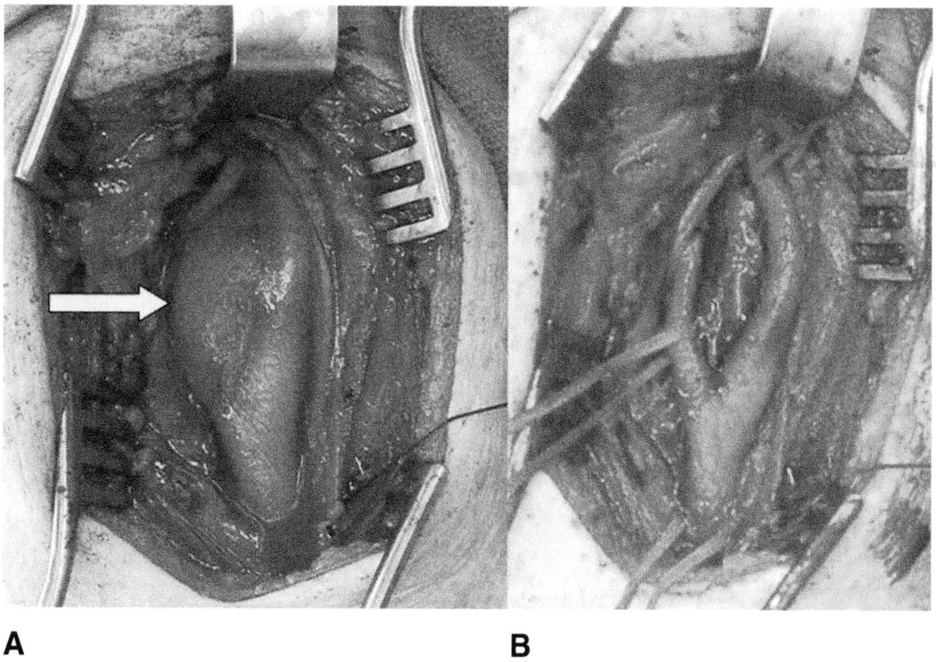

FIG. 23-6. **A.** A carotid body tumor (*arrow*) located adjacent to the carotid bulb. **B.** Following peri-adventitial dissection, the carotid body tumor is removed.

21. Fibromuscular dysplasia of the renal arteries
    A. Occurs more commonly in men
    B. Usually involves the proximal artery
    C. Affects the right renal artery more often than the left
    D. Is the most common cause of renovascular hypertension

Answer: C

The second most common cause of renal artery stenosis, after atherosclerosis, is fibromuscular dysplasia (FMD), which accounts for 20% of cases, and is most frequently encountered in young, often multiparous women. FMD of the renal artery represents a heterogeneous group of lesions that can produce histopathologic changes in the intima, media, or adventitia. The most common variety consists of medial fibroplasia, in which thickened fibromuscular ridges alternate with attenuated media producing the classic angiographic 'string of beads' appearance. The cause of medial fibroplasia remains unclear. Most common theories involve a modification of arterial smooth muscle cells in response to estrogenic stimuli during the reproductive years, unusual traction forces on affected vessels, and mural ischemia from impairment of vasa vasorum blood flow. Fibromuscular hyperplasia usually affects the distal two thirds of the main renal artery, and the right renal artery is affected more frequently than the left. (See Schwartz 9th ed., p 737, and Fig. 23-7.)

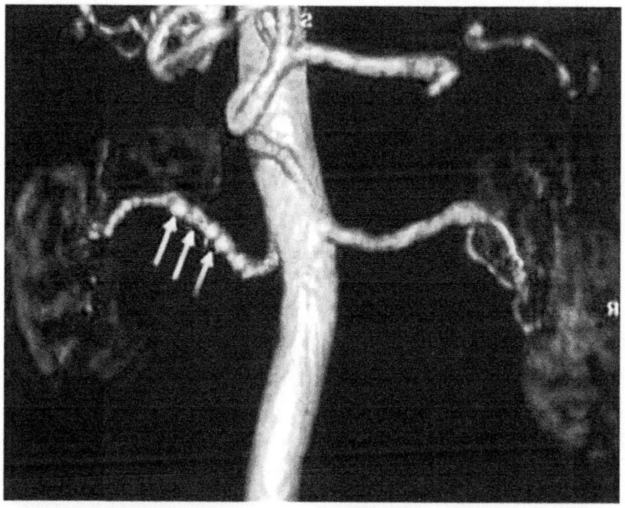

FIG. 23-7. Magnetic resonance angiography of the abdominal aorta revealed the presence of a left renal artery fibromuscular dysplasia (*arrows*).

22. Patients with chronic mesenteric ischemia may experience
    A. Pain out of proportion to physical findings
    B. Bloody diarrhea
    C. Fever
    D. "Food fear"

Answer: D

Abdominal pain out of proportion to physical findings is the classic presentation in patients with acute mesenteric ischemia and occurs following an embolic or thrombotic ischemic event of the SMA. Other manifestations include sudden onset of abdominal cramps in patients with underlying cardiac or atherosclerotic disease, often associated with bloody diarrhea, as a result of mucosal sloughing secondary to ischemia. Fever, nausea, vomiting, and abdominal distention are some common but nonspecific manifestations. Diffuse abdominal tenderness, rebound, and rigidity are late signs and usually indicate bowel infarction and necrosis.

Clinical manifestations of chronic mesenteric ischemia are more subtle owing to the extensive collateral development. However, when intestinal blood flow is unable to meet the physiologic GI demands, mesenteric insufficiency ensues. The classic symptoms include postprandial abdominal pain, "food fear," and weight loss. Persistent nausea, and occasionally diarrhea, may coexist. Diagnosis remains challenging, and most of the patients will undergo an extensive and expensive GI tract work-up for the above symptoms before referral to a vascular service. (See Schwartz 9th ed., p 732.)

23. Which of the following is the best initial treatment for a patient with severe acute limb ischemia?
    A. Endovascular thrombolysis
    B. Systemic thrombolysis
    C. Surgical embolectomy
    D. Anticoagulation

Answer: D

In the absence of any significant contraindication, the patient with an ischemic LE should be immediately anticoagulated. This will prevent propagation of the clot into unaffected vascular beds. IV fluid should be started and a Foley catheter inserted to monitor urine output. Baseline labs should be obtained and creatinine levels noted. A hypercoagulable work-up should be performed before initiation of heparin if there is sufficient suspicion. According to results from randomized trials, there is no clear superiority for thrombolysis over surgery in terms of 30-day limb salvage or mortality. Access to each treatment option is a major issue in the decision-making process, as time is often critical. National registry data from the United States reveal that surgery is used three- to fivefold more frequently than thrombolysis. (See Schwartz 9th ed., p 755.)

24. Which of the following ankle-brachial index would be expected in a patient with claudication?
    A. 1.0
    B. 0.8
    C. 0.6
    D. 0.4

Answer: C

There is increasing interest in the use of the ankle-brachial index (ABI) to evaluate patients at risk for cardiovascular events (Figure 23-1). An ABI <0.9 correlates with increased risk of myocardial infarction and indicates significant, although perhaps asymptomatic, underlying peripheral vascular disease. Normal is more than 1. Patients with claudication typically have an ABI in the 0.5 to 0.7 range, and those with rest pain are in the 0.3 to 0.5 range. Those with gangrene have an ABI of <0.3. These ranges can vary depending on the degree of compressibility of the vessel. The test is less reliable in patients with heavily calcified vessels. Due to noncompressibility, some patients such as diabetics and those with end-stage renal disease may have an ABI of 1.40 or greater and require additional noninvasive diagnostic testing to evaluate for peripheral arterial disease (PAD). (See Schwartz 9th ed., p 704.)

25. Which of the following is the most common type of endoleak after endovascular repair of an abdominal aortic aneurysm?
    A. Type I
    B. Type II
    C. Type III
    D. Type IV

Answer: B

Four types of endoleaks have been described (Table 23-8). *Type I endoleak* refers to fixation-related leaks that occur at the proximal or distal attachment sites. These represent less than 5% of all endoleaks and are seen as an early blush of contrast into the aneurysm sac from the proximal or distal ends of the device during completion angiography.

Type II endoleak refers to retrograde flow originating from a lumbar, inferior mesenteric, accessory renal, or hypogastric artery. They are the most common type of endoleak, accounting for 20 to 30% of all cases, and about one half resolve spontaneously.

Type III endoleaks refer to a failure of device integrity or component separation from modular systems. If detected intraoperatively or in the early perioperative period, it is usually from inadequate overlap between two stent grafts, while in the late period, it may be from a fabric tear or junctional separation from conformational changes of the aneurysm. Regardless of the etiology or timing, these should be promptly repaired.

Type IV endoleak refers to the diffuse, early blush seen during completion angiography due to graft porosity and/or suture holes of some Dacron-based devices. It does not have any clinical significance and usually cannot be seen after 48 hours and heparin reversal. (See Schwartz 9th ed., p 730, and Fig. 23-8.)

TABLE 23-8 Endoleak classification

Classification	Description
Type I endoleak	Attachment site leak
Type II endoleak	Side branch leak caused by lumbar or inferior mesenteric artery
Type III endoleak	Junctional leak (of overlapping endograft components)
Type IV endoleak	Endograft fabric or porosity leak

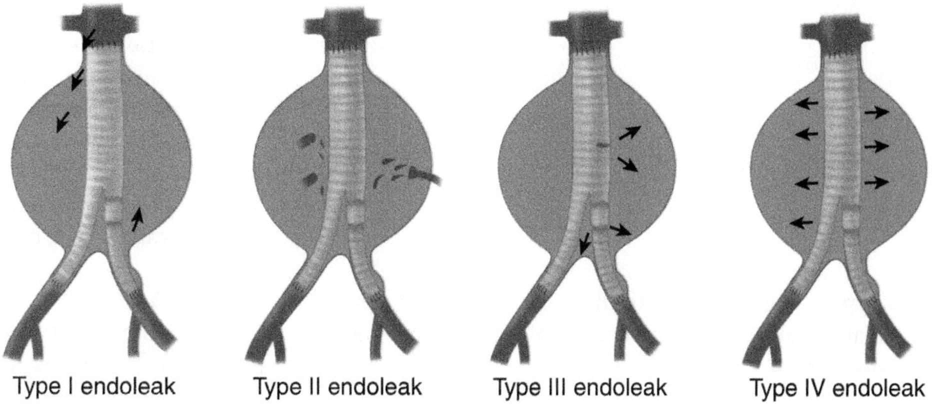

FIG. 23-8. Four types of endoleak that include: type I endoleak = attachment site leak; type II endoleak = side branch leak caused by lumbar or side branches; type III endoleak = endograft junctional leak due to overlapping device components; type IV endoleak = endograft fabric or porosity leak.

26. The 10-year patency rate for aortobifemoral bypass grafts is approximately
    A. 30%
    B. 50%
    C. 70%
    D. 90%

Answer: C

Surgical options for treatment of aortoiliac occlusive diseases consist of various configurations of aortobifemoral bypass (ABF) grafting, various types of extra-anatomic bypass grafts, and aortoiliac endarterectomy. The procedure performed is determined by several factors, including anatomic distribution of the disease, clinical condition of the patient, and personal preference of the surgeon. In most cases, ABF is performed because patients usually have disease in both iliac systems. Although one side may be more severely affected than the other, progression does occur, and bilateral bypass does not complicate the procedure or add to the physiologic stress of the operation. ABF reliably relieves symptoms, has excellent long-term patency (approximately 70 to 75% at 10 years), and can be completed with a tolerable perioperative mortality (2 to 3%). (See Schwartz 9th ed., p 745.)

27. The procedure of choice for acute thrombotic mesenteric ischemia is
    A. Endovascular clot lysis and balloon angioplasty
    B. Endovascular clot lysis and stenting of the superior mesenteric artery
    C. Open thrombectomy with patch angioplasty
    D. Open bypass of the superior mesenteric artery

Answer: D

Thrombotic mesenteric ischemia usually involves a severely atherosclerotic vessel, typically the proximal celiac artery (CA) and superior mesenteric artery (SMA). Therefore, these patients require a reconstructive procedure to the SMA to bypass the proximal occlusive lesion and restore adequate mesenteric flow. The saphenous vein is the graft material of choice, and prosthetic materials should be avoided in patients with nonviable bowel, due to the risk of bacterial contamination if resection of necrotic intestine is performed. The bypass graft may originate from either the aorta or iliac artery. (See Schwartz 9th ed., p 734.)

There are two main drawbacks with regard to thrombolytic therapy in mesenteric ischemia. Percutaneous, catheter-directed thrombolysis (CDT) does not allow the possibility to inspect the potentially ischemic intestine following restoration of the mesenteric flow. Additionally, a prolonged period of time may be necessary to achieve successful CDT, due in part to serial angiographic surveillance to document thrombus resolution. An incomplete or unsuccessful thrombolysis may lead to delayed operative revascularization, which may further necessitate bowel resection for irreversible intestinal necrosis. Therefore, catheter-directed thrombolytic therapy for acute mesenteric ischemia should only be considered in selected patients under a closely scrutinized clinical protocol. (See Schwartz 9th ed., p 735.)

28. Approximately what percentage of patients with peripheral vascular disease also have significant coronary artery disease?
    A. 20%
    B. 40%
    C. 60%
    D. 80%

Answer: B

The most important and controversial aspect of preoperative evaluation in patients with atherosclerotic disease requiring surgical intervention is the detection and subsequent management of associated coronary artery disease (CAD). Several studies have documented the existence of significant CAD in 40 to 50% or more of patients requiring peripheral vascular reconstructive procedures, 10 to 20% of whom may be relatively asymptomatic largely because of their inability to exercise. Myocardial infarction is responsible for the majority of both early and late postoperative deaths in patients with peripheral vascular disease. (See Schwartz 9th ed., p 708.)

CHAPTER 24

Venous and Lymphatic Disease

BASIC SCIENCE QUESTIONS

1. Which of the following veins does not have valves?
   A. Cranial sinuses
   B. Portal vein
   C. Iliac veins
   D. All of the above

Answer: D

The inferior vena cava (IVC), common iliac veins, portal venous system, and cranial sinuses are valveless. (See Schwartz 9th ed., p 778.)

2. Heparin induces anticoagulation primarily by
   A. Increasing production of antithrombin
   B. Increasing the activity of antithrombin
   C. Increasing conversion of factor X to Xa
   D. Increasing conversion of factor XI to XIa

Answer: B

Unfractionated heparin (UFH) binds to antithrombin via a specific 18-saccharide sequence, which increases its activity over 1000-fold. This antithrombin-heparin complex primarily inhibits factor IIa (thrombin) and factor Xa and, to a lesser degree, factors IXa, XIa, and XIIa. In addition, UFH also binds to tissue factor pathway inhibitor, which inhibits the conversion of factor X to Xa, and factor IX to IXa. Finally, UFH catalyzes the inhibition of thrombin by heparin cofactor II via a mechanism that is independent of antithrombin. (See Schwartz 9th ed., p 784.)

3. The Cockett perforator veins are located in the
   A. Medial thigh
   B. Lateral thigh
   C. Medial lower leg
   D. Lateral lower leg

Answer: C

Multiple perforator veins traverse the deep fascia to connect the superficial and deep venous systems. Clinically important perforator veins are the Cockett and Boyd perforators. The Cockett perforator veins drain the medial lower leg and are relatively constant. They connect the posterior arch vein (a tributary to the great saphenous vein (GSV)) and the posterior tibial vein. They may become varicose or incompetent in venous insufficiency states. The Boyd perforator veins connect the GSV to the deep veins approximately 10 cm below the knee and 1 to 2 cm medial to the tibia. (See Schwartz 9th ed., p 778.)

4. Warfarin inhibits γ-carboxylation of which of the following?
   A. Factor III
   B. Factor VII
   C. Factor VIII
   D. Factor XI

Answer: B

Vitamin K antagonists, which include warfarin and other coumarin derivatives, are the mainstay of long-term antithrombotic therapy in patients with venous thromboembolism (VTE). Warfarin inhibits the γ-carboxylation of vitamin K–dependent procoagulants (factors II, VII, IX, X) and anticoagulants (proteins C and S), which results in the formation of less functional proteins. (See Schwartz 9th ed., p 785.)

5. Thrombolytic drugs work by
   A. Converting plaminogen to plasmin
   B. Increasing the activity of plasmin
   C. Converting thrombin to fibrin
   D. Decreasing the activity of thrombin

Answer: A
Several thrombolysis preparations are available, including streptokinase, urokinase, alteplase (recombinant tissue plasminogen activator), reteplase, and tenecteplase. All these agents share the ability to convert plasminogen to plasmin, which leads to the degradation of fibrin. They differ with regard to their half-lives, their potential for inducing fibrinogenolysis (generalized lytic state), their potential for antigenicity, and their FDA-approved indications for use. (See Schwartz 9th ed., p 786.)

6. One of the factors which prevents thrombosis in the normal venous system is
   A. Smooth muscle contraction in the wall of the vein
   B. Distention of the vein as volume increases in diastole
   C. Endothelial production of prostaglandin
   D. Endothelial production of endothelial relaxing factor

Answer: D
Veins are thin-walled, highly distensible, and collapsible structures. Their structure specifically supports their two primary functions of transporting blood toward the heart and serving as a reservoir to prevent intravascular volume overload. The venous intima is composed of a nonthrombogenic endothelium with an underlying basement membrane and an elastic lamina. The endothelium produces endothelium-derived relaxing factor and prostacyclin, which help maintain a nonthrombogenic surface through inhibition of platelet aggregation and promotion of platelet disaggregation. (See Schwartz 9th ed., p 778.)

CLINICAL QUESTIONS

1. Anticoagulation with heparin requires monitoring which of the following?
   A. Thromboelastogram (TEG)
   B. Bleeding time
   C. PT
   D. PTT

Answer: D
The level of antithrombotic therapy after giving heparin should be monitored every 6 hours using the activated partial thromboplastin time (aPTT), with the goal range of 1.5 to 2.5 times control values.

This should correspond with plasma heparin anti-Xa activity levels of 0.3 to 0.7 IU/mL. (See Schwartz 9th ed., p 784.)

2. Which of the following is NOT a risk factor for venous thromboembolism?
   A. Factor XI elevation
   B. Protein C elevation
   C. Nephrotic syndrome
   D. Travel >6 hours

Answer: B
Protein C deficiency is a risk factor for thromboembolism. (See Schwartz 9th ed., p 781, and Table 24-1.)

TABLE 24-1 Risk factors for venous thromboembolism

Acquired	Inherited
Advanced age	Factor V Leiden
Hospitalization/immobilization	Prothrombin 20210A
Hormone replacement therapy and oral contraceptive use	Antithrombin deficiency
Pregnancy and puerperium	Protein C deficiency
Prior venous thromboembolism	Protein S deficiency
Malignancy	Factor XI elevation
Major surgery	Dysfibrinogenemia
Obesity	**Mixed Etiology**
Nephrotic syndrome	Homocysteinemia
Trauma or spinal cord injury	Factor VII, VIII, IX, XI elevation
Long-haul travel (>6 h)	Hyperfibrinogenemia
Varicose veins	Activated protein C resistance without factor V Leiden
Antiphospholipid antibody syndrome	
Myeloproliferative disease	
Polycythemia	

3. Full anticoagulation (steady state) when using warfarin is achieved in
   A. 24 hours
   B. 48 hours
   C. 4-5 days
   D. 7-10 days

Answer: C
Warfarin usually requires several days to achieve its full effect, because normal circulating coagulation proteins must first undergo their normal degradation. Factors X and II have the longest half-lives, in the range of 36 and 72 hours, respectively. In addition, the steady-state concentration of warfarin is usually not reached for 4 to 5 days. (See Schwartz 9th ed., p 785.)

4. The most effective therapy for lymphedema is
   A. Compression garments
   B. Surgical excision of the involved area
   C. Surgical bypass of the obstructed lymphatics
   D. Combined excision of affected areas with bypass of the obstructed lymphatics

Answer: A
An important aspect of the management of lymphedema is patient understanding that there is no cure for lymphedema. The primary goals of treatment are to minimize swelling and to prevent recurrent infections. Controlling the chronic limb swelling can improve discomfort, heaviness, and tightness, and potentially reduce the progression of disease.

Graded compression stockings are widely used in the treatment of lymphedema. The stockings reduce the amount of swelling in the involved extremity by preventing the accumulation of edema while the extremity is dependent. When worn daily, compression stockings have been associated with long-term maintenance of reduced limb circumference. They may also protect the tissues against chronically elevated intrinsic pressures, which lead to thickening of the skin and subcutaneous tissue. Compression stockings also offer a degree of protection against external trauma. (See Schwartz 9th ed., p 798.)

5. *Phlegmasia cerulea dolens* is caused by
   A. Obliteration of the major deep venous channels of the leg
   B. Obliteration of the major deep venous channels and the collateral veins of the leg
   C. Reperfusion injury following an isolated injury to the femoral vein
   D. Reperfusion injury following injury to both the femoral vein and artery

Answer: B
Massive DVT that obliterates the major deep venous channel of the extremity with relative sparing of collateral veins causes a condition called *phlegmasia alba dolens*. This condition is characterized by pain, pitting edema, and blanching. There is no associated cyanosis. When the thrombosis extends to the collateral veins, massive fluid sequestration and more significant edema ensues, resulting in a condition known as *phlegmasia cerulea dolens*. Phlegmasia cerulea dolens is preceded by phlegmasia alba dolens in 50 to 60% of patients. The affected extremity in phlegmasia cerulea dolens is extremely painful, edematous, and cyanotic, and arterial insufficiency or compartment syndrome may be present. If the condition is left untreated, venous gangrene can ensue, leading to amputation. (See Schwartz 9th ed., p 782.)

6. The incidence of deep vein thrombosis (DVT) in patients undergoing repair of a hip fracture who do NOT receive prophylaxis is greater than
   A. 10%
   B. 20%
   C. 30%
   D. 40%

Answer: D
Patients who undergo major general surgical, gynecologic, urologic, and neurosurgical procedures without thromboprophylaxis have a significant incidence of perioperative DVT (15 to 40%). The incidence is even higher with major trauma (40 to 80%), hip and knee replacement surgery (40 to 60%), and spinal cord injury (60 to 80%). (See Schwartz 9th ed., p 787, and Table 24-2.)

TABLE 24-2 Thromboembolism risk and recommended thromboprophylaxis in surgical patients

Level of Risk	Approximate DVT Risk without Thromboprophylaxis (%)	Suggested Thromboprophylaxis Options
Low risk	<10	No specific thromboprophylaxis
Minor surgery in mobile patients		Early and "aggressive" ambulation
Moderate risk	10–40	LMWH (at recommended doses), LDUH bid or tid, fondaparinux
Most general, open gynecologic, or urologic surgery		Mechanical thromboprophylaxis
Moderate VTE risk plus high bleeding risk		
High risk	40–80	LMWH (at recommended doses), fondaparinux, oral vitamin K antagonist (INR 2–3)
Hip or knee arthroplasty, hip fracture surgery		Mechanical thromboprophylaxis
Major trauma, spinal cord injury		
High VTE risk plus high bleeding risk		

DVT = deep vein thrombosis; INR = International Normalized Ratio; LDUH = low-dose unfractionated heparin; LMWH = low molecular weight heparin; VTE = venous thromboembolism.
Source: Adapted with permission from Geerts WH, Bergqvist D, Pineo GF, et al: Prevention of venous thromboembolism: American College of Chest Physicians Evidence-Based Clinical Practice Guidelines (8th edition). *Chest* 133:381, 2008.

7. The most common form of lymphedema is
   A. Congenital lymphedema
   B. Lymphedema praecox
   C. Lymphedema tarda
   D. Secondary lymphedema

Answer: D

Secondary lymphedema is far more common than primary lymphedema. Secondary lymphedema develops as a result of lymphatic obstruction or disruption. Axillary node dissection leading to lymphedema of the arm is the most common cause of secondary lymphedema in the United States. Other causes of secondary lymphedema include radiation therapy, trauma, infection, and malignancy. Globally, filariasis (caused by *Wuchereria bancrofti*, *Brugia malayi*, and *Brugia timori*) is the most common cause of secondary lymphedema.

Congenital lymphedema may involve a single lower extremity, multiple limbs, the genitalia, or the face. The edema typically develops before 2 years of age and may be associated with specific hereditary syndromes (Turner syndrome, Milroy syndrome, Klippel-Trenaunay-Weber syndrome). *Lymphedema praecox* is the most common form of primary lymphedema, accounting for 94% of cases. Lymphedema praecox is far more common in women, with the gender ratio favoring women 10:1. The onset is during childhood or the teenage years, and the swelling involves the foot and calf. *Lymphedema tarda* is uncommon, accounting for <10% of cases of primary lymphedema. The onset of edema is after 35 years of age. (See Schwartz 9th ed., p 796.)

8. The initial dose of heparin given to anticoagulate a patient with deep venous thrombosis is
   A. 50 units/kg
   B. 80 units/kg
   C. 120 units/kg
   D. 200 units/kg

Answer: B

Unfractionated heparin (UFH) therapy is most commonly administered with an initial IV bolus of 80 units/kg or 5000 units. Weight-based UFH dosages have been shown to be more effective than standard fixed boluses in rapidly achieving therapeutic levels. The initial bolus is followed by a continuous IV drip, initially at 18 units/kg per hour or 1300 units per hour. The half-life of IV UFH ranges from 45 to 90 minutes and is dose dependent. The level of antithrombotic therapy should be monitored every 6 hours using the activated partial thromboplastin time (aPTT), with the goal range of 1.5 to 2.5 times control values. This should correspond with plasma heparin anti-Xa activity levels of 0.3 to 0.7 IU/mL. (See Schwartz 9th ed., p 784.)

9. In a patient with symptomatic varicose veins where the great saphenous vein has reflux and a diameter of 1 cm, the preferred surgical treatment is
   A. Sclerotherapy
   B. RFA or laser ablation
   C. Vein valvuloplasty
   D. Surgical bypass

Answer: B

Patients with symptomatic great or small saphenous vein reflux may be treated with endovenous ablation techniques or surgical removal. Endovenous laser treatment and radiofrequency ablation (RFA) have gained in popularity in the past several years.

Injection sclerotherapy can be successful in varicose veins <3 mm in diameter and in telangiectatic vessels.

Saphenous vein ligation and stripping is still the more commonly performed procedure worldwide, and it may be the preferred therapy for patients with GSVs of very large diameter (>2 cm). (See Schwartz 9th ed., p 791.)

10. The preferred initial therapy of chronic venous insufficiency with ulceration is
   A. Compression therapy with Unna's boot or elastic stockings
   B. Saphenous vein high ligation and stripping or endovenous ablation
   C. Open ligation of perforator veins
   D. Reconstruction of the saphenofemoral junction

Answer: A

Compression therapy is most commonly achieved with graduated elastic compression stockings. Graduated elastic compression stockings, initially developed by Conrad Jobst in the 1950s, were made to simulate the gradient of hydrostatic forces exerted by water in a swimming pool. (See Schwartz 9th ed., p 793.)

Another method of compression was developed by the German dermatologist Paul Gerson Unna in 1896. Unna's boot has been used for many years to treat venous ulcers and is available in many versions. A typical Unna's boot consists of a three-layer dressing and requires application by trained personnel. A rolled gauze bandage impregnated with calamine, zinc oxide, glycerin, sorbitol, gelatin, and magnesium aluminum silicate is first applied with graded compression from the forefoot to just below the knee. The next layer consists of a 4-in-wide continuous gauze dressing followed by an outer layer of elastic wrap, also applied with graded compression. The bandage becomes stiff after drying and the rigidity may aid in preventing edema formation. Unna's boot is changed weekly, or sooner if the patient experiences significant drainage from the ulcer bed. (See Schwartz 9th ed., p 794.)

Incompetence of the perforating veins connecting the superficial and deep venous systems of the lower extremities has been implicated in the development of venous ulcers. The classic open technique described by Linton in 1938 for perforator vein ligation has a largely been abandoned. (See Schwartz 9th ed., p 795.)

11. Heparin-induced thrombocytopenia (HIT) occurs most commonly
    A. Within 24 hours of starting therapy
    B. 3 days after starting therapy
    C. 7 days after starting therapy
    D. 14 days after starting therapy

Answer: D

Heparin-induced thrombocytopenia (HIT) results from heparin-associated antiplatelet antibodies (HAAbs) directed against platelet factor 4 complexed with heparin. HIT occurs in 1 to 5% of patients being treated with heparin. In patients with repeat heparin exposure (such as vascular surgery patients), the incidence of HAAb may be as high as 21%. HIT occurs most frequently in the second week of therapy and may lead to disastrous venous or arterial thrombotic complications. Therefore, platelet counts should be monitored periodically in patients receiving continuous heparin therapy. (See Schwartz 9th ed., p 785.)

12. Indications to place an inferior vena cava (IVC) filter include
    A. Recurrent deep vein thrombosis (DVT) despite adequate anticoagulation
    B. Contraindication for anticoagulation in a patient with proximal DVT
    C. Pulmonary hypertension with recurrent pulmonary embolism
    D. All of the above

Answer: D

Placement of an IVC filter is indicated for patients who develop recurrent DVT (significant propagation of the original thrombus or proximal DVT at a new site) or pulmonary embolism (PE) despite adequate anticoagulation therapy and for patients with pulmonary hypertension who experience recurrent PE. In patients who receive IVC filters for these indications, therapeutic anticoagulation should be continued. The duration of anticoagulation is determined by the underlying venous thromboembolism (VTE) and not by the presence of the IVC filter itself. Practically speaking, however, many patients who require an IVC filter for recurrent VTE are the same ones who would benefit most from indefinite anticoagulation. The other major indication for placement of an IVC filter is a contraindication to, or complication of, anticoagulation therapy in the presence of an acute proximal DVT. (See Schwartz 9th ed., p 787.)

13. Initial therapy of a professional baseball player with acute venous thoracic outlet syndrome includes
    A. Observation
    B. Immobilization
    C. Thrombolytic therapy
    D. Surgical embolectomy and correction of the underlying anomaly

Answer: C

Patients with primary axillary-subclavian vein thrombosis (ASVT) often give a history of performing prolonged, repetitive motion activities, which results in damage to the subclavian vein, usually where it passes between the head of the clavicle and the first rib. This condition is also known as *venous thoracic outlet syndrome*, *effort thrombosis*, and *Paget-Schroetter syndrome*. Anticoagulation therapy should be initiated once ASVT is diagnosed to prevent PE and decrease symptoms. Patients presenting with acute symptomatic primary ASVT may be candidates for catheter-directed thrombolytic therapy. (See Schwartz 9th ed., p 790.)

14. A patient develops a first episode of deep venous thrombosis following a colon resection. How long should he be treated with anticoagulation?
    A. 2 weeks
    B. 4-6 weeks
    C. 3 months
    D. 1 year

Answer: C

The recommended duration of warfarin antithrombotic therapy is increasingly being stratified based on whether the deep vein thrombosis (DVT) was provoked or unprovoked, whether it was the first or a recurrent episode, where the DVT is located, and whether malignancy is present. Current American College of Chest Physicians (ACCP) recommendations for duration of warfarin therapy are summarized in Table 24-3. In patients with proximal DVT, several randomized clinical trials have demonstrated that shorter-term antithrombotic therapy (4 to 6 weeks) is associated with a higher rate of recurrence than 3 to 6 months of anticoagulation. (See Schwartz 9th ed., p 786.)

TABLE 24-3 Summary of American College of Chest Physicians recommendations regarding duration of long-term antithrombotic therapy for deep vein thrombosis (DVT)

Clinical Subgroup	Antithrombotic Treatment Duration
First episode DVT/transient risk	VKA for 3 mo
First episode DVT/unprovoked	VKA for at least 3 mo Consider for long-term therapy if: • Proximal DVT • Minimal bleeding risk • Stable coagulation monitoring
Distal DVT/unprovoked	VKA for 3 mo
Second episode DVT/unprovoked	VKA long-term therapy
DVT and cancer	LMWH 3–6 mo Then VKA or LMWH indefinitely until cancer resolves

LMWH = low molecular weight heparin; VKA = vitamin K antagonist.
Data from Kearon C, Kahn SR, Agnelli G, et al: Antithrombotic therapy for venous thromboembolic disease: American College of Chest Physicians Evidence-Based Clinical Practice Guidelines (8th edition). *Chest* 133:454S, 2008.

CHAPTER 25

Esophagus and Diaphragmatic Hernia

BASIC SCIENCE QUESTIONS

1. The esophagus has three normal points of narrowing. Which of the following is NOT one of the normal points of narrowing?
   A. At the cricopharyngeus muscle
   B. At the level of the aortic arch
   C. At the level of the carina
   D. At the level of the diaphragm

Answer: C

Three normal areas of esophageal narrowing are evident on the barium esophagogram or during esophagoscopy. The uppermost narrowing is located at the entrance into the esophagus and is caused by the cricopharyngeal muscle. Its luminal diameter is 1.5 cm, and it is the narrowest point of the esophagus. The middle narrowing is due to an indentation of the anterior and left lateral esophageal wall caused by the crossing of the left main stem bronchus and aortic arch. The luminal diameter at this point is 1.6 cm. The lowermost narrowing is at the hiatus of the diaphragm and is caused by the gastroesophageal sphincter mechanism. The luminal diameter at this point varies somewhat, depending on the distention of the esophagus by the passage of food, but has been measured at 1.6 to 1.9 cm. (See Schwartz 9th ed., p 805.)

2. The geometry of the circular muscle in the esophagus is
   A. Segmental
   B. Longitudinal
   C. Oblique
   D. Helical

Answer: D

The circular muscle layer of the esophagus is thicker than the outer longitudinal layer. In situ, the geometry of the circular muscle is helical and makes the peristalsis of the esophagus assume a wormlike drive, as opposed to segmental and sequential squeezing. As a consequence, severe motor abnormalities of the esophagus assume a corkscrew-like pattern on the barium swallow radiogram. (See Schwartz 9th ed., p 808.)

3. The components that contribute to the function of the LES include all of the following EXCEPT
   A. Length of the intra-abdominal esophagus
   B. Width of the diaphragmatic hiatus
   C. Resting pressure (tone) in the lower esophageal muscle
   D. Length of the area of increased tone in the lower esophageal muscle

Answer: B

As defined by esophageal manometry, there are three characteristics of the LES that work in unison to maintain its barrier function. These characteristics include the resting LES pressure, its overall length, and the intra-abdominal length that is exposed to the positive pressure environment of the abdomen.

Therefore, a permanently defective sphincter is defined by one or more of the following characteristics: An LES with a mean resting pressure of less than 6 mmHg, an overall sphincter length of <2 cm, and intra-abdominal sphincter length of <1 cm. When compared to normal subjects without GERD these values are below the 2.5 percentile for each parameter. The most common cause of a defective sphincter is an inadequate abdominal length. (See Schwartz 9th ed., p 828, and Table 25-1.)

TABLE 25-1 Normal manometric values of the distal esophageal sphincter, $n = 50$

Parameter	Median Value	2.5th Percentile	97.5th Percentile
Pressure (mmHg)	13	5.8	27.7
Overall length (cm)	3.6	2.1	5.6
Abdominal length (cm)	2	0.9	4.7

4. The primary reason that reflux is common after a big meal is
   A. Shortening of the LES
   B. Increased acid production
   C. Hyperperistalsis of the stomach
   D. Increased gastrin production

Answer: A

The resistance to gastroesophageal reflux is a function of both the resting LES pressure and length over which this pressure is exerted. Thus, as the sphincter becomes shorter, a higher pressure will be required in order to prevent a given amount of reflux. Much like the neck of a balloon as it is inflated, as the stomach fills and distends, sphincter length decreases. Therefore, if the overall length of the sphincter is permanently short from repeated distention of the fundus secondary to large volume meals, then with minimal episodes of gastric distention and pressure, there will be insufficient sphincter length for the barrier to remain competent, and reflux will occur. (See Schwartz 9th ed., p 851, and Fig. 25-1.)

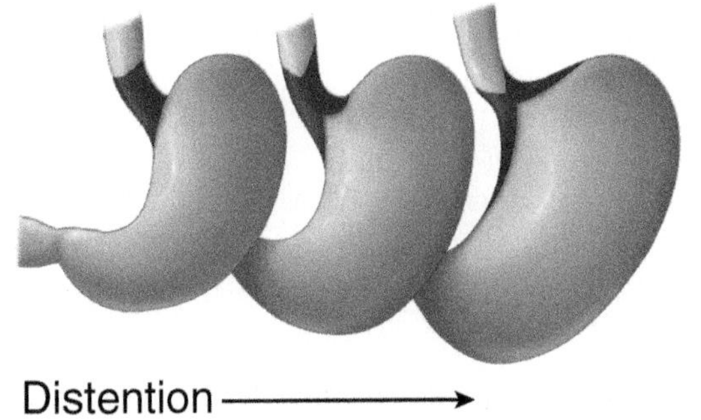

FIG. 25-1. A graphic illustration of the shortening of the lower esophageal sphincter that occurs as the sphincter is "taken up" by the cardia as the stomach distends.

5. Which of the following INCREASES lower esophageal sphincter (LES) pressure?
   A. Glucagon
   B. Gastrin
   C. Somatostatin
   D. Secretin

Answer: B

The LES has intrinsic myogenic tone, which is modulated by neural and hormonal mechanisms. Alpha-adrenergic neurotransmitters or beta blockers stimulate the LES, and alpha blockers and beta stimulants decrease its pressure. It is not clear to what extent cholinergic nerve activity controls LES pressure. The vagus nerve carries both excitatory and inhibitory fibers to the esophagus and sphincter. The hormones gastrin and motilin have been shown to increase LES pressure; and cholecystokinin, estrogen, glucagon, progesterone, somatostatin, and secretin decrease LES pressure. The peptides bombesin, l-enkephalin, and substance P increase LES pressure; and calcitonin gene-related peptide, gastric inhibitory peptide, neuropeptide Y, and vasoactive intestinal polypeptide decrease LES pressure. Some pharmacologic agents such as antacids, cholinergics, agonists, domperidone, metoclopramide, and prostaglandin F2 are known to increase LES pressure; and anticholinergics, barbiturates, calcium channel blockers, caffeine, diazepam, dopamine, meperidine, prostaglandin E_1 and E_2, and theophylline decrease LES pressure. Peppermint, chocolate, coffee, ethanol, and fat are all associated with decreased LES pressure and may be responsible for esophageal symptoms after a sumptuous meal. (See Schwartz 9th ed., p 812.)

6. Which of the following is NOT part of the arterial blood supply to the esophagus?
   A. Inferior thyroid artery
   B. Bronchial arteries
   C. Inferior phrenic artery
   D. Right gastric artery

Answer: D

The cervical portion of the esophagus receives its main blood supply from the inferior thyroid artery. The thoracic portion receives its blood supply from the bronchial arteries, with 75% of individuals having one right-sided and two left-sided branches. Two esophageal branches arise directly from the aorta. The abdominal portion of the esophagus receives its blood supply from the ascending branch of the left gastric artery and from inferior phrenic arteries. On entering the wall of the esophagus, the arteries assume a T-shaped division to form a longitudinal plexus, giving rise to an intramural vascular network in the muscular and submucosal layers. As a consequence, the esophagus can be mobilized from the stomach to the level of the aortic arch without fear of devascularization and ischemic necrosis. Caution should be exercised as to the extent of esophageal mobilization in patients who have had a previous thyroidectomy with ligation of the inferior thyroid arteries proximal to the origin of the esophageal branches. (See Schwartz 9th ed., p 808, and Fig. 25-2.)

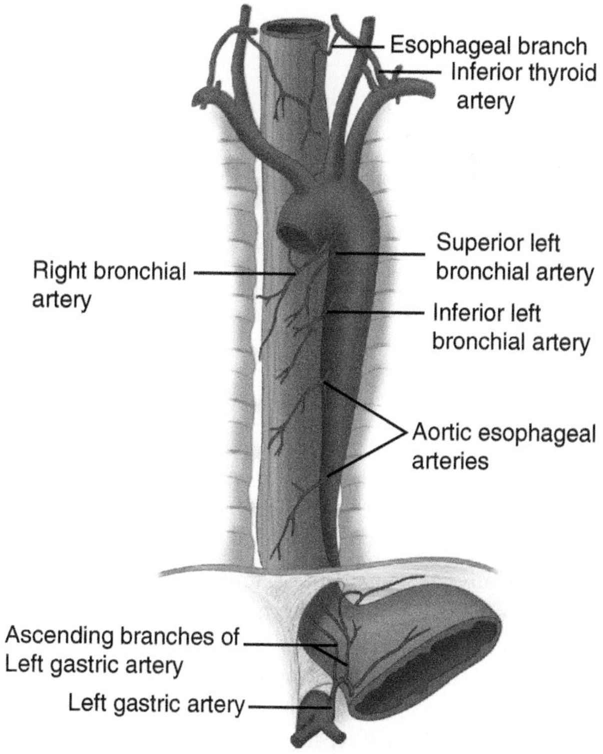

FIG. 25-2. Arterial blood supply of the esophagus. (Reproduced with permission from Rothberg M, DeMeester TR: Surgical anatomy of the esophagus, in Shields TW (ed): *General Thoracic Surgery*, 3rd ed. Philadelphia: Lea & Febiger, 1989, p 84.)

CLINICAL QUESTIONS

1. In a patient with Barrett's esophagitis, a fundoplication will
   A. Heal the mucosal injury
   B. Prevent Barrett's progression
   C. Improve symptoms
   D. All of the above

Answer: D

The long-term relief of symptoms remains the primary reason for performing antireflux surgery in patients with BE. Healing of esophageal mucosal injury and the prevention of disease progression are important secondary goals. In this regard, patients with BE are no different from the broader population of patients with gastroesophageal reflux. They should be considered for antireflux surgery when patient data suggest severe disease or predict the need for long-term medical management. Most patients with BE are symptomatic. Although it has been argued that some patients with BE may not have symptoms, careful history taking will reveal the presence of symptoms in most, if not all, patients. (See Schwartz 9th ed., p 831.)

2. Which of the following manometic findings is indicative of an incompetent lower esophageal sphincter (LES)?
   A. Average LES pressure <20 mmHg
   B. Average intra-abdominal esophagus <4 cm
   C. Average sphincter length <2 cm
   D. Average peak pressure <25 mmHg

Answer: C

A mechanically defective sphincter is identified by having one or more of the following characteristics: an average LES pressure of <6 mmHg, an average length exposed to the positive-pressure environment in the abdomen of 1 cm or less, and/or an average overall sphincter length of 2 cm or less. Compared with the normal volunteers, these values are below the 2.5 percentile for sphincter pressure and overall length and for abdominal length. (See Schwartz 9th ed., p 816, and Table 25-2.)

TABLE 25-2 Normal manometric values of the distal esophageal sphincter, $n = 50$

		Percentile	
	Median	**2.5**	**97.5**
Pressure (mmHg)	13	5.8	27.7
Overall length (cm)	3.6	2.1	5.6
Abdominal length (cm)	2	0.9	4.7
	Mean	**Mean − 2 SD**	**Mean +2 SD**
Pressure (mmHg)	13.8 ± 4.6	4.6	23.0
Overall length (cm)	3.7 ± 0.8	2.1	5.3
Abdominal length (cm)	2.2 ± 0.8	0.6	3.8

SD = standard deviation.
Source: Reproduced with permission from DeMeester TR, et al: Gastroesophageal reflux disease, in Moody FG, Carey LC, et al (eds): *Surgical Treatment of Digestive Disease.* Chicago: Year Book Medical, 1990, p 89. Copyright © Elsevier.

3. Nonoperative management of an esophageal perforation can be considered in patients who
   A. Have mild symptoms
   B. Show drainage of extravasated contrast back into the esophagus
   C. Have mild signs of sepsis
   D. All of the above

Answer: D

Conservative management [of esophageal perforation] should not be used in patients who have free perforations into the pleural space. Cameron proposed three criteria for the nonoperative management of esophageal perforation: (a) The barium swallow must show the perforation to be contained within the mediastinum and drain well back into the esophagus (Fig. 25-3), (b) symptoms should be mild, and (c) there should be minimal evidence of clinical sepsis. If these conditions are met, it is reasonable to treat the patient with hyperalimentation, antibiotics, and cimetidine to decrease acid secretion and diminish pepsin activity. Oral intake is resumed in 7 to 14 days, dependent on subsequent radiographic examinations. (See Schwartz 9th ed., p 876.)

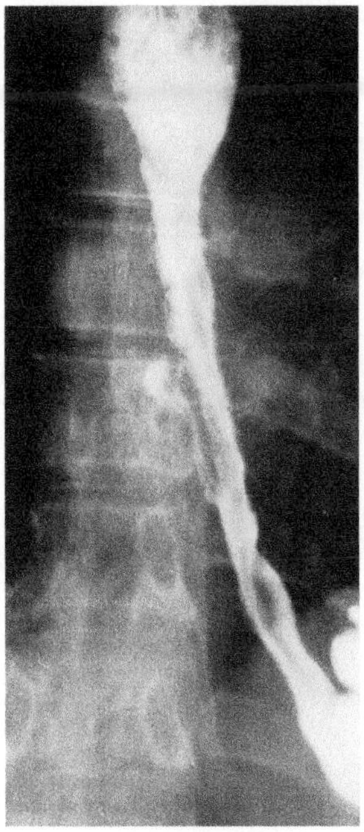

FIG. 25-3. Barium esophagogram showing a stricture and a contained perforation following dilation. The injury meets Cameron criteria: It is contained within the mediastinum and drawn back into the esophagus, the patient had mild symptoms, and there was no evidence of clinical sepsis. Nonoperative management was successful.

4. The initial pathologic change that leads to the clinical findings of achalasia is
   A. Hypertension of the LES
   B. Relaxation of the LES
   C. Hypertension of the body of the esophagus
   D. Diffuse relaxation of the body of the esophagus

Answer: A

The pathogenesis of achalasia is presumed to be a neurogenic degeneration, which is either idiopathic or due to infection. In experimental animals, the disease has been reproduced by destruction of the nucleus ambiguus and the dorsal motor nucleus of the vagus nerve. In patients with the disease, degenerative changes have been shown in the vagus nerve and in the ganglia in the myenteric plexus of the esophagus itself. This degeneration results in hypertension of the LES, a failure of the sphincter to relax on swallowing, elevation of intraluminal esophageal pressure, esophageal dilatation, and a subsequent loss of progressive peristalsis in the body of the esophagus. The esophageal dilatation results from the combination of a nonrelaxing sphincter, which causes a functional retention of ingested material in the esophagus, and elevation of intraluminal pressure from repetitive pharyngeal air swallowing (Fig. 25-4). With time, the functional disorder results in anatomic alterations seen on radiographic studies, such as a dilated esophagus with a tapering, 'bird's beak'–like narrowing of the distal end (Fig. 25-5). (See Schwartz 9th ed., p 851.)

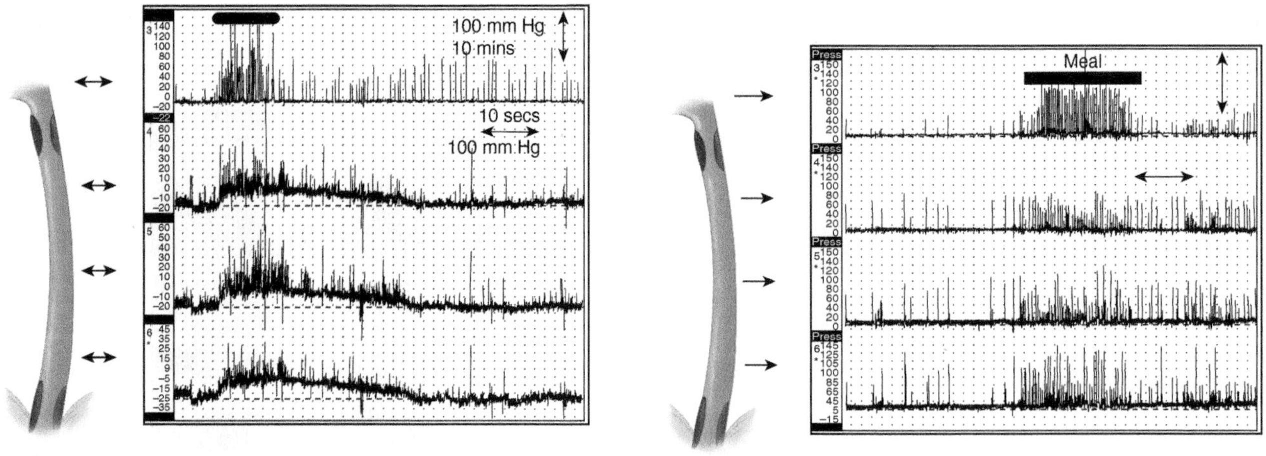

A B

FIG. 25-4. Pressurization of esophagus: Ambulatory motility tracing of a patient with achalasia. A. Before esophageal myotomy. B. After esophageal myotomy. The tracings have been compressed to exaggerate the motility spikes and baseline elevations. Note the rise in esophageal baseline pressure during a meal represented by the rise off the baseline to the left of panel A. No such rise occurs postmyotomy (panel B).

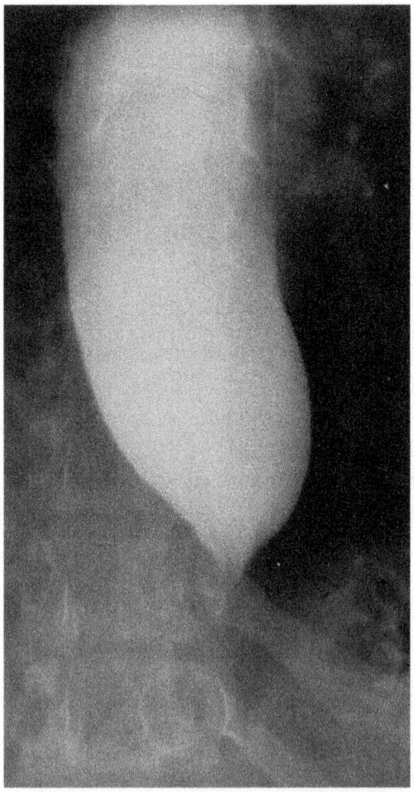

FIG. 25-5. Barium esophagogram showing a markedly dilated esophagus and characteristic "bird's beak" in achalasia. (Reproduced with permission from Waters PF, DeMeester TR: Foregut motor disorders and their surgical management. *Med Clin North Am* 65:1244, 1981. Copyright © Elsevier.)

5. The treatment of choice for an asymptomatic Schatzki's ring is
   A. Observation
   B. Dilation
   C. Incision (division of the ring)
   D. Resection with end-to-end anastomosis

Answer: A

Schatzki's ring is a thin submucosal circumferential ring in the lower esophagus at the squamocolumnar junction, often associated with a hiatal hernia.

The best form of treatment of a symptomatic Schatzki's ring in patients who do not have reflux consists of esophageal dilation for relief of the obstructive symptoms. In patients with a ring who have proven reflux and a mechanically defective sphincter, an antireflux procedure is necessary to obtain relief and avoid repeated dilation. (See Schwartz 9th ed., p 846, and Fig. 25-6.)

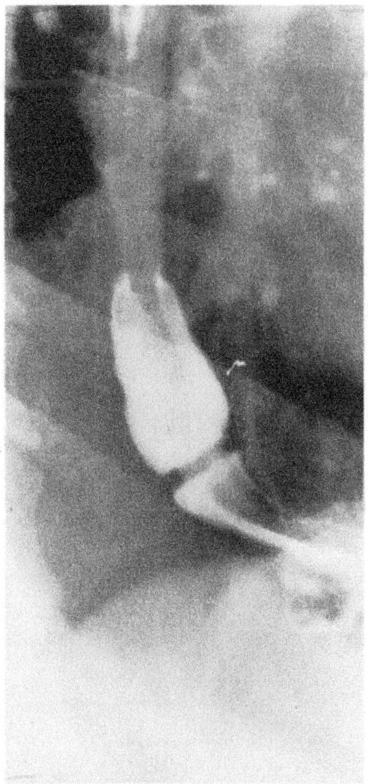

FIG. 25-6. Barium esophagogram showing Schatzki's ring (i.e., a thin circumferential ring in the distal esophagus at the squamocolumnar junction). Below the ring is a hiatal hernia.

6. Which of the following is NOT one of the five principles of surgical correction of gastroesophageal reflux?
   A. The fundoplication should be maintained in the abdomen by a crural repair
   B. The operation should restore the pressure of the LES to 10 times the resting gastric pressure
   C. An adequate amount of intra-abdominal esophagus must be obtained (approximately 2 cm)
   D. The fundoplication should not increase the resistance above what the peristalsis of the esophagus can overcome (approximately 2-cm wrap)

Answer: B

First, the operation should restore the pressure of the distal esophageal sphincter to a level twice the resting gastric pressure (i.e., 12 mmHg for a gastric pressure of 6 mmHg), and its length to at least 3 cm.

Second, the operation should place an adequate length of the distal esophageal sphincter in the positive-pressure environment of the abdomen by a method that ensures its response to changes in intra-abdominal pressure. The permanent restoration of 1.5 to 2 cm of abdominal esophagus in a patient whose sphincter pressure has been augmented to twice resting gastric pressure will maintain the competency of the cardia over various challenges of intra-abdominal pressure.

Third, the operation should allow the reconstructed cardia to relax on deglutition. In normal swallowing, a vagally mediated relaxation of the distal esophageal sphincter and the gastric fundus occurs. The relaxation lasts for approximately 10 seconds and is followed by a rapid recovery to the former tonicity. To ensure relaxation of the sphincter, three factors are important: (a) Only the fundus of the stomach should be used to buttress the sphincter, because it is known to relax in concert with the sphincter; (b) the gastric wrap should be properly placed around the sphincter and not incorporate a portion of the stomach or be placed around the stomach itself, because the body of the stomach does not relax with swallowing; and (c) damage to the vagal nerves during dissection of the thoracic esophagus should be avoided because it may result in failure of the sphincter to relax.

Fourth, the fundoplication should not increase the resistance of the relaxed sphincter to a level that exceeds the peristaltic power of the body of the esophagus. The resistance of the relaxed sphincter depends on the degree, length, and diameter of the gastric fundic wrap, and on the variation in intra-abdominal pressure. A 360° gastric wrap should be no longer than 2 cm and constructed over a 60F bougie. This will ensure that the relaxed sphincter will have an adequate diameter with minimal resistance.

Fifth, the operation should ensure that the fundoplication can be placed in the abdomen without undue tension, and maintained there by approximating the crura of the diaphragm above the repair. (See Schwartz 9th ed., p 836.)

7. Traction diverticula in the esophagus are the result of
   A. A congenital defect
   B. Infection or inflammation
   C. Motility disorders
   D. Trauma, usually iatrogenic

Answer: B

Diverticula of the esophagus may be characterized by their location in the esophagus (proximal, mid-, or distal esophagus), or by the nature of concomitant pathology. Diverticula associated with motor disorders are termed *pulsion diverticula* and those associated with inflammatory conditions are termed *traction diverticula*. Pulsion diverticula occur most commonly with nonspecific motility disorders, but can occur with all of the primary motility disorders. In the latter situation, the motility disorder is usually diagnosed before the development of the diverticulum. (See Schwartz 9th ed., p 853, and Fig. 25-7.)

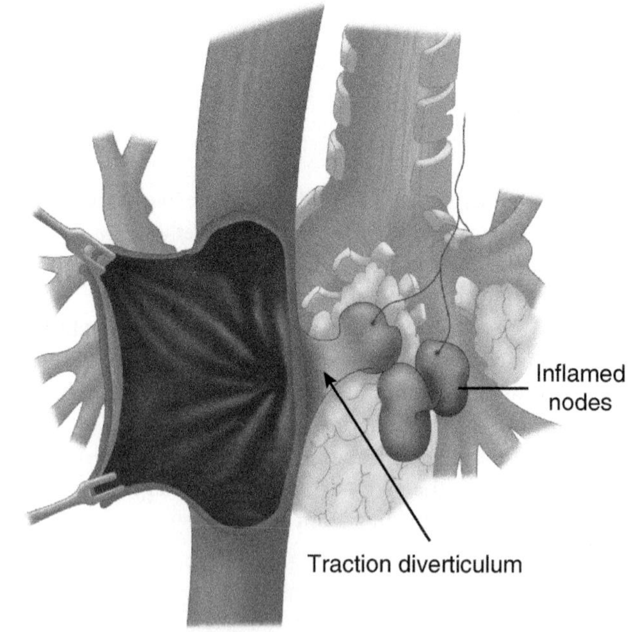

FIG. 25-7. Illustration of the pathophysiology of midesophageal diverticulum showing traction on the esophageal wall from adhesions to inflamed subcarinal lymph nodes.

8. Which of the following is the treatment of choice in a patient with scleroderma and multiple symptomatic strictures of the esophagus?
   A. Medical therapy alone (PPIs)
   B. Dilation and PPI's
   C. Toupet fundoplication, if dilation and PPI are ineffective
   D. Nissen fundoplication, if dilation and PPI are ineffective

Answer: C

Traditionally, esophageal symptoms [in patients with scleroderma] have been treated with PPIs, antacids, elevation of the head of the bed, and multiple dilations for strictures, with generally unsatisfactory results. The degree of esophagitis is usually severe and may lead to marked esophageal shortening as well as stricture. Scleroderma patients have frequently had numerous dilations before they are referred to the surgeon. The surgical management is somewhat controversial, but the majority of opinion suggests that a partial fundoplication (anterior or posterior) performed laparoscopically is the procedure of choice. The need for a partial fundoplication is dictated by the likelihood of severe dysphagia if a total fundoplication is performed in the presence of aperistalsis. Esophageal shortening may require a Collis gastroplasty in combination with a partial fundoplication. (See Schwartz 9th ed., p 847.)

9. Which of the following treatments should be considered in a patient with dysphagia and a T4N1M0 esophageal cancer of the gastroesophageal junction?
   A. Neoadjuvant chemotherapy, esophagectomy
   B. Esophagectomy, postoperative chemotherapy
   C. Palliative intraluminal stent
   D. Palliative radiation therapy

Answer: D

Therapy of esophageal cancer is dictated by the stage of the cancer at the time of diagnosis. Put simply, one needs to determine if the disease is confined to the esophagus (T1–T2, N0), locally advanced (T1–3, N1), or disseminated (any T, any N, M1). If cancer is confined to the esophagus, removal of the tumor with adjacent lymph nodes (LNs) may be curative. Very early tumors confined to the mucosa (T in situ, T1a, intramucosal cancer) may be addressed with endoscopic treatment. When the tumor is locally aggressive, modern therapy dictates a multimodality approach in a surgically fit patient. Multimodality therapy is either chemotherapy followed by surgery or radiation and chemotherapy followed by surgery. When given before surgery, these treatments are referred to as *neoadjuvant* or *induction therapy*. For disseminated cancer, treatment is aimed at palliation of symptoms. If the patient has dysphagia, as many do, the most rapid form of palliation is the placement of an expandable esophageal stent, endoscopically. For palliation of gastroesophageal junction (GEJ) cancer, radiation may be the first choice, as stents placed across the GEJ create a great deal of gastroesophageal reflux. (See Schwartz 9th ed., p 863.)

10. Patients with Barrett's esophagitis have a risk for adenocarcinoma of the esophagus that is
   A. 5 times the general population
   B. 40 times the general population
   C. 90 times the general population
   D. 200 times the general population

Answer: B

Adenocarcinoma developing in Barrett's mucosa was considered a rare tumor before 1975. Today, it occurs in approximately one in every 100 patient-years of follow-up, which represents a risk 40 times that of the general population. Most, if not all, cases of adenocarcinoma of the esophagus arise in Barrett's epithelium. (See Schwartz 9th ed., p 832.)

11. The most common type of hiatal hernia is
   A. Type I
   B. Type II
   C. Type III
   D. Type IV

Answer: A

With the advent of clinical radiology, it became evident that a diaphragmatic hernia was a relatively common abnormality and was not always accompanied by symptoms. Three types of esophageal hiatal hernia were identified: (a) the sliding hernia, type I, characterized by an upward dislocation of the cardia in the posterior mediastinum (Fig. 25-8A); (b) the rolling or paraesophageal hernia (PEH), type II, characterized by an upward dislocation of the gastric fundus alongside a normally positioned cardia (Fig. 25-8B); and (c) the combined sliding-rolling or mixed hernia, type III, characterized by an upward dislocation of both the cardia and the gastric fundus (Fig. 25-8C). The end stage of type I and type II hernias occurs when the whole stomach migrates up into the chest by rotating 180° around its longitudinal axis, with the cardia and pylorus as fixed points. In this situation the abnormality is usually referred to as an intrathoracic stomach (Fig. 25-8D). In some taxonomies, a type IV hiatal hernia is declared when an additional organ, usually the colon, herniates as well.

When radiographic examinations are done in response to GI symptoms, the incidence of a sliding hiatal hernia is seven times higher than that of a PEH. The PEH is also known as the *giant hiatal hernia*. Over time the pressure gradient between the abdomen and chest enlarges the hiatal hernia. In many cases the type 1 sliding hernia will evolve into a type III mixed hernia. Type II hernias are quite rare. (See Schwartz 9th ed., p 842.)

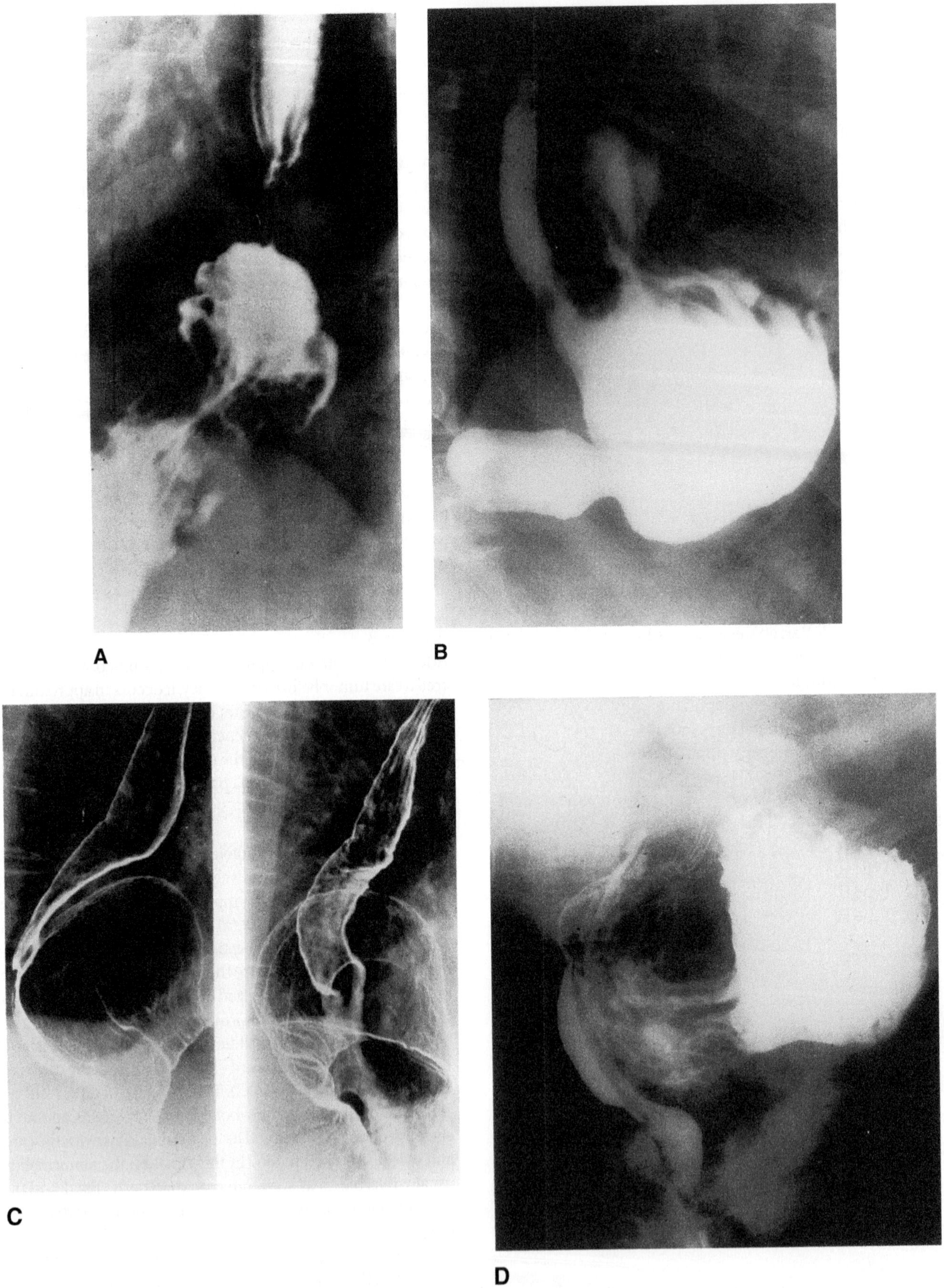

FIG. 25-8. A. Radiogram of a type I (sliding) hiatal hernia. B. Radiogram of a type II (rolling or paraesophageal) hernia. C. Radiogram of a type III (combined sliding-rolling or mixed) hernia. D. Radiogram of an intrathoracic stomach. This is the end stage of a large hiatal hernia regardless of its initial classification. Note that the stomach has rotated 180° around its longitudinal axis, with the cardia and pylorus as fixed points. (Reproduced with permission from DeMeester TR, Bonavina L: Paraesophageal hiatal hernia, in Nyhus LM, Condon RE (eds): *Hernia*, 3rd ed. Philadelphia: Lippincott, 1989, p 684.)

12. Which of the following is the best initial treatment for a patient with achalasia and a small hiatal hernia?
    A. Balloon dilation
    B. Botulinum toxin
    C. Myotomy of the LES
    D. Long esophageal myotomy

Answer: C

Long-term follow-up studies have shown that pneumatic dilation achieves adequate relief of dysphagia and pharyngeal regurgitation in 50 to 60% of patients with achalasia. Close follow-up is required, and if dilation fails, myotomy is indicated. For those patients who have a dilated and tortuous esophagus or an associated hiatal hernia, balloon dilation is dangerous and surgery is the better option. The outcome of the one controlled randomized study (38 patients) comparing the two modes of therapy suggests that surgical myotomy as a primary treatment gives better long-term results. Several randomized trials comparing laparoscopic cardiomyotomy with balloon dilation or botulinum toxin injection have favored the surgical approach as well. (See Schwartz 9th ed., p 857.)

In performing a surgical myotomy of the lower esophageal sphincter (LES), there are four important principles: (a) complete division of all circular and collarsling muscle fibers, (b) adequate distal myotomy to reduce outflow resistance, (c) "undermining" of the muscularis to allow wide separation of the esophageal muscle, and (d) prevention of postoperative reflux. In the past, the drawback of a surgical myotomy was the need for an open procedure, which often deterred patients from choosing the best treatment option for achalasia. With the advent of minimally invasive surgical techniques two decades ago, laparoscopic cardiomyotomy (Heller myotomy) has become the treatment of choice for most patients with achalasia. (See Schwartz 9th ed., p 859.)

13. Which of the following increases the risk of esophagitis in a patient with gastroesophageal reflux?
    A. Total time the esophageal mucosa is exposed to fluid with a pH <4
    B. Total time the esophageal mucosa is exposed to fluid with a pH >7
    C. Total time the esophageal mucosa is exposed to bile salts
    D. All of the above

Answer: D

Complications of gastroesophageal reflux such as esophagitis, stricture, and Barrett's metaplasia occur in the presence of two predisposing factors: a mechanically defective LES and an increased esophageal exposure to fluid with a pH of <4 and >7. (See Schwartz 9th ed., p 830.)

There is a considerable body of experimental evidence to indicate that maximal epithelial injury occurs during exposure to bile salts combined with acid and pepsin. These studies have shown that acid alone does minimal damage to the esophageal mucosa, but the combination of acid and pepsin is highly deleterious. Similarly, the reflux of duodenal juice alone does little damage to the mucosa, although the combination of duodenal juice and gastric acid is particularly noxious. (See Schwartz 9th ed., p 829.)

14. Which of the following makes curative resection of an esophageal cancer unlikely?
    A. Tumor length >6 cm
    B. Weight loss >10%
    C. Recurrent laryngeal nerve palsy
    D. >2 abnormal lymph nodes on CT scan

Answer: C

Clinical factors that indicate an advanced stage of carcinoma and exclude surgery with curative intent are recurrent nerve paralysis, Horner's syndrome, persistent spinal pain, paralysis of the diaphragm, fistula formation, and malignant pleural effusion. Factors that make surgical cure unlikely include a tumor >8 cm in length, abnormal axis of the esophagus on a barium radiogram, more than four enlarged lymph nodes (LNs) on CT, a weight loss more than 20%, and loss of appetite. Studies indicate that there are several favorable parameters associated with tumors <4 cm in length, there are fewer with tumors between 4 and 8 cm, and there are no favorable criteria for tumors >8 cm in length. Consequently, the finding of a tumor >8 cm in length should exclude curative resection; the finding of a smaller tumor should encourage an aggressive approach. (See Schwartz 9th ed., p 865.)

15. Following a cricopharyngeal myotomy, what is the best option to treat an associated 3-cm-long Zenker's diverticulum?
    A. Nothing, the diverticulum should be left in place
    B. Diverticulopexy
    C. Plication of the diverticulum
    D. Diverticulectomy

Answer: D
If a diverticulum is present and is large enough to persist after a myotomy, it may be sutured in the inverted position to the prevertebral fascia using a permanent suture (i.e., diverticulopexy) (Fig. 25-9). If the diverticulum is excessively large so that it would be redundant if suspended, or if its walls are thickened, a diverticulectomy should be performed. (See Schwartz 9th ed., p 849.)

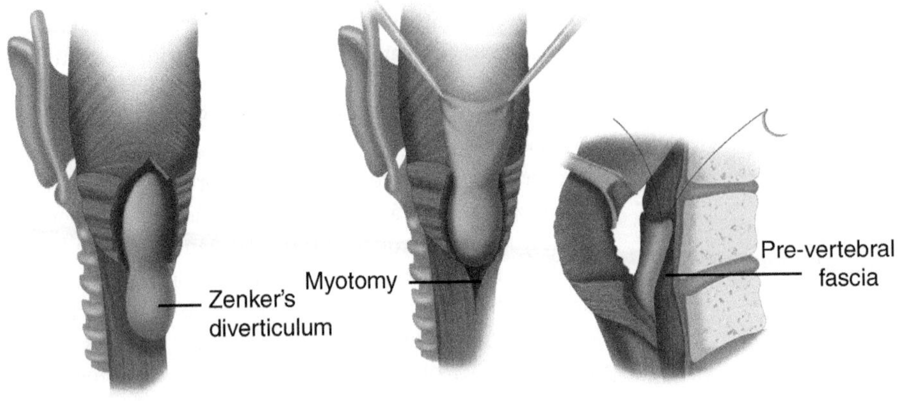

FIG. 25-9. Posterior of the anatomy of the pharynx and cervical esophagus showing pharyngoesophageal myotomy and pexing of the diverticulum to the prevertebral fascia.

16. A patient presents with dysphagia and undergoes a barium swallow. Based on the image in Fig. 25-10, the most likely diagnosis is
    A. Adenocarcinoma
    B. Adenoma
    C. Sarcoma
    D. Leiomyoma

Answer: D
A barium swallow is the most useful method to demonstrate a leiomyoma of the esophagus (Fig. 25-10). In profile, the tumor appears as a smooth, semilunar, or crescent-shaped filling defect that moves with swallowing, is sharply demarcated, and is covered and surrounded by normal mucosa. (See Schwartz 9th ed., p 874.)

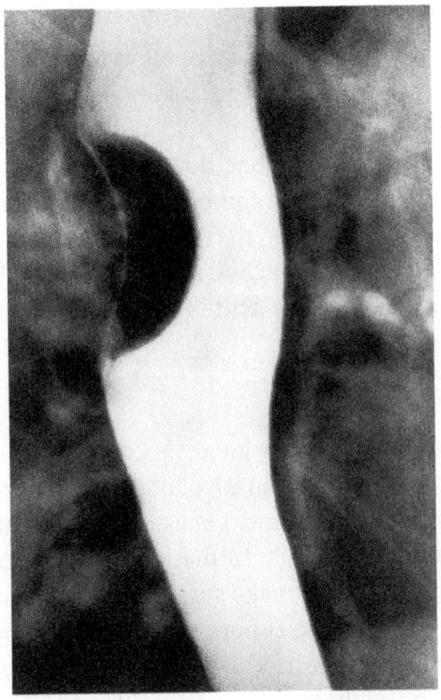

FIG. 25-10.

17. The most appropriate initial treatment for a patient with symptomatic nutcracker esophagus is
   A. Acid reducing agents
   B. Calcium channel blockers
   C. Nitroglycerin
   D. Dilation

Answer: A

At the lower end of peak pressure, it is unclear whether nutcracker esophagus causes any symptoms. In fact, chest pain symptoms in nutcracker esophagus patients may be related to GERD rather than intraluminal hypertension. Treatment in these patients should be aimed at the treatment of GERD. (See Schwartz 9th ed., p 852.)

18. In a patient with scleroderma, which of the following would be expected on a barium swallow?
   A. Dilated esophageal lumen
   B. Narrowed esophageal lumen
   C. "Beaking" of the distal esophagus
   D. Multiple strictures of the proximal esophagus

Answer: A

The diagnosis of scleroderma can be made manometrically by the observation of normal peristalsis in the proximal striated esophagus, with absent peristalsis in the distal smooth muscle portion. The LES pressure is progressively weakened as the disease advances. Because many of the systemic sequelae of the disease may be nondiagnostic, the motility pattern is frequently used as a specific diagnostic indicator. Gastroesophageal reflux commonly occurs in patients with scleroderma, because they have both hypotensive sphincters and poor esophageal clearance. This combined defect can lead to severe esophagitis and stricture formation. The typical barium swallow shows a dilated, barium-filled esophagus, stomach, and duodenum, or a hiatal hernia with distal esophageal stricture and proximal dilatation. (See Schwartz 9th ed., p 846.)

19. Esophageal adenocarcinoma occurs most commonly in the
   A. Cervical esophagus
   B. Upper thoracic esophagus
   C. Mid thoracic esophagus
   D. Lower thoracic esophagus

Answer: C

Tumors of the lower esophagus and cardia are usually adenocarcinomas. (See Schwartz 9th ed., p 865, and Fig. 25-11.)

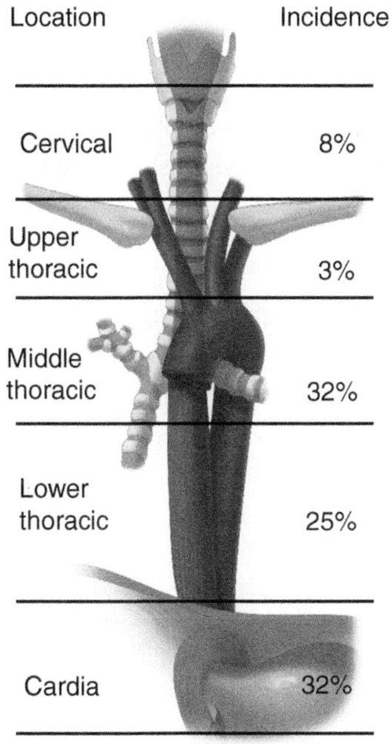
Location
Incidence
Cervical
8%
Upper thoracic
3%
Middle thoracic
32%
Lower thoracic
25%
Cardia
32%

FIG. 25-11. Incidence of carcinoma of the esophagus and cardia based on tumor location.

20. What is the appropriate treatment for a patient with a type III (mixed) hiatal hernia and iron deficiency anemia?
   A. Observation
   B. Acid reducing agents
   C. Repair of the hiatal hernia alone
   D. Repair of the hiatal hernia and fundoplication

Answer: D

Many patients with sliding hernias and reflux symptoms will lose the reflux symptoms when the hernia evolves into the paraesophageal variety. This can be explained by the re-creation of the cardiophrenic angle when the stomach herniates alongside the GEJ or becomes twisted in the sac. Repair of the hernia without addressing the reflux can create extremely bothersome heartburn. (See Schwartz 9th ed., p 843.)

21. A patient with dysphagia undergoes a barium swallow. Based on the image in Fig. 25-12, the most likely diagnosis is
    A. Achalasia
    B. Diffuse esophageal spasm
    C. Nutcracker esophagus
    D. Ineffective esophageal motility disorder

Answer: B
(See Schwartz 9th ed., p 852, and Fig. 25-12.)

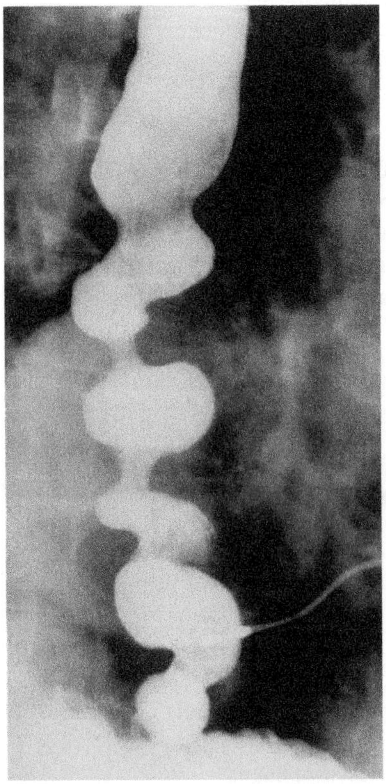

FIG. 25-12. Barium esophagogram of patient with diffuse spasm showing the corkscrew deformity.

22. In a patient undergoing curative resection for an adenocarcinoma of the gastroesophageal junction, how much proximal normal esophagus should be resected?
    A. 3 cm
    B. 5 cm
    C. 8 cm
    D. The entire thoracic esophagus (cervical division)

Answer: D
Because of the propensity of GI tumors to spread for long distances submucosally, long lengths of grossly normal GI tract should be resected. The longitudinal lymph flow in the esophagus can result in skip areas, with small foci of tumor above the primary lesion, which underscores the importance of a wide resection of esophageal tumors. Wong has shown that local recurrence at the anastomosis can be prevented by obtaining a 10-cm margin of normal esophagus above the tumor. Anatomic studies have also shown that there is no submucosal lymphatic barrier between the esophagus and the stomach at the cardia, and Wong has shown that 50% of the local recurrences in patients with esophageal cancer who are resected for cure occur in the intrathoracic stomach along the line of the gastric resection. Considering that the length of the esophagus ranges from 17 to 25 cm, and the length of the lesser curvature of the stomach is approximately 12 cm, a curative resection requires a cervical division of the esophagus and a >50% proximal gastrectomy in most patients with carcinoma of the distal esophagus or cardia. (See Schwartz 9th ed., p 865.)

23. Which of the following disorders is characterized by absent peristalsis in the esophageal body?
    A. Diffuse esophageal spasm
    B. Nutcracker esophagus
    C. Achalasia
    D. Hypertensive lower esophageal sphincter

Answer: C
(See Schwartz 9th ed., p 851, and Table 25-3.)

TABLE 25-3 Manometric characteristics of the primary esophageal motility disorders
Achalasia
Incomplete lower esophageal sphincter (LES) relaxation (<75% relaxation)
Aperistalsis in the esophageal body
Elevated LES pressure ≤26 mmHg
Increased intraesophageal baseline pressures relative to gastric baseline
Diffuse esophageal spasm (DES)
Simultaneous (nonperistaltic contractions) (>20% of wet swallows)
Repetitive and multipeaked contractions
Spontaneous contractions
Intermittent normal peristalsis
Contractions may be of increased amplitude and duration
Nutcracker esophagus
Mean peristaltic amplitude (10 wet swallows) in distal esophagus ≥180 mmHg
Increased mean duration of contractions (>7.0 s)
Normal peristaltic sequence
Hypertensive lower esophageal sphincter
Elevated LES pressure (≥26 mmHg)
Normal LES relaxation
Normal peristalsis in the esophageal body
Ineffective esophageal motility disorders
Decreased or absent amplitude of esophageal peristalsis (<30 mmHg)
Increased number of nontransmitted contractions

Source: Reproduced with permission from DeMeester TR, et al: Physiologic diagnostic studies, in Zuidema GD, Orringer MB (eds): *Shackelford's Surgery of the Alimentary Tract*, 3rd ed, Vol. I. Philadelphia: W.B. Saunders, 1991, p 115. Copyright © Elsevier.

24. A patient presents after vomiting 500 ml of bright red blood. Endoscopy shows a tear in the mucosa at the gastroesophageal junction (Mallory-Weiss syndrome). The most appropriate treatment is
    A. Observation
    B. Administration of anti-emetics
    C. Placement of a Sengstaken-Blakemore tube
    D. Surgical gastrotomy and oversewing of the tear

Answer: B
In the majority of patients [with Mallory-Weiss syndrome], the bleeding will stop spontaneously with nonoperative management. In addition to blood replacement, the stomach should be decompressed and antiemetics administered, as a distended stomach and continued vomiting aggravate further bleeding. A Sengstaken-Blakemore tube will not stop the bleeding, as the pressure in the balloon is not sufficient to overcome arterial pressure. Endoscopic injection of epinephrine may be therapeutic if bleeding does not stop spontaneously. Only occasionally will surgery be required to stop blood loss. The procedure consists of laparotomy and high gastrotomy with oversewing of the linear tear. Mortality is uncommon, and recurrence is rare. (See Schwartz 9th ed., p 876.)

25. Which of the following is NOT a risk factor for squamous carcinoma of the esophagus?
    A. Barrett's esophagitis
    B. Tylosis
    C. Human papillomavirus
    D. Zinc deficiency

Answer: A

Barrett's esophagitis is a risk factor for adenocarcinoma of the esophagus.

Squamous carcinoma accounts for the majority of esophageal carcinomas worldwide. Its incidence is highly variable, ranging from approximately 20 per 100,000 in the United States and Britain, to 160 per 100,000 in certain parts of South Africa and the Honan Province of China, and even 540 per 100,000 in the Guriev district of Kazakhstan. The environmental factors responsible for these localized high-incidence areas have not been conclusively identified, though additives to local foodstuffs (nitroso compounds in pickled vegetables and smoked meats) and mineral deficiencies (zinc and molybdenum) have been suggested. In Western societies, smoking and alcohol consumption are strongly linked with squamous carcinoma. Other definite associations link squamous carcinoma with long-standing achalasia, lye strictures, tylosis (an autosomal dominant disorder characterized by hyperkeratosis of the palms and soles), and human papillomavirus. (See Schwartz 9th ed., p 862.)

CHAPTER 26

Stomach

BASIC SCIENCE QUESTIONS

1. The majority of parietal cells are in the
   A. Fundus
   B. Cardia
   C. Body
   D. Antrum

Answer: C

The body of the stomach contains most of the parietal (oxyntic) cells, some of which are also present in the cardia and fundus. The normal human stomach contains approximately 1 billion parietal cells, and total gastric acid production is proportional to parietal cell mass. (See Schwartz 9th ed., p 890, and Fig. 26-1.)

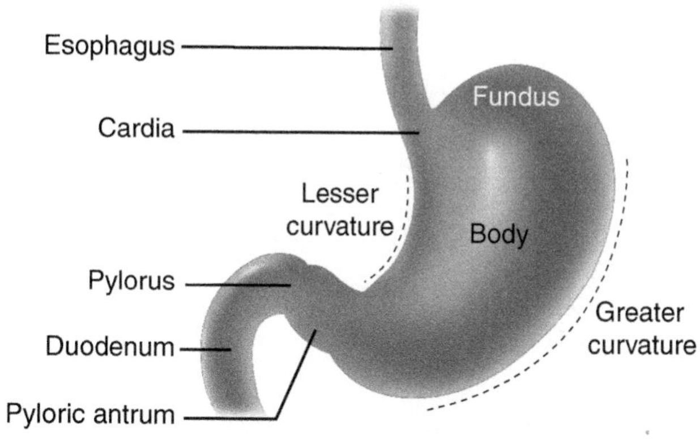

FIG. 26-1. Anatomic regions of the stomach. (Reproduced with permission from Mercer DW, Liu TH, Castaneda A: Anatomy and physiology of the stomach, in Zuidema GD, Yeo CJ (eds): *Shackelford's Surgery of the Alimentary Tract*, 5th ed., Vol. II. Philadelphia: Saunders, 2002, p 3. Copyright © Elsevier.)

2. Which of the following is consistently the largest artery to the stomach?
   A. Left gastric artery
   B. Right gastric artery
   C. Left gastroepiploic artery
   D. Right gastroepiploic artery

Answer: A

The consistently largest artery to the stomach is the left gastric artery, which usually arises directly from the celiac trunk and divides into an ascending and descending branch along the lesser gastric curvature. Approximately 15% of the time, the left gastric artery supplies an aberrant vessel that travels in the gastrohepatic ligament (lesser omentum) to the left side of the liver. Rarely, this is the only arterial blood supply to this part of the liver, and inadvertent ligation may lead to clinically significant hepatic ischemia in this unusual circumstance. The more common smaller aberrant left hepatic artery may usually be ligated without significant consequences. (See Schwartz 9th ed., p 890, and Fig. 26-2.)

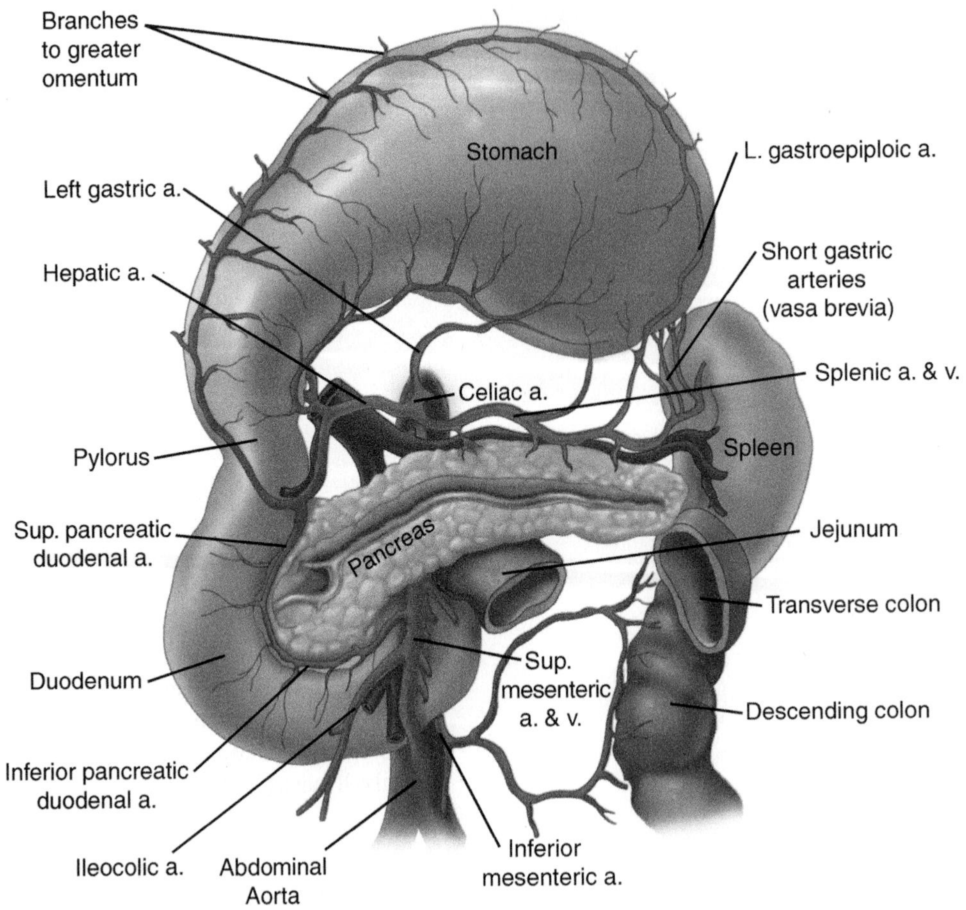

FIG. 26-2. Arterial blood supply to the stomach. a. = artery; v. = vein. (Reproduced with permission from Mercer DW, Liu TH, Castaneda A: Anatomy and physiology of the stomach, in Zuidema GD, Yeo CJ (eds): *Shackelford's Surgery of the Alimentary Tract*, 5th ed., Vol. II. Philadelphia: Saunders, 2002, p 3. Copyright © Elsevier.)

3. Which of the following gastric cells secrete intrinsic factor?
   A. Chief cells
   B. Parietal cells
   C. G cells
   D. D cells

Answer: B

Activated parietal cells secrete intrinsic factor in addition to hydrochloric acid. Presumably the stimulants are similar, but acid secretion and intrinsic factor secretion may not be linked. Intrinsic factor binds to luminal vitamin B_{12}, and the complex is absorbed in the terminal ileum via mucosal receptors. Vitamin B_{12} deficiency can be life threatening, and patients with total gastrectomy or pernicious anemia (i.e., patients with no parietal cells) require B_{12} supplementation by a nonenteric route. Some patients develop vitamin B_{12} deficiency following gastric bypass, presumably because there is insufficient intrinsic factor present in the small proximal gastric pouch. Under normal conditions, a significant excess of intrinsic factor is secreted, and acid-suppressive medication does not appear to inhibit intrinsic factor production and release.

Chief cells secrete pepsinogen, G cells secrete gastric, and D cells secrete somatostatin. (See Schwartz 9th ed., p 898.)

4. One of the important mediators of the gastric phase of acid secretion is
   A. The hypothalamus
   B. The vagal nerves
   C. Gastrin production by the antral G cells
   D. Hormonal stimulation by the small intestine

Answer: C

The acid secretory response that occurs after a meal is traditionally described in three phases: cephalic, gastric, and intestinal. The cephalic or vagal phase begins with the thought, sight, smell, and/or taste of food. These stimuli activate several cortical and hypothalamic sites (e.g., tractus solitarius, dorsal motor nucleus, and dorsal vagal complex), and signals are transmitted to the stomach by the vagal nerves. (See Schwartz 9th ed., p 897.)

When food reaches the stomach, the gastric phase of acid secretion begins. This phase lasts until the stomach is empty, and accounts for about 60% of the total acid secretion in response to a meal. The gastric phase of acid secretion has several components. Amino acids and small peptides directly stimulate antral G cells to secrete gastrin, which is carried in the bloodstream to the parietal cells and stimulates acid secretion in an endocrine fashion. In addition, proximal gastric distention stimulates acid secretion via a vagovagal reflex arc, which is abolished by truncal or HSV. Antral distention also stimulates antral gastrin secretion. Acetylcholine stimulates gastrin release and gastrin stimulates histamine release from ECL cells.

The intestinal phase of gastric secretion is poorly understood. It is thought to be mediated by a hormone yet to be discovered that is released from the proximal small bowel mucosa in response to luminal chyme. (See Schwartz 9th ed., p 898.)

5. The primary function of leptin is
   A. To stimulate acid production in the stomach
   B. To decrease acid production in the stomach
   C. To decrease appetite
   D. To increase appetite

Answer: C

Leptin is a protein primarily synthesized in adipocytes. It is also made by chief cells in the stomach, the main source of leptin in the GI tract. Leptin works at least in part via vagally mediated pathways to decrease food intake in animals. Not surprisingly, leptin, a satiety signal hormone, and ghrelin, a hunger signal hormone, are both primarily synthesized in the stomach, an organ increasingly recognized as central to the mechanisms of appetite control.

Ghrelin is a potent secretagogue of pituitary growth hormone (but not adrenocorticotropic hormone, follicle-stimulating hormone, luteinizing hormone, prolactin, or thyroid-stimulating hormone). Ghrelin appears to be an orexigenic regulator of appetite (i.e., when ghrelin is elevated, appetite is stimulated, and when it is suppressed, appetite is suppressed). Resection of the primary source of this hormone (i.e., the stomach) may partly account for the anorexia and weight loss seen in some patients following gastrectomy

(Fig. 26-3). The gastric bypass operation, a very effective treatment for morbid obesity, has been shown by some investigators to be associated with suppression of plasma ghrelin levels (and appetite) in humans (Fig. 26-4A). Other groups have failed to show a significant decrease in ghrelin levels following gastric bypass but have found such decreases following sleeve gastrectomy, another effective weight loss operation (Fig. 26-4B). Obviously appetite control is complex with redundant and overlapping orexigenic and anorexigenic pathways and signals.

Recently, it has been noted that the anorexigenic hormone leptin, secreted mostly by fat but also by gastric mucosa, inhibits gastric emptying, perhaps through the same pathway as CCK (which also has properties of a satiety hormone). The orexigenic hormone ghrelin has the opposite effect. (See Schwartz 9th ed., pp 899-900.)

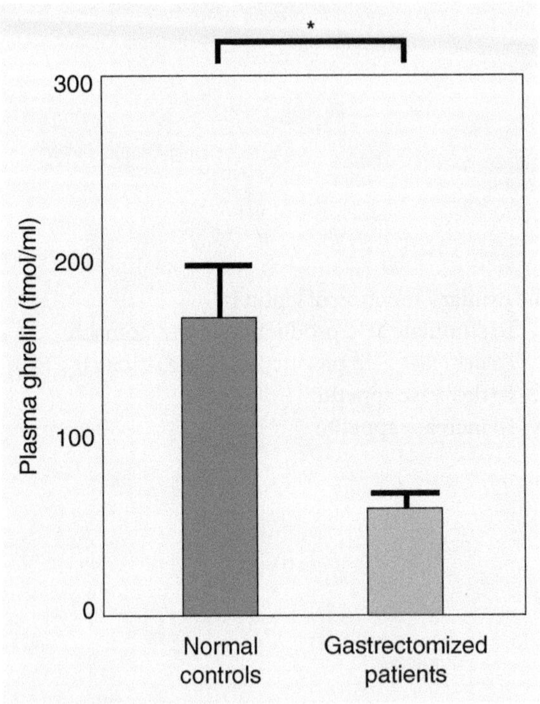

FIG. 26-3. Ghrelin levels are decreased after gastrectomy. (Reproduced with permission from Ariyasu H, Takaya K, Tagami T, et al: Stomach is a major source of circulating ghrelin, and feeding state determines plasma ghrelin-like immunoreactivity levels in humans. *J Clin Endocrinol Metab* 86:4753, 2001.)

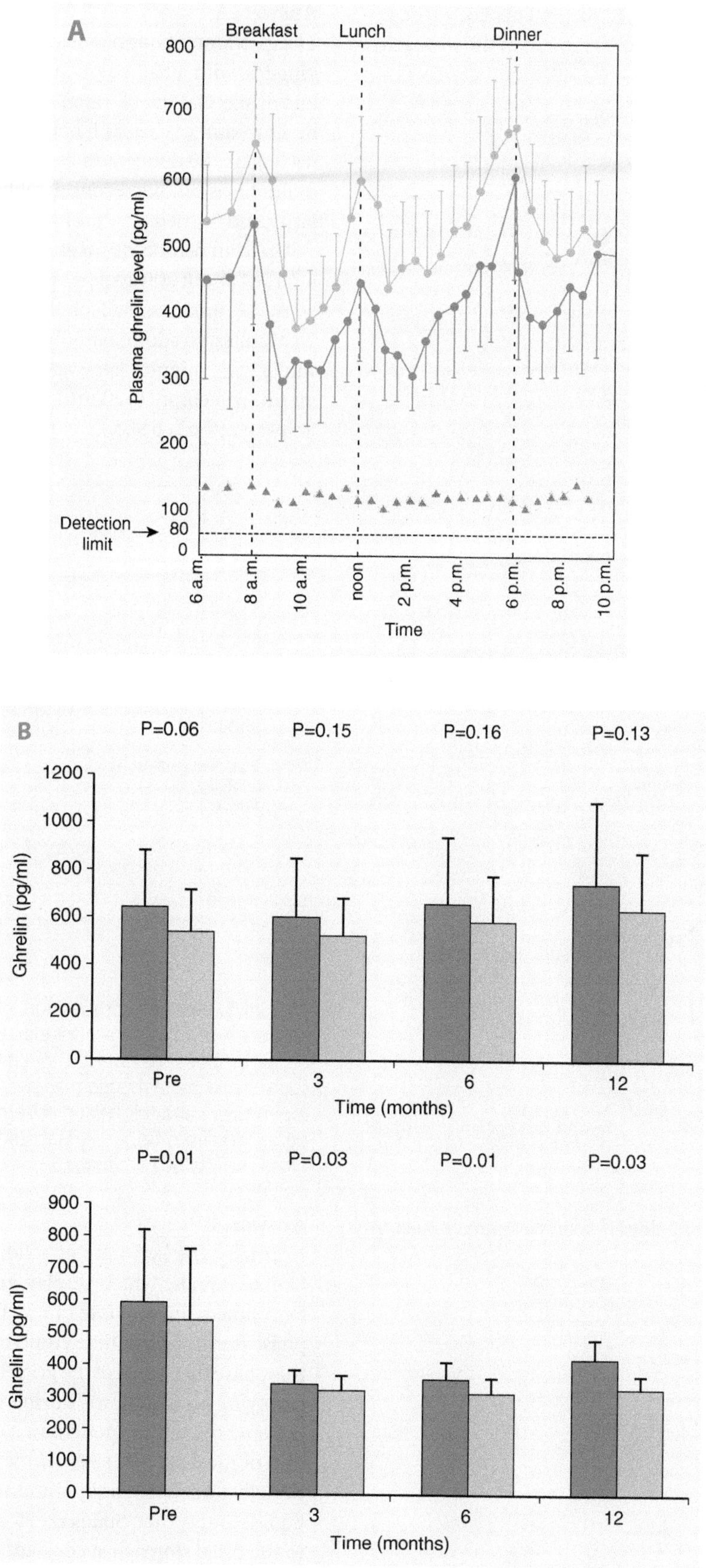

FIG. 26-4. A and B. Ghrelin secretion after bariatric surgery. Some investigators have suggested that ghrelin secretion is dramatically decreased after gastric bypass. Other groups have shown statistically insignificant changes in ghrelin levels after gastric bypass, but significant decreases after sleeve gastrectomy. (Fig. 26-4A reproduced with permission from Cummings DE, et al: Plasma ghrelin levels after diet-induced weight loss or gastric bypass surgery. *N Engl J Med* 346:1623, 2002. Copyright © 2002 Massachusetts Medical Society. All rights reserved. Fig. 26-4B reproduced with permission from Karamanakos SN, et al: Weight loss, appetite suppression, and changes in fasting and postprandial ghrelin and peptide-YY levels after Roux-en-Y gastric bypass and sleeve gastrectomy: A prospective, double blind study. *Ann Surg* 247:401, 2008.)

6. Thirty minutes after drinking 12 oz (360 mL) of water, approximately how much water will remain in the stomach?
   A. 70 mL
   B. 110 mL
   C. 180 mL
   D. 250 mL

Answer: A

The gastric emptying of water or isotonic saline follows first-order kinetics, with a half emptying time around 12 minutes. Thus, if one drinks 200 mL of water, about 100 mL enters the duodenum by 12 minutes, whereas if one drinks 400 mL of water, about 200 mL enters the duodenum by 12 minutes. This emptying pattern of liquids is modified considerably as the caloric density, osmolarity, and nutrient composition of the liquid changes (Fig. 26-5).

Up to an osmolarity of about 1 M, liquid emptying occurs at a rate of about 200 kcal per hour.

At 12 minutes, half of the 360 mL will remain (180). At 24 minutes, an additional 50% (or 90 mL) will have emptied, leaving 90. Six minutes later, approximately 25% of the remaining 90 mL will empty (~20 mL), leaving approximately 70 mL. (See Schwartz 9th ed., p 903.)

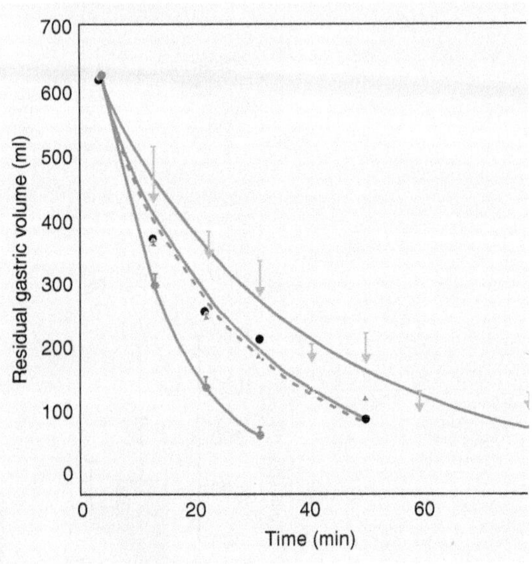

FIG. 26-5. Nutrient composition and caloric density affect liquid gastric emptying. Glucose solution (solid circles), the least calorically dense, emptied the fastest. Other more calorically dense solutions, such as milk protein (solid triangles) and peptide hydrolysates (open circles and solid triangles), emptied slower. (Reproduced with permission from Calbet JA, MacLean DA: Role of caloric content on gastric emptying in humans. *J Physiol* 498:533, 1997.)

7. Approximately how long does it take the stomach to empty half of a solid meal?
   A. <1 hour
   B. <2 hours
   C. 2-3 hours
   D. 3-4 hours

Answer: B

Normally, the half-time of solid gastric emptying is <2 hours. Unlike liquids, which display an initial rapid phase followed by a slower linear phase of emptying, solids have an initial lag phase during which little emptying of solids occurs. It is during this phase that much of the grinding and mixing occurs. A linear emptying phase follows, during which the smaller particles are metered out to the duodenum. Solid gastric emptying is a function of meal particle size, caloric content, and composition (especially fat). When liquids and solids are ingested together, the liquids empty first. Solids are stored in the fundus and delivered to the distal stomach at constant rates for grinding. Liquids also are sequestered in the fundus, but they appear to be readily delivered to the distal stomach for early emptying. The larger the solid component of the meal, the slower the liquid emptying. Patients bothered by dumping syndrome are advised to limit the amount of liquid consumed with the solid meal, taking advantage of this effect. (See Schwartz 9th ed., p 904.)

8. Which of the following agents is a motilin agonist?
   A. Metaclopramide
   B. Cisapride
   C. Erythromycin
   D. Domperidone

Answer: C
(See Schwartz 9th ed., p 904, and Table 26-1.)

TABLE 26-1 Drugs that accelerate gastric emptying

Agent	Typical Adult Dose	Mechanism of Action
Metoclopramide	10 mg PO qid	Dopamine antagonist
Erythromycin	250 mg PO qid	Motilin agonist
Domperidone	10 mg PO qid	Dopamine antagonist

9. What percentage of the world's population is infected with *Helicobacter pylori*?
   A. 5%
   B. 20%
   C. 35%
   D. 50%

Answer: D
With specialized flagella and a rich supply of urease, *H. pylori* is uniquely equipped for survival in the hostile environment of the stomach. Fifty percent of the world's population is infected with *H. pylori*, a major cause of chronic gastritis. The same sequence of inflammation to metaplasia to dysplasia to carcinoma, that is well known to occur in the esophagus from reflux-induced inflammation (and in the colon from inflammatory bowel disease), is now increasingly well recognized to occur in the stomach with *Helicobacter*-induced gastritis. The influence of prolonged acid suppression with PPIs or H_2RAs on these esophagogastric processes is largely unknown. *Helicobacter* also clearly has an etiologic role in the development of gastric lymphoma. (See Schwartz 9th ed., p 908.)

10. *Helicobacter pylori* causes increased acid production in the stomach by
   A. Stimulation of parietal cells
   B. Inhibition of D cells
   C. Stimulation of cells of Cajal
   D. Inhibition of G cells

Answer: B
One of the mechanisms by which *Helicobacter* causes gastric injury may be through a disturbance in gastric acid secretion. This is due, in part, to the inhibitory effect that *H. pylori* exerts on antral D cells that secrete somatostatin, a potent inhibitor of antral G-cell gastrin production. *H. pylori* infection is associated with decreased levels of somatostatin, decreased somatostatin messenger RNA production, and fewer somatostatin-producing D cells. These effects are probably mediated by *H. pylori*–induced local alkalinization of the antrum (antral acidification is the most potent antagonist to antral gastrin secretion), and *H. pylori*–mediated increases in other local mediators and cytokines. The end result is hypergastrinemia and acid hypersecretion. (See Schwartz 9th ed., pp 908-909, and Fig. 26-6.)

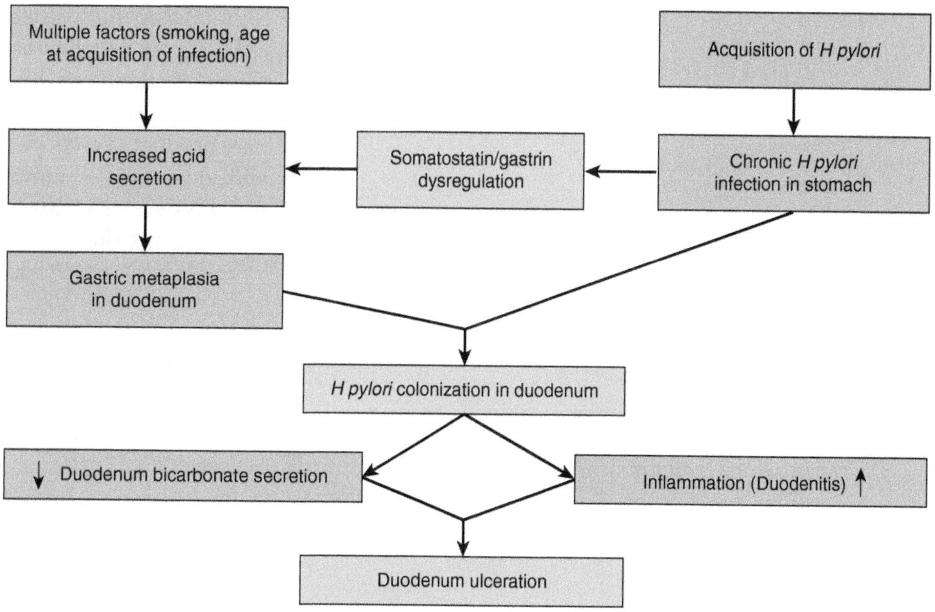

FIG. 26-6. Model of *Helicobacter* effects on duodenal ulcer pathogenesis. (Reproduced with permission from Peek RM Jr., Blaser MJ: Pathophysiology of *Helicobacter pylori*-induced gastritis and peptic ulcer disease. *Am J Med* 102:200, 1997. Copyright © Elsevier.)

11. Which of the following is a risk factor for gastric cancer?
    A. Blood group A
    B. Blood group B
    C. Blood group AB
    D. Blood group O

Answer: A

Gastric cancer is more common in patients with pernicious anemia, blood group A, or a family history of gastric cancer. When patients migrate from a high-incidence region to a low-incidence region, the risk of gastric cancer decreases in the subsequent generations born in the new region. This strongly suggests an environmental influence on the development of gastric cancer. Environmental factors appear to be more related etiologically to the intestinal form of gastric cancer than the more aggressive diffuse form. The commonly accepted risk factors for gastric cancer are listed in Table 26-2. (See Schwartz 9th ed., p 927.)

TABLE 26-2 Factors increasing or decreasing the risk of gastric cancer

Increase risk
Family history
Diet (high in nitrates, salt, fat)
Familial polyposis
Gastric adenomas
Hereditary nonpolyposis colorectal cancer
Helicobacter pylori infection
Atrophic gastritis, intestinal metaplasia, dysplasia
Previous gastrectomy or gastrojejunostomy (>10 y ago)
Tobacco use
Ménétrier's disease
Decrease risk
Aspirin
Diet (high fresh fruit and vegetable intake)
Vitamin C

12. The cell of origin of gastrointestinal stromal tumors (GIST) is
    A. Smooth muscle
    B. G cell
    C. D cell
    D. Interstitial cell of Cajal

Answer: D

GISTs arise from interstitial cells of Cajal (ICC) and are distinct from leiomyoma and leiomyosarcoma, which arise from smooth muscle.

Almost all GISTs (and almost no smooth muscle tumors) express *c-kit* (CD117) or the related PDGFRA, as well as CD34; almost all smooth muscle tumors (and almost no GISTs) express actin and desmin. These markers can often be detected on specimens obtained by fine-needle aspiration and are useful in differentiating between GIST and smooth muscle tumor histopathologically.

GISTs are usually positive for the protooncogene, *c-kit*, a characteristic shared with the ICC. Imatinib (Gleevec), a chemotherapeutic agent that blocks the activity of the tyrosine kinase product of c-*kit*, yields excellent results in many patients with metastatic or unresectable GIST. Up to 50% of treated patients develop resistance to imatinib by 2 years, and several newer agents show promise for patients with refractory disease. (See Schwartz 9th ed., p 937.)

AC

13. Calcium absorption occurs in
    A. The body of the stomach
    B. The antrum of the stomach
    C. The duodenum
    D. The proximal jejunum

Answer: C

Gastric surgery sometimes disturbs calcium and vitamin D metabolism. Calcium absorption occurs primarily in the duodenum, which is bypassed with gastrojejunostomy. (See Schwartz 9th ed., p 946.)

CLINICAL QUESTIONS

1. Long-term suppression of gastric acid with proton pump inhibitors (PPIs) has been associated with
   A. More virulent strains of *Salmonella*
   B. Increased incidence of gastric ulcer
   C. Higher risk for *Clostridium difficile* colitis
   D. Macrocytic anemia

Answer: C

Long-term acid suppression with proton pump inhibitors (PPIs) has been associated with an increased risk of community acquired *Clostridium difficile* colitis and other gastroenteritides, presumably because of the absence of this protective germicidal barrier. (See Schwartz 9th ed., p 897.)

2. A patient with a vagotomy and pyloroplasty returns with a recurrent ulcer. The best method for determining if there was an inadequate vagotomy performed is
   A. Direct vagal stimulation
   B. Stimulated gastric analysis
   C. Stimulated PPI (pancreatic polypeptide) levels
   D. None of the above—there is no good test to determine inadequate vagotomy

Answer: C

Historically, gastric analysis was performed most commonly to test for the adequacy of vagotomy in postoperative patients with recurrent or persistent ulcer. Now this can be done by assessing peripheral pancreatic polypeptide levels in response to sham feeding. A 50% increase in pancreatic polypeptide within 30 minutes of sham feeding suggests vagal integrity. (See Schwartz 9th ed., p 906.)

3. Which of the following is the best test to confirm eradication of *Helicobacter pylori*?
   A. Negative histology after biopsy during EGD
   B. Negative fecal antigen
   C. Negative urea breath test
   D. Negative urea blood test

Answer: C

A variety of tests can help the clinician to determine whether the patient has active *H. pylori* infection. The predictive value (positive and negative) of any of these tests when used as a screening tool depends on the prevalence of *H. pylori* infection in the screened population. *A positive test is quite accurate in predicting* H. pylori *infection, but a negative test is characteristically unreliable*. Thus, in the appropriate clinical setting, treatment for *H. pylori* should be initiated on the basis of a positive test, but not necessarily withheld if the test is negative.

A positive serologic test is presumptive evidence of active infection if the patient has never been treated for *H. pylori*. Histologic examination of an antral mucosal biopsy using special stains is the gold standard test. Other sensitive tests include commercially available rapid urease tests, which assay for the presence of urease in mucosal biopsies (strong presumptive evidence of infection). Urease is an omnipresent enzyme in *H. pylori* strains that colonize the gastric mucosa. The labeled carbon-13 urea breath test has become the standard test to confirm eradication of *H. pylori* following appropriate treatment. In this test, the patient ingests urea labeled with nonradioactive ^{13}C. The labeled urea is acted upon by the urease present in the *H. pylori* and converted into ammonia and carbon dioxide. The radiolabeled carbon dioxide is excreted from the lungs and can be detected in the expired air. It also can be detected in a blood sample. The fecal antigen test also is quite sensitive and specific for active *H. pylori* infection and may prove more practical in confirming a cure. (See Schwartz 9th ed., p 906.)

4. Which of the following locations of gastric ulcers is associated with increased acid production?
   A. Cardia
   B. Fundus
   C. Angularis Iincisiura
   D. Pylorus

Answer: D
In patients with gastric ulcer, acid secretion is variable. Currently, five types of gastric ulcer are described, although the original Johnson classification contained three types (Fig. 26-7). The most common, Johnson type I gastric ulcer, is typically located near the angularis incisura on the lesser curvature, close to the border between the antrum and the body of the stomach. Patients with type I gastric ulcer usually have normal or decreased acid secretion. Type II gastric ulcer is associated with active or quiescent duodenal ulcer disease, and type III gastric ulcer is prepyloric ulcer disease. Both type II and type III gastric ulcers are associated with normal or increased gastric acid secretion. Type IV gastric ulcers occur near the GE junction, and acid secretion is normal or below normal. Type V gastric ulcers are medication induced and may occur anywhere in the stomach. (See Schwartz 9th ed., p 909.)

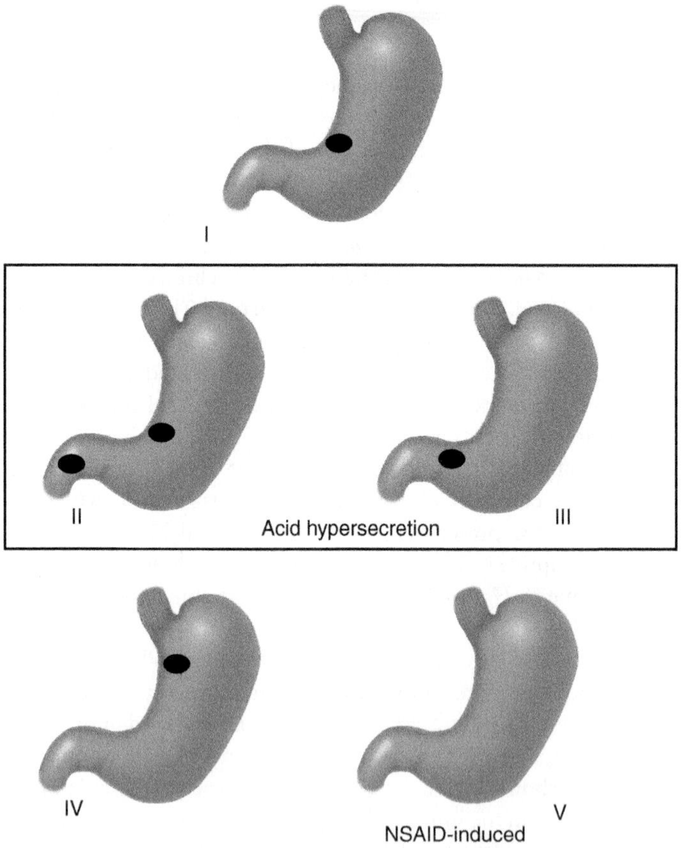
I
II
Acid hypersecretion
III
IV
V
NSAID-induced

FIG. 26-7. Modified Johnson classification for gastric ulcer. I. Lesser curve, incisura. II. Body of stomach, incisura + duodenal ulcer (active or healed). III. Prepyloric. IV. High on lesser curve, near gastroesophageal junction. V. Medication-induced (NSAID/acetylsalicylic acid), anywhere in stomach. (Reproduced with permission from Fisher WE, Brunicardi FC: Benign gastric ulcer, in Cameron JL (ed): *Current Surgical Therapy*, 9th ed. Philadelphia: Mosby Elsevier, 2008, p 81. Copyright © Elsevier.)

5. Which of the following variables confers the highest risk of mortality for a patient with a bleeding duodenal ulcer?
   A. Systolic blood pressure <90 mmHg
   B. BUN (blood urea nitrogen) 10-25 mmol/L
   C. Hg <10.0 g/dL
   D. Cardiac disease

Answer: C
The Blatchford score provides the highest weight to a BUN >25 mmol/L and a Hg <10 gm/dL. (See Schwartz 9th ed., p 914, and Table 26-3.)

TABLE 26-3 Risk-stratification tools for upper gastrointestinal hemorrhage[a]

A. Blatchford Score

At Presentation	Points
Systolic blood pressure	
100–109 mmHg	1
90–99 mmHg	2
<90 mmHg	3
Blood urea nitrogen	
6.5–7.9 mmol/L	2
8.0–9.9 mmol/L	3
10.0–24.9 mmol/L	4
≥25 mmol/L	6
Hemoglobin for men	
12.0–12.9 g/dL	1
10.0–11.9 g/dL	3
<10.0 g/dL	6
Hemoglobin for women	
10.0–11.9 g/dL	1
<10.0 g/dL	6
Other variables at presentation	
Pulse ≥100 beats/min	1
Melena	1
Syncope	2
Hepatic disease	2
Cardiac failure	2

B. Rockall Score

		Variable	Points
Complete Rockall Score	Clinical Rockall Score	Age	
		<60 y	0
		60–79 y	1
		≥80 y	2
		Shock	
		Heart rate >100 beats/min	1
		Systolic blood pressure <100 mmHg	2
		Coexisting illness	
		Ischemic heart disease, congestive heart failure, other major illness	2
		Renal failure, hepatic failure, metastatic cancer	3
		Endoscopic diagnosis	
		No lesions observed, Mallory-Weiss syndrome	0
		Peptic ulcer, erosive disease, esophagitis	1
		Cancer of the upper GI tract	2
		Endoscopic stigmata of recent hemorrhage	
		Clean base ulcer, flat pigmented spot	0
		Blood in upper GI tract, active bleeding, visible vessel, clot	2

[a]Panel A shows the values used in the Blatchford risk-stratification score, which ranges from 0 to 23, with higher scores indicating higher risk. Panel B shows the Rockall score, with point values assigned for each of three clinical variables (age and the presence of shock and coexisting illnesses) and two endoscopic variables (diagnosis and stigmata of recent hemorrhage). The complete Rockall score ranges from 0 to 11, with higher scores indicating higher risk. Patients with a clinical Rockall score of 0 or a complete Rockall score of 2 or less are considered to be at low risk for rebleeding or death.

Source: Reproduced with permission from Gralnek IM et al: Management of acute bleeding from peptic ulcer. *N Engl J Med* 359:928, 2008. Copyright © 2008 Massachusetts Medical Society. All rights reserved.

6. Which of the following procedures for peptic ulcer disease has the highest incidence of postoperative diarrhea?
   A. Graham patch
   B. Parietal cell vagotomy
   C. Truncal vagotomy and pyloroplasty
   D. Distal gastrectomy without vagotomy

Answer: C
(See Schwartz 9th ed., p 916, and Table 26-4.)

TABLE 26-4 Clinical results of surgery for duodenal ulcer	Parietal Cell Vagotomy	Truncal Vagotomy and Pyloroplasty	Truncal Vagotomy and Antrectomy
Operative mortality rate (%)	0	<1	1
Ulcer recurrence rate (%)	5–15	5–15	<2
Dumping (%)			
Mild	<5	10	10–15
Severe	0	1	1–2
Diarrhea (%)			
Mild	<5	25	20
Severe	0	2	1–2

Source: Modified with permission from Mulholland MW, Debas HT: Chronic duodenal and gastric ulcer. *Surg Clin North Am* 67:489, 1987. Copyright © Elsevier.

7. Which of the following is the procedure of choice in a low-risk patient with a perforated duodenal ulcer who is known to be *Helicobacter pylori* negative, and does not use NSAID's?
   A. Graham patch only
   B. Graham patch with highly selective vagotomy
   C. Truncal vagotomy and pyloroplasty
   D. Truncal vagotomy and antrectomy

Answer: B

See Table 26-5. The options for surgical treatment of perforated duodenal ulcer are simple patch closure, patch closure and HSV, or patch closure and V+D. Simple patch closure alone should be done in patients with hemodynamic instability and/or exudative peritonitis signifying a perforation >24 hours old. In all other patients, the addition of HSV may be considered because numerous studies have reported a negligible mortality with this approach. However, in the United States and Western Europe, there is clearly a trend away from definitive operation for perforated duodenal ulcer, probably because of the ready availability of PPI, and surgeon unfamiliarity with definitive operation in this setting. (See Schwartz 9th ed., p 921.)

TABLE 26-5 Surgical options in the treatment of duodenal and gastric ulcer

Indication	Duodenal	Gastric
Bleeding	1. Oversew[a] 2. Oversew, V+D 3. V+A	1. Oversew and biopsy[a] 2. Oversew, biopsy, V+D 3. Distal gastrectomy[b]
Perforation	1. Patch[a] 2. Patch, HSV[b] 3. Patch, V+D	1. Biopsy and patch[a] 2. Wedge excision, V+D 3. Distal gastrectomy[b]
Obstruction	1. HSV + GJ 2. V+A	1. Biopsy; HSV + GJ 2. Distal gastrectomy[b]
Intractability/nonhealing	1. HSV[b] 2. V+D 3. V+A	1. HSV and wedge excision 2. Distal gastrectomy

[a]Unless the patient is in shock or moribund, a definitive procedure should be considered.
[b]Operation of choice in low-risk patient.
GJ = gastrojejunostomy; HSV = highly selective vagotomy; V+A = vagotomy and antrectomy; V+D = vagotomy and drainage.

8. Which of the following gastric polyps is considered premalignant?
   A. Hamartomatous
   B. Heterotopic
   C. Inflammatory
   D. Adenomatous

Answer: D

There are five types of gastric epithelial polyps: inflammatory, hamartomatous, heterotopic, hyperplastic, and adenoma. The first three types have negligible malignant potential. Adenomas can lead to carcinoma, just like in the colon, and should be removed when diagnosed. Occasionally, hyperplastic polyps can be associated with carcinoma. Patients with familial adenomatous polyposis have a high prevalence of gastric adenomatous polyps (about 50%), and are 10 times more likely to develop adenocarcinoma of the stomach than the general population.

Screening EGD is indicated in these families. Patients with hereditary nonpolyposis colorectal cancer may also be at risk for gastric cancer. (See Schwartz 9th ed., p 928.)

9. The most common premalignant lesion of the stomach is
   A. Adenoma
   B. Chronic gastric ulcer
   C. Atrophic gastritis
   D. Verrucous gastritis

Answer: C
(See Schwartz 9th ed., p 930, and Figure 26-8.)

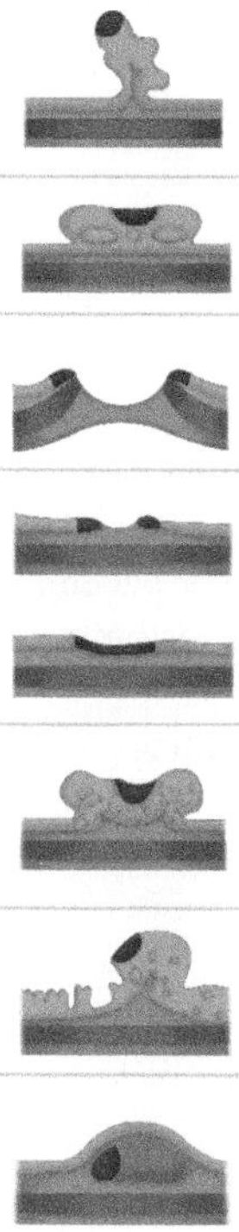

1900 Cases		
Precancerous lesion	Number of cases	%
Hyperplastic polyp	10	0.53
Adenoma	47	2.47
Chronic ulcer	13	0.68
Atrophic gastritis	1802	94.84
Verrucous gastritis	26	1.37
Stomach remnant	2	0.11
Aberrant pancreas	0	0
	Total 1900	100

N.C.C.H., Tokyo April 1988

FIG. 26-8. Precancerous lesions of the stomach. (Reproduced with permission from Ming S-C, Hirota T: Malignant epithelial tumors of the stomach, in Ming S-C, Goldman H (eds): *Pathology of the Gastrointestinal Tract*, 2nd ed. Baltimore: Williams & Wilkins, 1998, p 607.)

10. Prophylactic total gastrectomy may be indicated in
    A. Ménétrier's disease
    B. Familial mutation of the E-cadherin gene
    C. Hx of a first-degree relative with gastric cancer
    D. Hereditary nonpolyposis colorectal carcinoma

Answer: B
A mutated E-cadherin gene is associated with hereditary diffuse gastric cancer. Prophylactic total gastrectomy should be considered. Obviously, a myriad of genetic and environmental factors will affect members of the same family, and up to 10% of gastric cancer cases appear to be familial without a clear-cut genetic diagnosis. First-degree relatives of patients with gastric cancer have a two- to threefold increased risk of developing the disease. Patients with hereditary nonpolyposis colorectal cancer have a 10% risk of developing gastric cancer, predominantly the intestinal subtype. The mucous cell hyperplasia of Ménétrier's disease is generally considered to carry a 5 to 10% risk of adenocarcinoma. Periodic surveillance EGD is prudent in all the above conditions. The glandular hyperplasia associated with gastrinoma is not premalignant, but ECL hyperplasia and/or carcinoid tumors can occur. (See Schwartz 9th ed., p 930.)

11. In resecting a gastric adenocarcinoma, what is considered a minimum gross margin?
    A. 2 cm
    B. 3 cm
    C. 4 cm
    D. 5 cm

Answer: D

The goal of curative surgical treatment is resection of all tumor (i.e., R0 resection). Thus, all margins (proximal, distal, and radial) should be negative and an adequate lymphadenectomy performed. Generally, the surgeon strives for a grossly negative margin of at least 5 cm. Some gastric tumors, particularly the diffuse variety, are quite infiltrative and tumor cells can extend well beyond the tumor mass; thus, gross margins beyond 5 cm may be desirable. Frozen section confirmation of negative margins is important when performing operation for cure, but it is less important in patients with nodal metastases beyond the N1 nodal basin. (See Schwartz 9th ed., p 933.)

12. What is the minimal number of lymph nodes considered to be adequate for staging when resecting an adenocarcinoma of the stomach?
    A. 10
    B. 15
    C. 20
    D. 25

Answer: B

It should be strongly emphasized that many patients with positive lymph nodes are cured by adequate surgery. It should also be stressed that often lymph nodes that appear to be grossly involved with tumor turn out to be benign or reactive on pathologic examination. More than 15 resected lymph nodes are required for adequate staging. (See Schwartz 9th ed., p 933.)

13. The most appropriate initial treatment for a diabetic patient with gastroparesis is
    A. Implantation of a gastric pacemaker
    B. Gastrostomy and jejunostomy
    C. Gastric resection
    D. Enhanced diabetes control

Answer: D

Surgeons need to understand the role of surgery in primary gastroparesis. If appropriate, the patient with severe diabetic gastroparesis should be evaluated for pancreas transplant before any invasive abdominal procedure, because some patients improve substantially after pancreas transplant. If the diabetic gastroparetic patient is not a candidate for pancreas transplant, both gastrostomy (for decompression) and jejunostomy tubes (for feeding and prevention of hypoglycemia) can be effective. Infection and wound problems are more common in diabetics with transabdominal tubes than in nondiabetics. Other surgical options include implantation of a gastric pacemaker, and gastric resection. Generally, gastric resection should be done infrequently, if at all, for primary gastroparesis. (See Schwartz 9th ed., p 939.)

14. The most appropriate treatment for chronic bleeding from watermelon stomach is
    A. Beta blockers
    B. Oral nitrates
    C. Estrogen
    D. Total gastrectomy

Answer: C

The parallel red stripes atop the mucosal folds of the distal stomach give this rare entity its sobriquet. Histologically, gastric antral vascular ectasia is characterized by dilated mucosal blood vessels that often contain thrombi, in the lamina propria. Mucosal fibromuscular hyperplasia and hyalinization often are present. The histologic appearance can resemble portal hypertensive gastropathy, but the latter usually affects the proximal stomach, whereas watermelon stomach predominantly affects the distal stomach. Beta blockers and nitrates, useful in the treatment of portal hypertensive gastropathy, are ineffective in patients with gastric antral vascular ectasia. Patients with the latter diagnosis are usually elderly women with chronic GI blood loss requiring transfusion. Most have an associated autoimmune connective tissue disorder, and at least 25% have chronic liver disease. Nonsurgical treatment options include estrogen and progesterone, and endoscopic treatment with the neodymium yttrium-aluminum garnet (Nd:YAG) laser or argon plasma coagulator. Antrectomy may be required to control blood loss, and this operation is quite effective but carries increased morbidity in this elderly patient group. Patients with portal hypertension and antral vascular ectasia should be considered for transjugular intrahepatic portosystemic shunt. (See Schwartz 9th ed., p 940.)

15. Dumping is characterized by
    A. Tachycardia
    B. Crampy abdominal pain and diarrhea
    C. Diaphoresis
    D. All of the above

Answer: D

Clinically significant dumping occurs in 5 to 10% of patients after pyloroplasty, pyloromyotomy, or distal gastrectomy, and consists of a constellation of postprandial symptoms ranging in severity from annoying to disabling. The symptoms are thought to be the result of the abrupt delivery of a hyperosmolar load into the small bowel. This usually is due to ablation of the pylorus, but decreased gastric compliance with accelerated emptying of liquids (e.g., after highly selective vagotomy) is another accepted mechanism. About 15 to 30 minutes after a meal, the patient becomes diaphoretic, weak, light-headed, and tachycardic. These symptoms may be ameliorated by recumbence or saline infusion. Crampy abdominal pain is not uncommon and diarrhea often follows. This is referred to as *early dumping*, and should be distinguished from postprandial (reactive) hypoglycemia, also called *late dumping*, which usually occurs later (2 to 3 hours following a meal), and is relieved by the administration of sugar. (See Schwartz 9th ed., p 942.)

CHAPTER 27

The Surgical Management of Obesity

BASIC SCIENCE QUESTIONS

1. Which of the following has been directly implicated as a cause of obesity?
   A. Lack of early childhood exposure to fruits and vegetables
   B. Lack of early childhood exposure to exercise
   C. Increased appetite and drive to eat
   D. Decreased sensation of satiety

Answer: D

The increase in obesity is multifactorial. Genetics plays an important role in the development of obesity. Although the children of parents of normal weight have a 10% chance of becoming obese, the children of two obese parents have an 80 to 90% chance of developing obesity by adulthood. The weight of adopted children correlates strongly with the weight of their birth parents. Furthermore, concordance rates for obesity in monozygotic twins are double those in dizygotic twins.

Diet and culture are important factors as well. These environmental factors contribute significantly to the epidemic of obesity in the United States, because the rapid increase in obesity during the past two decades cannot be explained by any genetic cause. Other factors appear to contribute significantly to severe obesity.

Intermittent or consistent excessive caloric intake occurs. The lack of satiety, on a consistent or intermittent basis, appears to be strongly correlated with such episodes of excessive caloric ingestion. As yet the physiologic basis for such a lack of satiety is not understood.

Other factors commonly suggested to play a role in the disease of obesity include decreased energy expenditure from reduced metabolic activity, reduction in the thermogenic response to meals, an abnormally high set point for body weight, and a decrease in the loss of heat energy. Another factor that may influence absorption of ingested food is the composition of the intraluminal bacteria of the intestinal tract. Recent studies have documented a difference in the composition of the intestinal flora of obese individuals compared with those of normal weight. (See Schwartz 9th ed., p 951.)

2. Losing weight requires creating a calorie deficit. How much deficit is required to lose 1 pound weekly?
   A. 1000 calories
   B. 2250 calories
   C. 3500 calories
   D. 4200 calories

Answer: C

Lifestyle changes involving diet, exercise, and behavior modification constitute the first tier of therapy for obesity. Dietary restriction and exercise can each independently create a caloric deficit. A daily energy deficit so created of 500 kcal/d, resulting in a weekly deficit of 3500 kcal, results in the loss of 1 lb of fat weekly. It has been shown that low-calorie diets (800 to 1500 kcal/d) are as effective as very-low calorie diets at 1 year but result in a lower rate of nutritional deficiencies. Such diets may produce an average of 8% body weight loss over a 6-month period. Longer follow-up shows recidivism. Moderate daily physical activity can produce a 2 to 3% body weight loss. (See Schwartz 9th ed., p 952.)

CLINICAL QUESTIONS

1. A patient with a BMI of 38 is considered
   A. Overweight
   B. Obese
   C. Severely obese
   D. Superobese

Answer: C
(See Schwartz 9th ed., p 950, and Table 27-1.)

TABLE 27-1 Classification of obesity by body mass index (BMI)

Classification	BMI Range (kg/m^2)
Normal weight	20–25
Overweight	26–29
Obese	30–34
Severely obese	35–49
Superobese	≥50

2. Which of the following is associated with or caused by obesity?
   A. Cluster headaches
   B. Pseudotumor cerebri
   C. Liposarcoma
   D. Fat embolism

Answer: B
Significant comorbidities, defined as medical problems associated with or caused by obesity, are numerous. The most prevalent and acknowledged of these include degenerative joint disease, low back pain, hypertension, obstructive sleep apnea, gastroesophageal reflux disease (GERD), cholelithiasis, type 2 diabetes, hyperlipidemia, hypercholesterolemia, asthma, hypoventilation syndrome of obesity, fatal cardiac arrhythmias, right-sided heart failure, migraine headaches, pseudotumor cerebri, venous stasis ulcers, deep vein thrombosis, fungal skin rashes, skin abscesses, stress urinary incontinence, infertility, dysmenorrhea, depression, abdominal wall hernias, and an increased incidence of various cancers such as those of the uterus, breast, colon, and prostate.

Although migraines are associated with morbid obesity, cluster headaches are not. Uterine, breast, colon, and prostate cancers have an increased incidence in patients with morbid obesity, and liposarcoma does not. Fat embolism, seen after fractures, is not more common in morbidly obese patients. (See Schwartz 9th ed., p 951.)

3. What percent of morbidly obese patients are able to successfully lose weight and maintain that weight loss by eating fewer calories and increasing the amount of exercise they do?
   A. <5%
   B. 5-10%
   C. 10-15%
   D. >15%

Answer: A
Medical treatment for severe obesity is aimed at reducing body weight through a combination of decreased caloric intake and accompanying increases in energy expenditure from moderate exercise. This method of weight loss is the safest possible and may work well for obese individuals who have modest amounts of weight to lose to regain normal body weight or to return to being simply overweight instead of obese. For the severely obese individual, however, who usually must lose at least 75 lb or more to achieve elimination of obesity, this is a daunting and extremely difficult task. The success rate among severely obese patients who try dieting and exercise as a means of losing enough weight to no longer be obese and maintaining that weight loss is only approximately 3%. (See Schwartz 9th ed., p 951.)

4. Which of the following drugs is approved by the FDA for weight loss?
   A. Phentermine
   B. Nuphedragen
   C. Ambislim
   D. Sibutramine

Answer: D

Currently there are only two drugs approved by the U.S. Food and Drug Administration for the treatment of obesity that promote weight loss. Sibutramine is a noradrenaline and 5-hydroxytryptamine reuptake inhibitor that works as an appetite suppressant. Orlistat inhibits gastric and pancreatic lipase enzymes that promote lipid absorption in the intestine. Either of these drugs may produce a weight loss of between 6 and 10% of body weight after 1 year, but cessation of the drug usually results in prompt regaining of lost weight.

Phentermine is an appetite suppressant, similar to amphetamines chemically. In combination with fenfluramine (Phen-Fen), it can cause pulmonary hypertension. Phentermine is not approved by the FDA. Nuphedragen is sold as a "fat burner." There are no data on safety or efficacy and this is not approved by the FDA. Ambislim is an herbal mixture, also untested, that is not approved by the FDA. (See Schwartz 9th ed., p 952.)

5. A bilipancreatic diversion (BPD) with duodenal switch is primarily a
   A. Restrictive procedure
   B. Malabsorptive procedure
   C. Combination restrictive and malabsorptive procedure
   D. None of the above

Answer: C

The BPD is a combination restrictive and malabsorptive procedure. (See Schwartz 9th ed., p 953, and Table 27-2.)

TABLE 27-2 Types of commonly performed bariatric operations by mechanism of action

Restrictive	
	Laparoscopic adjustable gastric banding (LAGB)
	Sleeve gastrectomy (SG)
	Vertical banded gastroplasty (VBG)[a]
Malabsorptive	
	Biliopancreatic diversion (BPD)
	Jejunoileal bypass (JIB)[a]
Combined restrictive and malabsorptive	
	Roux-en-Y gastric bypass (RYGB)
	BPD with duodenal switch (DS)

[a]Now rarely performed and of historic interest only.

6. Which of the following patients would be considered a candidate for bariatric surgery?
   A. 70 year old, BMI 39, with no comorbidities
   B. 22 year old, BMI 34, with brittle (uncontrollable) diabetes
   C. 35 year old, BMI 38, with no comorbidities
   D. 56 year old, BMI 42, with no comorbidities

Answer: D

The indications for bariatric surgery have been clearly defined and are listed in Table 27-3. Of the patients listed, only D is the correct answer. (See Schwartz 9th ed., p 954.)

TABLE 27-3 Indications for bariatric surgery

Patient must:
1. Have body mass index (weight in kilograms/height in square meters) of ≥40 with or without comorbid medical conditions associated with obesity
2. Have body mass index of 35–40 with comorbid medical conditions

In addition it is expected that patients:
3. Have failed attempt at other weight loss treatments
4. Be psychologically stable

Source: Adapted from National Institutes of Health Consensus Conference. Gastrointestinal surgery for severe obesity. Consensus Development Conference Panel. *Ann Intern Med* 115:956, 1991.

7. Which group of patients has a poor outcome following placement of an adjustable gastric band?
   A. Overweight
   B. Obese
   C. Morbidly obese
   D. Superobese

Answer: D

Superobese patients have less weight loss than the obese or morbidly obese patients undergoing placement of an adjustable gastric band. Overweight people are not candidates for any bariatric procedure.

Efficacy of the operation in the superobese (body mass index (BMI) >50 kg/m^2) is less impressive, with average BMI remaining >40 kg/m^2 after 5- to 8-year follow-up. It has been our impression that optimal results occur with this operation in patients who are motivated, need to lose <50 kg to achieve a BMI of <30 kg/m^2, are willing and able to exercise regularly, are amenable to changing eating patterns as recommended, and live within a geographic area close enough for easy follow-up. Patients who are impatient to lose weight, are immobile, are unable to exercise, are confirmed 'grazers' or nibblers on high-calorie sweets, and expect to be able to continue their dietary habits without great alteration are not good candidates for this operation. Similarly, patients who have had previous upper gastric surgery, such as a Nissen fundoplication, are relatively poor candidates for laparoscopic adjustable gastric banding (LAGB) due to the potential tissue compromise in taking down the wrap to place the band. (See Schwartz 9th ed., p 959.)

8. Which of the following procedures has the highest rate of nutritional complications?
   A. Laparoscopic adjustable banding
   B. Roux-en-Y gastric bypass
   C. Sleeve gastrectomy
   D. Duodenal switch

Answer: D

The duodenal switch, also called the biliopancreatic diversion with duodenal switch, has the highest rate of nutritional complications. (See Schwartz 9th ed., pp 961; 968, and Table 27-4.)

TABLE 27-4 Outcomes for bariatric operations

	LAGB	RYGB	BPD/DS
Excess weight loss (%)	47.5	61.6	70.1
Mortality (%)	0.1	0.5	1.1
Morbidity (%)	10–25	13–38	27–33
Nutritional morbidity (%)	0–10	15–25	40–77

BPD/DS = biliopancreatic diversion with duodenal switch; LAGB = laparoscopic adjustable gastric banding; RYGB = Roux-en-Y gastric bypass.
Source: Data from Buchwald H, Avidor Y, Braunwald E, et al: Bariatric surgery. A systematic review and meta-analysis. *JAMA* 292:1724, 2004.

9. Which of the following is the most common emergent complication of laparoscopic adjustable gastric bands?
   A. Band slippage
   B. Dysfunction or leak from the reservoir or tubing
   C. Prolapse
   D. Erosion

Answer: C

Prolapse is perhaps the most common emergent complication that requires reoperation after laparoscopic adjustable gastric banding (LAGB). The incidence is generally in the 3% range. Postoperative vomiting predisposes to this problem, because the lower stomach can be pushed upward and trapped within the lumen of the band. Typical patient symptoms include immediate dysphagia, vomiting, and inability to take oral food or liquid. Either anterior or posterior prolapse may occur. Reoperation laparoscopically to reduce the prolapse and resuture the band imbrication is indicated. (See Schwartz 9th ed., p 961.)

10. Which of the following is a component of the Roux-en-Y gastric bypass?
    A. Creation of a gastric pouch approximately 100 mL in volume
    B. A proximal (biliopancreatic) limb >100 cm in length
    C. A Roux (alimentary) limb 75-150 cm in length
    D. Placing the Roux limb in a retrocolic position

Answer: C

The major feature of the operation is the creation of a proximal gastric pouch of small size (often <20 mL) that is totally separated from the stomach. A Roux limb of proximal jejunum is brought up and anastomosed to the pouch. The pathway of that limb can be anterior to the colon and stomach, posterior to both, or posterior to the colon and anterior to the stomach. The length of the biliopancreatic limb from the ligament of Treitz to the distal enteroenterostomy is from 20 to 50 cm, and the length of the Roux limb is 75 to 150 cm. (See Schwartz 9th ed., p 962.)

11. Patients undergoing Roux-en-Y gastric bypass are known to be at increased risk for developing gallstones. The current recommended management for patients with a negative ultrasound (no cholelithiasis) prior to surgery is
    A. Prophylactic cholecystectomy at the time of surgery
    B. Serial ultrasounds every 3 months after surgery for 2 years
    C. Ultrasounds after surgery only if the patient develops symptoms
    D. Oral ursodiol to prevent gallstone formation after surgery

Answer: D

We routinely perform screening ultrasound of the abdomen in patients planning to undergo LRYGB who have an intact gallbladder to rule out the presence of gallstones. Should gallstones be discovered, we currently recommend simultaneous laparoscopic cholecystectomy. Another approach is to defer cholecystectomy until after LRYGB if the patient is symptomatic. When a patient does not have gallstones as determined by preoperative ultrasound, we have followed the recommendations of a previous study which showed that prophylactic administration of ursodiol at a dosage of 300 mg bid will decrease the incidence of gallstone formation after RYGB to approximately 4%. (See Schwartz 9th ed., p 955.)

12. Which of the following is a relative contraindication to a Roux-en-Y gastric bypass?
    A. Spherocytosis
    B. Severe iron deficiency anemia
    C. B_{12} deficiency
    D. von Willebrand's disease

Answer: B

Laparoscopic adjustable Roux-en-Y gastric bypass (LRYGB) is an appropriate operation to consider for most patients eligible for bariatric surgery. Relative contraindications to LRYGB include previous gastric surgery, previous antireflux surgery, severe iron deficiency anemia, distal gastric or duodenal lesions that require ongoing future surveillance, and Barrett's esophagus with severe dysplasia.

Postoperative nutritional complications after LRYGB include iron deficiency in 20 to 40% of patients, iron deficiency anemia in 20%, vitamin B_{12} deficiency in 15%, and vitamin D deficiency in at least 15%, which usually is present preoperatively.

Because of the risk of postoperative iron deficiency anemia, the presence of severe iron deficiency preoperatively is a relative contraindication for surgery. (See Schwartz 9th ed., p 965.)

13. What percent of excess body weight do patients lose in the first year following Roux-en-Y gastric bypass?
    A. 20-30%
    B. 40-50%
    C. 60-70%
    D. 80-90%

Answer: C

Patients undergoing LRYGB usually lose between 60 and 80% of excess body weight during the first year after surgery. This has held true since the earliest large series of this operation was reported. Resolution of comorbidities varies depending on the disease but is >90% for GERD and venous stasis ulcers, and >80% for type 2 diabetes of <5 years' duration. Hyperlipidemias are almost always improved and resolve totally in approximately 70% of cases. Hypertension is resolved in 50 to 65% of cases (Table 27-5). Even superobese patients who do not achieve an ultimate BMI of <35 kg/m^2 can experience significant improvements in comorbidities after LRYGB or open RYGB. (See Schwartz 9th ed., pp 962, 965.)

TABLE 27-5 Effect of bariatric surgery on comorbid medical conditions

Condition	% Resolved	% Improved
Diabetes	76.8	85.4
Hypertension	61.7	78.5
Sleep apnea	83.6	85.7
Hyperlipidemia	70.0	96.9

Source: Data from Buchwald H, Avidor Y, Braunwald E, et al: Bariatric surgery. A systematic review and meta-analysis. *JAMA* 292:1724, 2004.

14. A 42-year-old man who is one year status post Roux-en-Y bypass presents with a 24-hour history of intermittent vomiting. He is stable and well hydrated and his electrolytes are normal. A CT scan confirms the clinical suspicion of a partial small bowel obstruction. The appropriate initial treatment for this patient is
    A. IV hydration and observation
    B. IV hydration, NG tube
    C. IV hydration, NG tube, and repeat CT in 24 hours
    D. Immediate surgical exploration

Answer: D

Several complications that are specific to the laparoscopic adjustable Roux-en-Y gastric bypass (LRYGB) procedure must be emphasized. The most important is small-bowel obstruction. This complication must be treated differently from obstruction in the average general surgery patient, in whom it is usually caused by adhesions and often will resolve with conservative, nonoperative therapy. Patients who have undergone LRYGB who have symptoms of obstruction *require surgical therapy on an emergent basis* (see Table 27-6). This is because the cause of the bowel obstruction after LRYGB is often an internal hernia from inadequate closure or nonclosure of the mesenteric defects by the surgeon at the time of operation. Treatment for these patients therefore differs from that for most patients with small-bowel obstruction. The *single most important point* made in this chapter is to caution general surgeons to be aware of the need to operate emergently on patients who present with small-bowel obstruction after LRYGB. Currently centers that perform small-bowel transplantation are finding that the leading patient group referred for that procedure is patients who had small-bowel obstruction after LRYGB, developed infarction of most of the bowel from the internal hernia, and have short-gut syndrome. (See Schwartz 9th ed., p 966.)

TABLE 27-6	Complications for which patients undergoing laparoscopic Roux-en-Y gastric bypass require urgent surgical intervention
Small-bowel obstruction	
Early postoperative vomiting with signs and symptoms suggesting obstruction	
Early postoperative hematemesis with signs and symptoms suggesting obstruction	

15. A postoperative marginal ulcer in a patient who has undergone a Roux-en-Y gastric bypass is best treated by
    A. Triple therapy for *Helicobacter pylori*
    B. Proton pump inhibitors
    C. Endoscopic dilation with post-dilation proton pump inhibitors
    D. Resection of the ulcer with surgical revision of the gastrojejunostomy

Answer: B

Marginal ulcers are another complication relatively specific to Roux-en-Y gastric bypass (RYGB), either laparoscopic adjustable Roux-en-Y gastric bypass (LRYGB) or open RYGB. The patient presents with pain in the epigastric region that is not altered by eating. Diagnosis is by endoscopy. Treatment is medical with administration of proton pump inhibitors, which are effective in 90% of cases. Only those with a gastrogastric fistula to the distal stomach or severe stenosis of the lumen of the gastrojejunostomy or non-healing ulcers require surgical therapy. (See Schwartz 9th ed., p 966.)

16. Which of the following is a component of a biliopancreatic diversion?
    A. Creation of a gastric pouch approximately 20 mL in volume
    B. Oversewing of the distal duodenum
    C. Creation of a Roux limb at least 150 cm in length
    D. Prophylactic cholecystectomy

Answer: D

The operation, which is pictured in Fig. 27-1, involves resection of the distal half to two thirds of the stomach and creation of an alimentary tract of the most distal 200 cm of ileum, which is anastomosed to the stomach. The biliopancreatic limb is anastomosed to the alimentary tract either 75 or 100 cm proximal to the ileocecal valve, depending on the protein content of the patient's diet. This operation met with limited international popularity, probably due to the technical difficulty of performing it combined with the significant percentage of nutritional complications that arise postoperatively.

The biliopancratic diversion (BPD) operation begins with performance of a distal subtotal gastrectomy. A residual 200-mL gastric pouch is created for superobese patients and a slightly larger pouch for patients with a BMI of <50 kg/m^2. The terminal ileum is identified and divided 250 cm proximal to the ileocecal valve. The distal end of that divided ileum is then anastomosed to the stomach, creating a 2- to 3-cm stoma. The proximal end of the ileum is then anastomosed side to side to the terminal ileum approximately 100 cm proximal to the ileocecal valve. Some surgeons perform the anastomosis only 50 cm proximal to the valve, but in these patients the likelihood of good protein intake postoperatively should be high. Prophylactic cholecystectomy is performed due to the high incidence of gallstone formation with the malabsorption of bile salts. (See Schwartz 9th ed., pp 969, 968.)

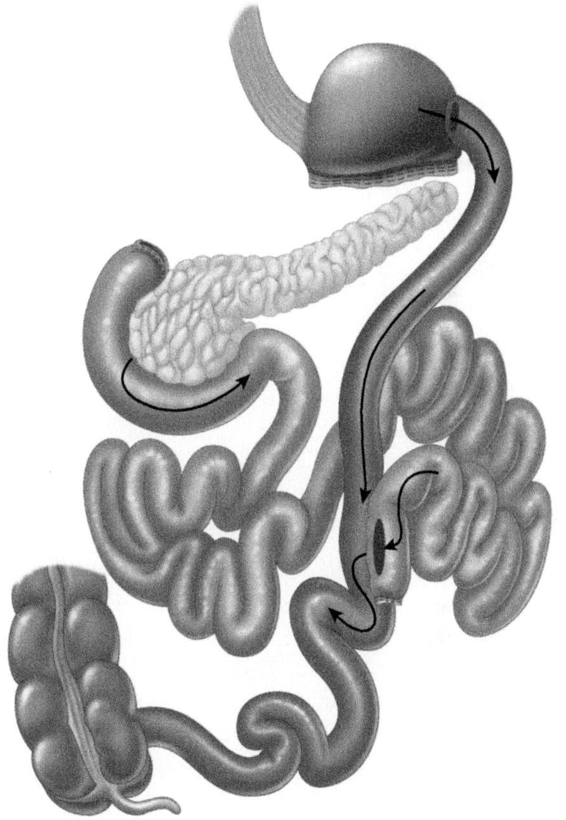

FIG. 27-1. Configuration of biliopancreatic diversion. (Reproduced with permission from Austrheim-Smith I, et al: Evolution of bariatric minimally invasive surgery, in Schauer PR, et al (eds): *Minimally Invasive Bariatric Surgery*, 1st ed. New York: Springer, 2007, p 21.)

17. Which component of the biliopancreatic diversion is different from a duodenal switch procedure?
   A. The size of the remaining stomach
   B. The length of the alimentary limb
   C. The length of the biliopancreatic limb
   D. None of the above—it is the same operation

Answer: A

The deuodenal switch (DS) procedure differs from BPD only in the proximal gut portion of the operation. Instead of a distal gastrectomy, a resection of all the stomach except for a narrow lesser curvature tube is performed. The diameter of this tube is calibrated with a dilator and, if limited to an approximately 32F (11-mm) diameter, produces the optimal amount of weight loss while still allowing adequate oral intake. The duodenum is now divided in its first portion and an approximately 2-cm length of duodenum is left intact beyond the pylorus. This end of the duodenum is then anastomosed to the distal 250 cm of ileum. (See Schwartz 9th ed., pp 969, 968, and Fig. 27-2.)

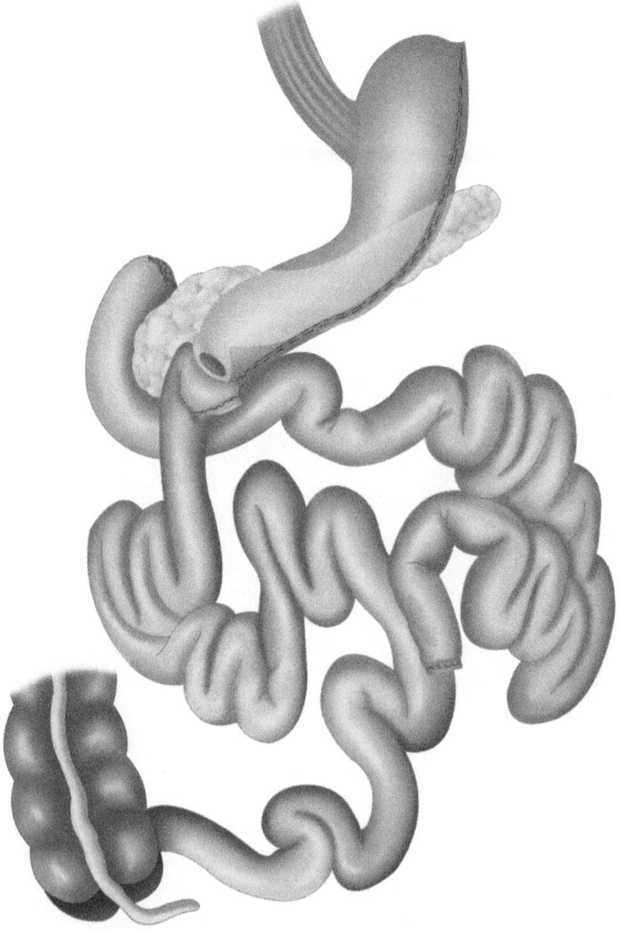

FIG. 27-2. Configuration of the duodenal switch. (Reproduced with permission from Austrheim-Smith I, et al: Evolution of bariatric minimally invasive surgery, in Schauer PR, et al (eds): *Minimally Invasive Bariatric Surgery*, 1st ed. New York: Springer, 2007, p 22.)

CHAPTER 28

Small Intestine

BASIC SCIENCE QUESTIONS

1. Calcium is primarily absorbed in the
   A. Stomach
   B. Duodenum
   C. Jejunum
   D. Ileum

Answer: B

Calcium is absorbed through both transcellular transport and paracellular diffusion. The duodenum is the major site for transcellular transport; paracellular transport occurs throughout the small intestine. A key step in transcellular calcium transport is mediated by calbindin, a calcium-binding protein located in the cytoplasm of enterocytes. Regulation of calbindin synthesis is the principal mechanism by which vitamin D regulates intestinal calcium absorption. (See Schwartz 9th ed., p 985.)

2. Which of the following distinguishes jejunum from ileum?
   A. Less prominent plica circularis
   B. Smaller diameter
   C. Thinner wall
   D. Longer vasa recta

Answer: D

No distinct anatomic landmark demarcates the jejunum from the ileum; the proximal 40% of the jejunoileal segment is arbitrarily defined as the jejunum and the distal 60% as the ileum. The ileum is demarcated from the cecum by the ileocecal valve. The small intestine contains mucosal folds known as *plicae circulares* or *valvulae conniventes* that are visible upon gross inspection. These folds are also visible radiographically and help in the distinction between small intestine and colon, which does not contain them, on abdominal radiographs. These folds are more prominent in the proximal intestine than in the distal small intestine. Other features evident on gross inspection that are more characteristic of the proximal than distal small intestine include a larger circumference, thicker wall, less fatty mesentery, and longer vasa recta (Fig. 28-1). (See Schwartz 9th ed., p 980.)

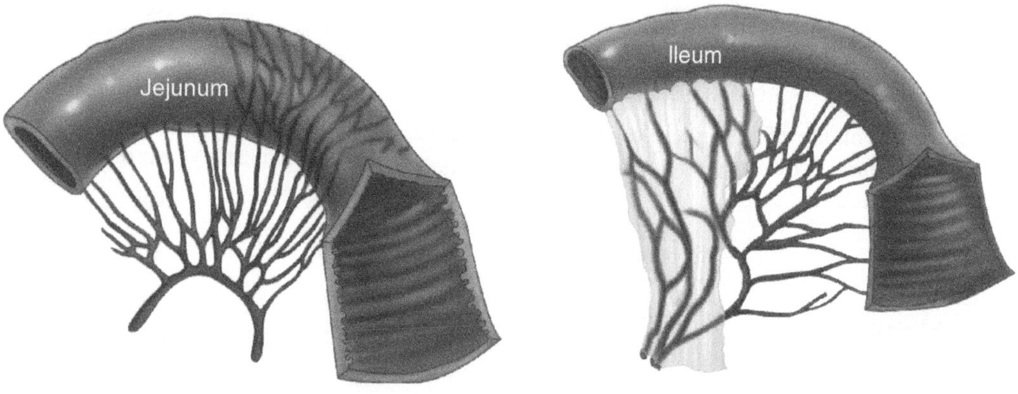

FIG. 28-1. Gross features of jejunum contrasted with those of ileum. Relative to the ileum, the jejunum has a larger diameter, thicker wall, more prominent plicae circulares, a less fatty mesentery, and longer vasa recta.

3. There are four cell types which originate in the crypts of the small bowel mucosa. Which one of these cell types completes differentiation in the crypt instead of during migration to the villus?
   A. Enterocyte
   B. Goblet cell
   C. Enteroendocrine cell
   D. Paneth cell

Answer: D

Intestinal, epithelial cellular proliferation is confined to the *crypts*, each of which carries an average census of 250 to 300 cells. All epithelial cells in each crypt are derived from an unknown number of the yet uncharacterized multipotent stem cells located at or near the crypt's base. Their immediate descendants are amplified by undergoing several cycles of rapid division. These descendants then make a commitment to differentiate along one of four pathways that ultimately yield *enterocytes* and *goblet, enteroendocrine*, and *Paneth* cells. With the exception of Paneth cells, these lineages complete their terminal differentiation during an upward migration from each crypt to adjacent villi.

Paneth cells are located at the base of the crypt and contain secretory granules containing growth factors, digestive enzymes, and antimicrobial peptides. (See Schwartz 9th ed., p 981.)

4. The first hormone discovered in the human body was
   A. Insulin
   B. Secretin
   C. Vasoactive intestinal peptide
   D. Somatostatin

Answer: B

Endocrinology as a discipline was born with the discovery of secretin, an intestinal regulatory peptide that was the first hormone to be identified. The small intestine is now recognized to be the largest hormone-producing organ in the body, both with respect to the number of hormone-producing cells and the number of individual hormones produced. Over 30 peptide hormone genes have been identified as being expressed in the GI tract. (See Schwartz 9th ed., p 987.)

5. Somatostatin causes
   A. Stimulation of intestinal secretion
   B. Stimulation of intestinal motility
   C. Inhibition of splanchnic perfusion
   D. Stimulation of intestinal mucosal growth

Answer: C

(See Schwartz 9th ed., p 987, and Table 28-1.)

TABLE 28-1 Representative regulatory peptides produced in the small intestine

Hormone	Source[a]	Actions
Somatostatin	D cell	Inhibits GI secretion, motility, and splanchnic perfusion
Secretin	S cell	Stimulates exocrine pancreatic secretion Stimulates intestinal secretion
Cholecystokinin	I cell	Stimulates pancreatic exocrine secretion Stimulates gallbladder emptying Inhibits sphincter of Oddi contraction
Motilin	M cell	Simulates intestinal motility
Peptide YY	L cell	Inhibits intestinal motility and secretion
Glucagon-like peptide 2	L cell	Stimulates intestinal epithelial proliferation
Neurotensin	N cell	Stimulates pancreatic and biliary secretion Inhibits small bowel motility Stimulates intestinal mucosal growth

[a]This table indicates which enteroendocrine cell types located in the intestinal epithelium produce these peptides. These peptides are also widely expressed in nonintestinal tissues.

6. The total volume of fluid secreted daily by the salivary glands, stomach, liver, and pancreas in a normal adult is approximately
   A. 2 liters
   B. 4 liters
   C. 6 liters
   D. 8 liters

Answer: C

(See Schwartz 9th ed., p 983, and Fig. 28-2.)

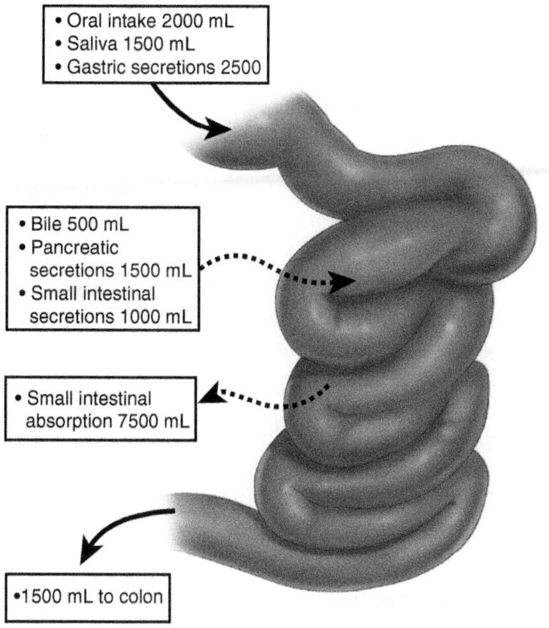

• Oral intake 2000 mL
• Saliva 1500 mL
• Gastric secretions 2500
• Bile 500 mL
• Pancreatic secretions 1500 mL
• Small intestinal secretions 1000 mL
• Small intestinal absorption 7500 mL
•1500 mL to colon

FIG. 28-2. Small intestinal fluid fluxes. Typical quantities (in volume per day) of fluid entering and leaving the small intestinal lumen in a healthy adult are shown.

7. Mutation in the *NOD2* gene is associated with an increased risk of
   A. Crohn's disease
   B. Cholera
   C. Adenocarcinoma of the small bowel
   D. Pseudo-obstruction

Answer: A

Specific genetic defects associated with Crohn's disease in human patients are beginning to be defined. For example, the presence of a locus on chromosome 16 (the so-called *IBD1 locus*) has been linked to Crohn's disease. The IBD1 locus has been identified as the *NOD2* gene. Persons with allelic variants on both chromosomes have a 40-fold relative risk of Crohn's disease compared to those without variant *NOD2* genes. The relevance of this gene to the pathogenesis of Crohn's disease is biologically plausible, as the protein product of the *NOD2* gene mediates the innate immune response to microbial pathogens. Other putative IBD loci have been identified on other chromosomes (IBD2 on chromosome 12q, and IBD3 on chromosome 6), and are under investigation. (See Schwartz 9th ed., p 994.)

8. Which of the following statements about gut-associated lymphoid tissue (GALT) is NOT true?
   A. GALT contains approximately 20% of the body's immune cells
   B. Peyer's patches are part of the GALT and function as an inductive site (to process foreign antigens)
   C. IgA is produced by plasma cells in the lamina propria of the small bowel
   D. IgA dimmers bound to secretory components are resistant to degradation in the lumen of the gut by proteolytic enzymes

Answer: A

The intestinal component of the immune system, known as the *gut-associated lymphoid tissue* (GALT), contains over 70% of the body's immune cells. The GALT is conceptually divided into inductive and effector sites. Inductive sites include Peyer's patches, mesenteric lymph nodes, and smaller isolated lymphoid follicles scattered throughout the small intestine (Fig. 28-3).

Effector lymphocytes are distributed into distinct compartments. IgA-producing plasma cells are derived from B cells and are located in the lamina propria. $CD4^+$ T cells are also located in the lamina propria. $CD8^+$ T cells migrate preferentially to the epithelium, but are also found in the lamina propria. These T cells are central to immune regulation; in addition the $CD8^+$ T cells have potent cytotoxic T lymphocyte activity. IgA is transported through the intestinal epithelial cells into the lumen, where it exists in the form of a dimer complexed with a secretory component. This configuration renders IgA resistant to proteolysis by digestive enzymes. IgA is believed to both help prevent the entry of microbes through the epithelium and to promote excretion of antigens or microbes that have already penetrated into the lamina propria. (See Schwartz 9th ed., pp 985, 986.)

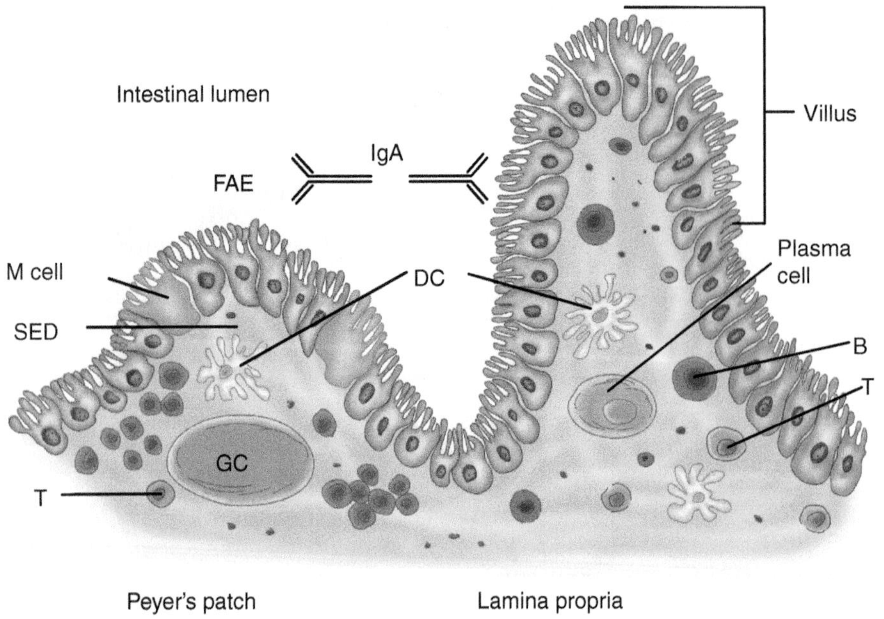
Intestinal lumen
Villus
IgA
FAE
Plasma cell
M cell
DC
SED
B
T
GC
T
Peyer's patch
Lamina propria

FIG. 28-3. Gut-associated lymphoid tissue. Select components of the gut-associated lymphoid tissue are schematically represented. Peyer's patches consist of a specialized follicle-associated epithelium (FAE) containing M cells, a subepithelial dome (SED) rich in dendritic cells (DC), and B-cell follicle containing germinal centers (GC). Plasma cells in the lamina propria produce immunoglobulin A (IgA), which is transported to the intestinal lumen where it serves as the first line of defense against pathogens. Other components of the gut-associated lymphoid tissue include isolated lymphoid follicles, mesenteric lymph nodes, and regulatory and effector lymphocytes. B = B cell; T = T cell.

9. The digestion of proteins in healthy individuals is initiated by
   A. Pepsin
   B. Trypsin
   C. Chymotrypsin
   D. Carboxypeptidase

Answer: A

Protein digestion begins in the stomach with action of pepsins. This is not, however, an essential step, because surgical patients who are achlorhydric, or have lost part or all of their stomach, are still able to successfully digest proteins. Digestion continues in the duodenum with the actions of a variety of pancreatic peptidases. These enzymes are secreted as inactive proenzymes. This is in contrast to pancreatic amylase and lipase, which are secreted in their active forms. In response to the presence of bile acids, enterokinase is liberated from the intestinal brush border membrane to catalyze the conversion of trypsinogen to active trypsin. (See Schwartz 9th ed., p 984, and Fig. 28-4.)

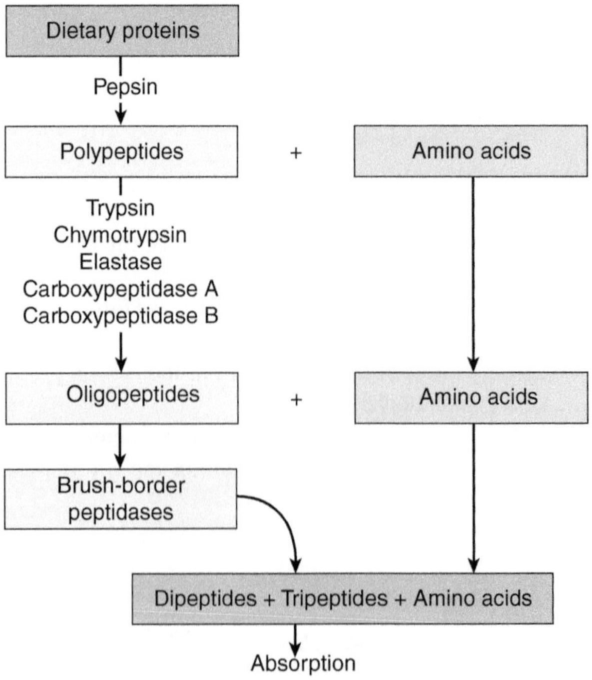
Dietary proteins
Pepsin
Polypeptides
+
Amino acids
Trypsin
Chymotrypsin
Elastase
Carboxypeptidase A
Carboxypeptidase B
Oligopeptides
+
Amino acids
Brush-border peptidases
Dipeptides + Tripeptides + Amino acids
Absorption

FIG. 28-4. Protein digestion. Dietary proteins must undergo hydrolysis into constituent single amino acids and di- and tripeptides before being absorbed by the intestinal epithelium. These hydrolytic reactions are catalyzed by pancreatic peptidases (e.g., trypsin) and by enterocyte brush border peptidases.

10. Contraction of the inner circular layer of the bowel wall
    A. Shortens the bowel
    B. Narrows the bowel lumen
    C. Promotes villus motility but doesn't affect peristalsis
    D. Promotes mixing of the luminal contents but doesn't affect peristalsis

Answer: B

Contraction of the outer longitudinal muscle layer results in bowel shortening; contraction of the inner circular layer results in luminal narrowing. Contractions of the muscularis mucosa contribute to mucosal or villus motility, but not to peristalsis. (See Schwartz 9th ed., p 986.)

11. Which of the following is an excitatory transmitter for small bowel motility?
    A. Nitric oxide
    B. Vasoactive intestinal peptide
    C. Adenosine triphosphate
    D. Acetylcholine

Answer: D

This intrinsic contractile mechanism is subject to neural and hormonal regulation. The enteric motor system (ENS) provides both inhibitory and excitatory stimuli. The predominant excitatory transmitters are acetylcholine and substance P, and the inhibitory transmitters include nitric oxide, vasoactive intestinal peptide, and adenosine triphosphate. In general, the sympathetic motor supply is inhibitory to the ENS; therefore, increased sympathetic input into the intestine leads to decreased intestinal smooth muscle activity. The parasympathetic motor supply is more complex, with projections to both inhibitory and excitatory ENS motor neurons. Correspondingly, the effects of parasympathetic inputs into intestinal motility are more difficult to predict. (See Schwartz 9th ed., pp 986, 987.)

12. Which cells are responsible for generating the basic rhythm of peristalsis in the bowel?
    A. Paneth cells
    B. Cells of Cajal
    C. Ganglion cells in Auerbach's plexus
    D. Ganglion cells in Meissner's plexus

Answer: B

The interstitial cells of Cajal are pleomorphic mesenchymal cells located within the muscularis propria of the intestine that generate the electrical slow wave (basic electrical rhythm or pacesetter potential) that plays a pacemaker role in setting the fundamental rhythmicity of small intestinal contractions. (See Schwartz 9th ed., p 986.)

13. Which of the following is the most prevalent fat consumed in a Western diet?
    A. Long-chain triglycerides
    B. Medium-chain triglycerides
    C. Short-chain triglycerides
    D. Cholesterol

Answer: A

Approximately 40% of the average Western diet consists of fat. Over 95% of dietary fat is in the form of long-chain triglycerides; the remainder includes phospholipids such as lecithin, fatty acids, cholesterol, and fat-soluble vitamins. Over 94% of the ingested fats are absorbed in the proximal jejunum. (See Schwartz 9th ed., p 985.)

14. Which of the following is the origin of the epithelium of the small bowel?
    A. Ectoderm
    B. Mesoderm
    C. Endoderm
    D. Neural crest

Answer: C

The first recognizable precursor of the small intestine is the embryonic gut tube, formed from the endoderm during the fourth week of gestation. The gut tube is divided into foregut, midgut, and hindgut. Other than duodenum, which is a foregut structure, the rest of the small intestine is derived from the midgut. The gut tube initially communicates with the yolk sac; however, the communication between these two structures narrows by the sixth week to form the vitelline duct. The yolk sac and vitelline duct usually undergo obliteration by the end of gestation. Incomplete obliteration of the vitelline duct results in the spectrum of defects associated with Meckel's diverticula. (See Schwartz 9th ed., p 981.)

15. Digestion of dietary starches is initiated by
    A. Amylase
    B. Sucrase
    C. Maltase
    D. Brush border hydrolases

Answer: A

Pancreatic amylase is the major enzyme of starch digestion, although salivary amylase initiates the process. The terminal products of amylase-mediated starch digestion are oligosaccharides, maltotriose, maltose, and alpha-limit dextrins (Fig. 28-5). (See Schwartz 9th ed., p 983.)

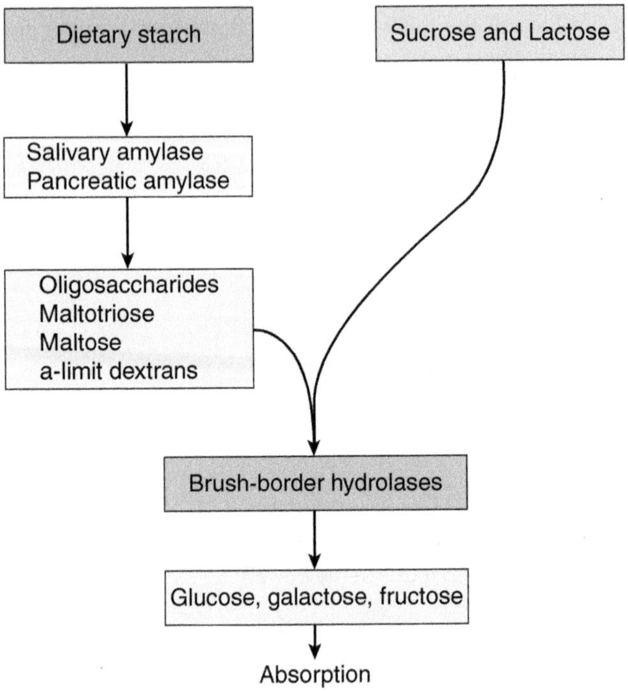

FIG. 28-5. Carbohydrate digestion. Dietary carbohydrates, including starch and the disaccharides sucrose and lactose, must undergo hydrolysis into constituent monosaccharides glucose, galactose, and fructose before being absorbed by the intestinal epithelium. These hydrolytic reactions are catalyzed by salivary and pancreatic amylase and by enterocyte brush border hydrolases.

16. Meissner's plexus is located in which layer of the bowel wall?
    A. Mucosa
    B. Submucosa
    C. Muscularis
    D. Serosa

Answer: B

The submucosa consists of dense connective tissue and a heterogeneous population of cells, including leukocytes and fibroblasts. The submucosa also contains an extensive network of vascular and lymphatic vessels, nerve fibers, and ganglion cells of the submucosal (Meissner's) plexus. The muscularis propria consists of an outer, longitudinally oriented layer and an inner, circularly oriented layer of smooth muscle fibers. Located at the interface between these two layers are ganglion cells of the myenteric (Auerbach's) plexus. (See Schwartz 9th ed., p 981.)

CLINICAL QUESTIONS

1. Which of the following decreases absorption of intraluminal water in the small bowel?
    A. Dopamine
    B. Somatostatin
    C. Glucosteroids
    D. Vasopressin

Answer: D

Dopamine, somatostatin, and glucosteroids all increase the absorption of water from the small bowel. Vasopressin decreases absorption of water. (See Schwartz 9th ed., p 983, and Table 28-2.)

TABLE 28-2	Regulation of intestinal absorption and secretion
Agents that stimulate absorption or inhibit secretion of water	
Aldosterone	
Glucocorticoids	
Angiotensin	
Norepinephrine	
Epinephrine	
Dopamine	
Somatostatin	
Neuropeptide Y	
Peptide YY	
Enkephalin	
Agents that simulate secretion or inhibit absorption of water	
Secretin	
Bradykinin	
Prostaglandins	
Acetylcholine	
Atrial natriuretic factor	
Vasopressin	
Vasoactive intestinal peptide	
Bombesin	
Substance P	
Serotonin	
Neurotensin	
Histamine	

2. What is the approximate clinical recurrence rate (return of symptoms) 5 years after surgery for Crohn's disease?
   A. 10%
   B. 35%
   C. 60%
   D. 95%

Answer: C

Most patients whose disease is resected eventually develop recurrence. If recurrence is defined endoscopically, 70% recur within 1 year of a bowel resection and 85% by 3 years. Clinical recurrence, defined as the return of symptoms confirmed as being due to Crohn's disease, affects 60% of patients by 5 years and 94% by 15 years after intestinal resection. Reoperation becomes necessary in approximately one third of patients by 5 years after the initial operation, with a median time to reoperation of 7 to 10 years. (See Schwartz 9th ed., p 997.)

3. Which of the following is NOT a known cause of chronic intestinal pseudo-obstruction?
   A. Scleroderma
   B. Parkinson's disease
   C. Hyperthyroidism
   D. Familial visceral myopathy (type I)

Answer: C

Chronic intestinal pseudo-obstruction can be caused by a large number of specific abnormalities affecting intestinal smooth muscle, the myenteric plexus, or the extraintestinal nervous system (Table 28-3). Visceral myopathies constitute a group of diseases characterized by degeneration and fibrosis of the intestinal muscularis propria. Visceral neuropathies encompass a variety of degenerative disorders of the myenteric and submucosal plexuses. Both sporadic and familial forms of visceral myopathies and neuropathies exist. Systemic disorders involving the smooth muscle, such as progressive systemic sclerosis and progressive muscular dystrophy, and neurologic diseases such as Parkinson's disease also can be complicated by chronic intestinal pseudo-obstruction. In addition, viral infections such as those associated with cytomegalovirus (CMV) and Epstein-Barr virus can cause intestinal pseudo-obstruction. (See Schwartz 9th ed., p 992.)

TABLE 28-3	Chronic intestinal pseudo-obstruction: Etiologies

Primary causes
- Familial types
  - Familial visceral myopathies (types I, II, and III)
  - Familial visceral neuropathies (types I and II)
  - Childhood visceral myopathies (types I and II)
- Sporadic types
  - Visceral myopathies
  - Visceral neuropathies

Secondary causes
- Smooth muscle disorders
  - Collagen vascular diseases (e.g., scleroderma)
  - Muscular dystrophies (e.g., myotonic dystrophy)
  - Amyloidosis
- Neurologic disorders
  - Chagas' disease, Parkinson's disease, spinal cord injury
- Endocrine disorders
  - Diabetes, hypothyroidism, hypoparathyroidism
- Miscellaneous disorders
  - Radiation enteritis
- Pharmacologic causes
  - (e.g., phenothiazines and tricyclic antidepressants)
- Viral infections

4. B_{12} deficiency can occur after
   A. Gastrectomy
   B. Gastric bypass
   C. Ileal resection
   D. All of the above

Answer: D

Vitamin B_{12} (cobalamin) malabsorption can result from a variety of surgical manipulations. The vitamin is initially bound by saliva-derived R protein. In the duodenum, R protein is hydrolyzed by pancreatic enzymes, allowing free cobalamin to bind to gastric parietal cell-derived intrinsic factor. The cobalamin-intrinsic factor complex is able to escape hydrolysis by pancreatic enzymes, allowing it to reach the terminal ileum, which expresses specific receptors for intrinsic factor. Subsequent events in cobalamin absorption are poorly characterized, but the intact complex probably enters enterocytes through translocation. Because each of these steps is necessary for cobalamin assimilation, gastric resection, gastric bypass, and ileal resection can each result in vitamin B_{12} insufficiency. (See Schwartz 9th ed., p 985.)

5. Which of the following is NOT true about imaging a patient with suspected bowel obstruction?
   A. Imaging has poor sensitivity for detecting intestinal ischemia
   B. Water-soluble enteral contrasts are preferred for CT imaging in cases of bowel obstruction
   C. Bowel greater than 3 cm on a plain film is suggestive of a small bowel obstruction
   D. The specificity of plain films and CT scans in diagnosing small bowel obstruction is the same (approximately 80%)

Answer: D

The finding most specific for small bowel obstruction on abdominal radiographs is the triad of dilated small bowel loops (>3 cm in diameter), air-fluid levels seen on upright films, and a paucity of air in the colon. The sensitivity of abdominal radiographs in the detection of small bowel obstruction ranges from 70 to 80%. Specificity is low because ileus and colonic obstruction can be associated with findings that mimic those observed with small bowel obstruction. False-negative findings on radiographs can result when the site of obstruction is located in the proximal small bowel and when the bowel lumen is filled with fluid but no gas, thereby preventing visualization of air-fluid levels or bowel distention. The latter situation is associated with closed-loop obstruction. (See Schwartz 9th ed., p 989.)

Computed tomographic (CT) scanning is 80 to 90% sensitive and 70 to 90% specific in the detection of small bowel obstruction. The findings of small bowel obstruction include a discrete transition zone with dilation of bowel proximally, decompression of bowel distally, intraluminal contrast that does not pass beyond the transition zone, and a colon containing little gas or fluid (Fig. 28-6). CT scanning may also provide evidence for the presence of closed-loop obstruction and strangulation. Closed-loop obstruction is suggested by the presence of a U-shaped or C-shaped dilated bowel loop associated with a radial distribution of mesenteric vessels converging toward a torsion point. (See Schwartz 9th ed., p 989.)

Strangulation is suggested by thickening of the bowel wall, pneumatosis intestinalis (air in the bowel wall), portal venous gas, mesenteric haziness, and poor uptake of IV contrast into the wall of the affected bowel (Fig. 28-7). CT scanning also offers a global evaluation of the abdomen and may therefore reveal the etiology of obstruction. (See Schwartz 9th ed., p 988.)

The CT scan usually is performed after administration of oral water soluble contrast, or diluted barium. The water soluble contrast has been shown to have prognostic and therapeutic values too. Several studies and a subsequent meta-analysis have shown that appearance of the contrast in the colon within 24 hours is predictive of nonsurgical resolution of bowel obstruction. Although use of oral contrast did not alter the rate of surgical intervention, it did reduce the overall length of hospital stay in those presenting with small bowel obstruction.

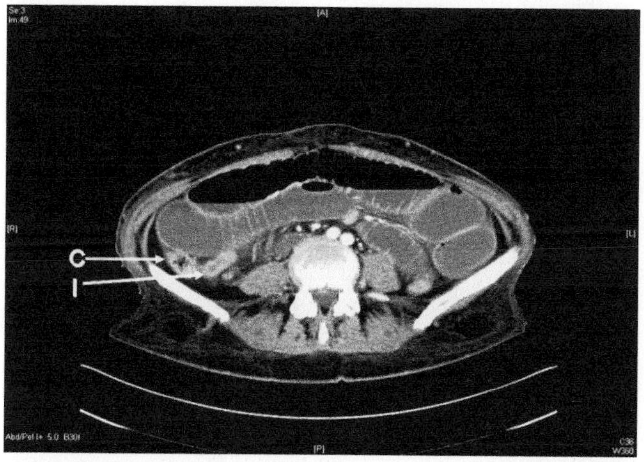

FIG. 28-6. Small bowel obstruction. A computed tomographic scan of a patient presenting with signs and symptoms of bowel obstruction. Image shows grossly dilated loops of small bowel, with decompressed terminal ileum (I) and ascending colon (C), suggesting a complete distal small bowel obstruction. At laparotomy, adhesive bands from a previous surgery were identified and divided.

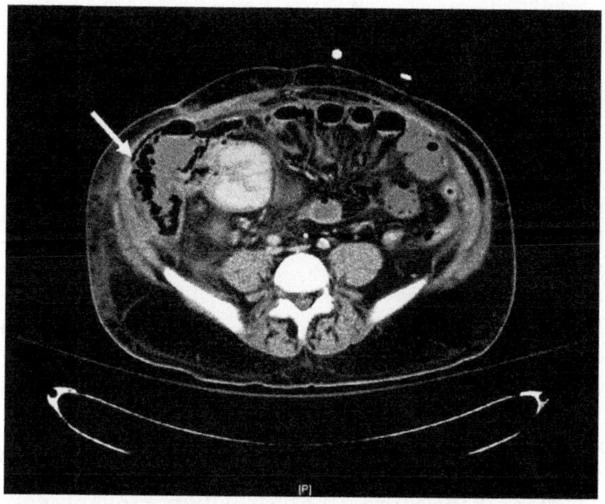

FIG. 28-7. Intestinal pneumatosis. This computed tomographic scan shows intestinal pneumatosis (*arrow*). The cause of this radiologic finding was intestinal ischemia. Patient was taken emergently to the operating room and underwent resection of an infarcted segment of small bowel.

6. Which of the following is the most common indication for surgery in a patient with Crohn's disease?
   A. Intestinal obstruction
   B. Intestinal perforation
   C. Gastrointestinal hemorrhage
   D. Growth retardation

Answer: A

Fifty to 70% of patients with Crohn's disease will ultimately require at least one surgical intervention for their disease. Surgery generally is reserved for patients whose disease is unresponsive to aggressive medical therapy or who develop complications of their disease (Table 28-4). Failure of medical management may be the indication for surgery if symptoms persist despite aggressive therapy for several months or if symptoms recur whenever aggressive therapy is tapered. Surgery should be considered if medication-induced complications arise, specifically corticosteroid-related complications, such as cushingoid features, cataracts, glaucoma, systemic hypertension, compression fractures, or aseptic necrosis of the femoral head. Growth retardation constitutes an indication for surgery in 30% of children with Crohn's disease.

One of the most common indications for surgical intervention is intestinal obstruction. Abscesses and fistulas frequently are encountered during operations performed for intestinal obstruction in these patients, but are rarely the only indication for surgery. Most abscesses are amenable to percutaneous drainage and fistulas unless associated with symptoms or metabolic derangements do not require surgical intervention. Less common complications that require surgical intervention are acute GI hemorrhage, perforations, and development of cancer. (See Schwartz 9th ed., p 996.)

TABLE 28-4 Indications for surgical intervention in Crohn's disease

Acute onset of severe disease
Crohn's colitis ± toxic megacolon (rare)
Failure of medical therapy
Persistent symptoms despite long-term steroid use
Recurrence of symptoms when high-dose steroids are tapered
Drug induced complications (Cushing's disease, hypertension)
Development of disease complications
Obstruction
Perforation
Complicated fistulas
Hemorrhage
Malignancy risk

7. The most common location for a primary adenocarcinoma of the small bowel is
   A. Duodenum
   B. Jejunum
   C. Ileum
   D. None of the above—the distribution is roughly equal

Answer: A

Adenocarcinomas, as well as adenomas (from which most are believed to arise), are most commonly found in the duodenum, except in patients with Crohn's disease, in whom most are found in the ileum. Lesions in the periampullary location can cause obstructive jaundice or pancreatitis. Adenocarcinomas located in the duodenum tend to be diagnosed earlier in their progression than those located in the jejunum or ileum, which are rarely diagnosed before the onset of locally advanced or metastatic disease. (See Schwartz 9th ed., p 1000.)

8. Following a gastric bypass, which form of calcium should be used as a supplement?
   A. Calcium carbonate
   B. Calcium chloride
   C. Calcium gluconate
   D. Calcium citrate

Answer: D

Abnormal calcium levels are increasingly seen in surgical patients who have undergone a gastric bypass. Although usual calcium supplementation is in the form of calcium carbonate, which is cheap, in such patients with low acid exposure, calcium citrate is a better formulation for replacement therapy.

Calcium chloride and calcium gluconate are used as food additives but are not used as calcium supplements. (See Schwartz 9th ed., p 985.)

9. The most common cause of acute mesenteric ischemia is
   A. Arterial embolus
   B. Arterial thrombosis
   C. Vasospasm (nonocclusive mesenteric ischemia)
   D. Venous thrombosis

Answer: A

Four distinct pathophysiologic mechanisms can lead to acute mesenteric ischemia:

1. Arterial embolus
2. Arterial thrombosis
3. Vasospasm (also known as nonocclusive mesenteric ischemia)
4. Venous thrombosis

Embolus is the most common cause of acute mesenteric ischemia, and is responsible for more than 50% of cases. The embolic source is usually in the heart; most often the left atrial or ventricular thrombi or valvular lesions. Indeed, up to 95% of patients with acute mesenteric ischemia due to emboli will have a documented history of cardiac disease. Embolism to the superior mesenteric artery accounts for 50% of cases; most of these emboli become wedged and cause occlusion at branch points in the mid- to distal superior mesenteric artery, usually distal to the origin of the middle colic artery. In contrast, acute occlusions due to thrombosis tend to occur in the proximal mesenteric arteries, near their origins. Acute thrombosis is usually superimposed on pre-existing atherosclerotic lesions at these sites. Nonocclusive mesenteric ischemia is the result of vasospasm and usually is diagnosed in critically ill patients receiving vasopressor agents. (See Schwartz 9th ed., p 1006.)

10. Which of the following factors is associated with poor spontaneous enterocutaneous fistulae closure rate?
    A. Radiation
    B. Albumin level >4
    C. Long (>2 cm) fistula tract
    D. Absence of epithelialization in fistula tract

Answer: A

Fistulas have the potential to close spontaneously. Factors inhibiting spontaneous closure, however, include malnutrition, sepsis, inflammatory bowel disease, cancer, radiation, obstruction of the intestine distal to the origin of the fistula, foreign bodies, high output, short fistulous tract (<2 cm), and epithelialization of the fistula tract (Table 28-5). (See Schwartz 9th ed., p 998.)

A useful mnemonic designates factors that inhibit spontaneous closure of intestinal fistulas: 'FRIEND'(*F*oreign body within the fistula tract, *R*adiation enteritis, *I*nfection/*I*nflammation at the fistula origin, *E*pithelialization of the fistula tract, *N*eoplasm at the fistula origin, *D*istal obstruction of the intestine). (See Schwartz 9th ed., p 998.)

TABLE 28-5 Factors negatively impacting enteric fistula closure

Patient factors
Poor nutrition
Medications such as steroids
Etiologic factors
Malignant fistula
Fistula related to Crohn's disease
Fistula in radiated fields
Fistula site
Gastric
Duodenal
Local factors
Persistence of local inflammation and sepsis
Presence of a foreign body (e.g., meshes or sutures)
Epithelialization of fistula tract
Fistula tract <2 cm
Distal obstruction to the fistula site

11. Which of the following has been shown to be effective in reducing the duration of postoperative ileus?
    A. NG suction
    B. Aggressive fluid administration
    C. Early enteral feeding
    D. Rectal suppository

Answer: C

Given the frequency of postoperative ileus and its financial impact, a large number of investigations have been conducted to define strategies to reduce its duration. Although often recommended, the use of early ambulation and routine NG intubation has not been demonstrated to be associated with earlier resolution of postoperative ileus. There is some evidence that early postoperative feeding protocols are generally well tolerated, reduce postoperative ileus, and can result in a shorter hospital stay. The administration of NSAIDs such as ketorolac and concomitant reductions in opioid dosing have been shown to reduce the duration of ileus in most studies. Similarly, the use of perioperative thoracic epidural anesthesia/analgesia with regimens containing local anesthetics combined with limitation or elimination of systemically administered opioids have been shown to reduce duration of postoperative ileus, although they have not reduced the overall length of hospital stay. Interestingly, recent data have suggested that limiting intra and postoperative fluid administration can also result in reduction of postoperative ileus, and shortened hospital stay. Table 28-6 summarizes some of the measures used to minimize postoperative ileus. (See Schwartz 9th ed., p 993.)

TABLE 28-6 Measures to reduce postoperative ileus
Intraoperative measures
Minimize handling of the bowel
Laparoscopic approach, if possible
Avoid excessive intraoperative fluid administration
Postoperative measures
Early enteral feeding
Epidural anesthesia, if indicated
Avoid excessive IV fluid administration
Correct electrolyte abnormalities
Consider m-opioid antagonists

12. Which of the following is a recognized risk factor for Crohn's disease?
    A. Male gender
    B. Having been breastfed as an infant
    C. Low socioeconomic status
    D. Smoking

Answer: D

The incidence of Crohn's disease varies among ethnic groups within the same geographic region. For example, members of the Eastern European Ashkenazi Jewish population are at two- to fourfold higher risk of developing Crohn's disease than members of other populations living in the same location. Most studies suggest that Crohn's disease is slightly more prevalent in females than in males.

Both genetic and environmental factors appear to influence the risk for developing Crohn's disease. The relative risk among first-degree relatives of patients with Crohn's disease is 14 to 15 times higher than that of the general population. Approximately one in five patients with Crohn's disease will report having at least one affected relative. The concordance rate among monozygotic twins is as high as 67%; however, Crohn's disease is not associated with simple mendelian inheritance patterns. Although there is a tendency within families for either ulcerative colitis or Crohn's disease to be present exclusively, mixed kindreds also occur, suggesting the presence of some shared genetic traits as a basis for both diseases.

Higher socioeconomic status is associated with an increased risk of Crohn's disease. Most studies have found breastfeeding to be protective against the development of Crohn's disease. Crohn's disease is more prevalent among smokers.

Furthermore, smoking is associated with the increased risk for both the need for surgery and the risk of relapse after surgery for Crohn's disease. (See Schwartz 9th ed., p 993.)

13. A patient with an asymptomatic 4-cm duodenal diverticulum should be treated with
   A. Observation alone
   B. Endoscopic ablation of the diverticular mucosa
   C. Diverticulectomy
   D. Segmental duodenectomy

Answer: A
Asymptomatic acquired diverticula should be left alone. Bacterial overgrowth associated with acquired diverticula is treated with antibiotics. Other complications, such as bleeding and diverticulitis, are treated with segmental intestinal resection for diverticula located in the jejunum or ileum.

Bleeding and obstruction related to lateral duodenal diverticula generally are treated with diverticulectomy alone. These procedures can be technically difficult for medial duodenal diverticula that penetrate into the substance of the pancreas. Complications related to these medial duodenal diverticula should be managed nonoperatively if possible, using endoscopy. In emergent situations, bleeding related to medial duodenal diverticula can be controlled using a lateral duodenotomy and oversewing of the bleeding vessel. Similarly, perforation can be managed with wide drainage rather than complex surgery. Whether diverticulectomy should be done in patients with biliary or pancreatic symptoms is controversial and is not routinely recommended. (See Schwartz 9th ed., p 1006.)

14. The most common location for gastrointestinal stromal tumors (GIST) is
   A. Stomach
   B. Duodenum
   C. Jejunum
   D. Ileum

Answer: A
Sixty to 70% of GISTs are located in the stomach. The small intestine is the second most common site, containing 25 to 35% of GISTs. There appears to be no regional variation in the prevalence of GISTs within the small intestine. GISTs have a greater propensity to be associated with overt hemorrhage than the other small intestinal malignancies. (See Schwartz 9th ed., p 1000.)

15. Which of the following findings is virtually pathognomic for Crohn's disease?
   A. Terminal ileal inflammation
   B. Thickened ileal wall
   C. Fat wrapping
   D. Ulceration in the ileal mucosa

Answer: C
A feature of Crohn's disease that is grossly evident and helpful in identifying affected segments of intestine during surgery is the presence of *fat wrapping*, which represents encroachment of mesenteric fat onto the serosal surface of the bowel (Fig. 28-8). This finding is virtually pathognomonic of Crohn's disease. The presence of fat wrapping correlates well with the presence of underlying acute and chronic inflammation. (See Schwartz 9th ed., p 993.)

The other findings listed can be found in Crohn's disease but are not specific, as they can also be found in other causes of ileal inflammation, such as infection.

Acute ileitis caused by *Campylobacter* and *Yersinia* species can be difficult to distinguish from that caused by an acute presentation of Crohn's disease. Typhoid enteritis caused by *Salmonella typhosa* can lead to overt intestinal bleeding and perforation, most often affecting the terminal ileum. The distal ileum and cecum are the most common sites of intestinal involvement by infection due to *Mycobacterium tuberculosis*. This condition can result in intestinal inflammation, strictures, and fistula formation, similar to those seen in Crohn's disease. CMV can cause intestinal ulcers, bleeding, and perforation. (See Schwartz 9th ed., p 995.)

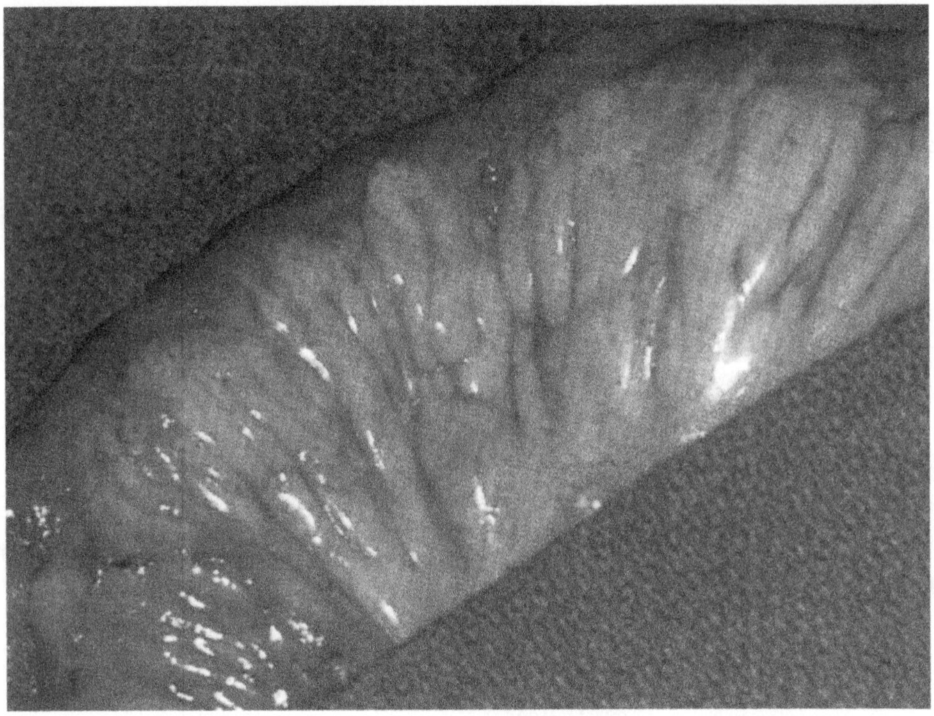

FIG. 28-8. Crohn's disease. This intraoperative photograph demonstrates encroachment of mesenteric fat onto the serosal surface of the intestine ("fat wrapping") that is characteristic of intestinal segments affected by active Crohn's disease.

16. Early postoperative obstruction following laparotomy
    A. Occurs in approximately 8% of patients undergoing laparotomy
    B. Is best treated surgically if signs of ischemia are detected
    C. Is most common after extensive retroperitoneal dissection
    D. Can be diagnosed with plain radiographs in >90% of patients

Answer: B

Obstruction presenting in *the early postoperative period* has been reported to occur in 0.7% patients undergoing laparotomy. Patients undergoing pelvic surgery, especially colorectal procedures, have the greatest risk for developing early postoperative small bowel obstruction. The presence of obstruction should be considered if symptoms of intestinal obstruction occur after the initial return of bowel function or if bowel function fails to return within the expected 3 to 5 days after abdominal surgery. Plain radiographs may demonstrate dilated loops of small intestine with air-fluid levels but are interpreted as normal or nonspecific in up to one third of patients with early postoperative obstruction. CT scanning or small bowel series is often required to make the diagnosis. Obstruction that occurs in the early postoperative period is usually partial and only rarely is associated with strangulation. Therefore, a period of extended nonoperative therapy (2 to 3 weeks) consisting of bowel rest, hydration, and total parenteral nutrition (TPN) administration is usually warranted. However, if complete obstruction is demonstrated or if signs suggestive of peritonitis are detected, expeditious reoperation should be undertaken without delay. (See Schwartz 9th ed., p 990.)

17. The presumed cell of origin for gastrointestinal stromal tumors (GIST) is
    A. Cell of Cajal
    B. Paneth cell
    C. Enteroendocrine cell
    D. Enterocyte

Answer: A

A defining feature of GISTs is their gain of function mutation of protooncogene KIT, a receptor tyrosine kinase. Pathologic KIT signal transduction is believed to be a central event in GIST pathogenesis. The majority of GISTs have activating mutations in the *c-kit* protooncogene, which cause KIT to become constitutively activated, presumably leading to persistence of cellular growth or survival signals. Because the interstitial cells of Cajal normally express KIT, these cells have been implicated as the cell of origin for GISTs. KIT expression is assessed by staining the tissues for CD117 antigen, which is part of the KIT receptor, and present in 95% of GISTs. (See Schwartz 9th ed., p 999.)

18. Which of the following is the LAST to recover from postoperative ileus?
    A. Stomach
    B. Small bowel
    C. Colon
    D. None of the above—the recovery is simultaneous

Answer: C

Following most abdominal operations or injuries, the motility of the GI tract is transiently impaired. Among the proposed mechanisms responsible for this dysmotility are surgical stress-induced sympathetic reflexes, inflammatory response mediator release, and anesthetic/analgesic effects; each of which can inhibit intestinal motility. The return of normal motility generally follows a characteristic temporal sequence, with small intestinal motility returning to normal within the first 24 hours after laparotomy and gastric and colonic motility returning to normal by 48 hours and 3 to 5 days, respectively. Because small bowel motility is returned before colonic and gastric motility, listening for bowel sounds is not a reliable indicator that ileus has fully resolved. Functional evidence of coordinated GI motility in the form of passing flatus or bowel movement is a more useful indicator. Resolution of ileus may be delayed in the presence of other factors capable of inciting ileus such as the presence of intra-abdominal abscesses or electrolyte abnormalities. (See Schwartz 9th ed., p 992.)

19. Which of the following is NOT a known cause of ileus?
    A. Pneumonia
    B. Hypomagnesemia
    C. Myocardial infarction
    D. Hyperkalemia

Answer: D

(See Schwartz 9th ed., p 992, and Table 28-7.)

TABLE 28-7 Ileus: Common etiologies
Abdominal surgery
Infection
Sepsis
Intra-abdominal abscess
Peritonitis
Pneumonia
Electrolyte abnormalities
Hypokalemia
Hypomagnesemia
Hypermagnesemia
Hyponatremia
Medications
Anticholinergics
Opiates
Phenothiazines
Calcium channel blockers
Tricyclic antidepressants
Hypothyroidism
Ureteral colic
Retroperitoneal hemorrhage
Spinal cord injury
Myocardial infarction
Mesenteric ischemia

20. A high output enterocutaneous fistula is defined as draining more than
    A. 100 mL/day
    B. 500 mL/day
    C. 1000 mL/day
    D. 2000 mL/day

Answer: B

Enterocutaneous fistulas that drain less than 200 mL of fluid per day are known as *low-output fistulas*, whereas those that drain more than 500 mL of fluid per day are known as *high-output fistulas*. (See Schwartz 9th ed., p 998.)

21. The most common complication seen in adults with a Meckel's diverticulum is
    A. Obstruction
    B. Meckel's diverticulitis
    C. Perforation
    D. Bleeding

Answer: A
Intestinal obstruction is the most common presentation in adults with Meckel's diverticula. Diverticulitis, present in 20% of patients with symptomatic Meckel's diverticula, is associated with a clinical syndrome that is indistinguishable from acute appendicitis. Neoplasms, most commonly carcinoid tumors, are present in 0.5 to 3.2% of symptomatic Meckel's diverticula that are resected.

Intestinal obstruction associated with Meckel's diverticulum can result from several mechanisms:

1. Volvulus of the intestine around the fibrous band attaching the diverticulum to the umbilicus
2. Entrapment of intestine by a mesodiverticular band (Fig. 28-9)
3. Intussusception with the diverticulum acting as a lead point
4. Stricture secondary to chronic diverticulitis

Meckel's diverticula can be found in inguinal or femoral hernia sacs (known as *Littre's hernia*). These hernias, when incarcerated, can cause intestinal obstruction.

Bleeding is the most common presentation in children with Meckel's diverticula, representing over 50% of Meckel's diverticulum-related complications among patients younger than 18 years of age. Bleeding associated with Meckel's diverticula is rare among patients older than 30 years of age. (See Schwartz 9th ed., p 1003.)

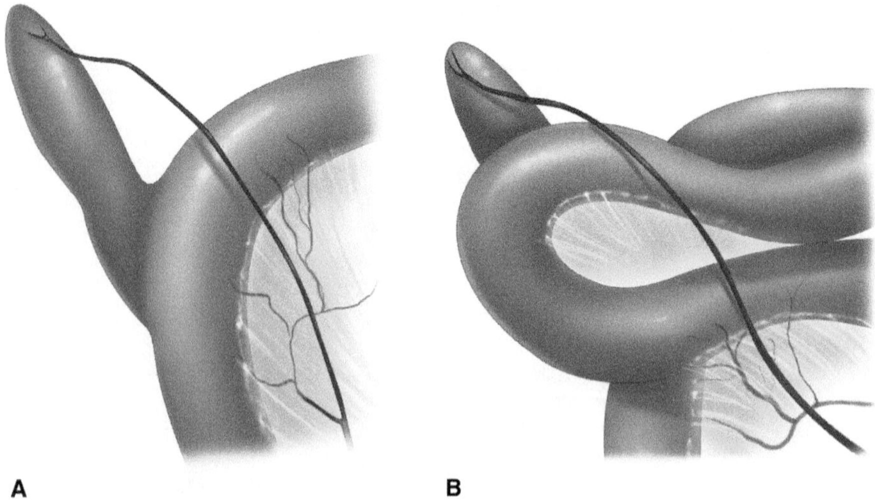

FIG. 28-9. A. Meckel's diverticulum with mesodiverticular band. B. One mechanism by which Meckel's diverticula can cause small bowel obstruction is entrapment of the intestine by a mesodiverticular band.

22. Which of the following is NOT an extraintestinal manifestation of Crohn's disease?
    A. Pyoderma gangrenosum
    B. Erythema nodosum
    C. Alopecia
    D. Arthritis

Answer: C
An estimated one fourth of all patients with Crohn's disease will have an extraintestinal manifestation of their disease. One fourth of those affected will have more than one manifestation. Many of these complications are common to both Crohn's disease and ulcerative colitis, although as a whole, they are more prevalent among patients with Crohn's disease than those with ulcerative colitis. The most common extraintestinal manifestations are listed in Table 28-8. The clinical severity of some of these manifestations, such as erythema nodosum and peripheral arthritis, is correlated with the severity of intestinal inflammation. The severity of other manifestations, such as pyoderma gangrenosum and ankylosing spondylitis, bears no apparent relationship to the severity of intestinal inflammation. (See Schwartz 9th ed., p 995.)

TABLE 28-8	Extraintestinal manifestations of Crohn's disease
Dermatologic	
Erythema nodosum	
Pyoderma gangrenosum	
Rheumatologic	
Peripheral arthritis	
Ankylosing spondylitis	
Sacroiliitis	
Ocular	
Conjunctivitis	
Uveitis/iritis	
Episcleritis	
Hepatobiliary	
Hepatic steatosis	
Cholelithiasis	
Primary sclerosing cholangitis	
Pericholangitis	
Urologic	
Nephrolithiasis	
Ureteral obstruction	
Miscellaneous	
Thromboembolic disease	
Vasculitis	
Osteoporosis	
Endocarditis, myocarditis, pleuropericarditis	
Interstitial lung disease	
Amyloidosis	
Pancreatitis	

23. Stricturoplasty is contraindicated in a patient with Crohn's disease who, at the time of surgery, is found to have
    A. Multiple areas of stenosis
    B. Stricture(s) >12 cm in length
    C. A fistula at the level of the stricture
    D. A stricture proximal to severe ileocecal disease

Answer: C

An alternative to segmental resection for obstructing lesions is stricturoplasty (Fig. 28-10). This technique allows for preservation of intestinal surface area and is especially well suited to patients with extensive disease and fibrotic strictures who may have undergone previous resection and are at risk for developing short bowel syndrome. In this technique, the bowel is opened longitudinally to expose the lumen. Any intraluminal ulcerations should be biopsied to rule out the presence of neoplasia. Depending on the length of the stricture, the reconstruction can be fashioned in a manner similar to the Heinecke-Mikulicz pyloroplasty (for strictures less than 12 cm in length) or the Finney pyloroplasty (for longer strictures as much as 25 cm in length). For longer strictures, variations on the standard stricturoplasty, namely the side-to-side isoperistaltic enteroenterostomy, have been advocated, and used for strictures with mean lengths of 50 cm. Stricturoplasty sites should be marked with metallic clips to facilitate their identification on radiographs and during subsequent operations. Stricturoplasty is associated with recurrence rates that are no different from those associated with segmental resection. Because the affected bowel is left in situ rather than resected, there is the potential for cancer developing at the stricturoplasty site. However, as data on this complication are limited to anecdotes, this risk remains a theoretical one. Stricturoplasty is contraindicated in patients with intra-abdominal abscesses or intestinal fistulas. The presence of a solitary stricture relatively close to a segment for which resection is planned is a relative contraindication. In general, stricturoplasty is performed in cases where single or multiple strictures are identified in diffusely involved segments of bowel, or where previous resections have been performed, and maintenance of intestinal length is of great importance. (See Schwartz 9th ed., p 997.)

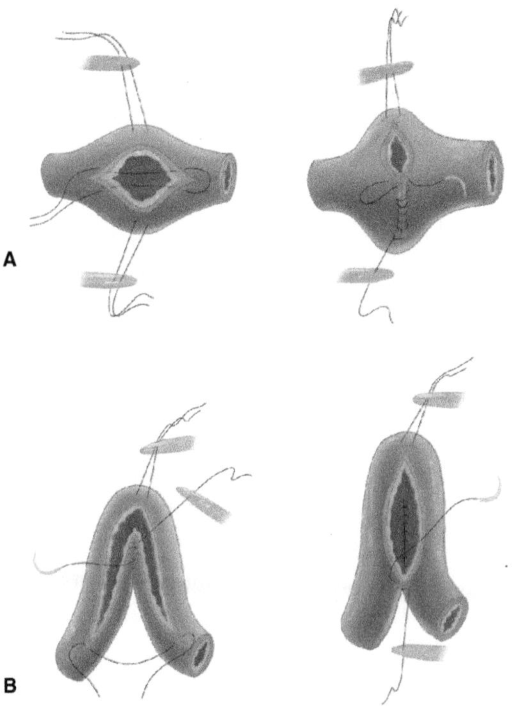

FIG. 28-10. Stricturoplasty. The wall of the strictured bowel is incised longitudinally. Reconstruction is performed by closing the defect transversely in a manner similar to the Heinecke-Mikulicz pyloroplasty for short strictures (A), or the Finney pyloroplasty for longer strictures (B).

24. The most common cause of small bowel obstruction is
    A. Adhesions
    B. Hernia
    C. Malignancy
    D. Crohn's disease

Answer: A

Intra-abdominal adhesions related to prior abdominal surgery account for up to 75% of the cases of small bowel obstruction. Over 300,000 patients are estimated to undergo surgery annually to treat adhesion-induced small bowel obstruction in the United States. Less prevalent etiologies for small bowel obstruction include hernias, malignant bowel obstruction, and Crohn's disease. (See Schwartz 9th ed., p 998, and Table 28-9.)

TABLE 28-9 Small bowel obstruction: Common etiologies
Adhesions
Neoplasms
Primary small bowel neoplasms
Secondary small bowel cancer (e.g., melanoma-derived metastasis)
Local invasion by intra-abdominal malignancy (e.g., desmoid tumors)
Carcinomatosis
Hernias
External (e.g., inguinal and femoral)
Internal (e.g., following Roux-en-Y gastric bypass surgery)
Crohn's disease
Volvulus
Intussusception
Radiation-induced stricture
Postischemic stricture
Foreign body
Gallstone ileus
Diverticulitis
Meckel's diverticulum
Hematoma
Congenital abnormalities (e.g., webs, duplications, and malrotation)

25. Which of the following is NOT associated with successful weaning of TPN in patients with short bowel syndrome?
    A. Length of small bowel >200 cm
    B. Presence of ileocecal valve
    C. Presence of colon
    D. Age >30 years

Answer: D

See Table 28-10. Pediatric patients adapt better than adult patients. (See Schwartz 9th ed., p 1010.)

TABLE 28-10 Risk factors for development of short bowel syndrome after massive small bowel resection

Small bowel length <200 cm
Absence of ileocecal valve
Absence of colon
Diseased remaining bowel (e.g., Crohn's disease)
Ileal resection

26. Which of the following agents has been shown to improve closure of enterocutaneous fistulae in Crohn's disease?
    A. Metotrexate
    B. 5-ASA
    C. Infliximab
    D. Corticosteroids

Answer: C

Infliximab is a chimeric monoclonal anti–tumor necrosis factor alpha antibody that has been shown to have efficacy in inducing remission and in promoting closure of enterocutaneous fistulas. It generally is used for patients resistant to standard therapy to help taper steroid dosage. Infliximab generally is well tolerated but should not be used in patients with ongoing septic processes, such as undrained intra-abdominal abscesses. (See Schwartz 9th ed., p 996.)

CHAPTER 29

Colon, Rectum, and Anus

BASIC SCIENCE QUESTIONS

1. Which of the following is a branch of the inferior mesenteric artery?
   A. Middle colic artery
   B. Ileocolic artery
   C. Sigmoidal arteries
   D. Right colic artery

Answer: C

The arterial supply to the colon is highly variable (Fig. 29-1). In general, the *superior mesenteric artery* branches into the *ileocolic artery* (absent in up to 20% of people), which supplies blood flow to the terminal ileum and proximal ascending colon, the *right colic artery*, which supplies the ascending colon, and the *middle colic artery*, which supplies the transverse colon. The *inferior mesenteric artery* branches into the *left colic artery*, which supplies the descending colon, several *sigmoidal branches*, which supply the sigmoid colon, and the *superior rectal artery*, which supplies the proximal rectum. The terminal branches of each artery form anastomoses with the terminal branches of the adjacent artery and communicate via the *marginal artery of Drummond*. This arcade is complete in only 15 to 20% of people. (See Schwartz 9th ed., p 1018.)

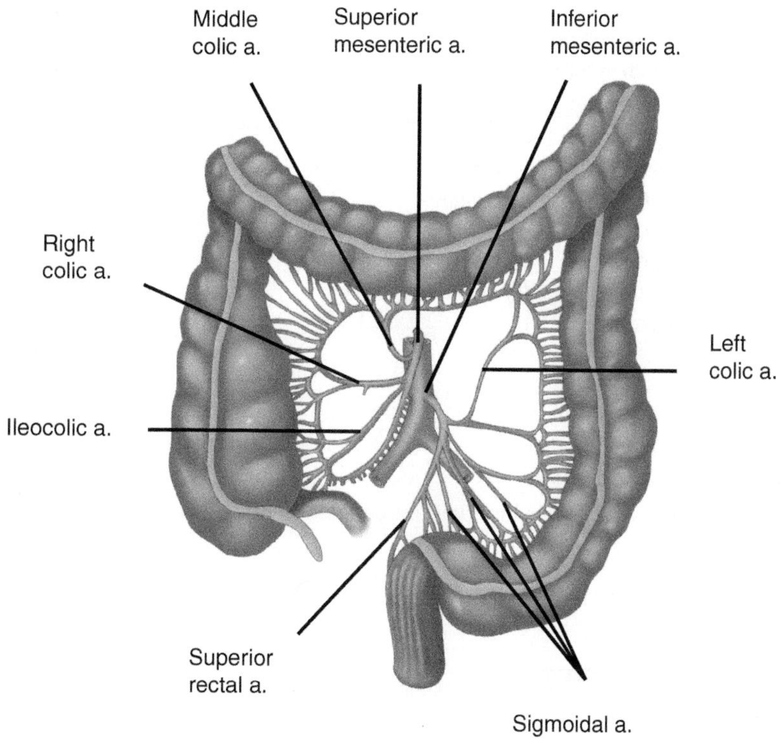

FIG. 29-1. Arterial blood supply to the colon. a. = artery.

2. Bacteria make up what percentage of the dry weight of feces?
   A. 10%
   B. 30%
   C. 50%
   D. 70%

Answer: B

Approximately 30% of fecal dry weight is composed of bacteria (1011 to 1012 bacteria/g of feces). Anaerobes are the predominant class of microorganism, and *Bacteroides* species are the most common (1011 to 1012 organisms/mL). *Escherichia coli* are the most numerous aerobes (108 to 1010 organisms/mL). (See Schwartz 9th ed., p 1019.)

3. Which of the following is associated with colorectal carcinoma?
   A. Activation of the K-ras gene
   B. Activation of APC
   C. Activation of DCC (deleted in colorectal carcinoma)
   D. Activation of p53

Answer: A

Over the past two decades, an intense research effort has focused on elucidating the genetic defects and molecular abnormalities associated with the development and progression of colorectal adenomas and carcinoma. Mutations may cause *activation of oncogenes* (K-ras) and/or *inactivation of tumor-suppressor genes* [APC, DCC (deleted in colorectal carcinoma), p53]. Colorectal carcinoma is thought to develop from adenomatous polyps by accumulation of these mutations (Fig. 29-2). (See Schwartz 9th ed., p 1041.)

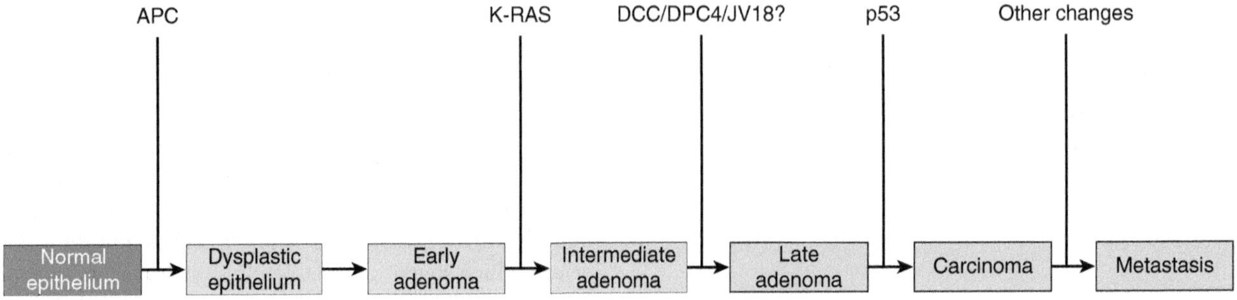

FIG. 29-2. Schematic showing progression from normal colonic epithelium to carcinoma of the colon.

4. Deletion in the tumor suppressor phosphatase and tensin homolog (PTEN) is associated with all of the following EXCEPT
   A. Familial adenomatous polyposis
   B. Peutz-Jeghers syndrome
   C. Juvenile polyposis
   D. Cowden syndrome

Answer: A

Deletion of the tumor suppressor phosphatase and tensin homolog (PTEN) appears to be involved in a number of hamartomatous polyposis syndromes. Deletions in PTEN have been identified in juvenile polyposis, Peutz-Jeghers syndrome, Cowden syndrome, and PTEN-hamartoma syndrome, in addition to multiple endocrine neoplasia IIB. (See Schwartz 9th ed., p 1042.)

5. Which of the following is important in maintaining the integrity of the colonic mucosa?
   A. Short-chain fatty acids
   B. Alanine
   C. Medium-chain fatty acids
   D. Glutamine

Answer: A

Short-chain fatty acids (acetate, butyrate, and propionate) are produced by bacterial fermentation of dietary carbohydrates. Short-chain fatty acids are an important source of energy for the colonic mucosa, and metabolism by colonocytes provides energy for processes such as active transport of sodium. Lack of a dietary source for production of short-chain fatty acids, or diversion of the fecal stream by an ileostomy or colostomy, may result in mucosal atrophy and diversion colitis. (See Schwartz 9th ed., p 1019.)

6. The parasympathetic innervations to the transverse colon are from
   A. T6-T12
   B. L1-L3
   C. S2-S4
   D. The vagus nerve

Answer: D

The colon is innervated by both *sympathetic* (inhibitory) and *parasympathetic* (stimulatory) nerves, which parallel the course of the arteries. Sympathetic nerves arise from T6–T12 and L1–L3. The parasympathetic innervation to the right and transverse colon is from the vagus nerve; the parasympathetic nerves to the left colon arise from sacral nerves S2–S4 to form the nervi erigentes. (See Schwartz 9th ed., p 1018.)

7. The origin of the middle rectal artery is the
   A. Inferior mesenteric artery
   B. Iliac artery
   C. Internal pudendal artery
   D. Inferior epigastric artery

Answer: B

The *superior rectal artery* arises from the terminal branch of the inferior mesenteric artery and supplies the upper rectum. The *middle rectal artery* arises from the internal iliac; the presence and size of these arteries are highly variable. The *inferior rectal artery* arises from the internal pudendal artery, which is a branch of the internal iliac artery. A rich network of collaterals connects the terminal arterioles of each of these arteries, thus making the rectum relatively resistant to ischemia (Fig. 29-3). (See Schwartz 9th ed., p 1018.)

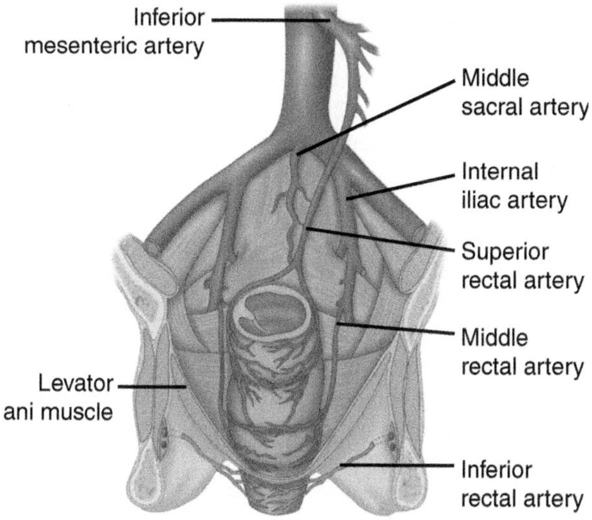

FIG. 29-3. Arterial supply to the rectum and anal canal.

8. Colorectal cancers which develop from defects in the RER (replication error repair) pathway when compared to tumors which develop from the LOH (loss of heterozygosity) pathway
   A. Occur more commonly in the left colon
   B. Have a worse prognosis
   C. Have chromosomal aneuploidy
   D. Express microsatellite instability

Answer: D

The RER pathway is associated with *microsatellite instability* (MSI). Microsatellites are regions of the genome in which short base-pair segments are repeated several times. These areas are particularly prone to RER. Consequently, a mutation in a mismatch repair gene produces variable lengths of these repetitive sequences, a finding that has been described as *microsatellite instability*. Approximately 15% of colorectal cancers are associated with MSI.

Tumors associated with MSI appear to have different biologic characteristics than do tumors that result from the LOH pathway. Tumors with MSI are more likely to be right sided, possess diploid DNA, and are associated with a better prognosis than tumors that arise from the LOH pathway that are microsatellite stable. Tumors arising from the LOH pathway tend to occur in the more distal colon, often have chromosomal aneuploidy, and are associated with a poorer prognosis. (See Schwartz 9th ed., p 1042.)

9. Extensive perianal condyloma accuminata is best treated with
   A. Topical steroids
   B. Topical podophyllin
   C. Topical imiquimod
   D. Surgical resection and fulguration

Answer: D

Treatment of anal condyloma depends on the location and extent of disease. Small warts on the perianal skin and distal anal canal may be treated in the office with topical application of bichloracetic acid or podophyllin. Although 60 to 80% of patients will respond to these agents, recurrence and reinfection are common. Imiquimod (Aldara) is an immunomodulator that recently was introduced for topical treatment of several viral infections, including anogenital condyloma. Initial reports suggest that this agent is highly effective in treating condyloma located on the perianal skin and distal anal canal. Larger and/or more numerous warts require excision and/or fulguration in the operating room. Excised warts should be sent for pathologic examination to rule out dysplasia or malignancy. It is important to note that prior use of podophyllin may induce histologic changes that mimic dysplasia. (See Schwartz 9th ed., p 1067.)

CLINICAL QUESTIONS

1. Which of the following manometric findings indicates dysfunction of the internal sphincter?
   A. Resting pressure 20 mmHg
   B. Squeeze pressure 60 mmHg
   C. High pressure zone 2 cm
   D. Presence of a rectoanal inhibitory reflex

Answer: A
The *resting pressure* in the anal canal reflects the function of the internal anal sphincter (normal: 40 to 80 mmHg), while the *squeeze pressure*, defined as the maximum voluntary contraction pressure minus the resting pressure, reflects function of the external anal sphincter (normal: 40 to 80 mmHg above resting pressure). The *high-pressure zone* estimates the length of the anal canal (normal: 2.0 to 4.0 cm). The *rectoanal inhibitory reflex* can be detected by inflating a balloon in the distal rectum; absence of this reflex is characteristic of Hirschsprung's disease. (See Schwartz 9th ed., p 1021.)

2. The treatment of choice for acute anal fissures is
   A. Excision and primary closure
   B. Lateral internal sphincterotomy
   C. Botulinum injection
   D. Laxatives and sitz baths

Answer: D
Therapy for an acute anal fissure focuses on breaking the cycle of pain, spasm, and ischemia thought responsible for development of fissure in ano. First-line therapy to minimize anal trauma includes bulk agents, stool softeners, and warm sitz baths. The addition of 2% lidocaine jelly or other analgesic creams can provide additional symptomatic relief. Botulinum toxin (Botox) causes temporary muscle paralysis by preventing acetylcholine release from presynaptic nerve terminals. Injection of botulinum toxin is used in some centers as an alternative to surgical sphincterotomy for chronic fissure. Surgical therapy traditionally has been recommended for chronic fissures that have failed medical therapy, and lateral internal sphincterotomy is the procedure of choice for most surgeons. (See Schwartz 9th ed., p 1060.)

3. A patient with obstipation and abdominal distention presents to the emergency room. Based on the results of the contrast enema shown in Fig. 29-4, the next step in management should be
   A. NG suction, bowel rest, and observation
   B. Enemas until the obstruction is relieved
   C. Proctoscopy
   D. Exploratory laparotomy

Answer: C
Sigmoid volvulus often can be differentiated from cecal or transversecolon volvulus by the appearance of plain x-rays of the abdomen. Sigmoid volvulus produces a characteristic *bent inner tube* or *coffee bean* appearance, with the convexity of the loop lying in the right upper quadrant (opposite the site of obstruction). Gastrografin enema shows a narrowing at the site of the volvulus and a pathognomonic *bird's beak* (See Fig. 29-4.).

Unless there are obvious signs of gangrene or peritonitis, the initial management of sigmoid volvulus is resuscitation followed by endoscopic detorsion. Detorsion is usually most easily accomplished by using a rigid proctoscope, but a flexible sigmoidoscope or colonoscope might also be effective. (See Schwartz 9th ed., p 1055.)

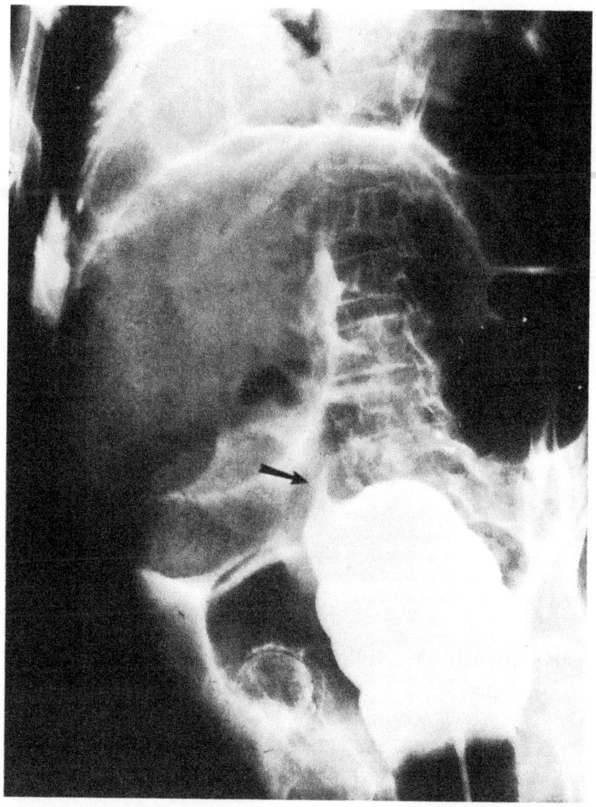

FIG. 29-4. Sigmoid volvulus: Gastrografin enema showing "bird-beak" sign (*arrow*). (Reproduced with permission from Nivatvongs S, Becker ER: Colon, rectum and anal canal, in James EC, Corry RJ, Perry JCF Jr. (eds): *Basic Surgical Practice*. Philadelphia: Hanley & Belfus, 1987. Copyright © Elsevier.)

4. Elective proctocolectomy should be advised for which of the following patients with ulcerative colitis?
   A. Low-grade dysplasia on biopsy
   B. Moderate dysplasia on biopsy
   C. Pancolonic disease for >20 years, independent of biopsy results
   D. All of the above

Answer: D

Although low-grade dysplasia was long thought to represent minimal risk, more recent studies show that invasive cancer may be present in up to 20% of patients with low-grade dysplasia. For this reason, any patient with dysplasia should be advised to undergo proctocolectomy. Controversy exists over whether prophylactic proctocolectomy should be recommended for patients who have had chronic ulcerative colitis for >10 years in the absence of dysplasia. Proponents of this approach note that surveillance colonoscopy with multiple biopsies samples only a small fraction of the colonic mucosa and dysplasia and carcinoma are often missed. Opponents cite the relatively low risk of progression to carcinoma if all biopsies have lacked dysplasia (approximately 2.4%). Neither approach has been definitively shown to decrease mortality from colorectal cancer.

Risk of malignancy increases with pancolonic disease and the duration of symptoms is approximately 2% after 10 years, 8% after 20 years, and 18% after 30 years. (See Schwartz 9th ed., p 1035.)

5. In order to avoid complications, output from an ileostomy should be kept below
   A. 500 mL/day
   B. 1000 mL/day
   C. 1500 mL/day
   D. 2000 mL/day

Answer: C

The creation of an ileostomy bypasses the fluid absorbing capability of the colon, and dehydration with fluid and electrolyte abnormalities is not uncommon. Ideally, ileostomy output should be maintained at less than 1500 mL/d to avoid this problem. Bulk agents and opioids (Lomotil, Imodium, tincture of opium) are useful. The somatostatin analogue, Octreotide, has been used with variable success in this setting. (See Schwartz 9th ed., p 1031.)

6. An internal hemorrhoid that prolapses past the dentate line with straining is a
   A. First-degree hemorrhoid
   B. Second-degree hemorrhoid
   C. Third-degree hemorrhoid
   D. Fourth-degree hemorrhoid

Answer: A
Internal hemorrhoids are located proximal to the dentate line and covered by insensate anorectal mucosa. Internal hemorrhoids may prolapse or bleed, but rarely become painful unless they develop thrombosis and necrosis (usually related to severe prolapse, incarceration, and/or strangulation). Internal hemorrhoids are graded according to the extent of prolapse. *First-degree hemorrhoids* bulge into the anal canal and may prolapse beyond the dentate line on straining. *Second-degree hemorrhoids* prolapse through the anus but reduce spontaneously. *Third-degree hemorrhoids* prolapse through the anal canal and require manual reduction. *Fourth-degree hemorrhoids* prolapse but cannot be reduced and are at risk for strangulation. (See Schwartz 9th ed., p 1058.)

7. In patients with inflammatory bowel disease, erythema nodosum
   A. Is seen more commonly in men
   B. May occur near a stoma
   C. Usually occurs on the lower legs
   D. All of the above

Answer: C
Erythema nodosum is seen in 5 to 15% of patients with inflammatory bowel disease and usually coincides with clinical disease activity. Women are affected three to four times more frequently than men. The characteristic lesions are raised, red, and predominantly on the lower legs. Pyoderma gangrenosum is an uncommon but serious condition that occurs almost exclusively in patients with inflammatory bowel disease. The lesion begins as an erythematous plaque, papule, or bleb, usually located on the pretibial region of the leg and occasionally near a stoma. The lesions progress and ulcerate, leading to a painful, necrotic wound. Pyoderma gangrenosum may respond to resection of the affected bowel in some patients. In others, this disorder is unaffected by treatment of the underlying bowel disease. (See Schwartz 9th ed., p 1034.)

8. Lymphoma of the colon is most commonly found in the
   A. Cecum
   B. Transverse colon
   C. Sigmoid colon
   D. Rectum

Answer: A
Lymphoma involving the colon and rectum is rare, but accounts for about 10% of all GI lymphomas. The cecum is most often involved, probably as a result of spread from the terminal ileum. Symptoms include bleeding and obstruction, and these tumors may be clinically indistinguishable from adenocarcinomas. Bowel resection is the treatment of choice for isolated colorectal lymphoma. Adjuvant therapy may be given based upon the stage of disease. (See Schwartz 9th ed., p 1052.)

9. Which of the following is the first test that should be performed in a patient with lower gastrointestinal bleeding?
   A. Nasogastric aspiration
   B. Anoscopy
   C. Proctoscopy
   D. Colonoscopy

Answer: A
Because the most common source of GI hemorrhage is esophageal, gastric, or duodenal, nasogastric aspiration should always be performed; return of bile suggests that the source of bleeding is distal to the ligament of Treitz. If aspiration reveals blood or nonbile secretions, or if symptoms suggest an upper intestinal source, esophagogastroduodenoscopy is performed. Anoscopy and/or limited proctoscopy can identify hemorrhoidal bleeding. If the patient is hemodynamically stable, a rapid bowel preparation (over 4 to 6 hours) can be performed to allow colonoscopy. (See Schwartz 9th ed., p 1022.)

10. In a patient with inflammatory colitis, which of the following would suggest the diagnosis of Crohn's colitis?
A. Ileitis
B. Crypt abscesses
C. Rectal sparing
D. Proctitis

Answer: C
Although ulcerative colitis and Crohn's colitis share many pathologic and clinical similarities, these conditions may be differentiated in 85% of patients. Ulcerative colitis is a mucosal process in which the colonic mucosa and submucosa are infiltrated with inflammatory cells. The mucosa may be atrophic and crypt abscesses are common. Endoscopically, the mucosa is frequently friable and may possess multiple inflammatory pseudopolyps. In long-standing ulcerative colitis, the colon may be foreshortened and the mucosa replaced by scar. In quiescent ulcerative colitis, the colonic mucosa may appear normal endoscopically and microscopically. Ulcerative colitis may affect the rectum (proctitis), rectum and sigmoid colon (proctosigmoiditis), rectum and left colon (left-sided colitis), or the rectum and entire colon (pancolitis). Ulcerative colitis does not involve the small intestine, but the terminal ileum may demonstrate inflammatory changes (backwash ileitis). A key feature of ulcerative colitis is the continuous involvement of the rectum and colon; rectal sparing or skip lesions suggest a diagnosis of Crohn's disease. (See Schwartz 9th ed., p 1034.)

11. Which of the following is the procedure of choice for a patient with Crohn's colitis involving the left colon who has rectal sparing?
A. Left colectomy with primary anastomosis
B. Left colectomy with colostomy
C. Total colectomy with primary anastomosis
D. Total colectomy with ileostomy

Answer: A
Unlike ulcerative colitis, Crohn's colitis may be segmental and rectal sparing often is observed. A segmental colectomy may be appropriate if the remaining colon and/or rectum appear normal. An isolated colonic stricture also may be treated by segmental colectomy. (See Schwartz 9th ed., p 1037.)

12. Approximately 5% of patients with complicated diverticulitis develop a fistula to an adjacent organ. The most commonly involved organ is
A. Small bowel
B. Skin
C. Bladder
D. Vagina

Answer: C
Approximately 5% of patients with complicated diverticulitis develop fistulas between the colon and an adjacent organ. *Colovesical* fistulas are most common, followed by *colovaginal* and *coloenteric* fistulas. *Colocutaneous* fistulas are a rare complication of diverticulitis. (See Schwartz 9th ed., p 1040.)

13. Azathioprine (which can be used in the treatment of inflammatory bowel disease)
A. Decreases the efficacy of leucocytes
B. Can be used instead of steroids in patients who are steroid refractory
C. Has an onset of action of 6-12 weeks
D. Requires intravenous administration

Answer: C
Azathioprine and 6-mercaptopurine are antimetabolite drugs that interfere with nucleic acid synthesis and thus decrease proliferation of inflammatory cells. These agents are useful for treating ulcerative colitis and Crohn's disease in patients who have failed salicylate therapy or who are dependent upon or refractory to corticosteroids. It is important to note, however, that the onset of action of these drugs takes 6 to 12 weeks, and concomitant use of corticosteroids almost always is required. (See Schwartz 9th ed., p 1035.)

14. The most common infectious cause for emergency laparotomy in a patient with AIDS is
A. Cytomegalovirus
B. Toxoplasmosis
C. Salmonella
D. Herpes simplex

Answer: A
Opportunistic infections with bacteria (*Salmonella, Shigella, Campylobacter, Chlamydia,* and *Mycobacterium* species), fungi (*Histoplasmosis, Coccidiosis, Cryptococcus*), protozoa (*Toxoplasmosis, Cryptosporidiosis, Isosporiasis*), and viruses (*CMV, herpes simplex virus*) can cause diarrhea, abdominal pain, and weight loss. CMV in particular

may cause severe enterocolitis and is the most common infectious cause of emergency laparotomy in AIDS patients. *C. difficile colitis* is a major concern in these patients, especially because many patients are maintained on suppressive antibiotic therapy. (See Schwartz 9th ed., p 1070.)

15. A microscopic focus of cancer is found in a polyp after endoscopic resection. Which of the following is an indication for colectomy in this patient?
    A. Focus of cancer 2 mm from the resection margin
    B. Polyp size >2 cm
    C. Lymphovascular invasion
    D. History of multiple polyps

Answer: C

Occasionally, a polyp that was thought to be benign will be found to harbor invasive carcinoma after polypectomy. Treatment of a *malignant polyp* is based upon the risk of local recurrence and the risk of lymph node metastasis. The risk of lymph node metastases depends primarily upon the depth of invasion. Invasive carcinoma in the head of a pedunculated polyp with no stalk involvement carries a low risk of metastasis (<1%) and may be completely resected endoscopically. However, lymphovascular invasion, poorly differentiated histology, or tumor within 1 mm of the resection margin greatly increases the risk of local recurrence and metastatic spread. Segmental colectomy is then indicated. Invasive carcinoma arising in a sessile polyp extends into the submucosa and is usually best treated with segmental colectomy (Fig. 29-5). (See Schwartz 9th ed., p 1048.)

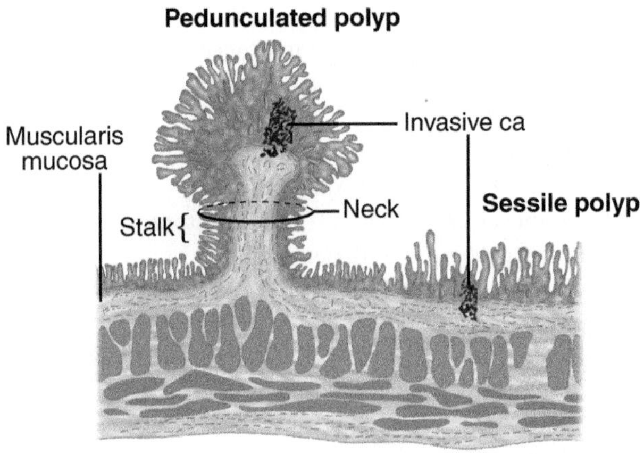

FIG. 29-5. Levels of invasive carcinoma in pedunculated and sessile polyps. ca = carcinoma.

16. The risk of cancer is highest in
    A. Tubular adenomas
    B. Villous adenomas
    C. Tubulovillous adenomas
    D. Hamartomatous adenomas

Answer: B

Adenomatous polyps are common, occurring in up to 25% of the population older than 50 years of age in the United States. By definition, these lesions are dysplastic. The risk of malignant degeneration is related to both the size and type of polyp. Tubular adenomas are associated with malignancy in only 5% of cases, whereas villous adenomas may harbor cancer in up to 40%. Tubulovillous adenomas are at intermediate risk (22%). (See Schwartz 9th ed., p 1042.)

In contrast to adenomatous polyps, hamartomatous polyps (juvenile polyps) usually are not premalignant. (See Schwartz 9th ed., p 1042.)

17. Which of the following is often effective in the treatment of a desmoid tumor of the mesentery in a patient with familial adenomatous polyposis?
    A. Tamoxifen
    B. Methotrexate
    C. Steroids
    D. Radiotherapy

Answer: A

Desmoid tumors in particular can make surgical management difficult and are a source of major morbidity and mortality in patients with FAP. Desmoid tumors are often hormone responsive and growth may be inhibited in some patients with tamoxifen. COX-2 inhibitors and NSAIDs also may be beneficial in this setting. (See Schwartz 9th ed., p 1044.)

18. Treatment of Ogilvie's syndrome includes
    A. Proctoscopy
    B. Sigmoid colectomy
    C. Intravenous neostigmine
    D. Saline enemas

Answer: C

Colonic pseudo-obstruction (Ogilvie's syndrome) is a functional disorder in which the colon becomes massively dilated in the absence of mechanical obstruction. Initial treatment consists of cessation of narcotics, anticholinergics, or other medications that may contribute to ileus. Strict bowel rest and IV hydration are crucial. Most patients will respond to these measures. In patients who fail to improve, colonoscopic decompression often is effective. However, this procedure is technically challenging and great care must be taken to avoid causing perforation. Recurrence occurs in up to 40% of patients. IV neostigmine (an acetylcholinesterase inhibitor) also is extremely effective in decompressing the dilated colon and is associated with a low rate of recurrence (20%). However, neostigmine may produce transient but profound bradycardia and may be inappropriate in patients with cardiopulmonary disease. Because the colonic dilatation typically is greatest in the proximal colon, placement of a rectal tube is rarely effective. (See Schwartz 9th ed., p 1056.)

19. Which of the following has the lowest recurrence rate after reduction and repair of a rectal prolapse?
    A. Perineal reefing of the rectal mucosa (Delorme procedure)
    B. Abdominal rectopexy (Ripstein procedure)
    C. Perineal rectosigmoidectomy (Altemeier procedure)
    D. Reduction of the perineal hernia and closure of the cul-de-sac (Moschcowitz procedure)

Answer: B

The primary therapy for rectal prolapse is surgery, and more than 100 different procedures have been described to treat this condition. Operations can be categorized as either *abdominal* or *perineal*. Abdominal operations have taken three major approaches: (a) reduction of the perineal hernia and closure of the cul-de-sac (*Moschcowitz's operation*); (b) fixation of the rectum, either with a prosthetic sling (*Ripstein* and *Wells rectopexy*) or by *suture rectopexy*; or (c) resection of redundant sigmoid colon. In some cases, resection is combined with rectal fixation (*resection rectopexy*). Abdominal rectopexy with or without resection also is increasingly performed laparoscopically. Perineal approaches have focused on tightening the anus with a variety of prosthetic materials, reefing the rectal mucosa (*Delorme procedure*), or resecting the prolapsed bowel from the perineum (*perineal rectosigmoidectomy* or *Altemeier procedure*) (Fig. 29-6).

Because rectal prolapse occurs most commonly in elderly women, the choice of operation depends in part upon the patient's overall medical condition. Abdominal rectopexy (with or without sigmoid resection) offers the most durable repair, with recurrence occurring in fewer than 10% of patients. Perineal rectosigmoidectomy avoids an abdominal operation and may be preferable in high-risk patients, but is associated with a higher recurrence rate. Reefing the rectal mucosa is effective for patients with limited prolapse. Anal encirclement procedures generally have been abandoned. (See Schwartz 9th ed., p 1054.)

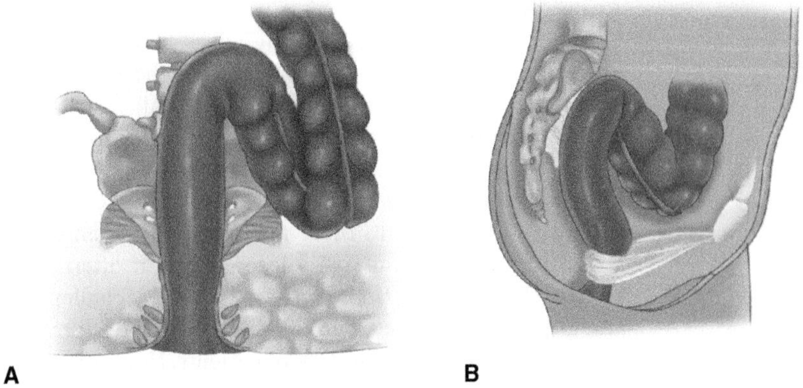

FIG. 29-6. Transabdominal proctopexy for rectal prolapse. The fully mobilized rectum is sutured to the presacral fascia. A. Anterior view. B. Lateral view. If desired, a sigmoid colectomy can be performed concomitantly to resect the redundant colon.

20. A 2-cm invasive cancer of the toproximal transverse colon carcinoma should be treated with which of the following procedures?
   A. Ileocecectomy
   B. Ascending colectomy
   C. Right hemicolectomy
   D. Extended right hemicolectomy

Answer: D

Curative resection of a colorectal cancer usually is accomplished best by performing a proximal mesenteric vessel ligation and radical mesenteric clearance of the lymphatic drainage basin of the tumor site with concomitant resection of the overlying omentum (Fig. 29-7). (See Schwartz 9th ed., p 1024, and Fig. 29-8.)

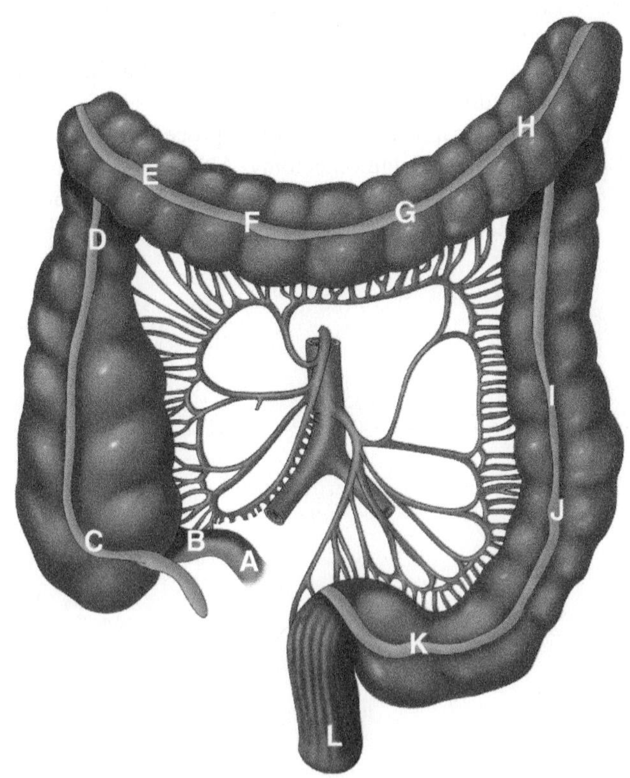

FIG. 29-7. Terminology of types of colorectal resections: A→C Ileocecectomy; + A + B→D Ascending colectomy; + A + B→F Right hemicolectomy; + A + B→G Extended right hemicolectomy; + E + F→G + H Transverse colectomy; G→I Left hemicolectomy; F→I Extended left hemicolectomy; J + K Sigmoid colectomy; + A + B→J Subtotal colectomy; + A + B→K Total colectomy; + A + B→L Total proctocolectomy. (Reproduced with permission from Fielding LP, Goldberg SM (eds): *Rob & Smith's Operative: Surgery of the Colon, Rectum, and Anus*. UK: Elsevier Science Ltd., 1993, p 349.)

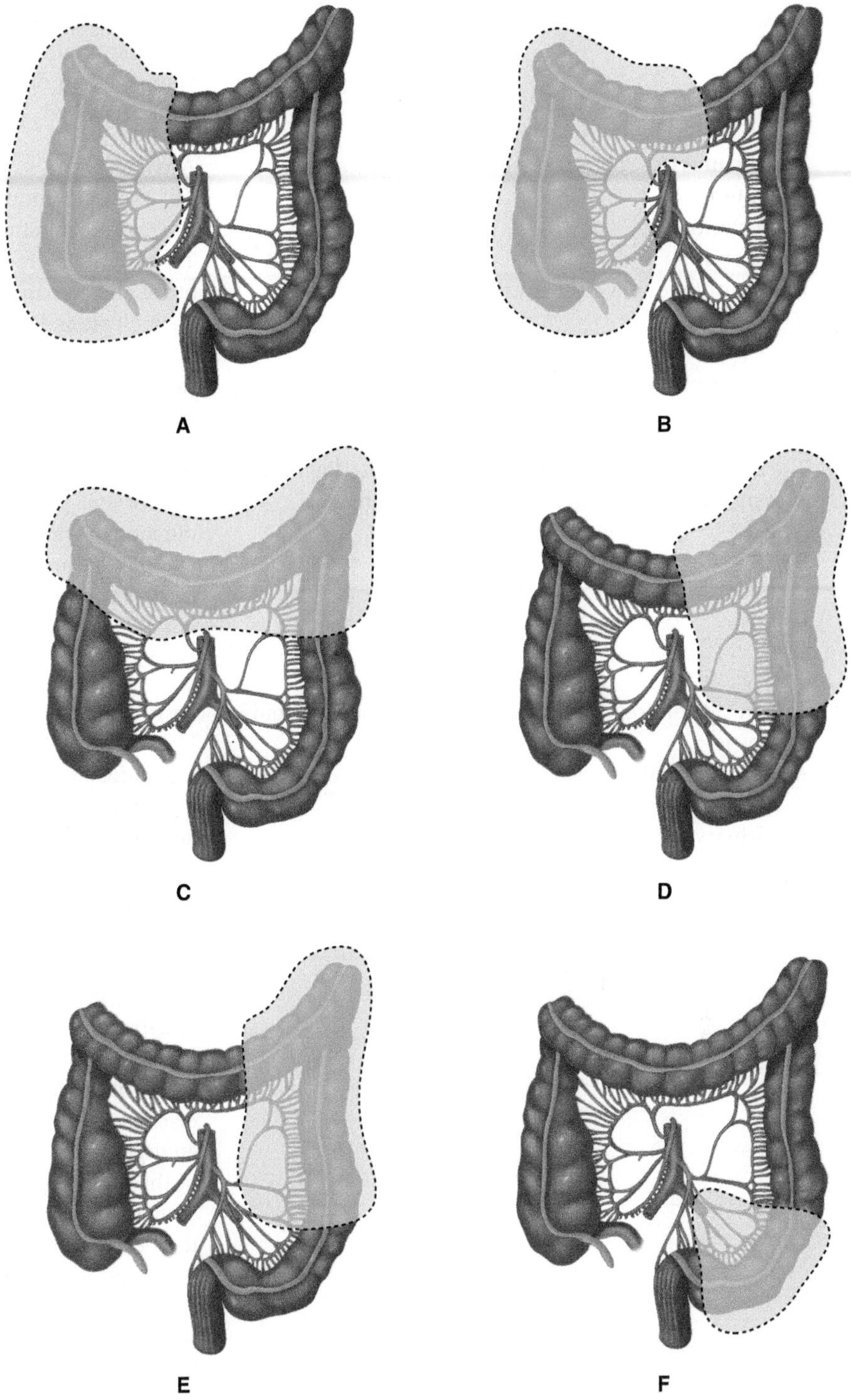

FIG. 29-8. Extent of resection for carcinoma of the colon. A. Cecal cancer. B. Hepatic flexure cancer. C. Transverse colon cancer. D. Splenic flexure cancer. E. Descending colon cancer. F. Sigmoid colon cancer.

21. Which of the following is an extraintestinal manifestation of inflammatory bowel disease?
    A. Hepatosteatosis
    B. Primary sclerosing cholangitis
    C. Pericholangitis
    D. All of the above

Answer: D

The liver is a common site of extracolonic disease in inflammatory bowel disease. Fatty infiltration of the liver is present in 40 to 50% of patients and cirrhosis is found in 2 to 5%. Fatty infiltration may be reversed by medical or surgical treatment of colonic disease, but cirrhosis is irreversible. Primary sclerosing cholangitis is a progressive disease characterized by intra- and extrahepatic bile duct strictures. Forty to 60% of patients with primary sclerosing cholangitis have ulcerative colitis. Colectomy will not reverse this disease, and the only effective therapy is liver transplantation. Pericholangitis also is associated with inflammatory bowel disease and may be diagnosed with a liver biopsy. Bile duct carcinoma is a rare complication of long-standing inflammatory bowel disease.

Patients who develop bile duct carcinoma in the presence of inflammatory bowel disease are, on average, 20 years younger than other patients with bile duct carcinoma. (See Schwartz 9th ed., p 1034.)

22. Anal fissures in Crohn's disease are most commonly
    A. Anterior
    B. Posterior
    C. Lateral
    D. None of the above: the distribution is equal

Answer: C

The most common perianal lesions in Crohn's disease are *skin tags* that are minimally symptomatic. *Fissures* also are common. Typically, a fissure from Crohn's disease is particularly deep or broad and perhaps better described as an anal ulcer. They often are multiple and located in a lateral position rather than anterior or posterior midline as seen in an idiopathic fissure in ano. A classic appearing fissure in ano located laterally should raise the suspicion of Crohn's disease. (See Schwartz 9th ed., p 1038.)

23. The risk of colon cancer in a patient who was diagnosed with ulcerative colitis 20 years ago is approximately
    A. 8%
    B. 18%
    C. 28%
    D. 38%

Answer: A

Risk of malignancy increases with pancolonic disease and the duration of symptoms is approximately 2% after 10 years, 8% after 20 years, and 18% after 30 years. Unlike sporadic colorectal cancers, carcinoma developing in the context of ulcerative colitis is more likely to arise from areas of *flat dysplasia* and may be difficult to diagnose at an early stage. (See Schwartz 9th ed., p 1036.)

24. The most common complication following hemorrhoidectomy is
    A. Fecal impaction
    B. Bleeding
    C. Urinary retention
    D. Infection

Answer: C

Urinary retention is a common complication following hemorrhoidectomy and occurs in 10 to 50% of patients. The risk of urinary retention can be minimized by limiting intraoperative and perioperative IV fluids, and by providing adequate analgesia. Pain also can lead to *fecal impaction*. Risk of impaction may be decreased by preoperative enemas or a limited mechanical bowel preparation, liberal use of laxatives postoperatively, and adequate pain control. Although a small amount of *bleeding*, especially with bowel movements, is to be expected, massive hemorrhage can occur after hemorrhoidectomy. Bleeding may occur in the immediate postoperative period (often in the recovery room) as a result of inadequate ligation of the vascular pedicle. This type of hemorrhage mandates an urgent return to the operating room where suture ligation of the bleeding vessel will often solve the problem. Bleeding may also occur 7 to 10 days after hemorrhoidectomy when the necrotic mucosa overlying the vascular pedicle sloughs. Although some of these patients may be safely observed, others will require an examination under anesthesia to ligate the bleeding vessel or to oversew the wounds if no specific site of bleeding is identified. *Infection* is uncommon after hemorrhoidectomy; however, necrotizing soft tissue infection can occur. (See Schwartz 9th ed., p 1059.)

25. A colorectal carcinoma that invades the submucosa and has two positive lymph nodes and no metastases is
    A. Stage I
    B. Stage II
    C. Stage III
    D. Stage IV

Answer: C

This is a T1, N1, M0 tumor, which makes it stage III. (See Schwartz 9th ed., p 1047, Tables 29-1 and 29-2.)

TABLE 29-1 TNM staging of colorectal carcinoma and 5-year survival

Stage	TNM	5-Y Survival (%)
I	T1–2, N0, M0	70–95
II	T3–4, N0, M0	54–65
III	Tany, N1–3, M0	39–60
IV	Tany, Nany, M1	0–16

Source: Data from Greene FL PD, Fleming ID, Fritz A, et al: *AJCC Cancer Staging Manual*, 6th ed. New York: Springer, 2002.

TABLE 29-2 TNM staging of colorectal carcinoma

Tumor stage (T)	Definition
TX	Cannot be assessed
T0	No evidence of cancer
Tis	Carcinoma in situ
T1	Tumor invades submucosa
T2	Tumor invades muscularis propria
T3	Tumor invades through muscularis propria into subserosa or into nonperitonealized pericolic or perirectal tissues
T4	Tumor directly invades other organs or tissues or perforates the visceral peritoneum of specimen
Nodal stage (N)	
NX	Regional lymph nodes cannot be assessed
N0	No lymph node metastasis
N1	Metastasis to one to three pericolic or perirectal lymph nodes
N2	Metastasis to four or more pericolic or perirectal lymph nodes
N3	Metastasis to any lymph node along a major named vascular trunk
Distant metastasis (M)	
MX	Presence of distant metastasis cannot be assessed
M0	No distant metastasis
M1	Distant metastasis present

Source: Data from Greene FL PD, Fleming ID, Fritz A, et al: *AJCC Cancer Staging Manual*, 6th ed. New York: Springer, 2002. Used with permission of the American Joint Committee on Cancer (AJCC), Chicago, Illinois. The original source for this material is the *AJCC Cancer Staging Manual*, Sixth Edition (2002) published by Springer Science and Business Media LLC, *www.springerlink.com*.

26. Treatment of severe *C. difficile* proctosigmoiditis which is unresponsive to intravenous antibiotics may include
   A. Saline enemas
   B. Steroid enemas
   C. Vancomycin enemas
   D. Probiotic enemas

Answer: C

Management [of *C. difficile* colitis] should include immediate cessation of the offending antimicrobial agent. Patients with mild disease (diarrhea but no fever or abdominal pain) may be treated as outpatients with a 10-day course of oral metronidazole. Oral vancomycin is a second-line agent used in patients allergic to metronidazole or in patients with recurrent disease. More severe diarrhea associated with dehydration and/or fever and abdominal pain is best treated with bowel rest, IV hydration, and oral metronidazole or vancomycin. Proctosigmoiditis may respond to vancomycin enemas. Recurrent colitis occurs in up to 20% of patients and may be treated by a longer course of oral metronidazole or vancomycin (up to 1 month). Reintroduction of normal flora by ingestion of *probiotics* has been suggested as a possible treatment for recurrent or refractory disease. Fulminant colitis, characterized by septicemia and/or evidence of perforation, requires emergent laparotomy. A total abdominal colectomy with end ileostomy may be lifesaving. (See Schwartz 9th ed., p 1057.)

27. Which of the following is an extraintestinal manifestation of familial adenomatous polyposis?
   A. Arthritis
   B. Uveitis
   C. Central nervous system tumors
   D. Erythema nodosum

Answer: C

FAP may be associated with extraintestinal manifestations such as congenital hypertrophy of the retinal pigmented epithelium, desmoid tumors, epidermoid cysts, mandibular osteomas (Gardner's syndrome), and central nervous system tumors (Turcot's syndrome). (See Schwartz 9th ed., p 1044.)

28. Which of the following is characterized by hamartomas formed from all three embryonic layers?
   A. Familial juvenile polyposis
   B. Peutz-Jeghers syndrome
   C. Cronkite-Canada syndrome
   D. Cowden syndrome

Answer: D

Cowden syndrome is an autosomal dominant disorder with hamartomas of all three embryonal cell layers. Facial trichilemmomas, breast cancer, thyroid disease, and GI polyps are typical of the syndrome. Patients should be screened for cancers. Treatment is otherwise based upon symptoms. (See Schwartz 9th ed., p 1043.)

29. How many distinct layers of the rectal wall can be seen on endorectal ultrasound?
   A. 2
   B. 3
   C. 4
   D. 5

Answer: D

Endorectal ultrasound is primarily used to evaluate the depth of invasion of neoplastic lesions in the rectum. The normal rectal wall appears as a five-layer structure (Fig. 29-9). Ultrasound can reliably differentiate most benign polyps from invasive tumors based upon the integrity of the submucosal layer. Ultrasound also can differentiate superficial T1–T2 from deeper T3–T4 tumors. Overall, the accuracy of ultrasound in detecting depth of mural invasion ranges between 81 and 94%. This modality also can detect enlarged perirectal lymph nodes, which may suggest nodal metastases; accuracy of detection of pathologically positive lymph nodes is 58 to 83%. Ultrasound may also prove useful for early detection of local recurrence after surgery. (See Schwartz 9th ed., p 1020.)

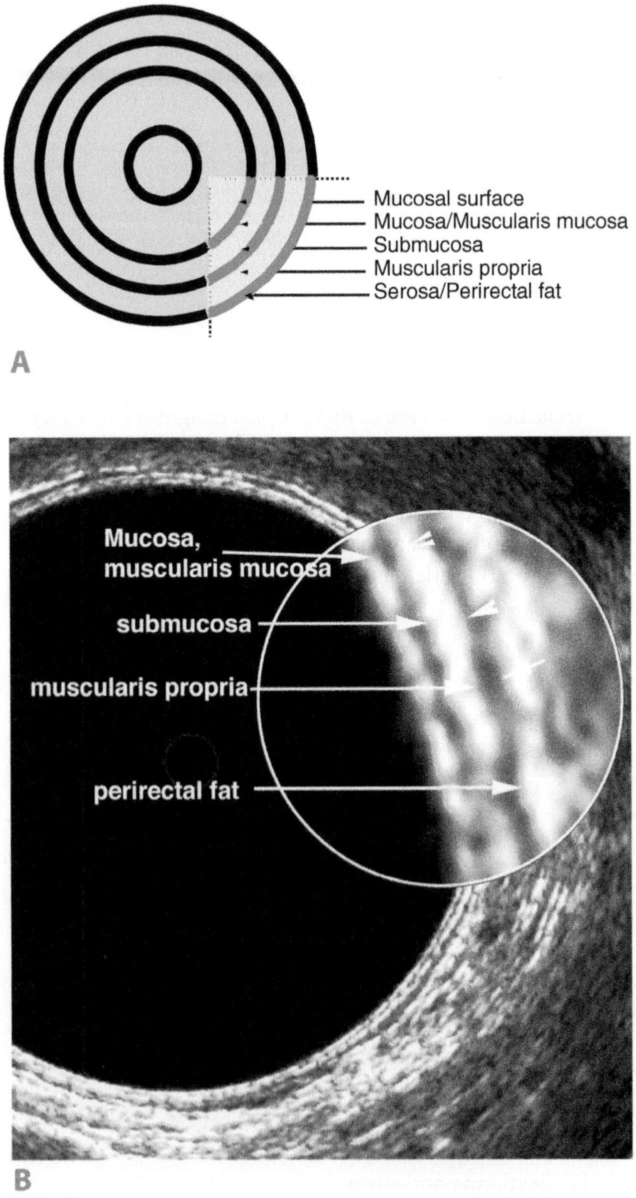

FIG. 29-9. A. Schematic of the layers of the rectal wall observed on endorectal ultrasonography. B. Normal endorectal ultrasonography. *(A. Courtesy of Charles O. Finne III, MD, Minneapolis, MN.)*

30. The initial treatment of symptomatic pouchitis includes
   A. Oral antibiotics
   B. Intravenous antibiotics
   C. Probiotic enemas
   D. Steroid enemas

Answer: A

Pouchitis is an inflammatory condition that affects both ileoanal pouches and continent ileostomy reservoirs. Incidence of pouchitis ranges from 30 to 55%. Symptoms include increased diarrhea, hematochezia, abdominal pain, fever, and malaise. Diagnosis is made endoscopically with biopsies. Differential diagnosis includes infection and undiagnosed Crohn's disease. The etiology of pouchitis is unknown. Some believe pouchitis results from fecal stasis within the pouch but emptying studies are not confirmatory. Antibiotics (metronidazole ± ciprofloxacin) are the mainstays of therapy and most patients will respond rapidly to either oral preparations or enemas. Some patients develop chronic pouchitis that necessitates ongoing suppressive antibiotic therapy. Salicylate and corticosteroid enemas also have been used with some success. Reintroduction of normal flora by ingestion of *probiotics* has been suggested as a possible treatment in refractory cases. Occasionally, pouch excision is necessary to control the symptoms of chronic pouchitis. (See Schwartz 9th ed., p 1032.)

CHAPTER 30

The Appendix

BASIC SCIENCE QUESTIONS

1. Which of the following is produced by the appendix?
   A. T cells
   B. B cells
   C. IgG
   D. IgA

Answer: D

For many years, the appendix was erroneously viewed as a vestigial organ with no known function. It is now well recognized that the appendix is an immunologic organ that actively participates in the secretion of immunoglobulins, particularly immunoglobulin IgA. (See Schwartz 9th ed., p 1073.)

2. Lymphoid tissue in the appendix
   A. Is present at birth
   B. Steadily increases in amount throughout life
   C. Is maximally present during puberty
   D. Disappears by the 5th decade of life

Answer: C

Lymphoid tissue first appears in the appendix approximately 2 weeks after birth. The amount of lymphoid tissue increases throughout puberty, remains steady for the next decade, and then begins a steady decrease with age. After the age of 60 years, virtually no lymphoid tissue remains within the appendix, and complete obliteration of the appendiceal lumen is common. (See Schwartz 9th ed., p 1074.)

3. The luminal capacity of a normal appendix is
   A. 0.1 mL
   B. 1 mL
   C. 5 mL
   D. 10 mL

Answer: A

The luminal capacity of the normal appendix is only 0.1 mL. Secretion of as little as 0.5 mL of fluid distal to an obstruction raises the intraluminal pressure to 60 cm H_2O. (See Schwartz 9th ed., p 1075.)

CLINICAL QUESTIONS

1. Appendectomy may decrease the risk of developing which of the following diseases?
   A. HIV
   B. Burkitt's lymphoma
   C. Ulcerative colitis
   D. Colon cancer

Answer: C

Although there is no clear role for the appendix in the development of human disease, recent studies demonstrate a potential correlation between appendectomy and the development of inflammatory bowel disease. There appears to be a negative age-related association between prior appendectomy and subsequent development of ulcerative colitis. In addition, comparative analysis clearly shows that prior appendectomy is associated with a more benign phenotype in ulcerative colitis and a delay in onset of disease. The association between Crohn's disease and appendectomy is less clear. Although earlier studies suggested that appendectomy increases the risk of developing Crohn's disease, more recent studies that carefully assessed the timing of appendectomy in relation to the onset of Crohn's disease demonstrated a negative correlation. These data suggest that appendectomy may protect against the subsequent development of inflammatory bowel disease; however, the mechanism is unclear. (See Schwartz 9th ed., p 1073.)

2. Cultures should be taken at the time of surgery
   A. For all patients with appendicitis
   B. For all (but only) patients with perforated appendicitis
   C. For immunocompromised patients with appendicitis
   D. Never

Answer: C

The routine culture of intraperitoneal samples in patients with either perforated or nonperforated appendicitis is questionable. By the time culture results are available, the patient often has recovered from the illness. In addition, the number of organisms cultured and the ability of a specific laboratory to culture anaerobic organisms vary greatly. Peritoneal culture should be reserved for patients who are immunosuppressed, as a result of either illness or medication, and for patients who develop an abscess after the treatment of appendicitis. (See Schwartz 9th ed., p 1076.)

3. Which of the following is a positive Rovsing sign?
   A. Pain with percussion of the right lower quadrant
   B. Pain in the right lower quadrant with compression of the left lower quadrant
   C. Cutaneous hyperesthesia in the T10-T12 distribution
   D. Suprapubic pain on rectal examination

Answer: B

The Rovsing sign—pain in the right lower quadrant when palpatory pressure is exerted in the left lower quadrant—also indicates the site of peritoneal irritation.

The other three choices are important physical findings in appendicitis but are not the Rovsing sign. Pain with percussion in the right lower quadrant is rebound tenderness.

Cutaneous hyperesthesia in the area supplied by the spinal nerves on the right at T10, T11, and T12 frequently accompanies acute appendicitis. In patients with obvious appendicitis, this sign is superfluous, but in some early cases, it may be the first positive sign. Hyperesthesia is elicited either by needle prick or by gently picking up the skin between the forefinger and thumb.

With a retrocecal appendix, the anterior abdominal findings are less striking, and tenderness may be most marked in the flank. When the inflamed appendix hangs into the pelvis, abdominal findings may be entirely absent, and the diagnosis may be missed unless the rectum is examined. As the examining finger exerts pressure on the peritoneum of Douglas' cul-de-sac, pain is felt in the suprapubic area as well as locally within the rectum. (See Schwartz 9th ed., p 1076.)

4. Which of the following is important to consider in the differential diagnosis of an HIV+ patient with right lower quadrant abdominal pain?
   A. Herpes type 1 enteritis
   B. Cytomegalovirus infection
   C. Cecal volvulus
   D. Small bowel diverticulitis

Answer: B

The differential diagnosis of right lower quadrant pain is expanded in HIV-infected patients compared with the general population. In addition to the conditions discussed elsewhere in this chapter, opportunistic infections should be considered as a possible cause of right lower quadrant pain. Such opportunistic infections include cytomegalovirus (CMV) infection, Kaposi's sarcoma, tuberculosis, lymphoma, and other causes of infectious colitis. CMV infection may be seen anywhere in the GI tract. CMV infection causes a vasculitis of blood vessels in the submucosa of the gut, which leads to thrombosis. Mucosal ischemia develops, leading to ulceration, gangrene of the bowel wall, and perforation. Spontaneous peritonitis may be caused by opportunistic pathogens, including CMV, *Mycobacterium avium-intracellulare* complex, *Mycobacterium tuberculosis*, *Cryptococcus neoformans*, and *Strongyloides*. Kaposi's sarcoma and non-Hodgkin's lymphoma may present with pain and a right lower quadrant mass. Viral and bacterial colitis occur with a higher frequency in HIV-infected patients than in the general population. Colitis should always be considered in HIV-infected patients presenting with right lower quadrant pain. Neutropenic enterocolitis (typhlitis) should also be considered in the differential diagnosis of right lower quadrant pain in HIV-infected patients. Herpes type 1 does not cause enteritis. Cecal volvulus and small bowel diverticulitis are very rare, and no more likely to occur in an HIV patient than in someone without HIV infection. (See Schwartz 9th ed., p 1083.)

5. Incidental appendectomy is indicated in which of the following patients?
   A. Otherwise healthy patients between the age of 16 and 30 years
   B. Patients with Crohn's disease with active disease in the appendix
   C. Patients undergoing surgery who will be traveling to remote locations
   D. Children between the age of 12 and 18 years with chronic recurring abdominal pain

Answer: C

Epidemiological data about appendicitis no longer supports incidental appendectomy in patients.

Although incidental appendectomy is generally neither clinically nor economically appropriate, there are some special patient groups in whom it should be performed during laparotomy or laparoscopy for other indications. These include children about to undergo chemotherapy, the disabled who cannot describe symptoms or react normally to abdominal pain, patients with Crohn's disease in whom the cecum is free of macroscopic disease, and individuals who are about to travel to remote places where there is no access to medical or surgical care. (See Schwartz 9th ed., p 1088.)

6. A patient with a 1.5-cm carcinoid tumor of the mid appendix should undergo
   A. Appendectomy only
   B. Partial cecectomy and lymph node sampling to confirm negative margins
   C. Resection of the cecum, terminal ileum, and adjacent mesentery (en bloc resection)
   D. Right hemicolectomy

Answer: A

Because this is a tumor <2 cm in size in the mid appendix, an appendectomy is adequate treatment. (See Schwartz 9th ed., p 1088, and Fig. 30-1.)

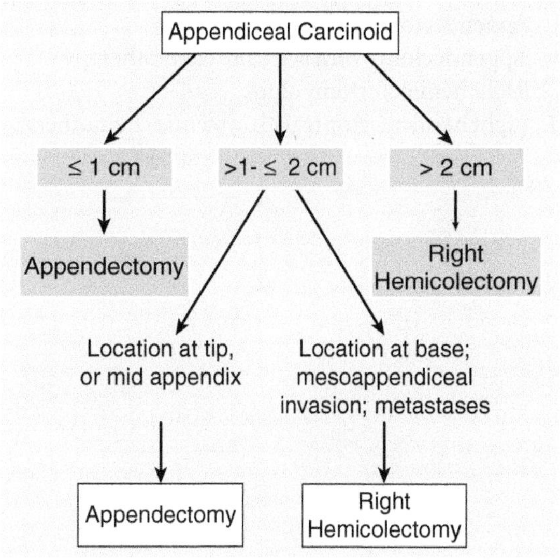

FIG. 30-1. Algorithm for the management of patients with appendiceal carcinoid.

7. At the time of laparoscopic surgery for presumed appendicitis, the patient is noted to have a mucous-filled, distended appendix measuring 3 cm in diameter. There is no acute inflammation or signs of perforation. The correct treatment for this patient is
   A. Diagnostic laparoscopy only (no resection) with CT scan staging before proceeding with further surgery
   B. Laparoscopic appendectomy with pathologic confirmation of a negative margin at the base of the appendix
   C. Conversion to open appendectomy with pathologic confirmation of a negative margin at the base of the appendix
   D. Right hemicolectomy

Answer: C

An intact mucocele presents no future risk for the patient; however, the opposite is true if the mucocele has ruptured and epithelial cells have escaped into the peritoneal cavity. As a result, when a mucocele is visualized at the time of laparoscopic examination, conversion to open laparotomy is recommended. Conversion from a laparoscopic approach to a laparotomy ensures that a benign process will not be converted to a malignant one through mucocele rupture. In addition, laparotomy allows for thorough abdominal exploration to rule out the presence of mucoid fluid accumulations. The presence of a mucocele of the appendix does not mandate performance of a right hemicolectomy. The principles of surgery include resection of the appendix, wide resection of the mesoappendix to include all the appendiceal lymph nodes, collection and cytologic examination of all intraperitoneal mucus, and careful inspection of the base of the appendix. Right hemicolectomy, or preferably cecectomy, is reserved for patients with a positive margin at the base of the appendix or positive periappendiceal lymph nodes. (See Schwartz 9th ed., p 1088.)

8. Which of the following is indicated in a patient with pseudomyxoma peritonei of appendiceal origin?
   A. Right hemicolectomy
   B. Hysterectomy with bilateral salgingo-oophorectomy
   C. Abdominal XRT
   D. Systemic chemotherapy

Answer: B

Pseudomyxoma is invariably caused by neoplastic mucus-secreting cells within the peritoneum. These cells may be difficult to classify as malignant because they may be sparse, widely scattered, and have a low-grade cytologic appearance.... Thorough surgical debulking is the mainstay of treatment. All gross disease and the omentum should be removed. If not done previously, appendectomy is routinely performed. Hysterectomy with bilateral salpingo-oophorectomy is performed in women. *Because 5-year survival of mucinous appendiceal neoplasms is only 30%,* adjuvant intraperitoneal hyperthermic chemotherapy is advocated as a standard adjunct to radical cytoreductive surgery. Abdominal XRT and systemic chemotherapy are not used in the treatment of pseudomyoxa peritonei. Right hemicolectomy is not indicated as a routine procedure. (See Schwartz 9th ed., pp 1088-89.)

9. The treatment for lymphoma confined to the appendix is
   A. Appendectomy alone
   B. Appendectomy with systemic chemotherapy
   C. Right hemicolectomy alone
   D. Right hemicolectomy with systemic chemotherapy

Answer: A

The management of appendiceal lymphoma confined to the appendix is appendectomy. Right hemicolectomy is indicated if tumor extends beyond the appendix onto the cecum or mesentery. A postoperative staging workup is indicated before initiating adjuvant therapy. Adjuvant therapy is not indicated for lymphoma confined to the appendix. (See Schwartz 9th ed., p 1089.)

CHAPTER 31

Liver

BASIC SCIENCE QUESTIONS

1. What is the average weight of an adult liver?
   A. 700 g
   B. 1100 g
   C. 1500 g
   D. 1900 g

Answer: C

The liver is the largest [intestinal] organ in the body, weighing approximately 1500 g. (See Schwartz 9th ed., p 1094.)

2. The falciform ligament divides
   A. Segments I and II
   B. Segments III and IV
   C. Segments V and VI
   D. Segments VII and VIII

Answer: B

The round ligament is the remnant of the obliterated umbilical vein and enters the left liver hilum at the front edge of the falciform ligament. The falciform ligament separates the left lateral and left medial segments along the umbilical fissure and anchors the liver to the anterior abdominal wall.

Couinaud divided the liver into eight segments, numbering them in a clockwise direction beginning with the caudate lobe as segment I. Segments II and III comprise the left lateral segment, and segment IV is the left medial segment. Thus, the left lobe is made up of the left lateral segment (Couinaud's segments II and III) and the left medial segment (segment IV). Segment IV can be subdivided into segment IVB and segment IVA. Segment IVA is cephalad and just below the diaphragm, spanning from segment VIII to the falciform ligament adjacent to segment II. Segment IVB is caudad and adjacent to the gallbladder fossa. The right lobe is comprised of segments V, VI, VII, and VIII, with segments V and VIII making up the right anterior lobe, and segments VI and VII the right posterior lobe. (See Schwartz 9th ed., p 1095, and Fig. 31-1.)

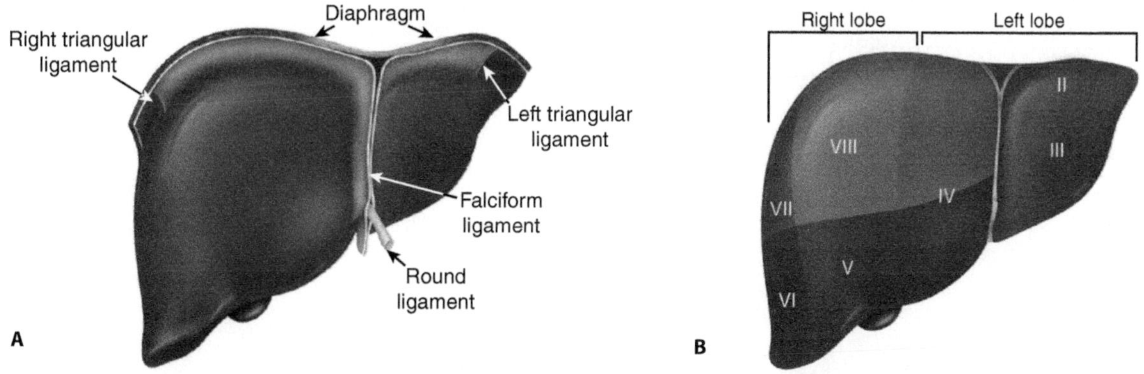

FIG. 31-1. A. Hepatic ligaments suspending the liver to the diaphragm and anterior abdominal wall. B. Couinaud's liver segments (I through VIII) numbered in a clockwise manner. The left lobe includes segments II to IV, the right lobe includes segments V to VIII, and the caudate lobe is segment I. IVC = inferior vena cava.

3. Approximately what percentage of the blood supply to the liver is provided by the hepatic artery?
   A. <10%
   B. 25%
   C. 50%
   D. 75%

Answer: B

The liver has a dual blood supply consisting of the hepatic artery and the portal vein. The hepatic artery delivers approximately 25% of the blood supply, and the portal vein approximately 75%. (See Schwartz 9th ed., p 1096.)

4. The hepatic artery usually arises from the celiac trunk and divides into the right and left hepatic artery after giving off the gastroduodenal artery. Which of the following is the most common variant of this normal anatomy?
   A. More proximal bifurcation of the common hepatic artery (near the celiac) into right and left hepatic arteries
   B. More distal bifurcation of the common hepatic artery (near the liver) into right and left hepatic arteries
   C. Replaced right hepatic artery (origin from the SMA)
   D. Replaced left hepatic artery (origin from the SMA)

Answer: C

The hepatic artery arises from the celiac axis (trunk), which gives off the left gastric, splenic, and common hepatic arteries (Fig. 31-2). The common hepatic artery then divides into the gastroduodenal artery and the hepatic artery proper. The right gastric artery typically originates off of the hepatic artery proper, but this is variable. The hepatic artery proper divides into the right and left hepatic arteries. This 'classic' or standard arterial anatomy is present in only approximately 75% of cases, with the remaining 25% having variable anatomy.

The most common hepatic arterial variants are shown (Fig. 31-3). The right hepatic artery is replaced coming off the superior mesenteric artery (SMA) 18 to 22% of the time. When there is a replacement or accessory right hepatic artery, it traverses posterior to the portal vein and then takes up a right lateral position before diving into the liver parenchyma. (See Schwartz 9th ed., p 1096.)

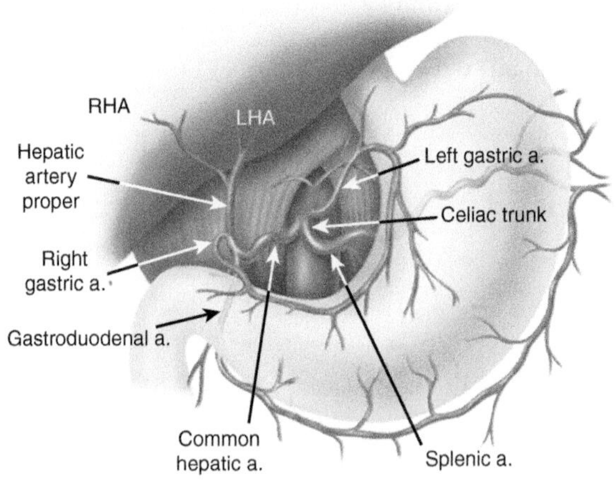

FIG. 31-2. Arterial anatomy of the upper abdomen and liver, including the celiac trunk and hepatic artery branches. a. = artery; LHA = left hepatic artery; RHA = right hepatic artery.

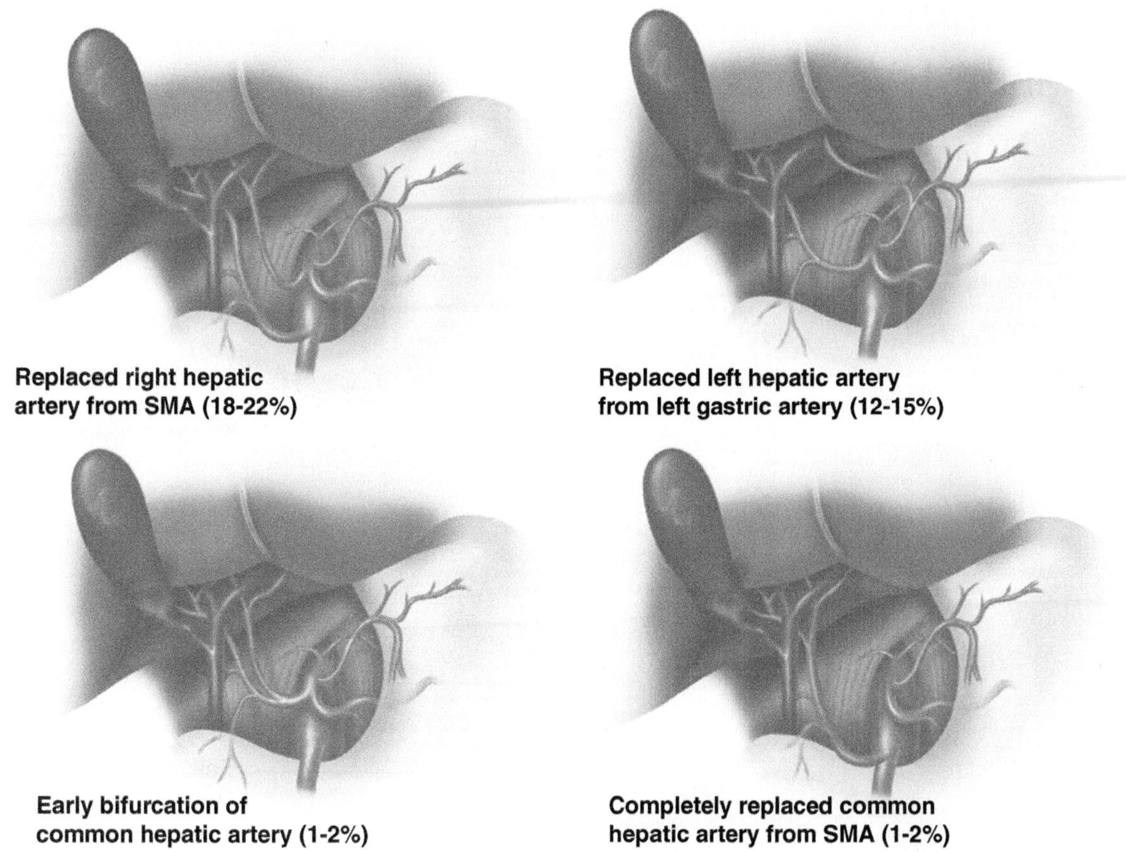
Replaced right hepatic artery from SMA (18-22%)
Replaced left hepatic artery from left gastric artery (12-15%)
Early bifurcation of common hepatic artery (1-2%)
Completely replaced common hepatic artery from SMA (1-2%)

FIG. 31-3. Common hepatic artery anatomic variants. SMA = superior mesenteric artery.

5. The right hepatic vein drains
   A. Segment I only
   B. Segment II-III
   C. Segment V-VIII
   D. Segment VIII only

Answer: C

There are three hepatic veins (right, middle, and left) that pass obliquely through the liver to drain the blood to the suprahepatic IVC and eventually the right atrium (Fig. 31-4). The right hepatic vein drains segments V to VIII; the middle hepatic vein drains segment IV as well as segments V and VIII; and the left hepatic vein drains segments II and III. The caudate lobe [segment I] is unique because its venous drainage feeds directly into the IVC. (See Schwartz 9th ed., p 1098.)

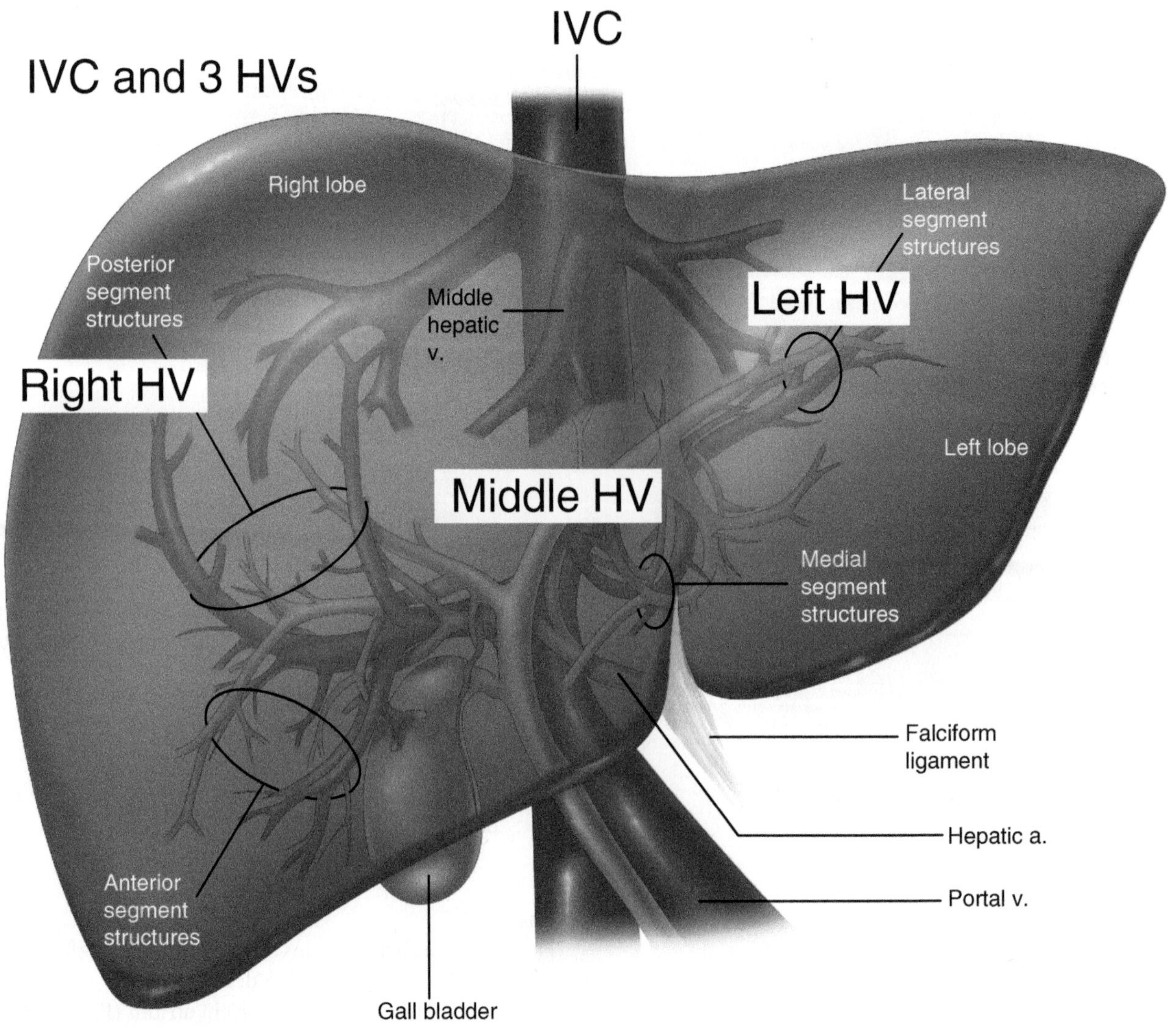

FIG. 31-4. Confluence of the three hepatic veins (HVs) and the inferior vena cava (IVC). Note that the middle and left hepatic veins (HVs) drain into a common trunk before entering the IVC. a. = artery; v. = vein. (Adapted with permission from Cameron JL (ed): *Atlas of Surgery*. Vol. I, *Gallbladder and Biliary Tract, the Liver, Portasystemic Shunts, the Pancreas*. Toronto: BC Decker, 1990, p 153.)

6. Bile acids produced in the liver are conjugated to which of the following amino acids before secretion in the bile?
   A. Alanine
   B. Glycine
   C. Tryptophan
   D. Valine

Answer: B

Bile salts, in conjunction with phospholipids, are responsible for the digestion and absorption of lipids in the small intestine. Bile salts are sodium and potassium salts of bile acids conjugated to amino acids. The bile acids are derivatives of cholesterol synthesized in the hepatocyte. Cholesterol, ingested from the diet or derived from hepatic synthesis, is converted into the bile acids cholic acid and chenodeoxycholic acid. These bile acids are conjugated to either glycine or taurine before secretion into the biliary system. Bacteria in the intestine can remove glycine and taurine from bile salts. They can also convert some of the primary bile acids into secondary bile acids by removing a hydroxyl group, producing deoxycholic from cholic acid, and lithocholic from chenodeoxycholic acid. (See Schwartz 9th ed., p 1100.)

7. Acetaminophen overdose causes liver damage by
   A. Creation of a toxic metabolite by the cytochrome P-450 system
   B. Creation of a toxic metabolite by conjugation
   C. Direct injury to the cell membrane of the hepatocyte
   D. Direct injury to the mitochondria of the hepatocyte

Answer: A

There are two main reactions that can occur in the liver important for drug metabolism. Phase I reactions include oxidation, reduction, and hydrolysis of molecules that result in metabolites that are more hydrophilic than the original chemicals. The cytochrome P-450 system is a family of hemoproteins important for oxidative reactions involving drug and toxic substances. Phase II reactions, also known as *conjugation reactions*, are synthetic reactions that involve addition of subgroups to the drug molecule. These subgroups include glucuronate, acetate, glutathione, glycine, sulfate, and methyl groups.

It is important to note that some drugs may be converted to active products by metabolism in the liver. An example is acetaminophen when taken in larger doses. Normally, acetaminophen is conjugated by the liver to harmless glucuronide and sulfate metabolites that are water soluble and eliminated in the urine. During an overdose, the normal metabolic pathways are overwhelmed, and some of the drug is converted to a reactive and toxic intermediate by the cytochrome P-450 system. Glutathione can normally bind to this intermediate and lead to the excretion of a harmless product. However, as glutathione stores are diminished, the reactive intermediate cannot be detoxified and it combines with lipid bilayers of hepatocytes, which results in cellular necrosis. Thus, treatment of acetaminophen overdoses consists of replacing glutathione with sulfhydryl compounds such as acetylcysteine. (See Schwartz 9th ed., p 1100.)

8. Which of the following is an acute phase protein?
   A. Albumin
   B. Pre-albumin
   C. Transferrin
   D. Ceruloplasmin

Answer: D

The liver is the site of synthesis of acute phase proteins that consist of a group of plasma proteins that are rapidly released in response to inflammatory conditions elsewhere in the body. The synthesis of these proteins in the liver is influenced by a number of inflammatory mediators. Cytokines such as tumor necrosis factor alpha (TNF-α),interferon-γ, interleukin-1 (IL-1), interleukin-6 (IL-6), and interleukin-8 (IL-8) are released by inflammatory cells into the circulation at sites of injury and modulate the acute phase response. In response to these cytokines, the liver increases synthesis and release of a wide variety of proteins, including ceruloplasmin, complement factors, C-reactive protein, D-dimer protein, alpha$_1$-antitrysin, and serum amyloid A. There are proteins such as serum albumin and transferring whose levels also decrease (negative acute phase proteins) in response to inflammation. (See Schwartz 9th ed., p 1102.)

9. Which hepatic cells provides the primary defense against lipopolysaccharide (LPS)?
   A. Hepatocytes
   B. Kupffer cells
   C. Bile duct epithelial cells
   D. Intrahepatic endothelial cells

Answer: B

The complications of gram-negative sepsis are initiated by endotoxin (lipopolysaccharide, or LPS). LPS is a glycolipid constituent of the outer membranes of gram-negative bacteria composed of a hydrophilic polysaccharide portion and a hydrophobic domain called *lipid A*. The lipid A structure is the LPS component responsible for the biologic effects of LPS. Mere nanogram amounts of LPS injected into humans can result in the manifestations of septic shock. The profound effects of LPS are caused not only by the direct effect of LPS itself but also by activation of LPS-sensitive cells, which results in the excessive release of cytokines and other inflammatory mediators.

The liver is the main organ involved in the clearance of LPS from the bloodstream and so plays a critical role in the identification and processing of LPS. Kupffer cells are the resident macrophages of the liver and have been shown to participate in LPS clearance. Studies have demonstrated that the majority of radiolabeled LPS injected IV is quickly cleared from the circulation and found in the liver, primarily localized to the Kupffer cells. Kupffer cells also contribute to the inflammatory cascade by producing cytokines in response to LPS. Interestingly, hepatocytes, the parenchymal cells of the liver, also have all the components required for LPS recognition and signaling and can participate in the response to LPS and process LPS for clearance. (See Schwartz 9th ed., p 1102.)

10. Heme is broken down by heme oxygenase to three products of metabolism. Which of the following is one of those three products of metabolism?
    A. Ferrous sulfate
    B. Carbon monoxide
    C. Conjugated bilirubin
    D. Ferritin

Answer: B

Heme oxygenase (HO) is the rate-limiting enzyme in the degradation of heme to yield biliverdin, carbon monoxide (CO), and free iron (Fig. 31-5). The HO system, which is activated in response to multiple cellular stresses, has been shown to be an endogenous cytoprotectant in a variety of inflammatory conditions. Currently three HO isozymes have been identified. HO-1 is the inducible form of HO, whereas HO-2 and HO-3 are constitutively expressed. The function of HO in heme degradation is essential due to the potentially toxic effects of heme. An excess of heme can cause cellular damage from oxidative stress due to its production of reactive oxygen species. Thus, the HO system is an important defense mechanism against free heme-mediated oxidative stress. (See Schwartz 9th ed., p 1104.)

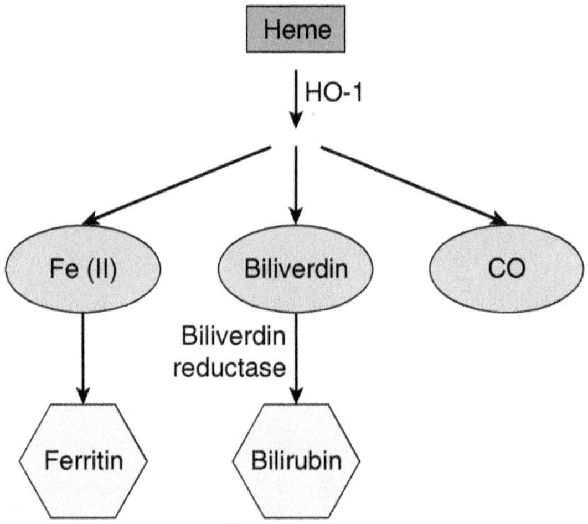

FIG. 31-5. Heme oxygenase 1 (HO-1) and carbon monoxide (CO) signaling. HO-1 is an enzyme involved in the degradation of heme. Its protective effects in settings of hepatic stress are mediated by the catalytic products of heme degradation: ferritin, bilirubin, and CO.

11. The primary function of toll-like receptors is
    A. Vasodilation
    B. Removal of oxygen free radicals
    C. Activation of the immune system
    D. Regulation of the calcium channel

Answer: C

The liver is a central regulator of the systemic immune response after acute insults to the body. Not only does it play a crucial role in modulating the systemic inflammatory response to infection or injury, it is also subject to injury and dysfunction from these same processes. Recent advances in the study of mechanisms for the activation of the innate immune system have pointed to the TLRs as a common pathway for immune recognition of microbial invasion and tissue injury. By recognizing either microbial products or endogenous molecules released from damaged sites, the TLR system is capable of alerting the host to danger by activating the innate immune system. (See Schwartz 9th ed., p 1105.)

12. Portosystemic shunts can occur in
    A. The rectum
    B. The pancreas
    C. The falciform ligament
    D. None of the above

Answer: C

The portal venous system is without valves and drains blood from the spleen, pancreas, gallbladder, and abdominal portion of the alimentary tract into the liver. Tributaries of the portal vein communicate with veins draining directly into the systemic circulation. These communications occur at the gastroesophageal junction, anal canal, falciform ligament, splenic venous bed and left renal vein, and retroperitoneum (Fig. 31-6). The normal portal venous pressure is 5 to 10 mmHg, and at this pressure very little blood is shunted from the portal venous system into the systemic circulation. As portal venous pressure increases, however, the communications with the systemic circulation dilate, and a large amount of blood may be shunted around the liver and into the systemic circulation. (See Schwartz 9th ed., p 1111.)

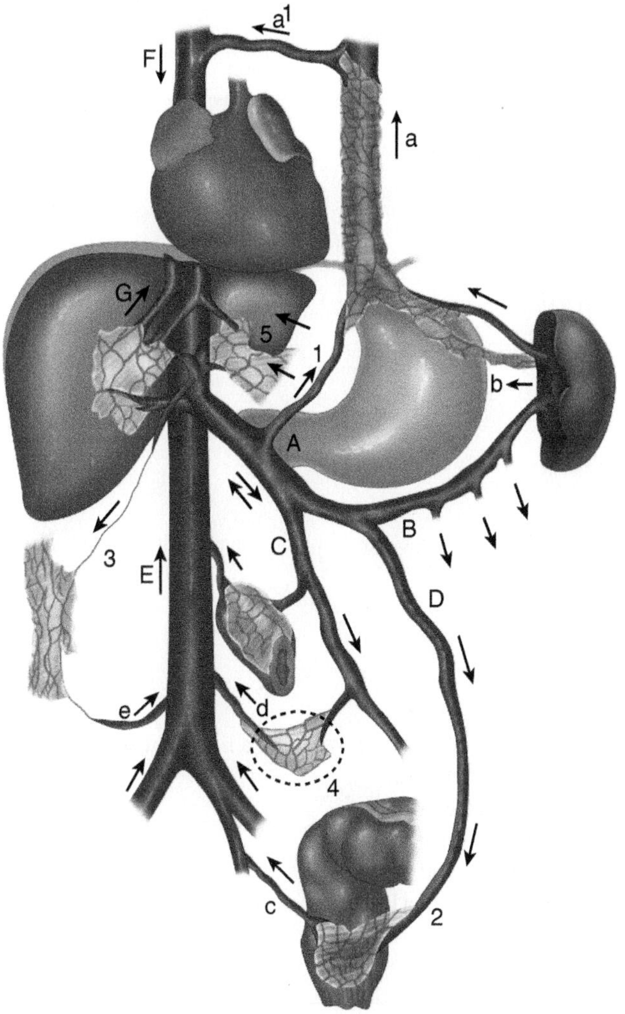

FIG. 31-6. Intra-abdominal venous flow pathways leading to engorged veins (varices) from portal hypertension. *1*, Coronary vein; *2*, superior hemorrhoidal veins; *3*, paraumbilical veins; *4*, Retzius' veins; *5*, veins of Sappey; *A*, portal vein; *B*, splenic vein; *C*, superior mesenteric vein; *D*, inferior mesenteric vein; *E*, inferior vena cava; *F*, superior vena cava; *G*, hepatic veins; *a*, esophageal veins; *a*[1], azygos system; *b*, vasa brevia; *c*, middle and inferior hemorrhoidal veins; *d*, intestinal; *e*, epigastric veins.

13. The most common gene mutation in adult polycystic liver disease is in which of the following genes?
   A. Polycystic kidney disease gene
   B. Bilirubin UDP-glucuronosyltransferase
   C. Alpha$_1$-antitrypsin
   D. ATP7B

Answer: A

Adult polycystic liver disease (ADPCLD) occurs as an autosomal dominant disease and usually presents in the third decade of life. Some 44 to 76% of affected families are found to have mutations of PKD1 and approximately 75% have mutations of PKD2.

Mutations in bilirubin UDP-glucuronosyltransferase are associated with Gilbert syndrome and Crigler-Najjar syndrome. Mutation in ATP7B cause's Wilson's disease.

Mutations in alpha$_1$-antitrypsin cause alpha$_1$-antitrypsin deficiency. (See Schwartz 9th ed., p 1119.)

CLINICAL QUESTIONS

1. Which of the following laboratory test is most specific for liver disease?
   A. AST
   B. ALT
   C. Alkaline phosphatase
   D. Albumin

Answer: B

Hepatocellular injury of the liver is usually indicated by abnormalities in levels of the liver aminotransferases AST and ALT. These enzymes participate in gluconeogenesis by catalyzing the transfer of amino groups from aspartic acid or alanine to ketoglutaric acid to produce oxaloacetic acid and pyruvic acid, respectively (these enzymes were formerly referred to as *glutamic-oxaloacetic transaminase* and *glutamic-pyruvic transaminase*). AST is found in the liver, cardiac muscle, skeletal muscle, kidney, brain, pancreas, lungs, and red blood cells and thus is less specific for disorders of the liver. ALT is predominately found in the liver and thus is more specific for liver disease.

Alkaline phosphatase is present in bone and kidney as well as the liver.

Albumin synthesis is an important function of the liver and thus can be measured to evaluate the liver's synthetic function. The liver produces approximately 10 g of albumin per day. However, albumin levels are dependent on a number of factors such as nutritional status, renal dysfunction, protein-losing enteropathies, and hormonal disturbances. In addition, level of albumin is not a marker of acute hepatic dysfunction due to albumin's long half-life of 15 to 20 days. (See Schwartz 9th ed., p 1101.)

2. Which of the following would be a likely cause of indirect hyperbilirubinemia?
   A. Biliary atresia
   B. Pancreatic cancer
   C. Mirizzi's syndrome
   D. Resorption of a large hematoma

Answer: D

Bilirubin is a breakdown product of hemoglobin metabolism. Unconjugated bilirubin is insoluble and thus is transported to the liver bound to albumin. In the liver, it is conjugated to allow excretion in bile. Measured total bilirubin levels can be low, normal, or high in patients with significant liver disease because of the liver's reserve ability to conjugate significant amounts of bilirubin. Thus, to help aid in the diagnosis of hyperbilirubinemia, fractionation of the total bilirubin is usually performed to distinguish between conjugated (direct) and unconjugated (indirect) bilirubin. Indirect bilirubin is a term frequently used to refer to unconjugated bilirubin in the circulation because the addition of another chemical is necessary to differentiate this fraction from the whole. Normally, >90% of serum bilirubin is unconjugated. The testing process for conjugated bilirubin, in contrast, is direct without the addition of other agents. The direct bilirubin test measures the levels of conjugated bilirubin and delta bilirubin (conjugated bilirubin bound to albumin). The patterns of elevation of the different fractions of bilirubin provide important diagnostic clues as to the cause of cholestasis. In general, an elevated indirect bilirubin level suggests intrahepatic cholestasis and an elevated direct bilirubin level suggests extrahepatic obstruction. Mechanisms that can result in increases in unconjugated bilirubin levels include increased bilirubin production (hemolytic disorders and resorption of hematomas) or defects (inherited or acquired) in hepatic uptake or conjugation. The rate-limiting step in bilirubin metabolism is the excretion of bilirubin from hepatocytes, so conjugated hyperbilirubinemia can be seen in inherited or acquired disorders of intrahepatic excretion or extrahepatic obstruction.

Biliary atresia, pancreatic cancer, and Mirizzi's syndrome all cause obstruction of the biliary system, which will result in conjugated (direct) hyperbilirubinemia. (See Schwartz 9th ed., p 1100.)

3. A patient with Gilbert syndrome presents to the ER with a mild flu-like illness and a bilirubin of 5.2. The most appropriate treatment is
   A. Discharge home, no treatment is needed
   B. IV hydration only
   C. IV hydration, transfusion for Hg <10 g/dL
   D. Plasmapheresis

Answer: A

Gilbert syndrome is a genetic variant characterized by diminished activity of the enzyme glucuronyltransferase, which results in decreased conjugation of bilirubin to glucuronide. It is a benign condition that affects approximately 4 to 7% of the population. Typically, the disease results in transient mild increases in unconjugated bilirubin levels and jaundice during episodes of fasting, stress, or illness. These episodes are self limited and usually do not require further treatment. (See Schwartz 9th ed., p 1102.)

4. The most common cause of acute liver failure (ALF) in the United States is
   A. Hepatitis C
   B. Hepatitis B
   C. Drug ingestion
   D. Trauma

Answer: C

Acute liver failure (ALF) occurs when the rate and extent of hepatocyte death exceeds the liver's regenerative capabilities. It was initially described as a specific disease entity in the 1950s. It also has been referred to as *fulminant hepatic failure*. ALF is a rare disorder affecting approximately 2000 patients annually in the United States.

In the East and developing portions of the world, the most common causes of ALF are viral infections, primarily hepatitis B, A, and E. In these areas there are a relatively small number of drug-induced cases. In contrast, 65% of cases of ALF in the West are thought to be due to drugs and toxins, with acetaminophen (paracetamol) being the most common etiologic agent in the United States, Australia, United Kingdom, and most of Europe. It is interesting that in France and Spain, where acetaminophen sales are restricted, the rate of acetaminophen-induced ALF is quite low. Acetaminophen-induced ALF is also uncommon in South America. The U.S. Acute Liver Failure Study Group identified several other causes of ALF, including autoimmune hepatitis, hypoperfusion of the liver (in cardiomyopathy or cardiogenic shock), pregnancy-related conditions, and Wilson's disease. Even with exhaustive efforts to identify a cause, approximately 20% of all cases of ALF remain indeterminate in origin.

If acetaminophen overdose is suspected to have occurred within a few hours of presentation, administration of activated charcoal may be useful to reduce the volume of acetaminophen present in the GI tract. *N*-acetylcysteine (NAC), the clinically effective antidote for acetaminophen overdose, should be administered as early as possible to any patient with suspected acetaminophen-associated ALF. NAC also should be administered to patients with ALF of unclear etiology, because glutathione stabilization may be beneficial in this patient population as well. (See Schwartz 9th ed., p 1107.)

5. Which of the following may be associated with improved prognosis for a patient with acute liver failure?
   A. Hypophosphatemia
   B. Hyperkalemia
   C. Hypokalemia
   D. Hypernatremia

Answer: A

The majority of patients with ALF need to be monitored in the intensive care unit (ICU) setting, and specific attention needs to be given to fluid management, ulcer prophylaxis, hemodynamic monitoring, electrolyte management, and surveillance for and treatment of infection. Surveillance cultures should be performed to identify bacterial and fungal infections as early as possible. Serum phosphorus levels need to be monitored. Hypophosphatemia, which may indicate a higher likelihood of spontaneous recovery, needs to be corrected via IV administration of phosphorus. (See Schwartz 9th ed., p 1108 .)

6. A patient with cirrhosis requires an elective segmental colon resection for a benign polyp. His bilirubin is 2.3, albumin is 2.4, and INR is 1.8 and he has no ascites or encephalopathy. His risk of dying from his colon resection is approximately
   A. 10%
   B. 30%
   C. 50%
   D. 80%

Answer: B

The Child-Turcotte-Pugh (CTP) score was originally developed to evaluate the risk of portocaval shunt procedures secondary to portal hypertension and subsequently has been shown to be useful in predicting surgical risks of other intra-abdominal operations performed on cirrhotic patients (Table 31-1). Numerous studies have demonstrated overall surgical mortality rates of 10% for patients with class A cirrhosis, 30% for those with class B cirrhosis, and 75 to 80% for those with class C cirrhosis.

This patient has a Child-Turcotte-Pugh score of 2 (bilirubin 2-3 mg/dL) + 3 (albumin <2.8 g/dL) + 2 (INR 1.7-2.2) = 7, which makes him a class B cirrhotic. (See Schwartz 9th ed., p 1111.)

TABLE 31-1 Child-Turcotte-Pugh (CTP) score

Variable	1 Point	2 Points	3 Points
Bilirubin level	<2 mg/dL	2–3 mg/dL	>3 mg/dL
Albumin level	>3.5 g/dL	2.8–3.5 g/dL	<2.8 g/dL
International normalized ratio	<1.7	1.7–2.2	>2.2
Encephalopathy	None	Controlled	Uncontrolled
Ascites	None	Controlled	Uncontrolled

Child-Turcotte-Pugh class

Class A = 5–6 points
Class B = 7–9 points
Class C = 10–15 points

7. The MELD score is calculated using
   A. Bilirubin, creatinine, INR
   B. Bilirubin, INR, ascites
   C. INR, ascites, encephalopathy
   D. None of the above

Answer: A

The Model for End-Stage Liver Disease (MELD) is a linear regression model based on objective laboratory values (INR, bilirubin level, and creatinine level). It was originally developed as a tool to predict mortality after transjugular intrahepatic portosystemic shunt (TIPS) but has been validated and has been used as the sole method of liver transplant allocation in the United States since 2002. The MELD formula is as follows: MELD score = $10\ [0.957\ \text{Ln(SCr)} + 0.378\ \text{Ln(Tbil)} + 1.12\ \text{Ln(INR)} + 0.643]$ where SCr is serum creatinine level (in milligrams per deciliter) and Tbil is serum bilirubin level (in milligrams per deciliter). (See Schwartz 9th ed., p 1111.)

8. Portal hypertension is defined as
   A. Wedged hepatic venous pressure >10 mmHg
   B. Splenic pressure >15 mmHg
   C. Wedged hepatic venous pressure >20 mmHg
   D. venous pressure (measured at surgery) >25 mmHg

Answer: B

The most accurate method of determining portal hypertension is hepatic venography. The most commonly used procedure involves placing a balloon catheter directly into the hepatic vein and measuring the free hepatic venous pressure (FHVP) with the balloon deflated and the wedged hepatic venous pressure (WHVP) with the balloon inflated to occlude the hepatic vein. The hepatic venous pressure gradient (HVPG) is then calculated by subtracting the free from the wedged venous pressure (HVPG = WHVP – FHVP). The HVPG represents the pressure in the hepatic sinusoids and portal vein and is a measure of portal venous pressure.

A WHVP or direct portal venous pressure that is >5 mmHg greater than the inferior vena cava (IVC) pressure, a splenic pressure of >15 mmHg, or a portal venous pressure measured at surgery of >20 mmHg is abnormal and indicates portal hypertension. A portal pressure of >12 mmHg is necessary for varices to form and subsequently bleed. (See Schwartz 9th ed., p 1112.)

9. Myeloproliferative disorders cause portal hypertension that is
   A. Presinusoidal (extrahepatic)
   B. Presinusoidal (intrahepatic)
   C. Intrahepatic
   D. Postsinusoidal

Answer: B

The causes of portal hypertension can be divided into three major groups: presinusoidal, sinusoidal, and postsinusoidal. Although multiple disease processes can result in portal hypertension (Table 31-2), in the United States the most common cause of portal hypertension is usually an intrahepatic one, namely, cirrhosis. (See Schwartz 9th ed., p 1112.)

TABLE 31-2 Etiology of portal hypertension

- Presinusoidal
  - Sinistral/extrahepatic
    - Splenic vein thrombosis
    - Splenomegaly
    - Splenic arteriovenous fistula
  - Intrahepatic
    - Schistosomiasis
    - Congenital hepatic fibrosis
    - Nodular regenerative hyperplasia
    - Idiopathic portal fibrosis
    - Myeloproliferative disorder
    - Sarcoid
    - Graft-versus-host disease
- Sinusoidal
  - Intrahepatic
    - Cirrhosis
      - Viral infection
      - Alcohol abuse
      - Primary biliary cirrhosis
      - Autoimmune hepatitis
      - Primary sclerosing cholangitis
      - Metabolic abnormality
- Postsinusoidal
  - Intrahepatic
    - Vascular occlusive disease
  - Posthepatic
    - Budd-Chiari syndrome
    - Congestive heart failure
    - Inferior vena caval web
    - Constrictive pericarditis

10. A patient with Child's B cirrhosis is admitted to the ICU with a massive acute variceal bleed. Initial orders should include
    A. Factor VIIa
    B. Transfusion of packed red blood cells (PRBCs) for Hg <12 g
    C. Ceftriaxone
    D. Dopamine tritrated to keep systolic BP ≥100 mmHg

Answer: C

The most significant manifestation of portal hypertension and the leading cause of morbidity and mortality associated with portal hypertension is variceal bleeding. Approximately 30% of patients with compensated cirrhosis and 60% of patients with decompensated cirrhosis have esophageal varices. One third of all patients with varices experience variceal bleeding. Each episode of bleeding is associated with a 20 to 30% risk of mortality. Seventy percent of patients who survive the initial bleed will experience recurrent variceal hemorrhage within 1 year if left untreated.

Patients with acute variceal hemorrhage should be admitted to an ICU for resuscitation and management. Blood resuscitation should be performed carefully to a hemoglobin level of approximately 8 g/dL. Over replacement of packed red blood cells and the overzealous administration of saline can lead to both rebleeding and increased mortality. Administration of fresh-frozen plasma and platelets can be considered in patients with severe coagulopathy. Use of recombinant factor VIIa has not been shown to be more beneficial than standard therapy and therefore is not recommended at this time. Cirrhotic patients with variceal bleeding have a high risk of developing bacterial infections, which are associated with rebleeding and a higher mortality rate. The use of short-term prophylactic antibiotics has been shown both to decrease the rate of bacterial infections and to increase survival. Therefore, their use is recommended, and ceftriaxone 1 g/day IV is often given. Pharmacologic therapy for the variceal hemorrhage can be initiated as soon as the diagnosis of variceal bleeding is made. Vasopressin, administered IV at a dose of 0.2 to 0.8 units/min, is the most potent vasoconstrictor. However, its use is limited by its large number of side effects, and it should be administered for only a short period of time at high doses to prevent ischemic complications. Somatostatin and its analogue octreotide (initial bolus of 50 μg IV followed by continuous infusion of 50 μg/h) also cause splanchnic vasoconstriction. Octreotide has the advantage that it can be administered for 5 days or longer, and it is currently the preferred pharmacologic agent for initial management of acute variceal bleeding. In addition to pharmacologic therapy EGD should be carried out as soon as possible and EVL should be performed. This combination of pharmacologic and EVL therapy has been shown both to improve the initial control of bleeding and to increase the 5-day hemostasis rate. (See Schwartz 9th ed., p 1113.)

11. The best initial therapy for bleeding greater curve (gastric) varices in a patient with a patent splenic vein is
    A. Embolism of the splenic vein
    B. Splenectomy
    C. Endoscopic variceal ablation
    D. Splenorenal shunt

Answer: C

Gastric varices that occur along the lesser curvature of the stomach should be considered an extension of the patient's esophageal varices and treated in a manner similar to esophageal varices. Gastric varices along the greater curvature, however, require the evaluation of the splenic vein to assure patency. In the presence of cirrhosis and a patent splenic vein, greater curvature gastric varices can be managed with gastric variceal obturation using N-butyl-cyanoacrylate if available. If gastric variceal obturation is unavailable or if endoscopic therapy fails, the patient should be considered for TIPS, which will control variceal bleeding in >90% of cases. (See Schwartz 9th ed., p 1113.)

12. Initial therapy for primary Budd-Chiari syndrome is
    A. Anticoagulation
    B. Symptomatic control of bleeding varices
    C. TIPS
    D. Portocaval shunt

Answer: A

Budd-Chiari syndrome (BCS) is an uncommon congestive hepatopathy characterized by the obstruction of hepatic venous outflow. Patients may present with acute signs and symptoms of abdominal pain, scites, and hepatomegaly or more chronic symptoms related to long-standing portal hypertension.

BCS is defined as primary when the obstructive process involves an endoluminal venous thrombosis. BCS is considered as a secondary process when the veins are compressed or invaded by a neighboring lesion originating outside the vein. A thorough evaluation demonstrates one or more thrombotic risk factors in approximately 75 to 90% of patients with primary BCS. Twenty-five percent of primary BCS patients have two or more risk factors. BCS remains poorly understood, however, and primary myeloproliferative disorders account for approximately 35 to 50% of the primary cases of BCS.

Initial treatment consists of diagnosing and medically managing the underlying disease process and preventing extension of the hepatic vein thrombosis through systemic anticoagulation. The BCS-associated portal hypertension and ascites are medically managed in a manner similar to that in most cirrhotic patients. Thrombolytic therapy alone for acute thrombosis may be attempted. However, the risk:benefit ratio is still unknown. Hepatic decompression aims to decrease sinusoidal pressure by restoring the outflow of blood from the liver via either medical therapy, recanalization of the obstructed hepatic veins, or side-to-side portacaval shunt. Radiographic and surgical intervention should be reserved for those patients whose condition is nonresponsive to medical therapy. (See Schwartz 9th ed., p 1114.)

13. The most common organism isolated from hepatic abscesses is
    A. *Escherichia coli*
    B. *Bacteroides fragilis*
    C. *Staphyloccus aureus*
    D. *Group A Streptococcus*

Answer: A

Approximately 40% of abscesses are monomicrobial, an additional 40% are polymicrobial, and 20% are culture negative. The most common infecting agents are gram-negative organisms. *Escherichia coli* is found in two thirds, and *Streptococcus faecalis*, *Klebsiella*, and *Proteus vulgaris* are also common. Anaerobic organisms such as *Bacteroides fragilis* are also seen frequently. *Staphylococcus* and *Streptococcus* are more common in patients with endocarditis and infected indwelling catheters. (See Schwartz 9th ed., p 1115.)

14. Which of the following is considered the current standard treatment of a 5 cm pyogenic abscess of the right hepatic lobe?
    A. Percutaneous aspiration
    B. Percutaneous drainage
    C. Laparoscopic drainage
    D. Open surgical drainage

Answer: A

The current cornerstones of treatment include correction of the underlying cause, needle aspiration, and IV antibiotic therapy. On presentation, percutaneous aspiration and culture of the aspirate may be beneficial to guide subsequent antibiotic therapy. Initial antibiotic therapy needs to cover gram-negative as well as anaerobic organisms. Aspiration and placement of a drainage catheter is beneficial for only a minority of pyogenic abscesses, because most are quite viscous and drainage is ineffective. Antibiotic therapy must be continued for at least 8 weeks. Aspiration and IV antibiotic therapy can be expected to be effective in 80 to 90% of patients. If this initial mode of therapy fails, the patients should undergo surgical therapy, including laparoscopic or open drainage. Anatomic surgical resection can be performed in patients with recalcitrant abscesses. (See Schwartz 9th ed., p 1115.)

15. Which of the following empiric medications should be added for patients with a liver abscess who have traveled extensively in South America?
   A. Metronidazole
   B. Albendazole
   C. Piperazine citrate
   D. Mebendazole

Answer: A

Entamoeba histolytica is a parasite that is endemic worldwide, infecting approximately 10% of the world's population. Amebiasis is most common in subtropical climates, especially in areas with poor sanitation. Amebiasis should be considered in patients who have traveled to an endemic area and present with right upper quadrant pain, fever, hepatomegaly, and hepatic abscess. Even though this disease process is secondary to a colonic infection, the presence of diarrhea is unusual. For most patients findings of the fluorescent antibody test for *E. histolytica* are positive, and results can remain positive for some time after a clinical cure. Amebiasis is unlikely to be present if the serologic test results are negative.

Metronidazole 750 mg tid for 7 to 10 days is the treatment of choice and is successful in 95% of cases. Defervescence usually occurs in 3 to 5 days. The time necessary for the abscess to resolve depends on the initial size at presentation and varies from 30 to 300 days.

Hydatid disease is most common in sheep-raising areas, where dogs have access to infected offal. These include South Australia, New Zealand, Africa, Greece, Spain, and the Middle East. The diagnosis of hydatid disease is based on the findings of an enzyme-linked immunosorbent assay (ELISA) for echinococcal antigens, and results are positive in approximately 85% of infected patients. The ELISA results may be negative in an infected patient if the cyst has not leaked or does not contain scolices, or if the parasite is no longer viable. Eosinophilia of >7% is found is approximately 30% of infected patients. Ultrasonography and CT scanning of the abdomen are both quite sensitive for detecting hydatid cysts. The appearance of the cysts on images depends on the stage of cyst development. Typically, hydatid cysts are well-defined hypodense lesions with a distinct wall. Ring-like calcifications of the pericysts are present in 20 to 30% of cases. As healing occurs, the entire cyst calcifies densely, and a lesion with this appearance is usually dead or inactive. Daughter cysts generally occur in a peripheral location and are typically slightly hypodense compared with the mother cyst. Unless the cysts are small or the patient is not a suitable candidate for surgical resection, the treatment of hydatid disease is surgically based because of the high risk of secondary infection and rupture. Medical treatment with albendazole relies on drug diffusion through the cyst membrane. The concentration of drug achieved in the cyst is uncertain but is better than that of mebendazole, and albendazole can be used as initial treatment for small, asymptomatic cysts.

Ascaris infection is particularly common in the Far East, India, and South Africa. Ova of the roundworm *Ascaris lumbricoides* arrive in the liver by retrograde flow in the bile ducts. The adult worm is 10 to 20 cm long and may lodge in the common bile duct, producing partial bile duct obstruction and secondary cholangitic abscesses. The ascaris may be a nucleus for the development of intrahepatic gallstones. The clinical presentation in an affected patient may include any of the following: biliary colic, acute cholecystitis, acute pancreatitis, or hepatic abscess. Plain abdominal radiographs, abdominal ultrasound, and endoscopic retrograde cholangiography (ERCP) all can demonstrate the ascaris as linear filling defects in the bile ducts. Occasionally worms can be seen moving into and out of the biliary tree from the duodenum. Treatment consists of administration of piperazine citrate, mebendazole, or albendazole in combination with ERCP extraction of the worms. (See Schwartz 9th ed., pp 1115-16.)

16. The best treatment for a symptomatic 6-cm simple hepatic cyst of the left lobe is
    A. Aspiration alone
    B. Aspiration and sclerotherapy
    C. Laparoscopic fenestration
    D. Left lobectomy

Answer: B

The preferred treatment for symptomatic cysts is ultrasound- or CT-guided percutaneous cyst aspiration followed by sclerotherapy. This approach is approximately 90% effective in controlling symptoms and ablating the cyst cavity. If percutaneous treatment is unavailable or ineffective, treatment may include either laparoscopic or open surgical cysts fenestration. The laparoscopic approach is being used more frequently and is 90% effective. The excised cyst wall is sent for pathologic analysis to rule out carcinoma, and the remaining cyst wall must be carefully inspected for evidence of neoplastic change. If such change is present, complete resection is required, either by enucleation or formal hepatic resection. (See Schwartz 9th ed., pp 1118-19.)

17. An isolated mass in the liver which has a central scar on CT scan is most likely
    A. An adenoma
    B. Focal nodular hyperplasia
    C. A hemangioma
    D. Hepatocellular carcinoma

Answer: B

A good-quality biphasic CT scan usually is diagnostic of FNH, on which such lesions appear well circumscribed with a typical central scar (see Fig. 31-7). They show intense homogeneous enhancement on arterial phase contrast images and are often isodense or invisible compared with background liver on the venous phase. On MRI scans, FNH lesions are hypointense on T1-weighted images and isointense to hyperintense on T2-weighted images. After gadolinium administration, lesions are hyperintense but become isointense on delayed images. The fibrous septa extending from the central scar are also more readily seen with MRI. If CT or MRI scans do not show the classic appearance, radionuclide sulfur colloid imaging may be used to diagnose FNH based on select uptake by Kupffer cells.

The majority of hemangiomas can be diagnosed by liver imaging studies. On biphasic contrast CT scan, large hemangiomas show asymmetrical nodular peripheral enhancement that is isodense with large vessels and exhibit progressive centripetal enhancement fill-in over time (Fig. 31-7). On MRI, hemangiomas are hypointense on T1-weighted images and hyperintense on T2-weighted images. With gadolinium enhancement, hemangiomas show a pattern of peripheral nodular enhancement similar to that seen on contrast CT scans.

On CT scan, adenomas usually have sharply defined borders and can be confused with metastatic tumors. With venous phase contrast, they can look hypodense or isodense in comparison with background liver, whereas on arterial phase contrast subtle hypervascular enhancement often is seen (see Fig. 31-7). On MRI scans, adenomas are hyperintense on T1-weighted images and enhance early after gadolinium injection. On nuclear medicine imaging, they typically appear as 'cold,' in contrast with FNH.

HCCs are typically hypervascular with blood supplied predominantly from the hepatic artery. Thus, the lesion often appears hypervascular during the arterial phase of CT studies (Fig. 31-8) and relatively hypodense during the delayed phases due to early washout of the contrast medium by the arterial blood. MRI imaging also is effective in characterizing HCC. HCC is variable on T1-weighted images and usually hyperintense on T2-weighted images. As with contrast CT, HCC enhances in the arterial phase after gadolinium injection because of its hypervascularity and becomes hypointense in the delayed phases due to contrast washout. HCC has a tendency to invade the portal vein, and the presence of an enhancing portal vein thrombus is highly suggestive of HCC. (See Schwartz 9th ed., p 1120.)

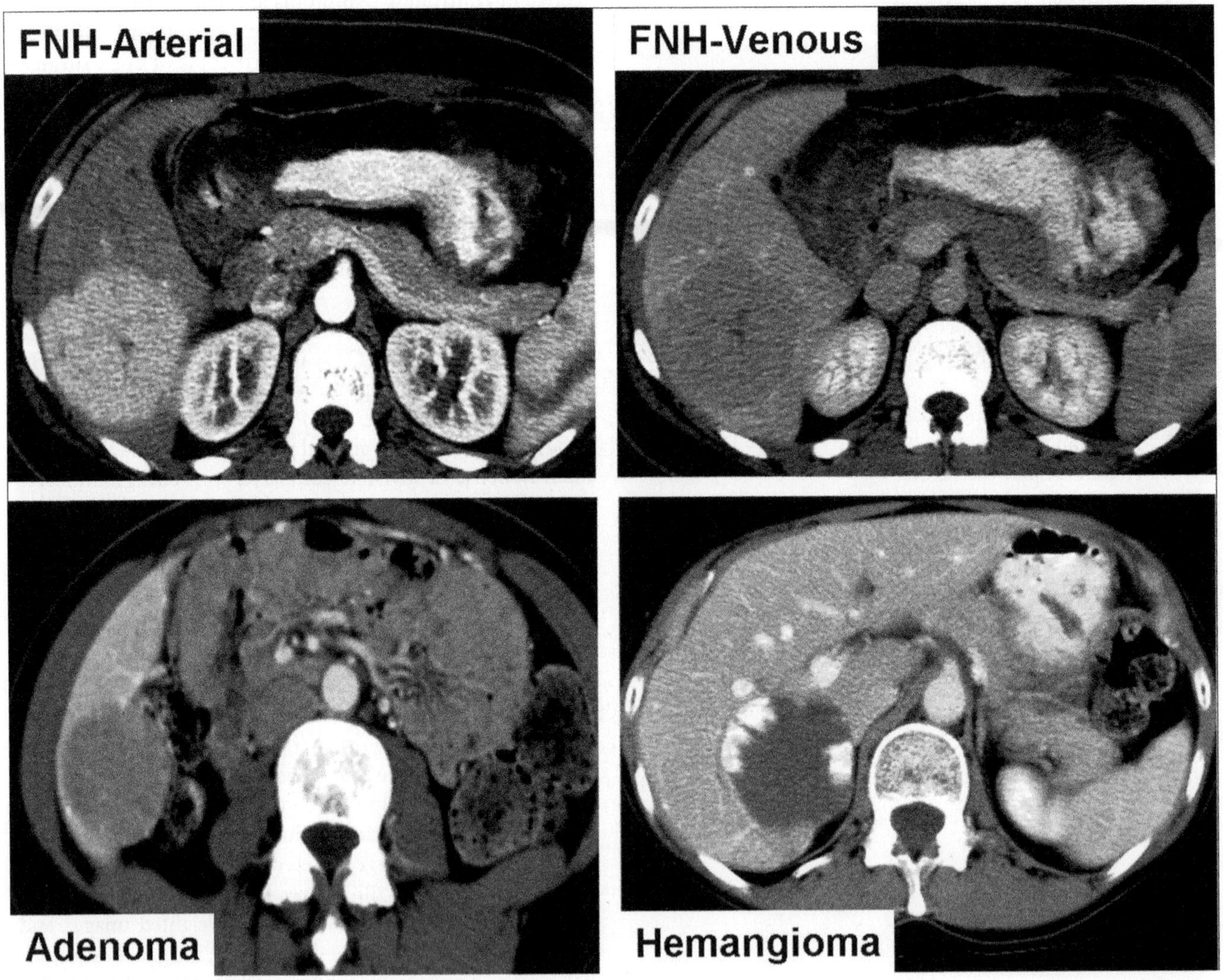

FIG. 31-7. Computed tomographic scans showing classic appearance of benign liver lesions. Focal nodular hyperplasia (FNH) is hypervascular on arterial phase, is isodense to liver on venous phase, and has a central scar (*upper panels*). Adenoma is hypovascular (*lower left panel*). Hemangioma shows asymmetrical peripheral enhancement (*lower right panel*).

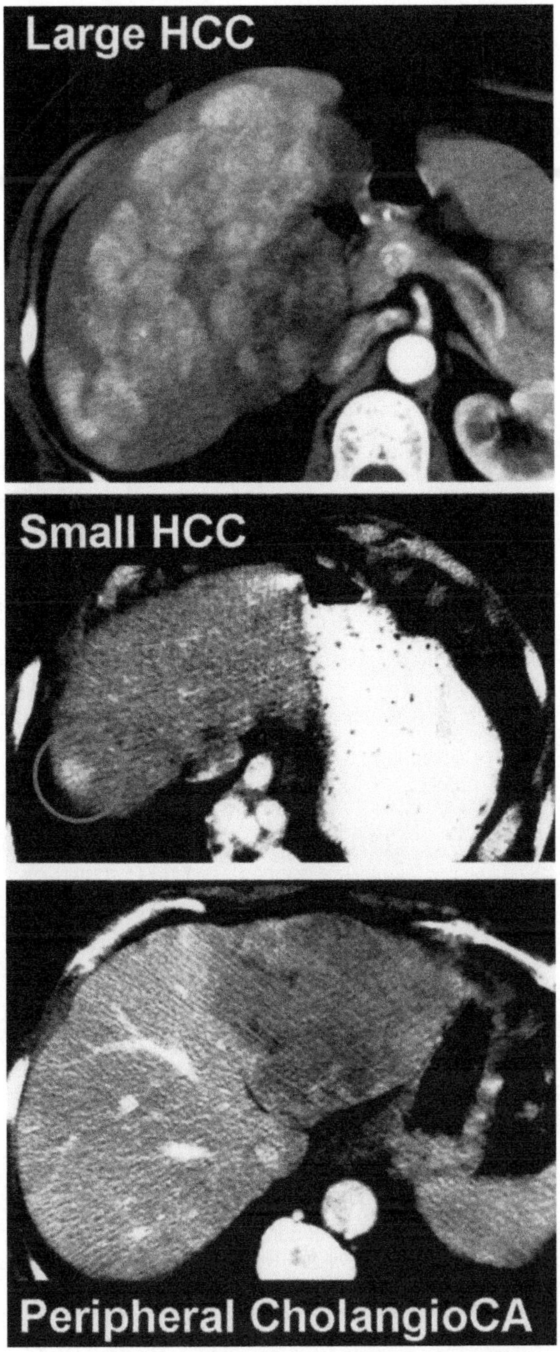

FIG. 31-8. Computed tomographic (CT) images of hepatocellular carcinoma (HCC) and peripheral cholangiocarcinoma. CT scans reveal a large (*upper panel*) and small (*middle panel*) hypervascular HCC. A hypovascular left lobe peripheral cholangiocarcinoma (Cholangio CA) is also shown (*lower panel*).

18. Standard therapy for a 4-cm right lobe hepatic adenoma is
    A. Observation only
    B. Arterial embolism to prevent further growth
    C. Laparoscopic ablation
    D. Surgical resection

Answer: D

Hepatic adenomas carry a significant risk of spontaneous rupture with intraperitoneal bleeding. The clinical presentation may be abdominal pain, and in 10 to 25% of cases hepatic adenomas present with spontaneous intraperitoneal hemorrhage. Hepatic adenomas also have a risk of malignant transformation to a well-differentiated HCC. Therefore, it usually is recommended that a hepatic adenoma (once diagnosed) be surgically resected. Oral contraceptive or estrogen use should be stopped when either FNH or adenoma is diagnosed. (See Schwartz 9th ed., p 1120.)

19. The best treatment for a 42-year-old patient with Child's B cirrhosis and a single 4-cm hepatocellular carcinoma in segment VI is
    A. Radiofrequency
    B. Segmental resection with 1-cm margins
    C. Right lobectomy
    D. Liver transplantation

Answer: D

For patients without cirrhosis who develop HCC, resection is the treatment of choice. For those patients with Child's class A cirrhosis with preserved liver function and no portal hypertension, resection also is considered. If resection is not possible because of poor liver function and the HCC meets the Milan criteria (one nodule <5 cm, or two or three nodules all <3 cm, no gross vascular invasion or extrahepatic spread), liver transplantation is the treatment of choice. (See Schwartz 9th ed., p 1121, and Fig. 31-9.)

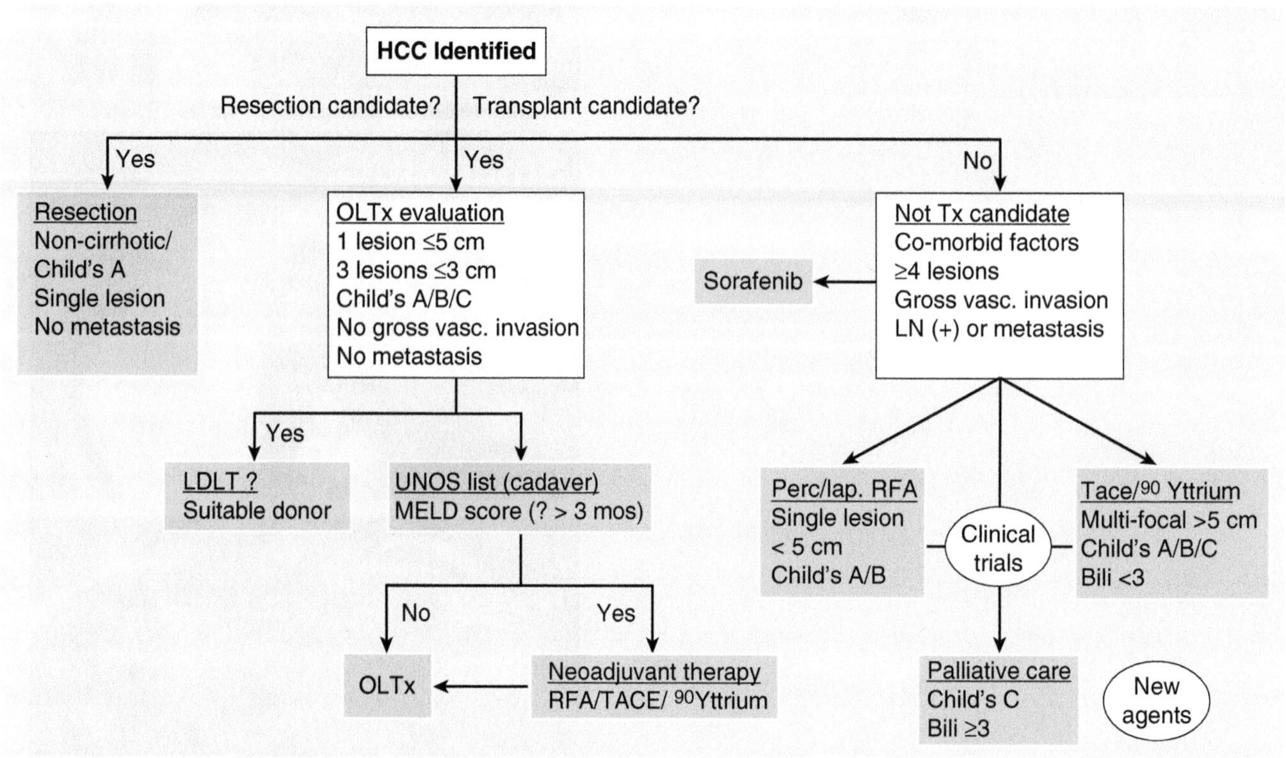

FIG. 31-9. Algorithm for the management of hepatocellular carcinoma (HCC). The treatment algorithm for HCC begins with determining whether the patient is a resection candidate or liver transplant candidate. Bili = bilirubin level (in milligrams per deciliter); Child's = Child-Turcotte-Pugh class; lap = laparoscopic; LDLT = living-donor liver transplantation; LN = lymph node; MELD = Model for End-Stage Liver Disease; OLTx = orthotopic liver transplantation; Perc = percutaneous; RFA = radiofrequency ablation; TACE = transarterial chemoembolization; Tx = transplantation; UNOS = United Network for Organ Sharing; vasc. = vascular.

CHAPTER 32

Gallbladder and the Extrahepatic Biliary System

BASIC SCIENCE QUESTIONS

1. The common bile duct and pancreatic duct merge to enter the duodenum as a single duct in what percentage of the population?
   A. 20%
   B. 30%
   C. 50%
   D. 70%

Answer: D
The union of the common bile duct and the main pancreatic duct follows one of three configurations. In about 70% of people, these ducts unite outside the duodenal wall and traverse the duodenal wall as a single duct. In about 20%, they join within the duodenal wall and have a short or no common duct, but open through the same opening into the duodenum. In about 10%, they exit via separate openings into the duodenum. (See Schwartz 9th ed., p 1138.)

2. How much bile does a healthy adult produce each day?
   A. 50-100 ml
   B. 200-300 ml
   C. 500-1000 ml
   D. 1200-1800 ml

Answer: C
The liver produces bile continuously and excretes it into the bile canaliculi. The normal adult consuming an average diet produces within the liver 500 to 1000 mL of bile a day. The secretion of bile is responsive to neurogenic, humoral, and chemical stimuli. Vagal stimulation increases secretion of bile, whereas splanchnic nerve stimulation results in decreased bile flow. Hydrochloric acid, partly digested proteins, and fatty acids in the duodenum stimulate the release of secretin from the duodenum that, in turn, increases bile production and bile flow. Bile flows from the liver through to the hepatic ducts, into the common hepatic duct, through the common bile duct, and finally into the duodenum. With an intact sphincter of Oddi, bile flow is directed into the gallbladder. (See Schwartz 9th ed., p 1138.)

3. Bile is normally a neutral pH or slightly alkaline. Consumption of large amounts of which of the following will decrease the pH of bile?
   A. Fat
   B. Carbohydrate
   C. Protein
   D. Ethanol

Answer: C
Bile is mainly composed of water, electrolytes, bile salts, proteins, lipids, and bile pigments. Sodium, potassium, calcium, and chlorine have the same concentration in bile as in plasma or extracellular fluid. The pH of hepatic bile is usually neutral or slightly alkaline, but varies with diet; an increase in protein shifts the bile to a more acidic pH. (See Schwartz 9th ed., p 1138.)

4. The cystic artery most commonly arises from the right hepatic artery (80-90%). The second most anatomic configuration of the cystic artery, which occurs in 10% of people, is
   A. Two cystic arteries, both arising from the right hepatic artery
   B. Two cystic arteries, one arising from the right hepatic artery and one arising from the left hepatic artery
   C. One cystic artery, arising from an aberrant right hepatic artery
   D. One cystic artery, arising from the gastroduodenal artery

Answer: C

The second most common anatomic configuration is one cystic artery, arising from an accessory, or aberrant right hepatic artery. (See Schwartz 9th ed., p 1139, and Fig. 32-1.)

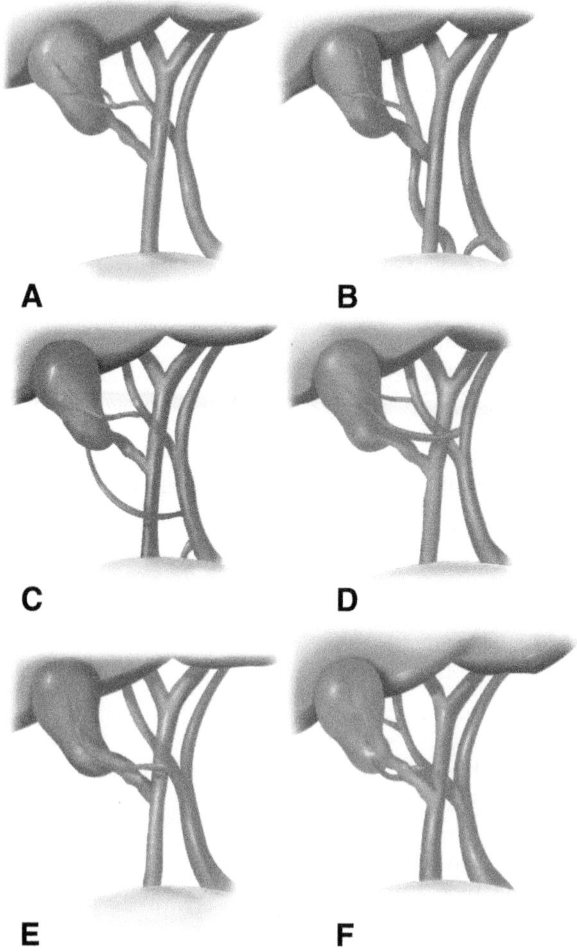

FIG. 32-1. Variations in the arterial supply to the gallbladder. **A.** Cystic artery from right hepatic artery, about 80–90%. **B.** Cystic artery from right hepatic artery (accessory or replaced) from superior mesenteric artery, about 10%. **C.** Two cystic arteries, one from the right hepatic, the other from the common hepatic artery, rare. **D.** Two cystic arteries, one from the right hepatic, the other from the left hepatic artery, rare. **E.** The cystic artery branching from the right hepatic artery and running anterior to the common hepatic duct, rare. **F.** Two cystic arteries arising from the right hepatic artery, rare.

5. The gallbladder is able to store only a small fraction of the bile produced by the liver. What is the primary mechanism used to keep the gallbladder from becoming distended (and developing high pressure) by this volume of bile?
   A. The bile is continuously secreted into the duodenum once the pressure in the gallbladder increases
   B. There is enough contraction of the gallbladder in response to eating to empty the large volume of bile
   C. The gallbladder concentrates the large volume of bile
   D. The liver decreases bile production when the pressure in the gallbladder increases

Answer: C

In the fasting state, approximately 80% of the bile secreted by the liver is stored in the gallbladder. This storage is made possible because of the remarkable absorptive capacity of the gallbladder, as the gallbladder mucosa has the greatest absorptive power per unit area of any structure in the body. It rapidly absorbs sodium, chloride, and water against significant concentration gradients, concentrating the bile as much as 10-fold and leading to a marked change in bile composition. This rapid absorption is one of the mechanisms that prevent a rise in pressure within the biliary system under normal circumstances. Gradual relaxation as well as emptying of the gallbladder during the fasting period also plays a role in maintaining a relatively low intraluminal pressure in the biliary tree. (See Schwartz 9th ed., p 1139.)

6. The primary mediator of gallbladder contraction is
   A. Vasoactive intestinal polypeptide
   B. Somatostatin
   C. Cholecystokinin
   D. Enkephalin

Answer: C

One of the main stimuli to gallbladder emptying is the hormone cholecystokinin (CCK). CCK is released endogenously from the duodenal mucosa in response to a meal. When stimulated by eating, the gallbladder empties 50 to 70% of its contents within 30 to 40 minutes. Over the following 60 to 90 minutes, the gallbladder gradually refills. This is correlated with a reduced CCK level.

Vasoactive intestinal polypeptide inhibits contraction and causes gallbladder relaxation. Somatostatin and its analogues are potent inhibitors of gallbladder contraction. Patients treated with somatostatin analogues and those with somatostatinoma have a high incidence of gallstones, presumably due to the inhibition of gallbladder contraction and emptying. Other hormones such as substance P and enkephalin affect gallbladder motility, but the physiologic role is unclear. (See Schwartz 9th ed., p 1139.)

7. The half-life of CCK is
   A. 2-3 minutes
   B. 20-30 minutes
   C. 2-3 hours
   D. 20-30 hours

Answer: A

CCK is a peptide that comes from epithelial cells of the upper GI tract and is found in the highest concentrations in the duodenum. CCK is released into the bloodstream by acid, fat, and amino acids in the duodenum. CCK has a plasma half-life of 2 to 3 minutes and is metabolized by both the liver and the kidneys. CCK acts directly on smooth muscle receptors of the gallbladder and stimulates gallbladder contraction. It also relaxes the terminal bile duct, the sphincter of Oddi, and the duodenum. CCK stimulation of the gallbladder and the biliary tree also is mediated by cholinergic vagal neurons. In patients who have had a vagotomy, the response to CCK stimulation is diminished and the size and the volume of the gallbladder are increased. (See Schwartz 9th ed., p 1139.)

CLINICAL QUESTIONS

1. The sensitivity of ultrasound in detecting gallstones is
   A. >99%
   B. 90-95%
   C. 85-90%
   D. 80-85%

Answer: B

An ultrasound is the initial investigation of any patient suspected of disease of the biliary tree. It is noninvasive, painless, does not submit the patient to radiation, and can be performed on critically ill patients. It is dependent upon the skills and the experience of the operator, and it is dynamic (i.e., static images do not give the same information as those obtained during the ultrasound investigation itself). Ultrasound will show stones in the gallbladder with sensitivity and specificity of >90%. Stones are acoustically dense and reflect the ultrasound waves back to the ultrasonic transducer. Because stones block the passage of sound waves to the region behind them, they also produce an acoustic shadow (Fig. 32-2). Stones move with changes in position. Polyps may be calcified and reflect shadows, but do not move with change in posture. Some stones form a layer in the gallbladder; others a sediment or sludge. (See Schwartz 9th ed., p 1140.)

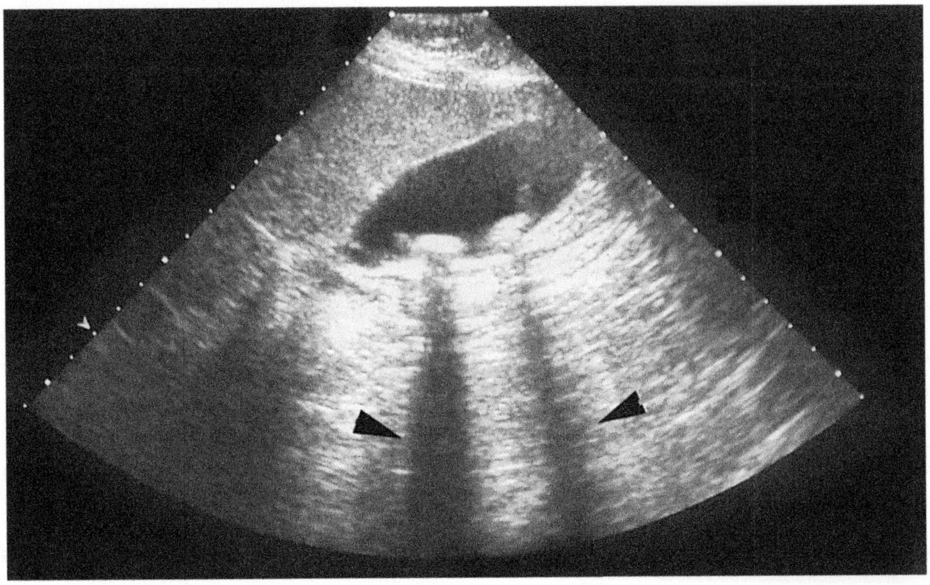

FIG. 32-2. An ultrasonography of the gallbladder. *Arrows* indicate the acoustic shadows from stones in the gallbladder.

2. Which of the following is associated with an increased risk for cholelithiasis?
   A. Ulcerative colitis
   B. Crohn's disease
   C. Jejunal resection
   D. Carcinoma of the colon

Answer: B

Certain conditions predispose to the development of gallstones. Obesity, pregnancy, dietary factors, Crohn's disease, terminal ileal resection, gastric surgery, hereditary spherocytosis, sickle cell disease, and thalassemia are all associated with an increased risk of developing gallstones. Women are three times more likely to develop gallstones than men, and first-degree relatives of patients with gallstones have a twofold greater prevalence. (See Schwartz 9th ed., p 1142.)

3. A 35-year-old woman has an incidental finding of cholelithiasis on a plain radiograph obtained following a minor car accident. Her risk of developing symptoms from these gallstones in the next 20 years is
   A. 7%
   B. 18%
   C. 33%
   D. 52%

Answer: C

Gallstones in patients without biliary symptoms are commonly diagnosed incidentally on ultrasonography, CT scans, or abdominal radiography or at laparotomy. Several studies have examined the likelihood of developing biliary colic or developing significant complications of gallstone disease. Approximately 3% of asymptomatic individuals become symptomatic per year (i.e., develop biliary colic). Once symptomatic, patients tend to have recurring bouts of biliary colic. Complicated gallstone disease develops in 3 to 5% of symptomatic patients per year. Over a 20-year period, about two thirds of asymptomatic patients with gallstones remain symptom free. (See Schwartz 9th ed., p 1143.)

4. Which of the following is an indication for cholecystectomy in an asymptomatic patient with an incidental finding of gallstones?
   A. Any history of abdominal pain
   B. Family history of complications of cholelithiasis
   C. Porcelain gallbladder
   D. Frequent travel out of the country

Answer: C

Because few patients develop complications without previous biliary symptoms, prophylactic cholecystectomy in asymptomatic persons with gallstones is rarely indicated. For elderly patients with diabetes, for individuals who will be isolated from medical care for extended periods of time, and in populations with increased risk of gallbladder cancer, a prophylactic cholecystectomy may be advisable. Porcelain gallbladder, a rare premalignant condition in which the wall of the gallbladder becomes calcified, is an absolute indication for cholecystectomy. (See Schwartz 9th ed., p 1143.)

5. Which of the following is one of the components of gallstones?
   A. Biliverdin
   B. Hemoglobin
   C. Lecithin
   D. Short chain fatty acids

Answer: C

Lecithin is a phospholipid that is one of the three major components of gallstones (see Fig. 32-3). Gallstones form as a result of solids settling out of solution. The major organic solutes in bile are bilirubin, bile salts, phospholipids, and cholesterol. Gallstones are classified by their cholesterol content as either cholesterol stones or pigment stones. Pigment stones can be further classified as either black or brown. In Western countries about 80% of gallstones are cholesterol stones and about 15 to 20% are black pigment stones. Brown pigment stones account for only a small percentage. Both types of pigment stones are more common in Asia. (See Schwartz 9th ed., p 1143.)

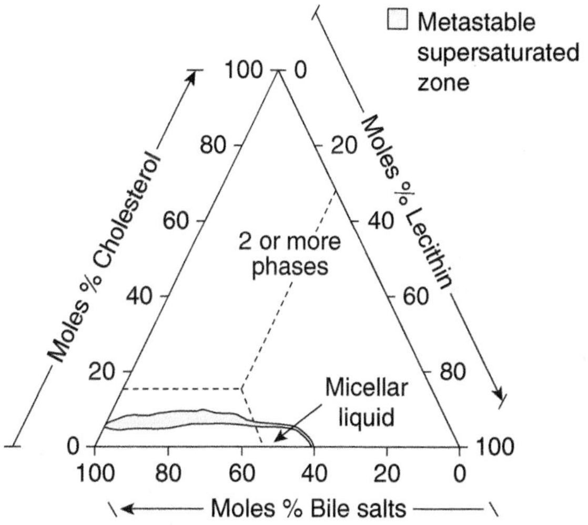

FIG. 32-3. The three major components of bile plotted on triangular coordinates. A given point represents the relative molar ratios of bile salts, lecithin, and cholesterol. The area labeled "micellar liquid" shows the range of concentrations found consistent with a clear micellar solution (single phase), where cholesterol is fully solubilized. The shaded area directly above this region corresponds to a metastable zone, supersaturated with cholesterol. Bile with a composition that falls above the shaded area has exceeded the solubilization capacity of cholesterol and precipitation of cholesterol crystals occurs. (Reproduced with permission from Holzbach RT: Pathogenesis and medical treatment of gallstones, in Slesinger MH, Fordtran JS, eds: *Gastrointestinal Diseases*. Philadelphia: WB Saunders, 1989, p 1672.)

6. Which of the following is the most common location for pain during an attack of biliary colic?
   A. Left periumbilical
   B. Right shoulder
   C. Epigastrium
   D. Scapula

Answer: C

The most common location for pain during an episode of biliary colic is the epigastrium (64%) followed by the right upper quadrant (50%).

Atypical presentation of gallstone disease is common. Association with meals is present in only about 50% of patients. Some patients report milder attacks of pain, but relate it to meals. The pain may be located primarily in the back or the left upper or lower right quadrant. Bloating and belching may be present and associated with the attacks of pain. In patients with atypical presentation, other conditions with upper abdominal pain should be sought out, even in the presence of gallstones. These include peptic ulcer disease, gastroesophageal reflux disease, abdominal wall hernias, irritable bowel disease, diverticular disease, liver diseases, renal calculi, pleuritic pain, and myocardial pain. Many patients with other conditions have gallstones. (See Schwartz 9th ed., p 1146, and Fig. 32-4.)

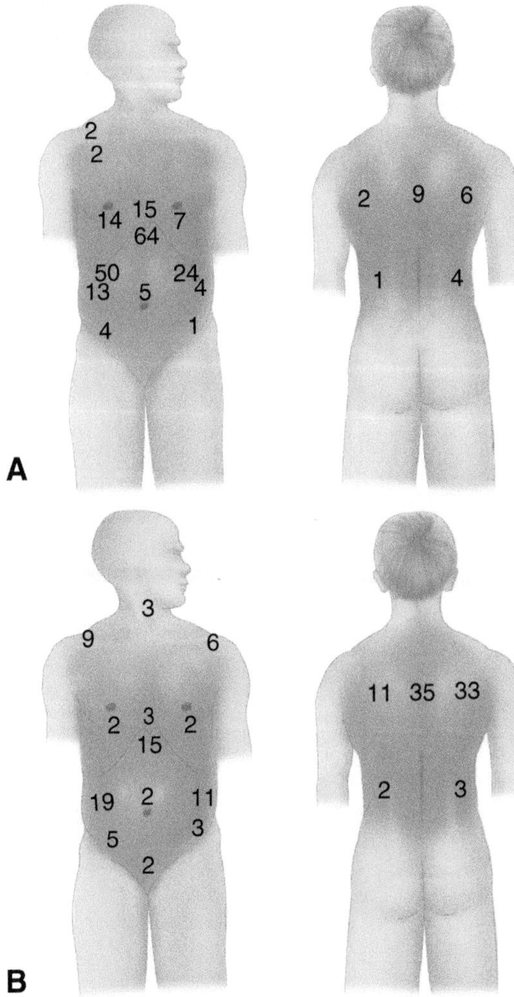

FIG. 32-4. A. Sites of the most severe pain during an episode of biliary pain in 107 patients with gallstones (% values add up to >100% because of multiple responses). The subxiphoid and right subcostal areas were the most common sites; note that the left subcostal area was not an unusual site of pain. B. Sites of pain radiation (%) during an episode of biliary pain in the same group of patients. (Reproduced with permission from Gunn A, Keddie N: Some clinical observations on patients with gallstones. *The Lancet* 300(7771):239–241, Copyright © 1972, with permission from Elsevier.)

7. Which of the following is the appropriate treatment for adenomyomatosis of the gallbladder?
   A. Observation only
   B. INH
   C. Serial exams with EGD and ultrasound every 12 months
   D. Cholecystectomy

Answer: D

Adenomyomatosis or cholecystitis glandularis proliferans is characterized on microscopy by hypertrophic smooth muscle bundles and by the ingrowths of mucosal glands into the muscle layer (epithelial sinus formation). Granulomatous polyps develop in the lumen at the fundus, and the gallbladder wall is thickened and septae or strictures may be seen in the gallbladder. In symptomatic patients, cholecystectomy is the treatment of choice. (See Schwartz 9th ed., p 1146.)

8. A 24-year-old woman in the 20th week of pregnancy experiences a single episode of biliary colic. The most appropriate initial management is
   A. Observation with plans to follow her after delivery for recurrent episodes
   B. Dietary changes
   C. Elective laparoscopic cholecystectomy during 2nd trimester
   D. Elective open cholecystectomy during 2nd trimester.

Answer: B

Patients with symptomatic gallstones should be advised to have elective laparoscopic cholecystectomy. While waiting for surgery, or if surgery has to be postponed, the patient should be advised to avoid dietary fats and large meals. Diabetic patients with symptomatic gallstones should have a cholecystectomy promptly, as they are more prone to develop acute cholecystitis that is often severe. Pregnant women with symptomatic gallstones who cannot be managed expectantly with diet modifications can safely undergo laparoscopic cholecystectomy during the second trimester. Laparoscopic cholecystectomy is safe and effective in children as well as in the elderly. (See Schwartz 9th ed., p 1146.)

9. A 53-year-old man is admitted with 24 hours of pain from acute cholecystitis. He is made npo, IV antibiotics are started, and analgesia is given. He should undergo cholecystectomy
   A. Urgently
   B. In 1-3 days
   C. In 7-10 days
   D. In 6-8 weeks

Answer: B

Patients who present with acute cholecystitis will need IV fluids, antibiotics, and analgesia. The antibiotics should cover gram-negative aerobes as well as anaerobes. A third-generation cephalosporin with good anaerobic coverage or a second-generation cephalosporin combined with metronidazole is a typical regimen. For patients with allergies to cephalosporins, an aminoglycoside with metronidazole is appropriate. Although the inflammation in acute cholecystitis may be sterile in some patients, more than one half will have positive cultures from the gallbladder bile. It is difficult to know who is secondarily infected; therefore, antibiotics have become a part of the management in most medical centers. Cholecystectomy is the definitive treatment for acute cholecystitis. In the past, the timing of cholecystectomy has been a matter of debate. Early cholecystectomy performed within 2 to 3 days of the illness is preferred over interval or delayed cholecystectomy that is performed 6 to 10 weeks after initial medical treatment and recuperation. Several studies have shown that unless the patient is unfit for surgery, early cholecystectomy should be recommended, as it offers the patient a definitive solution in one hospital admission, quicker recovery times, and an earlier return to work. Laparoscopic cholecystectomy is the procedure of choice. (See Schwartz 9th ed., p 1148.)

10. Primary choledochal stones are usually
   A. Cholesterol stones
   B. Black pigment stones
   C. Brown pigment stones
   D. Mulberry stones

Answer: C

The vast majority of ductal stones in Western countries are formed within the gallbladder and migrate down the cystic duct to the common bile duct. These are classified as secondary common bile duct stones, in contrast to the primary stones that form in the bile ducts. The secondary stones are usually cholesterol stones, whereas the primary stones are usually of the brown pigment type. The primary stones are associated with biliary stasis and infection and are more commonly seen in Asian populations. The causes of biliary stasis that lead to the development of primary stones include biliary stricture, papillary stenosis, tumors, or other (secondary) stones. (See Schwartz 9th ed., p 1148.)

11. A patient presents with biliary colic. On ultrasound there are multiple small gallstones in the gallbladder and the common bile duct measures 9 mm in diameter. No stone is visualized in the common bile duct. Which of the following is the most reasonable next step?
   A. Repeat ultrasound in 24-48 hours
   B. MRCP with contrast
   C. Percutaneous cholangiography
   D. Laparosopic cholecystectomy and intraopetrative cholangiography

Answer: D

For patients with symptomatic gallstones and suspected common bile duct stones, either preoperative endoscopic cholangiography or an intraoperative cholangiogram will document the bile duct stones. If an endoscopic cholangiogram reveals stones, sphincterotomy and ductal clearance of the stones is appropriate, followed by a laparoscopic cholecystectomy. An intraoperative cholangiogram at the time of cholecystectomy will also document the presence or absence of bile duct stones (Fig. 32-5). Laparoscopic common bile duct exploration via the cystic duct or with formal choledochotomy allows the stones to be retrieved in the same setting. If the expertise and/or the instrumentation for laparoscopic common bile duct exploration are not available, a drain should be left adjacent to the cystic duct and the patient scheduled for endoscopic sphincterotomy the following day. An open common bile duct exploration is an option if the endoscopic method has already been tried or is, for some reason, not feasible. (See Schwartz 9th ed., p 1148.)

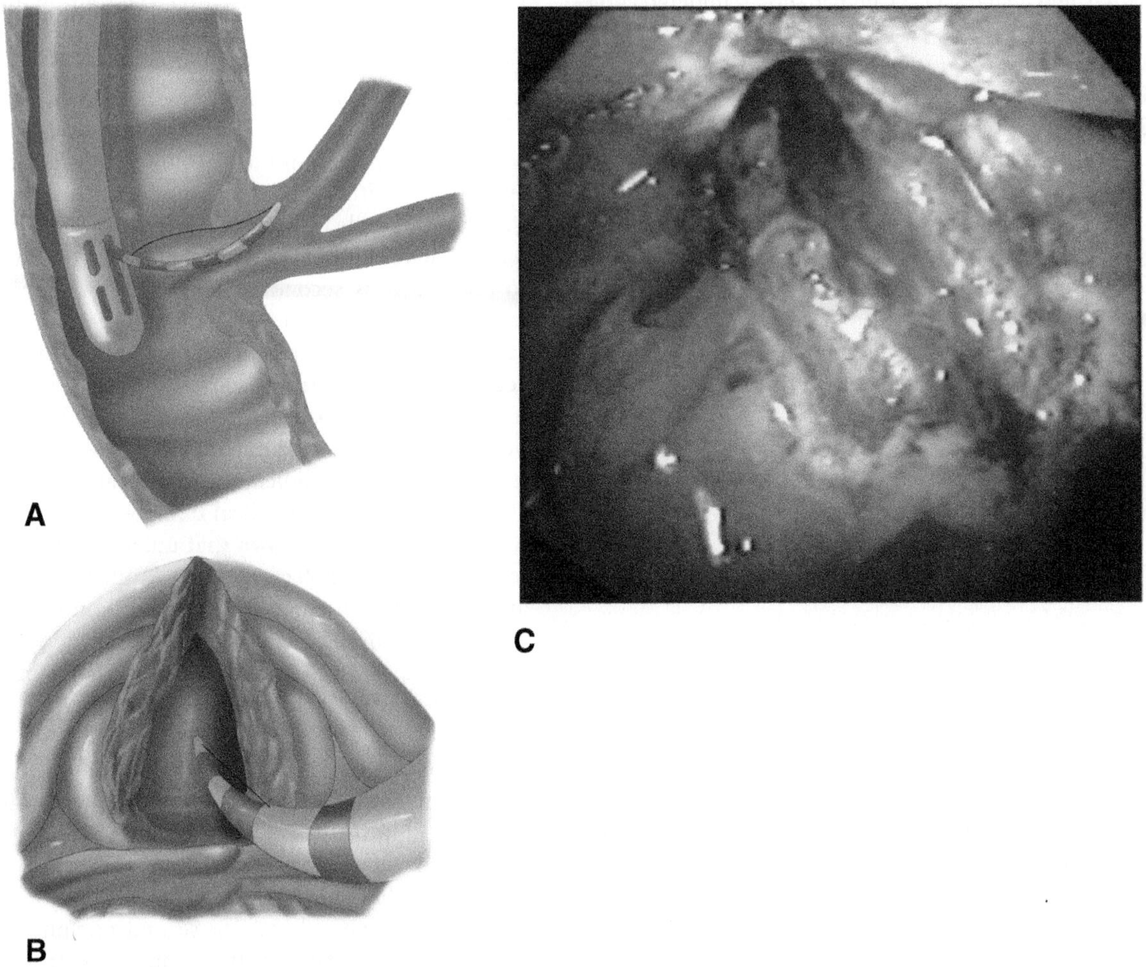

FIG. 32-5. An endoscopic sphincterotomy. A. The sphincterotome in place. B. Completed sphincterotomy. C. Endoscopic picture of completed sphincterotomy.

12. A 75-year-old man presents with cholangitis, symptomatic cholelithiasis, and choledocholithiasis. The best treatment for him is
    A. ERCP followed by cholecystectomy
    B. Cholecystectomy, flushing of the common bile duct with subsequent ERCP if necessary
    C. Laparoscopic cholecystectomy and common bile duct exploration
    D. ERC and endoscopic sphincterotomy

Answer: D

Patients >70 years old presenting with bile duct stones should have their ductal stones cleared endoscopically. Studies comparing surgery to endoscopic treatment have documented less morbidity and mortality for endoscopic treatment in this group of patients. They do not need to be submitted for a cholecystectomy, as only about 15% will become symptomatic from their gallbladder stones, and such patients can be treated as the need arises by a cholecystectomy. (See Schwartz 9th ed., p 1149.)

13. Which of the following is NOT part of Reynolds' pentad?
    A. Hypovolemic shock
    B. Jaundice
    C. Mental status changes
    D. Fever

Answer: A

The most common presentation [of cholangitis] is fever, epigastric or right upper quadrant pain, and jaundice.

These classic symptoms, well known as *Charcot's triad*, are present in about two thirds of patients. The illness may progress rapidly with septicemia and disorientation, known as *Reynolds' pentad* (e.g., fever, jaundice, right upper quadrant pain, septic shock, and mental status changes). However, the presentation may be atypical, with little if any fever, jaundice, or pain. This occurs most commonly in the elderly, who may have unremarkable symptoms until they collapse with septicemia. (See Schwartz 9th ed., p 1149.)

14. Cholangiohepatitis is seen most commonly in which of the following groups?
    A. Caucasian patients of Northern European descent
    B. Jewish patients of Ashkenazi descent
    C. Asian patients of Chinese descent
    D. Native American patients

Answer: C

Cholangiohepatitis, also known as *recurrent pyogenic cholangitis*, is endemic to the Orient. It also has been encountered in the Chinese population in the United States, as well as in Europe and Australia. It affects both sexes equally and occurs most frequently in the third and fourth decades of life. Cholangiohepatitis is caused by bacterial contamination (commonly *E. coli*, *Klebsiella* species, *Bacteroides* species, or *Enterococcus faecalis*) of the biliary tree, and often is associated with biliary parasites such as *Clonorchis sinensis*, *Opisthorchis viverrini*, and *Ascaris lumbricoides*. Bacterial enzymes cause deconjugation of bilirubin, which precipitates as bile sludge. The sludge and dead bacterial cell bodies form brown pigment stones. The nucleus of the stone may contain an adult *Clonorchis* worm, an ovum, or an ascarid. These stones are formed throughout the biliary tree and cause partial obstruction that contributes to the repeated bouts of cholangitis. Biliary strictures form as a result of recurrent cholangitis and lead to further stone formation, infection, hepatic abscesses, and liver failure (secondary biliary cirrhosis). (See Schwartz 9th ed., p 1151.)

15. The treatment of a type II choledochal cyst is
    A. Observation with annual ultrasound
    B. ERCP with sphincterotomy
    C. Drainage with a Roux-en-Y choledochojejunostomy
    D. Resection with a Roux-en-Y hepaticojejunostomy

Answer: D

For types I, II, and IV [choledochal cysts], excision of the extrahepatic biliary tree, including cholecystectomy, with a Roux-en-Y hepaticojejunostomy, are ideal. In type IV, additional segmental resection of the liver may be appropriate, particularly if intrahepatic stones, strictures, or abscesses are present, or if the dilatations are confined to one lobe. The risk of cholangiocarcinoma developing in choledochal cysts is as high as 15% in adults, and supports complete excision when they are diagnosed. For type III, sphincterotomy is recommended. (See Schwartz 9th ed., p 1155; 1158, and Fig. 32-6.)

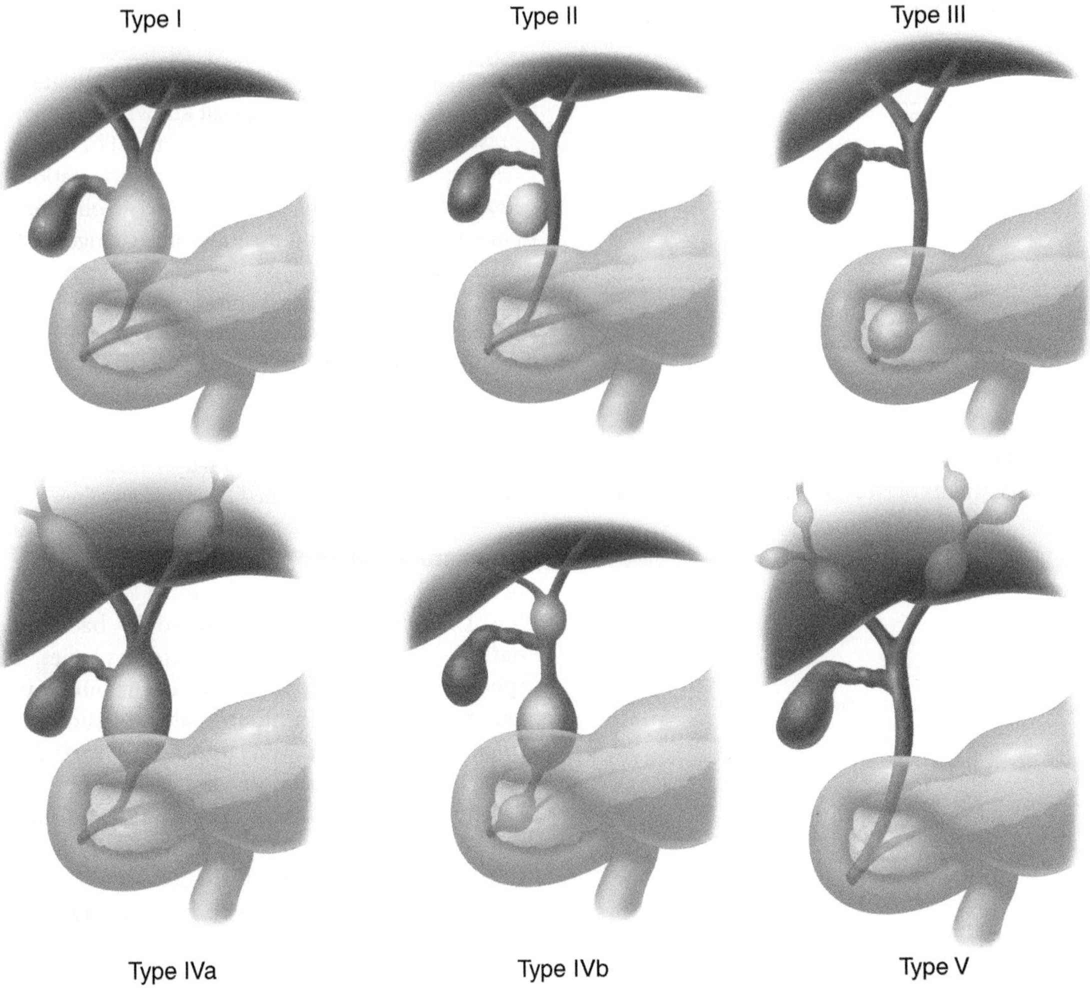
Type I
Type II
Type III
Type IVa
Type IVb
Type V

FIG. 32-6. Classification of choledochal cysts. Type I, fusiform or cystic dilations of the extrahepatic biliary tree, is the most common type, making up >50% of the choledochal cysts. Type II, saccular diverticulum of an extrahepatic bile duct. Rare, <5% of choledochal cysts. Type III, bile duct dilatation within the duodenal wall (choledochoceles), makes up about 5% of choledochal cysts. Type IVa and IVb, multiple cysts, make up 5–10% of choledochal cysts. Type IVa affects both extrahepatic and intrahepatic bile ducts while Type IVb cysts affect the extrahepatic bile ducts only. Type V, intrahepatic biliary cysts, is very rare and makes up 1% of choledochal cysts.

16. Primary sclerosing cholangitis is seen more commonly in patients with
    A. Ulcerative colitis
    B. Crohn's disease
    C. Rheumatoid arthritis
    D. Celiac sprue

Answer: A

[Primary sclerosing cholangitis] is associated with ulcerative colitis in about two thirds of patients. Other diseases associated with sclerosing cholangitis include Riedel's thyroiditis and retroperitoneal fibrosis. Autoimmune reaction, chronic lowgrade bacterial or viral infection, toxic reaction, and genetic factors have all been suggested to play a role in its pathogenesis. The human leukocyte antigen haplotypes HLA-B8, -DR3, -DQ2, and -DRw52A, commonly found in patients with autoimmune diseases, also are more frequently seen in patients with sclerosing cholangitis than in controls. (See Schwartz 9th ed., p 1156.)

17. In addition to regional lymphadenectomy, appropriate surgical treatment for a T2 carcinoma of the gallbladder is
    A. Cholecystectomy only
    B. Cholecystectomy with resection of liver segments IVB and V
    C. Cholecystectomy with limited right hepatectomy
    D. Cholecystectomy with extended right hepatectomy

Answer: B

Tumors limited to the muscular layer of the gallbladder (T1) are usually identified incidentally, after cholecystectomy for gallstone disease. There is near universal agreement that simple cholecystectomy is an adequate treatment for T1 lesions and results in a near 100% overall 5-year survival rate. When the tumor invades the perimuscular connective tissue without extension beyond the serosa or into the liver (T2 tumors), an extended cholecystectomy should be performed. That includes resection of liver segments IVB and V, and lymphadenectomy of the cystic duct, and pericholedochal, portal, right celiac, and posterior pancreatoduodenal lymph nodes. One half of patients with T2 tumors are found to have nodal disease on pathologic examination. Therefore, regional lymphadenectomy is an important part of surgery for T2 cancers. For tumors that grow beyond the serosa or invade the liver or other organs (T3 and T4 tumors), there is a high likelihood of intraperitoneal and distant spread. If no peritoneal or nodal involvement is found, complete tumor excision with an extended right hepatectomy (segments IV, V, VI, VII, and VIII) must be performed for adequate tumor clearance. An aggressive approach in patients who will tolerate surgery has resulted in an increased survival for T3 and T4 lesions. (See Schwartz 9th ed., p 1161.)

18. Cholangiocarcinoma most commonly occurs
    A. In the intrahepatic ducts
    B. In the common hepatic duct, at the bifurcation
    C. At the junction of the hepatic and common bile ducts
    D. In the distal common bile duct

Answer: B

Cholangiocarcinoma is a rare tumor arising from the biliary epithelium and may occur anywhere along the biliary tree. About two thirds are located at the hepatic duct bifurcation. Surgical resection offers the only chance for cure; however, many patients have advanced disease at the time of diagnosis. Therefore, palliative procedures aimed to provide biliary drainage to prevent liver failure and cholangitis are often the only therapeutic possibilities. Most patients with unresectable disease die within 1 year of diagnosis.

About two thirds of cholangiocarcinomas are located in the perihilar location. Perihilar cholangiocarcinomas, also referred to as Klatskin tumors, are further classified based on anatomic location by the Bismuth-Corlette classification (Fig. 32-7). Type I tumors are confined to the common hepatic duct, but type II tumors involve the bifurcation without involvement of the secondary intrahepatic ducts. Type IIIa and IIIb tumors extend into the right and left secondary intrahepatic ducts, respectively. Type IV tumors involve both the right and left secondary intrahepatic ducts. (See Schwartz 9th ed., p 1162.)

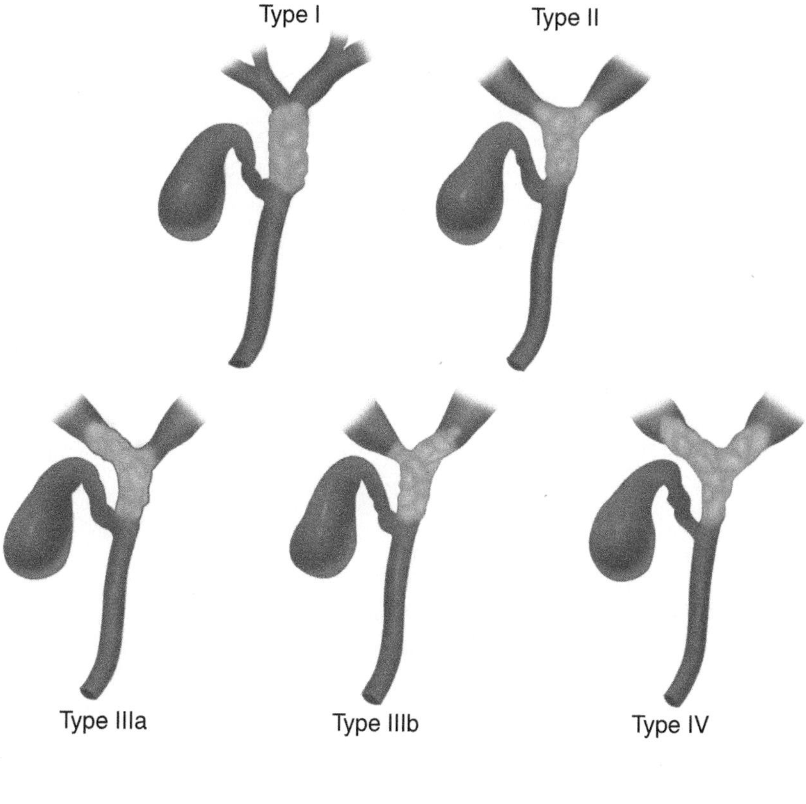
Type I
Type II
Type IIIa
Type IIIb
Type IV

FIG. 32-7. Bismuth-Corlette classification of bile duct tumors.

CHAPTER 33

Pancreas

BASIC SCIENCE QUESTIONS

1. The origin of the inferior pancreaticoduodenal artery is the
   A. Gastroduodenal artery
   B. Superior mesenteric artery
   C. Superior pancreaticoduodenal artery
   D. Common hepatic artery

Answer: B

The blood supply to the pancreas comes from multiple branches from the celiac and superior mesenteric arteries (Fig. 33-1). The common hepatic artery gives rise to the gastroduodenal artery before continuing toward the porta hepatis as the proper hepatic artery. The gastroduodenal artery becomes the superior pancreaticoduodenal artery as it passes behind the first portion of the duodenum and branches into the anterior and posterior superior pancreaticoduodenal arteries. As the superior mesenteric artery passes behind the neck of the pancreas, it gives off the inferior pancreaticoduodenal artery at the inferior margin of the neck of the pancreas. This vessel quickly divides into the anterior and posterior inferior pancreaticoduodenal arteries. The superior and inferior pancreaticoduodenal arteries join together within the parenchyma of the anterior and posterior sides of the head of the pancreas along the medial aspect of the C-loop of the duodenum to form arcades that give off numerous branches to the duodenum and head of the pancreas. Therefore, it is impossible to resect the head of the pancreas without devascularizing the duodenum, unless a rim of pancreas containing the pancreaticoduodenal arcade is preserved. (See Schwartz 9th ed., p 1171.)

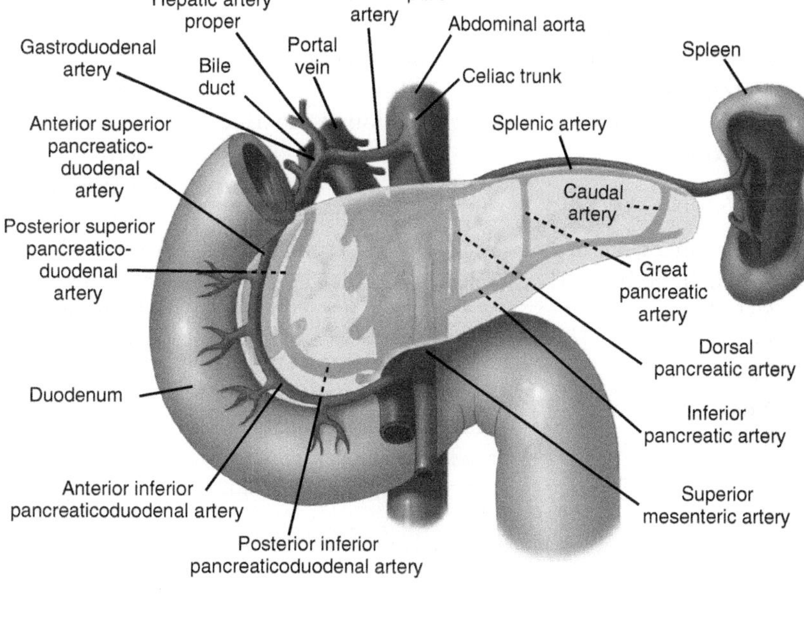

FIG. 33-1. Arterial supply to the pancreas. Multiple arcades in the head and body of the pancreas provide a rich blood supply. The head of the pancreas cannot be resected without devascularizing the duodenum unless a rim of pancreas containing the pancreaticoduodenal arcade is preserved.

2. Insulin secretion is stimulated by
   A. Lysine
   B. Somatostatin
   C. Amylin
   D. Alpha adrenergic stimulation

Answer: A

Oral glucose stimulates the release of enteric hormones such as gastric inhibitory peptide (also known as *glucose-dependent insulinotropic polypeptide* or *GIP*), glucagon-like peptide-1 (GLP-1), and CCK, that augment the secretion of insulin, and are therefore referred to as *incretins*.

Insulin secretion by the β-cell is also influenced by plasma levels of amino acids such as arginine, lysine, leucine, and free fatty acids. Glucagon, GIP, GLP-1, and CCK stimulate insulin release, while somatostatin, amylin, and pancreastatin inhibit insulin release. Cholinergic fibers and beta sympathetic fibers stimulate insulin release, while alpha sympathetic fibers inhibit insulin secretion. (See Schwartz 9th ed., p 1175.)

3. The highest concentration of PP (pancreatic polypeptide) cells is found in the
   A. Head of the pancreas
   B. Body of the pancreas
   C. Tail of the pancreas
   D. None of the above—they are equally distributed across the pancreas

Answer: A

The β- and δ-cells are evenly distributed throughout the pancreas, but islets in the head and uncinate process (ventral anlage) have a higher percentage of PP cells and fewer α-cells, whereas islets in the body and tail (dorsal anlage) contain the majority of α-cells and few PP cells. This is clinically significant because pancreatoduodenectomy removes 95% of the PP cells in the pancreas. This may partially explain the higher incidence of glucose intolerance after the Whipple procedure than after distal pancreatectomy. In addition, chronic pancreatitis, which disproportionately affects the pancreatic head, is associated with PP deficiency and pancreatogenic diabetes. (See Schwartz 9th ed., p 1177.)

4. Which of the following pancreatic enzymes is secreted in an active form?
   A. Amylase
   B. Chymotrypsinogen
   C. Tyrpsinogen
   D. Pepsin

Answer: A

Pancreatic amylase is secreted in its active form and completes the digestive process already begun by salivary amylase. Amylase is the only pancreatic enzyme secreted in its active form, and it hydrolyzes starch and glycogen to glucose, maltose, maltotriose, and dextrins.

The proteolytic enzymes are secreted as proenzymes that require activation. Trypsinogen is converted to its active form, trypsin, by another enzyme, enterokinase, which is produced by the duodenal mucosal cells. Trypsin, in turn, activates the other proteolytic enzymes. (See Schwartz 9th ed., p 1174.)

5. Sympathetic stimulation of the pancreas results in
   A. Stimulation of endocrine and exocrine secretion
   B. Inhibition of endocrine and exocrine secretion
   C. Stimulation of endocrine and inhibition of exocrine secretion
   D. Inhibition of endocrine and stimulation of exocrine secretion

Answer: B

The pancreas is innervated by the sympathetic and parasympathetic nervous systems. The acinar cells responsible for exocrine secretion, the islet cells responsible for endocrine secretion, and the islet vasculature are innervated by both systems. The parasympathetic system stimulates endocrine and exocrine secretion and the sympathetic system inhibits secretion. (See Schwartz 9th ed., p 1173.)

6. Somatostatin-28, one of the two active forms of somatostatin present in the human body, selectively binds to
   A. SSTR1
   B. SSTR3
   C. SSTR5
   D. None of the above

Answer: C

One gene encodes for a common precursor that is differentially processed to generate tissue-specific amounts of two bioactive products, somatostatin-14 and somatostatin-28. These peptides inhibit endocrine and exocrine secretion and affect neurotransmission, GI and biliary motility, intestinal absorption, vascular tone, and cell proliferation. Five different somatostatin receptors (SSTRs) have been cloned and the biologic properties of each are being unraveled. All five are G-protein-coupled receptors with seven highly conserved transmembrane domains and unique amino and carboxy termini. Phosphorylation sites located within the second and third intracellular loops and in the cytoplasmic C-terminal segment are thought to mediate receptor regulation. Although the naturally occurring peptides bind to all five receptors, somatostatin-28 is relatively selective for SSTR5. (See Schwartz 9th ed., p 1176.)

7. The most common gene mutation found in pancreatic cancer is
   A. HER2/*neu*
   B. K-*ras*
   C. *p53*
   D. *Smad 4*

Answer: B

Pancreatic carcinogenesis probably involves multiple mutations that are inherited and acquired throughout aging. The K-*ras* oncogene is currently thought to be the most commonly mutated gene in pancreatic cancer, with approximately 90% of tumors having a mutation. This prevalent mutation is present in precursor lesions and is therefore thought to occur early and be essential to pancreatic cancer development. K-*ras* mutations can be detected in DNA from serum, stool, pancreatic juice, and tissue aspirates of patients with pancreatic cancer, suggesting that the presence of this mutation may provide the basis for diagnostic testing in select individuals. The HER2/*neu* oncogene, homologous to the epidermal growth factor receptor (EGFr), is overexpressed in pancreatic cancers. This receptor is involved in signal transduction pathways that lead to cellular proliferation. Multiple tumor-suppressor genes are deleted and/or mutated in pancreatic cancer, and include *p53*, *p16*, and *DPC4* (*Smad 4*), and in a minority of cases, *BRCA2*. Most pancreatic cancers have three or more of the above mutations. (See Schwartz 9th ed., p 1220.)

8. Pancreatic delta cells produce
   A. Somatostatin
   B. Ghrelin
   C. Pancreatic polypeptide (PP)
   D. Glucagon

Answer: A

There are nearly 1 million islets of Langerhans in the normal adult pancreas. They vary greatly in size from 40 to 900 μm. Larger islets are located closer to the major arterioles and smaller islets are embedded more deeply in the parenchyma of the pancreas. Most islets contain 3000 to 4000 cells of five major types: alpha cells that secrete glucagon, β-cells that secrete insulin, delta cells that secrete somatostatin, epsilon cells that secrete ghrelin, and PP cells that secrete PP (Table 33-1). (See Schwartz 9th ed., p 1175.)

TABLE 33-1 Pancreatic islet peptide products

Hormones	Islet Cell	Functions
Insulin	β (beta cell)	Decreased gluconeogenesis, glycogenolysis, fatty acid breakdown, and ketogenesis Increased glycogenesis, protein synthesis
Glucagon	α (alpha cell)	Opposite effects of insulin; increased hepatic glycogenolysis and gluconeogenesis
Somatostatin	δ (delta cell)	Inhibits GI secretion Inhibits secretion and action of all GI endocrine peptides Inhibits cell growth
Pancreatic polypeptide	PP (PP cell)	Inhibits pancreatic exocrine secretion and section of insulin Facilitates hepatic effect of insulin
Amylin (IAPP)	β (beta cell)	Counterregulates insulin secretion and function
Pancreastatin	β (beta cell)	Decreases insulin and somatostatin release Increases glucagon release Decreases pancreatic exocrine secretion
Ghrelin	ε (epsilon cell)	Decreases insulin release and insulin action

IAPP = islet amyloid polypeptide.

9. Pancreatic acinar cells secrete
   A. Lipases
   B. Amylase
   C. Proteases
   D. All of the above

Answer: D

The acinar cells secrete amylase, proteases, and lipases, enzymes responsible for the digestion of all three food types: carbohydrate, protein, and fat. The acinar cells are pyramid-shaped, with their apices facing the lumen of the acinus. Near the apex of each cell are numerous enzyme-containing zymogen granules that fuse with the apical cell membrane. Unlike the endocrine pancreas, where islet cells specialize in the secretion of one hormone type, individual acinar cells secrete all types of enzymes. However, the ratio of the different enzymes released is adjusted to the composition of digested food through nonparallel regulation of secretion. (See Schwartz 9th ed., p 1174, and Table 33-2.)

TABLE 33-2 Pancreatic enzymes

Enzyme	Substrate	Product
Carbohydrate		
Amylase (active)	Starch, glycogen	Glucose, maltose, maltotriose, dextrins
Protein		
Endopeptidases	Cleave bonds between amino acids	Amino acids, dipeptides
Trypsinogen (inactive) —Enterokinase→ Trypsin (active)		
Chymotrypsinogen (inactive) —Enterokinase/Trypsin→ Chymotrypsin (active)		
Proelastase (inactive) —Enterokinase/Trypsin→ Elastase (active)		
Exopeptidases	Cleave amino acids from end of peptide chains	—
Procarboxy peptidase A&B (inactive) —Enterokinase→ Carboxypeptidase A&B (active)		
Fat		
Pancreatic lipase (active)	Triglycerides	2-Monoglycerides fatty acids
Phospholipase A2 (inactive) —Trypsin→ Phospholipase A2 (active)	Phospholipase	—
Cholesterol esterase	Neutral lipids	—

10. Which of the following is the primary stimulus for secretion of bicarbonate by the pancreas?
   A. CCK
   B. Gastrin
   C. Acetylcholine
   D. Secretin

Answer: D

The hormone secretin is released from cells in the duodenal mucosa in response to acidic chyme passing through the pylorus into the duodenum. Secretin is the major stimulant for bicarbonate secretion, which buffers the acidic fluid entering the duodenum from the stomach. CCK also stimulates bicarbonate secretion, but to a much lesser extent than secretin. CCK potentiates secretin-stimulated bicarbonate secretion. Gastrin and acetylcholine, both stimulants of gastric acid secretion, are also weak stimulants of pancreatic bicarbonate secretion. (See Schwartz 9th ed., p 1175.)

11. Approximately what percentage of the population has a replaced right hepatic artery?
   A. <2%
   B. 5%
   C. 10%
   D. 15%

Answer: D

Variations in the arterial anatomy occur in one out of five patients. The right hepatic artery, common hepatic artery, or gastroduodenal arteries can arise from the superior mesenteric artery. In 15 to 20% of patients, the right hepatic artery will arise from the superior mesenteric artery and travel upwards toward the liver along the posterior aspect of the head of the pancreas (referred to as a *replaced right hepatic artery*). It is important to look for this variation on preoperative computed tomographic (CT) scans and in the operating room so the replaced hepatic artery is recognized and injury is avoided. (See Schwartz 9th ed., p 1171.)

12. The veins of the head of the pancreas drain into the
    A. Anterior surface of the portal vein
    B. Posterolateral surface of the portal vein
    C. Right renal vein
    D. Inferior vena cava

Answer: B

Venous branches draining the pancreatic head and uncinate process enter along the right lateral and posterior sides of the portal vein. There are usually no anterior venous tributaries, and a plane can usually be developed between the neck of the pancreas and the portal and superior mesenteric veins during pancreatic resection, unless the tumor is invading the vein anteriorly. (See Schwartz 9th ed., p 1171, and Fig. 33-2.)

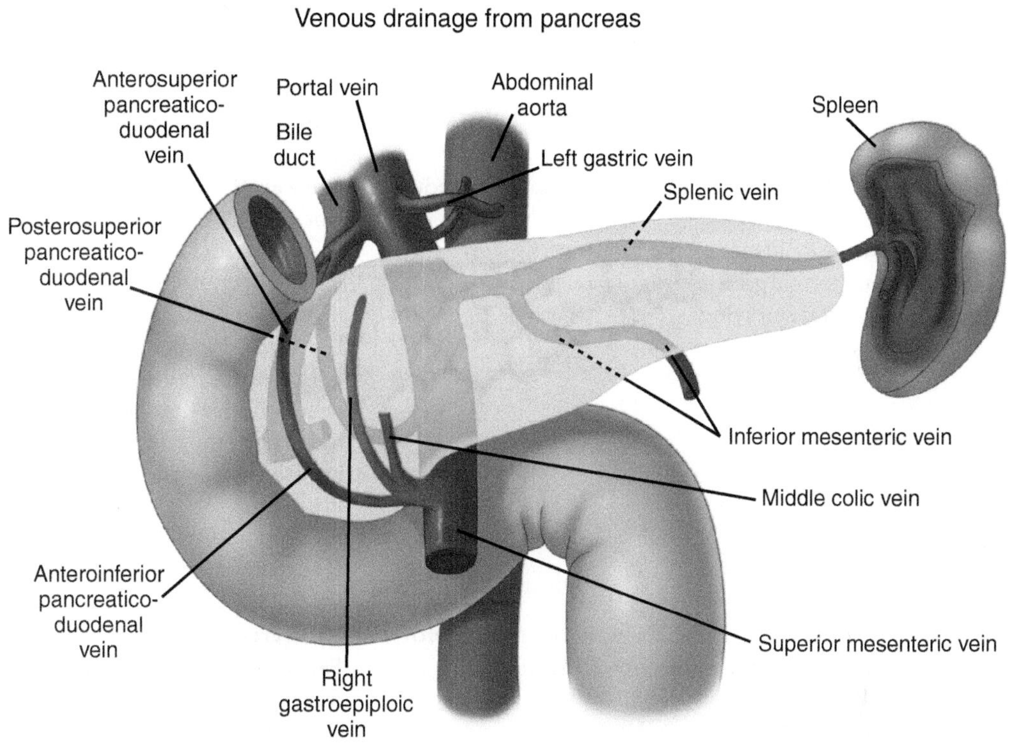

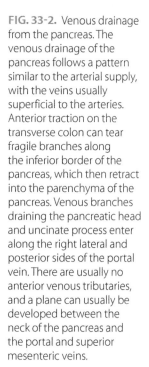

FIG. 33-2. Venous drainage from the pancreas. The venous drainage of the pancreas follows a pattern similar to the arterial supply, with the veins usually superficial to the arteries. Anterior traction on the transverse colon can tear fragile branches along the inferior border of the pancreas, which then retract into the parenchyma of the pancreas. Venous branches draining the pancreatic head and uncinate process enter along the right lateral and posterior sides of the portal vein. There are usually no anterior venous tributaries, and a plane can usually be developed between the neck of the pancreas and the portal and superior mesenteric veins.

CLINICAL QUESTIONS

1. Which of the following is NOT a cause of elevated gastrin?
   A. Proton pump inhibitors
   B. Gastric outlet obstruction
   C. Chronic pancreatitis
   D. Pernicious anemia

Answer: C

The diagnosis of [Zollinger-Ellison syndrome (due to excess gastrin secretion by a gastrinoma)] is made by measuring the serum gastrin level. It is important that patients stop taking proton pump inhibitors for this test. In most patients with gastrinomas, the level is >1000 pg/mL. Gastrin levels can be elevated in conditions other than ZES. Common causes of hypergastrinemia include pernicious anemia, treatment with proton pump inhibitors, renal failure, G-cell hyperplasia, atrophic gastritis, retained or excluded antrum, and gastric outlet obstruction. In equivocal cases, when the gastrin level is not markedly elevated, a secretin stimulation test is helpful. (See Schwartz 9th ed., p 1218.)

2. Which of the following should be ordered in a patient with a gastrinoma?
   A. Serum vitamin D level
   B. Serum calcium
   C. Serum B12 level
   D. Stool occult blood

Answer: B

It is important to rule out MEN1 syndrome by checking serum calcium levels before surgery because resection of the gastrinoma(s) in these patients rarely results in normalization of serum gastrin concentrations or a prolongation of survival. Only one fourth of gastrinomas occur in association with the MEN1 syndrome. One half of patients with gastrinomas will have solitary tumors while the remainder will have multiple gastrinomas. Multiple tumors are more common in patients with MEN1 syndrome. Aggressive surgical treatment is justified in patients with sporadic gastrinomas. If patients have MEN1 syndrome, the parathyroid hyperplasia is addressed with total parathyroidectomy and implantation of parathyroid tissue in the forearm. (See Schwartz 9th ed., p 1219.)

3. Preservation of the pylorus during the Whipple procedure may
   A. Increase the incidence of marginal ulcers
   B. Maintain normal gastric hormone release
   C. Impair gastric emptying
   D. Improve quality of life

Answer: B

The preservation of the pylorus has several theoretical advantages, including prevention of reflux of pancreaticobiliary secretions into the stomach, decreased incidence of marginal ulceration, normal gastric acid secretion and hormone release, and improved gastric function. Patients with pylorus-preserving resections have appeared to regain weight better than historic controls in some studies. Return of gastric emptying in the immediate postoperative period may take longer after the pylorus-preserving operation, and it is controversial whether there is any significant improvement in long-term quality of life with pyloric preservation. (See Schwartz 9th ed., p 1226.)

4. Which of the following drugs has been shown to improve outcome in patients with mild pancreatitis?
   A. H_2 blockers
   B. Somatostatin
   C. Glucagon
   D. None of the above

Answer: D

Pancreatitis is classified as mild when the patient has no systemic complications, low APACHE-II scores and Ransons signsand sustained clinical improvement and when a CT scan rules out necrotizing pancreatitis. The treatment then is mostly supportive and has the important aim of *resting the pancreas* through restriction of oral food and fluids. Nasogastric suction and H_2-blockers have routinely been used in this connection, based on the reasoning that even the smallest amount of gastric acid reaching the duodenum could stimulate pancreatic secretion. However, these measures are of little value. The following secretion-inhibiting drugs have also been tried without notable success: atropine, calcitonin, somatostatin, glucagon, and fluorouracil. (See Schwartz 9th ed., p 1184, and Fig. 33-3.)

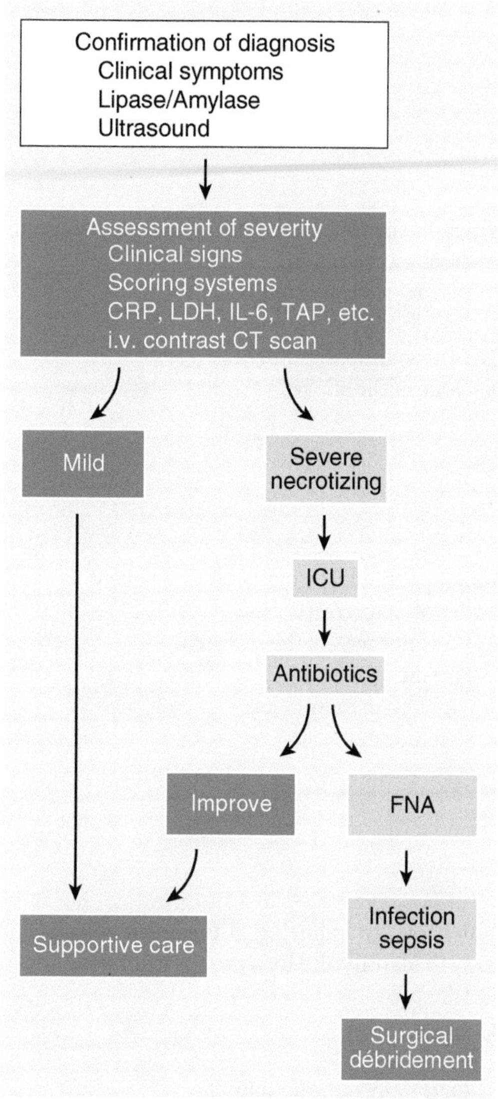

FIG. 33-3. Algorithm for managing acute pancreatitis. CRP = C-reactive protein; CT = computed tomography; FNA = fine-needle aspiration; ICU = intensive care unit; IL-6 = interleukin 6; LDH = lactate dehydrogenase; TAP = trypsinogen activation peptide.

5. Which of the following procedures is the best treatment for a 1.5-cm insulinoma located in the mid pancreas?
   A. Enucleation
   B. Wedge resection
   C. Distal pancreatectomy
   D. Duodenal sparing total pancreatectomy

Answer: A

Unlike most endocrine pancreatic tumors, the majority (90%) of insulinomas are benign and solitary, and only 10% are malignant. They are typically cured by simple enucleation. However, tumors located close to the main pancreatic duct and large (>2 cm) tumors may require a distal pancreatectomy or pancreaticoduodenectomy. Intraoperative US is useful to determine the tumor's relation to the main pancreatic duct and guides intraoperative decision making. Enucleation of solitary insulinomas and distal pancreatectomy for insulinoma can sometimes be performed using a minimally invasive technique. (See Schwartz 9th ed., p 1218.)

6. The most common type of pancreatic cancer is
   A. Ductal adenocarcinoma
   B. Adenosquamous carcinoma
   C. Acinar cell carcinoma
   D. Squamous cell carcinoma

Answer: A

In addition to ductal adenocarcinoma, which makes up about 75% of nonendocrine cancers of the pancreas, there are a variety of less common types of pancreatic cancer. Adenosquamous carcinoma is a variant that has both glandular and squamous differentiation. The biologic behavior of this lesion is unfortunately no better than the typical ductal adenocarcinoma. Acinar cell carcinoma is an uncommon type of pancreatic cancer that usually presents as a large tumor, often 10 cm in diameter or more, but the prognosis of patients with these tumors may be better than with ductal cancer. (See Schwartz 9th ed., p 1220.)

7. Which of the following techniques decreases the risk of pancreatic anastomotic leak in the Whipple procedure?
   A. End-to-side anastomosis
   B. Side-to-side anastomosis
   C. Duct to mucosa sutures
   D. None of the above

Answer: D

Techniques for the pancreaticojejunostomy include end-to-side or end-to-end and duct-to-mucosa sutures or invagination. Pancreaticogastrostomy has also been investigated. Some surgeons use stents, glue to seal the anastomosis, or octreotide to decrease pancreatic secretions. No matter what combination of these techniques is used, the pancreatic leakage rate is always about 10%. Therefore, the choice of techniques depends more on the surgeon's personal experience. (See Schwartz 9th ed., p 1227.)

8. Which of the following is often adjacent to the inferior border of a pancreatic pseudocyst?
   A. Posterior wall of the stomach
   B. Splenic vein
   C. Transverse mesocolon
   D. Left kidney

Answer: C

Pancreatic pseudocysts commonly develop in the area of the lesser sac, and the posterior aspect of the stomach can form the anterior wall of the pseudocyst, allowing drainage into the stomach. The base of the transverse mesocolon attaches to the inferior margin of the body and tail of the pancreas. The transverse mesocolon often forms the inferior wall of pancreatic pseudocysts or inflammatory processes allowing surgical drainage through the transverse mesocolon. (See Schwartz 9th ed., p 1168.)

9. Which of the following is the most sensitive imaging study to identify and localize a gastrinoma?
   A. CT scan
   B. MRI
   C. PET scan
   D. Octreotide scintigraphy

Answer: D

In 70 to 90% of patients, the primary gastrinoma is found in Passaro's triangle, an area defined by a triangle with points located at the junction of the cystic duct and common bile duct, the second and third portion of the duodenum, and the neck and body of the pancreas. However, because gastrinomas can be found almost anywhere, whole-body imaging is required. The test of choice is SSTR (octreotide) scintigraphy in combination with CT. The octreotide scan is more sensitive than CT, locating about 85% of gastrinomas and detecting tumors <1 cm. With the octreotide scan, the need for tedious and technically demanding selective angiography and measurement of gastrin gradients has declined. EUS is another new modality that assists in the preoperative localization of gastrinomas. It is particularly helpful in localizing tumors in the pancreatic head or duodenal wall, where gastrinomas are usually <1 cm in size. A combination of octreotide scan and EUS detects >90% of gastrinomas. (See Schwartz 9th ed., p 1218.)

10. Which of the following is suggestive of malignancy in a cystic lesion of the pancreas?
    A. Elevated LDH in the cyst fluid
    B. Cyst wall >3 mm in thickness
    C. Thick, mucinous fluid in the cyst cavity
    D. Hemorrhagic fluid in the cyst cavity

Answer: C

A cystic neoplasm needs to be considered when a patient presents with a fluid-containing pancreatic lesion. Cystic neoplasms of the pancreas may be more frequent than previously recognized and are being identified with increasing frequency as the use of abdominal CT scanning has increased. Most of these lesions are benign or slow growing, and the prognosis is significantly better than with pancreatic adenocarcinoma. However, some of these neoplasms slowly undergo malignant transformation and thus represent an opportunity for surgical cure, which is exceedingly uncommon in the setting of pancreatic adenocarcinoma. Cysts that contain thick fluid with mucin, elevated carcinoembryonic antigen (CEA), or atypical cells must be treated as potentially malignant (Fig. 33-4). (See Schwartz 9th ed., p 1232.)

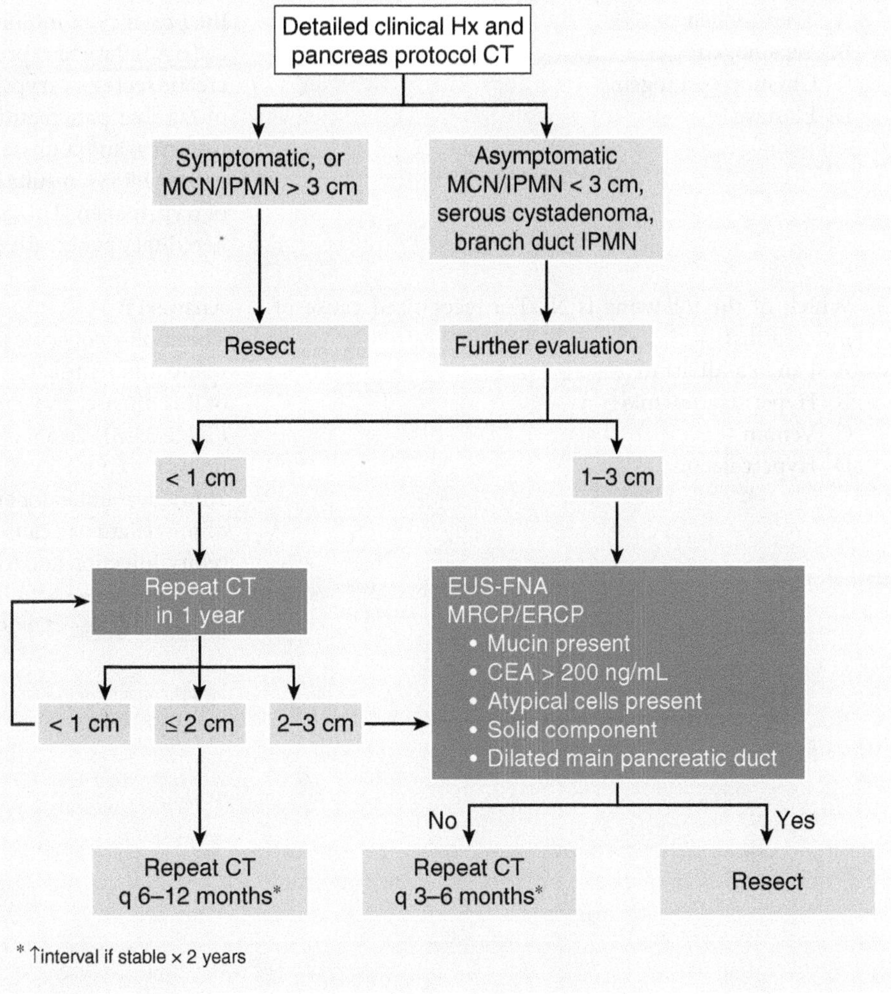

FIG. 33-4. Algorithm for management of pancreatic cystic neoplasms. CEA = carcinoembryonic antigen; CT = computed tomography; ERCP = endoscopic retrograde cholangiopancreatography; EUS = endoscopic ultrasound; FNA = fine-needle aspiration; Hx = history; IPMN = intraductal papillary mucinous neoplasm of the pancreas; MCN = mucinous cystic neoplasm; MRCP = magnetic resonance cholangiopancreatography.

11. The most common location for a VIPoma is
    A. Head of the pancreas
    B. Tail of the pancreas
    C. Passaro's triangle
    D. Duodenal wall

Answer: B

In 1958, Verner and Morrison first described the syndrome associated with a pancreatic neoplasm secreting VIP. The classic clinical syndrome associated with this pancreatic endocrine neoplasm consists of severe intermittent watery diarrhea leading to dehydration, and weakness from fluid and electrolyte losses. Large amounts of potassium are lost in the stool. The *vasoactive intestinal peptidesecreting tumor (VIPoma) syndrome* is also called the *WDHA syndrome* due to the presence of watery *d*iarrhea, *h*ypokalemia, and *a*chlorhydria. The massive (5 L/d) and episodic nature of the diarrhea associated with the appropriate electrolyte abnormalities should raise suspicion of the diagnosis. Serum VIP levels must be measured on multiple occasions because the excess secretion of VIP is episodic, and single measurements might be normal and misleading. A CT scan localizes most VIPomas, although as with all islet cell tumors, EUS is the most sensitive imaging method. Electrolyte and fluid balance is sometimes difficult to correct preoperatively and must be pursued aggressively. Somatostatin analogues are helpful in controlling the diarrhea and allowing replacement of fluid and electrolytes. VIPomas are more commonly located in the distal pancreas and most have spread outside the pancreas. (See Schwartz 9th ed., p 1219.)

12. Failure to inhibit activation of which of the following enzymes can cause familial pancreatitis?
    A. Trypsinogen
    B. Pepsinogen
    C. Chymotrypsinogen
    D. Elastase

Answer: A

Trypsinogen activation within the pancreas is prevented by the presence of inhibitors that are also secreted by the acinar cells. A failure to express a normal trypsinogen inhibitor, pancreatic secretory trypsin inhibitor (PSTI) or *SPINK1*, is a cause of familial pancreatitis. Trypsinogen is expressed in several isoforms, and a missense mutation on the cationic trypsinogen, or *PRSS1*, results in premature, intrapancreatic activation of trypsinogen. This accounts for about two-thirds of cases of hereditary pancreatitis. (See Schwartz 9th ed., p 1174.)

13. Which of the following is NOT a recognized cause of pancreatitis?
    A. Pancreas divisum
    B. Hypermagnesemia
    C. Venom
    D. Hypercalcemia

Answer: B

The etiology of acute pancreatitis is a complex subject because many different factors have been implicated in the causation of this disease, and sometimes there are no identifiable causes (Table 33-3). Two factors, biliary tract stone disease and alcoholism, account for 80 to 90% of the cases. The remaining 10 to 20% is accounted for either by idiopathic disease or by a variety of miscellaneous causes including trauma, surgery, drugs, heredity, infection and toxins. (See Schwartz 9th ed., p 1178.)

TABLE 33-3 Etiologies of acute pancreatitis

Alcohol
Biliary tract disease
Hyperlipidemia
Hereditary
Hypercalcemia
Trauma
External
Surgical
Endoscopic retrograde cholangiopancreatography
Ischemia
Hypoperfusion
Atheroembolic
Vasculitis
Pancreatic duct obstruction
Neoplasms
Pancreas divisum
Ampullary and duodenal lesions
Infections
Venom
Drugs
Idiopathic

Source: Reproduced with permission from Yeo CJ, Cameron JL: Exocrine pancreas, in Townsend CM et al (eds): *Sabiston's Textbook of Surgery*. Philadelphia: Saunders, 2000, p 1117. Copyright © Elsevier.

14. Which of the following CT findings is NOT considered a sign that a pancreatic tumor is unresectable?
    A. Enlarged lymph nodes outside the boundary of resection
    B. Ascites
    C. Invasion of the superior mesenteric vein
    D. Invasion of the superior mesenteric artery

Answer: C

CT findings that indicate a tumor is unresectable include invasion of the hepatic or superior mesenteric artery, enlarged lymph nodes outside the boundaries of resection, ascites, and distant metastases (e.g., liver). Invasion of the superior mesenteric vein or portal vein is not in itself a contraindication to resection as long as the veins are patent. In contrast, CT scanning is less accurate in predicting resectable disease. CT scanning will miss small liver metastases, and predicting arterial involvement is sometimes difficult. (See Schwartz 9th ed., p 1222.)

15. Serum amylase rises at the onset of pancreatitis and remains elevated for
   A. 24 hours
   B. 48 hours
   C. 3-5 days
   D. 7-10 days

Answer: C
Serum amylase concentration increases almost immediately with the onset of disease and peaks within several hours. It remains elevated for 3 to 5 days before returning to normal. There is no significant correlation between the magnitude of serum amylase elevation and severity of pancreatitis; in fact, a milder form of acute pancreatitis is often associated with higher levels of serum amylase as compared with that in a more severe form of the disease.

Other pancreatic enzymes also have been evaluated to improve the diagnostic accuracy of serum measurements. Specificity of these markers ranges from 77 to 96%, the highest being for lipase. Because serum levels of lipase remain elevated for a longer time than total or p-amylase, it is the serum indicator of highest probability of the disease. (See Schwartz 9th ed., p 1182.)

16. Which of the following is NOT a risk factor for pancreatic cancer?
   A. Age >60
   B. African American race
   C. Smoking
   D. Female gender

Answer: D
Pancreatic cancer is more common in the elderly with most patients being >60 years old. Pancreatic cancer is more common in African Americans and slightly more common in men than women. The risk of developing pancreatic cancer is two to three times higher if a parent or sibling had the disease. Another risk factor that is consistently linked to pancreatic cancer is cigarette smoking. Smoking increases the risk of developing pancreatic cancer by at least twofold due to the carcinogens in cigarette smoke. Coffee and alcohol consumption have been investigated as possible risk factors, but the data are inconsistent. As in other GI cancers, diets high in fat and low in fiber, fruits, and vegetables are thought to be associated with an increased risk of pancreatic cancer. (See Schwartz 9th ed., p 1220.)

17. The "fish eye" sign, or mucin extruding from the ampulla of Vater during ERCP, is virtually pathognomonic for
   A. Cystadenoma of the pancreas
   B. Mucinous cystadenoma
   C. Intraductal papillary mucinous neoplasm
   D. Mucinous adenocarcinoma of the pancreas

Answer: C
At ERCP, mucin can be seen extruding from the ampulla of Vater, a so-called *fish-eye lesion*, that is virtually diagnostic of IPMN.

Intraductal papillary mucinous neoplasms (IPMNs) usually occur within the head of the pancreas and arise within the pancreatic ducts. The ductal epithelium forms a papillary projection into the duct, and mucin production causes intraluminal cystic dilation of the pancreatic ducts. Patients are usually in their seventh to eighth decade of life and present with abdominal pain or recurrent pancreatitis, thought to be caused by obstruction of the pancreatic duct by thick mucin. Some patients (5 to 10%) have steatorrhea, diabetes, and weight loss secondary to pancreatic insufficiency. (See Schwartz 9th ed., p 1234.)

18. Which of the following analgesic drugs should NOT be used in a patient with pancreatitis?
   A. Meperidine
   B. Morphine
   C. Buprenorphine
   D. Pentazocine

Answer: B
The severe pain of acute pancreatitis prevents the patient from resting, and results in ongoing cholinergic discharge, which stimulates gastric and pancreatic secretion. Therefore, pain management is of great importance. Administration of buprenorphine, pentazocine, procaine hydrochloride, and meperidine are all of value in controlling abdominal pain. Morphine is to be avoided, due to its potential to cause sphincter of Oddi spasm. (See Schwartz 9th ed., p 1184.)

19. The most common complication of chronic pancreatitis is
    A. Hemorrhage
    B. Necrotizing infection
    C. Pseudocyst
    D. Duodenal obstruction

Answer: C

A chronic collection of pancreatic fluid surrounded by a nonepithelialized wall of granulation tissue and fibrosis is referred to as a *pseudocyst*. Pseudocysts occur in up to 10% of patients with acute pancreatitis, and in 20 to 38% of patients with chronic pancreatitis, and thus, they comprise the most common complication of chronic pancreatitis. (See Schwartz 9th ed., p 1200, and Table 33-4.)

TABLE 33-4 Complications of chronic pancreatitis

Intrapancreatic complications
Pseudocysts
Duodenal or gastric obstruction
Thrombosis of splenic vein
Abscess
Perforation
Erosion into visceral artery
Inflammatory mass in head of pancreas
Bile duct stenosis
Portal vein thrombosis
Duodenal obstruction
Duct strictures and/or stones
Ductal hypertension and dilatation
Pancreatic carcinoma
Extrapancreatic complications
Pancreatic duct leak with ascites or fistula
Pseudocyst extension beyond lesser sac into mediastinum, retroperitoneum, lateral pericolic spaces, pelvis, or adjacent viscera

20. Appropriate management of a patient with an asymptomatic 3-cm cystadenoma of the tail of the pancreas is
    A. Observation and serial CT scans
    B. Percutaneous cyst aspiration and sclerosis
    C. Enucleation
    D. Distal pancreatectomy

Answer: A

Serous cystadenomas are essentially considered benign tumors without malignant potential. Serous cystadenocarcinoma has been reported very rarely (<1%). Therefore, malignant potential should not be used as an argument for surgical resection, and the majority of these lesions can be safely observed in the absence of symptoms due to mass effect or rapid growth.

All regions of the pancreas are affected, with half of cystadenomas found in the head/uncinate process, and half in the neck, body, or tail of the pancreas. They have a spongy appearance, and multiple small cysts (microcystic) are more common than larger cysts (macrocystic or oligocystic). These lesions contain thin serous fluid that does not stain positive for mucin and is low in CEA (<200 ng/mL). Typical imaging characteristics include a well-circumscribed cystic mass, small septations, fluid close to water density, and sometimes, a central scar with calcification. If a conservative management is adopted, it is important to be sure of the diagnosis. EUS-FNA should yield nonviscous fluid with low CEA and amylase levels, and if cells are obtained, which is rare, they are cuboidal and have a clear cytoplasm. (See Schwartz 9th ed., p 1233.)

21. Which of the following is NOT an indication for diagnostic laparoscopy to determine respectability in a patient with pancreatic cancer?
    A. CT demonstrates respectable disease
    B. CA19-9 is high
    C. Tumor size <2 cm
    D. Ascites

Answer: C

Diagnostic laparoscopy is possibly best applied to patients with pancreatic cancer on a selective basis. Diagnostic laparoscopy will have a higher yield in patients with large tumors (>4 cm), tumors located in the body or tail, patients with equivocal findings of metastasis or CT scan, ascites, high CA 19-9, or marked weight loss. (See Schwartz 9th ed, pp 1223, 1224 and Fig. 33-5.)

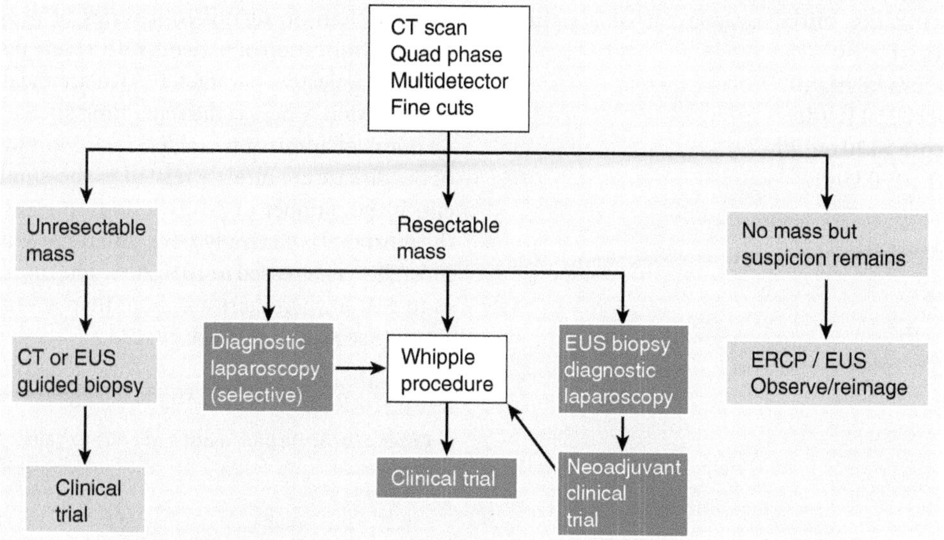

FIG. 33-5. Diagnostic and treatment algorithm for pancreatic cancer. If computed tomography (CT) scan demonstrates a potentially resectable tumor, patients are offered participation in a clinical trial after histologic confirmation by CT or endoscopic ultrasound (EUS)-guided biopsy. If CT scan demonstrates resectable disease, diagnostic laparoscopy is used selectively in patients with tumors in the body/tail, equivocal findings of metastasis or CT scan, ascites, high CA19-9, or marked weight loss. Patients also have diagnostic laparoscopy if they elect to participate in a neoadjuvant clinical trial. In cases where no mass is demonstrated on CT scan, but suspicion of cancer remains, EUS or endoscopic retrograde cholangiopancreatography (ERCP) with brushings are performed, and the CT may be repeated after an interval of observation.

22. Which of the following is the preferred treatment for a persistent pseudocyst after traumatic injury to the pancreas?
    A. External drainage
    B. Endoscopic stenting of the pancreatic duct
    C. Cystgastrostomy
    D. Cystjejunostomy

Answer: B

Because pseudocysts often communicate with the pancreatic ductal system, two newer approaches to pseudocyst management are based on main duct drainage, rather than pseudocyst drainage per se. Transpapillary stents inserted at the time of ERCP may be directed into a pseudocyst through the ductal communication itself, or can be left across the area of suspected duct leakage to facilitate decompression and cyst drainage, analogous to the use of common bile duct stents in the setting of a cystic duct leak. In a surgical series of patients with chronic pancreatitis, ductal dilatation, and a coexisting pseudocyst, Nealon and Walser showed that duct drainage alone, without a separate cystoenteric anastomosis, was as successful as a combined drainage procedure. Furthermore, the 'duct drainage only' group enjoyed a shorter hospital stay and fewer complications than the group who underwent a separate cystoenterostomy. These observations suggest that transductal drainage may be a safe and effective approach to the management of pseudocystic disease. The endoscopic approach seems logical in the treatment of postoperative or posttraumatic pseudocysts when duct disruption is documented or in those patients with pseudocysts that communicate with the duct. (See Schwartz 9th ed., p 1202.)

23. The most common endocrine tumor of the pancreas is
    A. Gastrinoma
    B. Glucagonoma
    C. Insulinoma
    D. Somatostatinoma

Answer: C

Insulinomas are the most common pancreatic endocrine neoplasms and present with a typical clinical syndrome known as Whipple's triad. The triad consists of symptomatic fasting hypoglycemia, a documented serum glucose level <50 mg/dL, and relief of symptoms with the administration of glucose. (See Schwartz 9th ed., p 1217.)

24. Which of the following is one of Ranson's criteria determined during the initial assessment of a patient with pancreatitis?
    A. Serum calcium <8 mg/dL
    B. Serum LDH >350 IU/dL
    C. Blood glucose >120 mg/dL
    D. Serum AST >150 U/dL

Answer: B

In 1974, Ranson identified a series of prognostic signs for early identification of patients with severe pancreatitis. Out of these 11 objective parameters, five are measured at the time of admission, whereas the remaining six are measured within 48 hours of admission (Table 33-5). Morbidity and mortality of the disease are directly related to the number of signs present. If the number of positive Ranson signs is less than two, the mortality is generally zero; with three to five positive signs, mortality is increased to 10 to 20%. The mortality rate increases to >50% when there are more than seven positive Ranson signs. (See Schwartz 9th ed., p 1183.)

TABLE 33-5 Ranson's prognostic signs of pancreatitis

Criteria for acute pancreatitis not due to gallstones	
At admission	During the initial 48 h
Age >55 y	Hematocrit fall >10 points
WBC >16,000/mm^3	BUN elevation >5 mg/dL
Blood glucose >200 mg/dL	Serum calcium <8 mg/dL
Serum LDH >350 IU/L	Arterial Po_2 <60 mm Hg
Serum AST >250 U/dL	Base deficit >4 mEq/L
	Estimated fluid sequestration >6 L
Criteria for acute gallstone pancreatitis	
At admission	During the initial 48 h
Age >70 y	Hematocrit fall >10 points
WBC >18,000/mm^3	BUN elevation >2 mg/dL
Blood glucose >220 mg/dL	Serum calcium <8 mg/dL
Serum LDH >400 IU/L	Base deficit >5 mEq/L
Serum AST >250 U/dL	Estimated fluid sequestration >4 L

AST = aspartate transaminase; BUN = blood urea nitrogen; LDH = lactate dehydrogenase; Po_2 = partial pressure of oxygen; WBC = white blood cell count.
Source: Data from Ranson JHC: Etiological and prognostic factors in human acute pancreatitis: A review. *Am J Gastroenterol* 77:633, 1982. From Macmillan Publishers Ltd. Ranson JH, Rifkind KM, Roses DF, et al: Prognostic signs and the role of operative management in acute pancreatitis. *Surg Gynecol Obstet* 139:69, 1974.

25. Which of the following is the most sensitive diagnostic test for chronic pancreatitis?
    A. Serum amylase
    B. Serum lipase
    C. Postprandial pancreatic polypeptide hormone
    D. Oral glucose tolerance test

Answer: C

The direct measurement of pancreatic enzymes (e.g., lipase and amylase) by blood test is highly sensitive and fairly specific in acute pancreatitis but is seldom helpful in the diagnosis of chronic pancreatitis. The pancreatic endocrine product that correlates most strongly with chronic pancreatitis is the PP response to a test meal. Severe chronic pancreatitis is associated with a blunted or absent PP response to feeding but, as with many other tests, a normal PP response does not rule out the presence of early disease. (See Schwartz 9th ed., p 1198.)

26. At the time of laparotomy, which of the following is a contraindication to proceeding with a Whipple resection?
    A. Duodenal invasion
    B. Pyloric invasion
    C. Clinically positive hilar lymph nodes
    D. Clinically positive peripancreatic nodes

Answer: C

Hepatic hilar node involvement is a contraindication to proceeding with the Whipple procedure (Table 33-6). Enlarged or firm lymph nodes that can be swept down toward the head of the pancreas with the specimen do not preclude resection. Invasion of the duodenum or pylorus is not a contraindication to resection. (See Schwartz 9th ed., p 1225.)

TABLE 33-6	Findings at exploration
Findings contraindicating resection	
Liver metastases (any size)	
Celiac lymph node involvement	
Peritoneal implants	
Hepatic hilar lymph node involvement	
Findings not contraindicating resection	
Invasion at duodenum or distal stomach	
Involved peripancreatic lymph nodes	
Involved lymph nodes along the porta hepatis that can be swept down with the specimen	

27. Patients with gallstone pancreatitis should undergo cholecystectomy
    A. Emergently (within the first 12-24 hours of admission)
    B. Within 48-72 hours of admission
    C. Following ERCP
    D. 4-6 weeks after resolution of symptoms

Answer: B

General consensus favors either urgent intervention (cholecystectomy) within the first 48 to 72 hours of admission, or briefly delayed intervention (after 72 hours, but during the initial hospitalization) to give an inflamed pancreas time to recover. Cholecystectomy and operative common duct clearance is probably the best treatment for otherwise healthy patients with obstructive pancreatitis. However, patients who are at high risk for surgical intervention are best treated by endoscopic sphincterotomy, with clearance of stones by ERCP. In the case of acute biliary pancreatitis in which chemical studies suggest that the obstruction persists after 24 hours of observation, emergency endoscopic sphincterotomy and stone extraction is indicated. Routine ERCP for examination of the bile duct is discouraged in cases of biliary pancreatitis, as the probability of finding residual stones is low, and the risk of ERCP-induced pancreatitis is significant. (See Schwartz 9th ed., p 1186.)

28. What percentage of patients who consume 100 to 150 g (7-10 drinks) of alcohol per day will develop pancreatitis?
    A. 1-3%
    B. 10-15%
    C. 20-30%
    D. 50-65%

Answer: B

The nature of alcohol consumed (i.e., beer, wine, or hard liquor) is less significant than a daily intake of between 100 and 150 g of ethanol. Between 10 and 15% of individuals with this degree of alcohol intake go on to develop pancreatitis, while a similar proportion develop cirrhosis of the liver. (See Schwartz 9th ed., p 1179.)

29. The most common cause of chronic pancreatitis is
    A. Alcohol consumption
    B. Hypertriglyceridemia
    C. Autoimmune pancreatitis
    D. Hereditary pancreatitis

Answer: A

Worldwide, alcohol consumption and abuse is associated with chronic pancreatitis in up to 70% of cases. In 1878, Friedreich proposed that 'a general chronic interstitial pancreatitis may result from excessive alcoholism (drunkard's pancreas).' Since that observation, numerous studies have shown that a causal relationship exists between alcohol and chronic pancreatitis, but the prevalence of this etiology of the disease in Western countries ranges widely, from 38 to 94%. Other major causes worldwide include tropical (nutritional) and idiopathic disease, as well as hereditary causes.

There is a linear relationship between exposure to alcohol and the development of chronic pancreatitis. The risk of disease is present in patients with even a low or occasional exposure to alcohol (1 to 20 g/d), so there is no threshold level of alcohol exposure below which there is no risk of developing chronic pancreatitis. Furthermore, although the risk of disease is dose related, and highest in heavy (150 g/d) drinkers, <15% of confirmed alcohol abusers suffer from chronic pancreatitis. (See Schwartz 9th ed., p 1186, and Table 33-7.)

TABLE 33-7	Etiology of chronic pancreatitis
Alcohol, 70%	
Idiopathic (including tropical), 20%	
Other, 10%	
Hereditary	
Hyperparathyroidism	
Hypertriglyceridemia	
Autoimmune pancreatitis	
Obstruction	
Trauma	
Pancreas divisum	

30. Which of the following is the most commonly used initial treatment for pancreatic ascites?
    A. Octreotide, bowel rest, TPN
    B. Endoscopic stenting of the pancreatic duct
    C. Roux-en-Y pancreaticojejunostomy
    D. Distal pancreatectomy

Answer: A
ERCP is most helpful to delineate the location of the pancreatic duct leak in patients with pancreatic ascites and to elucidate the underlying pancreatic ductal anatomy. Pancreatic duct stenting may be considered at the time of ERCP, but if nonsurgical therapy is undertaken and then abandoned, repeat imaging of the pancreatic duct is appropriate to guide surgical treatment. Antisecretory therapy with the somatostatin analogue octreotide acetate, together with bowel rest and parenteral nutrition, is successful in more than half of patients. Reapposition of serosal surfaces to facilitate closure of the leak is considered a part of therapy, and this is accomplished by complete paracentesis. For pleural effusions, a period of chest tube drainage may facilitate closure of the internal fistula. Surgical therapy is reserved for those who fail to respond to medical treatment. If the leak originates from the central region of the pancreas, a Roux-en-Y pancreaticojejunostomy is performed to the site of duct leakage. If the leak is in the tail, a distal pancreatectomy may be considered, or an internal drainage procedure can be performed. The results of surgical treatment are usually favorable if the ductal anatomy has been carefully delineated preoperatively. (See Schwartz 9th ed., p 1204.)

31. The median survival following pancreaticoduodenectomy (Whipple procedure) for pancreatic cancer is approximately
    A. 9 months
    B. 2 years
    C. 4 years
    D. 8 years

Answer: B
Median survival after pancreaticoduodenectomy is about 22 months. Even long-term (5-year) survivors often eventually die due to pancreatic cancer recurrence. Although pancreaticoduodenectomy may be performed with the hope of the rare cure in mind, the operation more importantly provides better palliation than any other treatment, and is the only modality that offers any meaningful improvement in survival. If the procedure is performed without major complications, many months of palliation are usually achieved. It is the surgeon's duty to make sure patients and their families have a realistic understanding of the true goals of pancreaticoduodenectomy in the setting of pancreatic cancer. (See Schwartz 9th ed., p 1230.)

32. Which of the following is the initial medication used to treat pain in patients with chronic pancreatitis?
    A. Enteric-coated pancreatic enzyme preparations
    B. Non–enteric-coated pancreatic enzyme preparations
    C. Octreotide
    D. Somatostatin

Answer: B
Conventional (non–enteric-coated) enzyme preparations are partially degraded by gastric acid but are available within the duodenal and jejunal regions to bind to CCK-releasing peptide, and downregulate the release of CCK. This theoretically reduces the enteric signal for pancreatic exocrine secretion, which reduces the pressure within a partially or completely obstructed pancreatic duct. Enteric-coated preparations result in little to no pain relief, presumably due to their reduced bioavailability in the proximal gut.

Somatostatin administration has been shown to inhibit pancreatic exocrine secretion and CCK release. The somatostatin analogue patients with chronic pancreatitis. In a double-blind, prospective, randomized 4-week trial, 65% of patients who received 200 μg of octreotide acetate subcutaneously three times daily reported pain relief, compared with 35% of placebo-treated subjects. Patients who had the best results were patients with chronic abdominal pain, suggestive of obstructive pancreatopathy. However, in another trial that used a 3-day duration of treatment, no significant pain relief was observed. None of the studies published thus far have examined the sustained-release formulation of octreotide, and it remains unclear what subgroups of patients, or what dose of octreotide, might be beneficial in the treatment of pain. (See Schwartz 9th ed., p 1206.)

33. In a patient with chronic pancreatitis, pancreatic stones, and a 6-mm pancreatic duct, which of the following treatments is most likely to result in symptomatic relief?
    A. Endoscopic stone retrieval and stenting of the pancreatic duct
    B. Transduodenal sphincteroplasty with retrieval of pancreatic stones
    C. Caudal Roux-en-Y pancreaticojejunostomy (Duval procedure)
    D. Longitudinal Roux-en-Y pancreaticojejunostomy (Puestow or Frey procedure)

Answer: D

Endoscopic removal of pancreatic duct stones is usually coupled to prolonged pancreatic duct stenting, which carries the risk of further inflammation. Despite the risk of perioperative complications, the surgical management of pancreatic duct stones and stenosis has been shown to be superior to endoscopic treatment in randomized clinical trials in which the long, side-to-side technique of pancreaticojejunostomy is used.

The effectiveness of decompression of the pancreatic duct is dependent on the extent to which ductal hypertension is the etiologic agent for the disease. Thus, the diameter of the pancreatic duct is a surrogate for the degree of ductal hypertension, and the Puestow procedure has been shown to be effective for pain relief when the maximum duct diameter is 6 mm.

Zollinger and associates described the caudal Roux-en-Y pancreaticojejunostomy for the treatment of chronic pancreatitis in 1954. The so-called Duval procedure was used for decades by some surgeons, but it almost invariably failed due to restenosis and segmental obstruction of the pancreas due to progressive scarring.

Successful pain relief after the Puestow-type decompression procedure has been reported in 75 to 85% of patients for the first few years after surgery, but pain recurs in >20% of patients after 5 years, even in patients who are abstinent from alcohol. (See Schwartz 9th ed., p 1210.)

34. Pancreas divisum occurs as a result of
    A. Pancreatitis
    B. Carcinoma of the pancreas
    C. Trauma
    D. Abnormal fusion of the pancreatic ducts

Answer: D

An understanding of embryology is required to appreciate the common variations in pancreatic duct anatomy. The pancreas is formed by the fusion of a ventral and dorsal bud. The duct from the smaller ventral bud, which arises from the hepatic diverticulum, connects directly to the common bile duct. The duct from the larger dorsal bud, which arises from the duodenum, drains directly into the duodenum. The duct of the ventral anlage becomes the duct of Wirsung, and the duct from the dorsal anlage becomes the duct of Santorini. With gut rotation, the ventral anlage rotates to the right and around the posterior side of the duodenum to fuse with the dorsal bud. The ventral anlage becomes the inferior portion of the pancreatic head and the uncinate process, while the dorsal anlage becomes the body and tail of the pancreas. The ducts from each anlage usually fuse together in the pancreatic head such that most of the pancreas drains through the duct of Wirsung, or main pancreatic duct, into the common channel formed from the bile duct and pancreatic duct.

In 10% of patients, the ducts of Wirsung and Santorini fail to fuse. This results in the majority of the pancreas draining through the duct of Santorini and the lesser papilla, while the inferior portion of the pancreatic head and uncinate process drains through the duct of Wirsung and major papilla. This normal anatomic variant, which occurs in one out of 10 patients, is referred to as *pancreas divisum* (Fig. 33-6). In a minority of these patients, the minor papilla can be inadequate to handle the flow of pancreatic juices from the majority of the gland. This relative outflow obstruction can result in pancreatitis and is sometimes treated by sphincteroplasty of the minor papilla. (See Schwartz 9th ed., p 1171.)

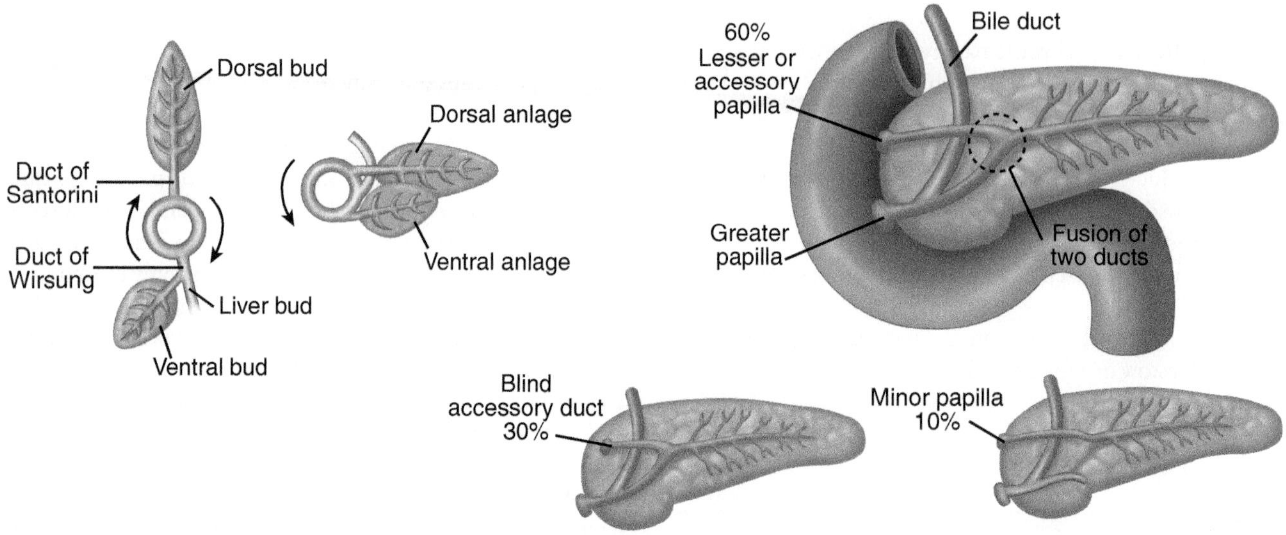

FIG. 33-6. Embryology of pancreas and duct variations. The duct of Wirsung from the ventral bud connects to the bile duct, while the duct of Santorini from the larger dorsal bud connects to the duodenum. With gut rotation, the two ducts fuse in most cases such that the majority of the pancreas drains through the duct of Wirsung to the major papilla. The duct of Santorini can persist as a blind accessory duct or drain through the lesser papilla. In a minority of patients, the ducts remain separate, and the majority of the pancreas drains through the duct of Santorini, a condition referred to as *pancreas divisum*.

CHAPTER 34

Spleen

BASIC SCIENCE QUESTIONS

1. More than 80% of accessory spleens are found in the splenic hilum. What is the second most common location for an accessory spleen?
   A. The greater omentum
   B. The gastrocolic ligament
   C. The tail of the pancreas
   D. The splenocolic ligament

Answer: B

The most common anomaly of splenic embryology is the accessory spleen. Present in up to 20% of the population, one or more accessory spleens may also occur in up to 30% of patients with hematologic disease. Over 80% of accessory spleens are found in the region of the splenic hilum and vascular pedicle. Other locations for accessory spleens in descending order of frequency are the gastrocolic ligament, the pancreas tail, the greater omentum, the stomach's greater curve, the splenocolic ligament, the small and large bowel mesentery, the left broad ligament in women, and the left spermatic cord in men. (See Schwartz 9th ed., p 1246.)

2. Which of the following is the primary function of the spleen in humans?
   A. Production of red cells
   B. Production of white cells
   C. Storage of blood
   D. Host defense

Answer: D

Many mammals have splenic capsules and trabeculae with abundant smooth muscle cells, which upon autonomic stimulation contract to expel large volumes of stored blood into the general circulation. Such spleens are descriptively characterized as *storage spleens*. The human splenic capsule and trabeculae, by contrast, contain few or no smooth muscle cells, and their function is largely related to immunologic protection. Thus the term *defense spleen* characterizes the human organ. Historically the four splenic functions have been accurately noted as (a) filtration, (b) host defense, (c) storage, and (d) cytopoiesis. For the adult human, the most important, dominant functions are filtration and host defense. (See Schwartz 9th ed., p 1248.)

3. Approximately what volume of aged red blood cells are removed by the spleen every day?
   A. 2 mL
   B. 20 mL
   C. 100 mL
   D. 250 mL

Answer: B

The spleen acts as the major site for clearance from the blood of damaged or aged red blood cells and in addition has a part in the removal of abnormal white blood cells and platelets. A minimum of 2 days of the erythrocyte's 120-day life cycle is spent sequestered in the spleen. Daily, approximately 20 mL of aged red blood cells are removed. (See Schwartz 9th ed., p 1248.)

4. In a normal patient what percentage of platelets are sequestered in the spleen?
   A. 2%
   B. 16%
   C. 33%
   D. 50%

Answer: C

The life cycles of cellular elements vary widely in human blood. A neutrophil in circulation has a normal half-life of approximately 6 hours. The spleen's role in the normal clearance of neutrophils is not well established. It is clear that hypersplenism may result in neutropenia through sequestration of normal white blood cells or the removal of abnormal ones. Platelets, on the other hand, generally survive in the circulation for 10 days. Under normal circumstances a third of the total platelet pool is sequestered in the spleen. Thrombocytopenia may result from excessive sequestration of platelets as well as accelerated platelet destruction in the spleen. Splenomegaly may result in sequestration of up to 80% of the platelet pool. (See Schwartz 9th ed., p 1248.)

5. Which of the following proteins is abnormal in patients with hereditary spherocytosis?
   A. Tuftsin
   B. Ankyrin
   C. Opsonin
   D. Properdin

Answer: B
Hereditary spherocytosis (HS) results from an inherited dysfunction or deficiency in one of the erythrocyte membrane proteins (*spectrin, ankyrin, band 3 protein*, or *protein 4.2*). The resulting destabilization of the membrane lipid bilayer allows a pathologic release of membrane lipids. The red blood cell assumes a more spherical, less deformable shape, and the spherocytic erythrocytes are sequestered and destroyed in the spleen. Hemolytic anemia ensues; in fact, HS is the most common hemolytic anemia for which splenectomy is indicated. The spleen produces opsonins, tuftsin, and properdin, which are all part of the humoral host defense and area not related to red blood cell membrane deformation. (See Schwartz 9th ed., p 1250.)

6. Transposition between the *bcr* gene on chromosome 9 and the *abl* gene on chromosome 22 is the hallmark of which of the following conditions?
   A. Chronic myeloid leukemia
   B. Chronic myelomonocytic leukemia
   C. Acute myeloid leukemia
   D. Polycythemia vera

Answer: A
Chronic myeloid leukemia (CML) is a disorder of the primitive pluripotent stem cell in the bone marrow that results in a significant increase in erythroid, megakaryotic, and pluripotent progenitors in the peripheral blood smear. The genetic hallmark is a transposition between the *bcr* gene on chromosome 9 and the *abl* gene on chromosome 22. CML accounts for 7 to 15% of all leukemias, with an incidence of 1.5 in 100,000 in the United States. It is often asymptomatic, but CML can cause fatigue, anorexia, sweating, and left upper quadrant pain and early satiety secondary to splenomegaly. Enlargement of the spleen is found in roughly one half of patients with CML. Splenectomy is indicated to ease pain and early satiety. (See Schwartz 9th ed., p 1254.)

7. Abnormal storage of sphingomyelin is found in
   A. Gaucher's disease
   B. Niemann-Pick disease
   C. Amyloidosis
   D. Felty's syndrome

Answer: B
Niemann-Pick disease is an inherited disorder of abnormal lysosomal storage of sphingomyelin and cholesterol in cells of the macrophage monocyte system. Four types of the disease (A, B, C, and D) exist, with unique clinical presentations. Types A and B result from a deficiency in lysosomal hydrolase and are the forms most likely to demonstrate splenomegaly with its concomitant symptoms.

Gaucher's disease is an inherited lipid storage disorder characterized by the deposition of glucocerebroside in cells of the macrophagemonocyte system. The underlying abnormality is a deficiency in the activity of a lysosomal hydrolase. Abnormal glycolipid storage results in organomegaly, particularly hepatomegaly and splenomegaly.

Amyloidosis is a disorder of abnormal extracellular protein deposition. There are multiple forms of amyloidosis, each with its own individual clinical presentation, and the severity of disease may range from asymptomatic to multiorgan failure. Patients with primary amyloidosis, associated with plasma cell dyscrasia, have splenic involvement in approximately 5% of cases.

The triad of rheumatoid arthritis, splenomegaly, and neutropenia is called *Felty's syndrome.* It exists in approximately 3% of all patients with rheumatoid arthritis, two thirds of whom are women. (See Schwartz 9th ed., p 1256.)

8. Which of the following is the most common cause of congenital hemolytic anemia?
   A. Glucose-6-phosphate dehydrogenase deficiency
   B. Pyruvate kinase deficiency
   C. Hereditary spherocytosis
   D. Hereditary elliptocytosis

Answer: B

The most common red blood cell enzyme deficiency to cause congenital chronic hemolytic anemia is pyruvate kinase (PK) deficiency. Its pathophysiology is unclear. PK deficiency affects people worldwide, with a slight preponderance among those of Northern European or Chinese descent. Clinical manifestations of the disease vary widely, from transfusion-dependent severe anemia in early childhood to well-compensated mild anemia in adolescents or adults. Diagnosis is made either by a screening test or by detection of specific mutations at the complementary DNA or genomic level. Splenomegaly is common, and in severe cases splenectomy can alleviate transfusion requirements.

Hereditary spherocytosis and elliptocytosis are disorders of the red blood cell membrane, and not enzymatic deficiencies. (See Schwartz 9th ed., p 1251.)

CLINICAL QUESTIONS

1. An 18-year-old otherwise healthy woman is incidentally found to have a 2-cm splenic aneurysm of the mid portion of the splenic artery. Which of the following is the treatment of choice for this patient?
   A. Observation only
   B. Embolization
   C. Ligation or resection of the aneurysm
   D. Splenectomy

Answer: C

Although splenic artery aneurysm is rare, it is the most common visceral artery aneurysm. Women are four times more likely to be affected than men. The aneurysm usually arises in the middle to distal portion of the splenic artery. In one series, mortality was significantly higher in patients with underlying portal hypertension (>50%) than in those without it (17%). Indications for treatment include presence of symptoms, pregnancy, intention to become pregnant, and presence of pseudoaneurysms associated with inflammatory processes. Aneurysm resection or ligation alone is acceptable for amenable lesions in the midsplenic artery, but distal lesions in close proximity to the splenic hilum should be treated with concomitant splenectomy. An excellent prognosis follows elective treatment. Splenic artery embolization has been used to treat splenic artery aneurysm, but painful splenic infarction and abscess may follow. (See Schwartz 9th ed., p 1256.)

2. A 48-year-old patient presents with isolated bleeding gastric varices, splenic vein thrombosis, and normal liver function. Which of the following is likely to be the treatment of choice?
   A. Beta blockers and banding
   B. Splenorenal bypass
   C. Splenic vein ligation
   D. Splenectomy

Answer: D

Portal hypertension secondary to splenic vein thrombosis is potentially curable with splenectomy. Patients with bleeding from isolated gastric varices who have normal liver function test results, especially those with a history of pancreatic disease, should be examined for splenic vein thrombosis and treated with splenectomy if findings are positive. (See Schwartz 9th ed., p 1256.)

3. Splenectomy is indicated in a child with sickle cell following
   A. 1 episode of sequestration
   B. 2 episodes of sequestration
   C. 3 episodes of sequestration
   D. None of the above

Answer: A

Sequestration occurs in the spleen, with splenomegaly resulting early in the disease course. In most patients subsequent infarction of the spleen and autosplenectomy occur at some later time. The most frequent indications for splenectomy in sickle cell disease are recurrent acute sequestration crises, hypersplenism, and splenic abscess. The occurrence of one major acute sequestration crisis characterized by rapid painful enlargement of the spleen and circulatory collapse, generally is considered sufficient grounds for splenectomy. Preoperative preparation should include special attention to adequate hydration and avoidance of hypothermia. (See Schwartz 9th ed., p 1251.)

4. Which of the following is associated with an increased risk for pulmonary hypertension following splenectomy?
   A. Sickle cell disease
   B. Warm antibody auto-immune hemolytic anemia
   C. Thalassemia
   D. Idiopathic thrombocytopenic purpura

Answer: C

Treatment for thalassemia involves red blood cell transfusions to maintain a hemoglobin level of >9 mg/dL, along with intensive parenteral chelation therapy with deferoxamine. Splenectomy is indicated for patients with excessive transfusion requirements (>200 mL/kg per year), discomfort due to splenomegaly, or painful splenic infarction. Careful assessment of the risk:benefit ratio is essential. Thalassemia patients are at high risk for pulmonary hypertension after splenectomy; the precise etiology of this sequela is under investigation. The increase in infectious complications is likely to be due to a coexisting immune deficiency, in large part brought about by iron overload, which may be associated both with the thalassemia itself and with transfusions. The disproportionately high rate of overwhelming postsplenectomy infection in thalassemia patients has led some investigators to consider partial splenectomy in children; some success in reducing mortality has been reported. However, splenectomy should be delayed until after the age of 4 years unless it is absolutely necessary. (See Schwartz 9th ed., p 1252.)

5. What percentage of patients referred for surgery for idiopathic thrombocytopenic purpura will have a permanent response (i.e., not need further steroids)?
   A. 15%
   B. 35%
   C. 55%
   D. 75%

Answer: D

The usual first line of therapy [for ITP] is oral prednisone at a dosage of 1.0 to 1.5 mg/kg per day. No consensus exists as to the optimal duration of steroid therapy, but most responses occur within the first 3 weeks. Response rates range from 50 to 75%, but relapses are common. IV immunoglobulin, given at 1.0 g/kg per day for 2 to 3 days, is indicated for internal bleeding when platelet counts remain <5000/mm^3 or when extensive purpura exists. IV immunoglobulin is thought to impair clearance of immunoglobulin G–coated platelets by competing for binding to tissue macrophage receptors. An immediate response is common but a sustained remission is not. Splenectomy is indicated for failure of medical therapy, for prolonged use of steroids with undesirable effects, or for most cases of first relapse.

Prolonged use of steroids can be defined in various ways, but a persistent need for more than 10 to 20 mg/d for 3 to 6 months to maintain a platelet count of >30,000/mm^3 generally prompts referral for splenectomy. Splenectomy provides a permanent response without subsequent need for steroids in 75 to 85% of patients. (See Schwartz 9th ed., p 1253, and Table 34-1.)

TABLE 34-1 Platelet response after laparoscopic splenectomy for idiopathic thrombocytopenic purpura

Study	*n*	No. Showing Initial Response (%)	No. Showing Long-Term Response (%)	Mean Follow-Up (mo)
Vianelli et al	402	86	66	57
Szold et al	104	NA	84	36
Balague et al	103	89	75	33
Katkhouda et al	67	84	78	38
Wu et al	67	83	74	23
Duperier et al	67	NA	64	22
Berends et al	50	86	64	35

(continued)

TABLE 34-1 (continued)

Study	*n*	No. Showing Initial Response (%)	No. Showing Long-Term Response (%)	Mean Follow-Up (mo)
Trias et al	48	NA	88	30
Tanoue et al	35	83	79	36
Friedman et al	31	NA	93	2
Stanton	30	89	89	30
Fass et al	29	90	80	43
Bresler et al	27	93	88	28
Harold et al	27	92	85	20
Lozano-Salazar et al	22	89	88	15
Meyer et al	16	NA	86	14
Watson et al	13	100	83	60
Total/mean	**1138**	**89**	**80**	**31**

NA = not available.

6. A patient who presents with altered mental status, thrombocytopenia, and lower extremity petechia will most likely benefit from
   A. Steroids
   B. Methotrexate
   C. Plasma exchange
   D. Splenectomy

Answer: C

TTP occurs in approximately 3.7 individuals per million, but this rare disorder's dramatic clinical sequelae and favorable response to early therapy demand an understanding of its clinical presentation to ensure an early diagnosis. Clinical features of the disorder include petechiae, fever, neurologic symptoms, renal failure, and, infrequently, cardiac symptoms such as heart failure or arrhythmias. Petechial hemorrhages in the lower extremities are the most common presenting sign. Along with fever, patients may experience flulike symptoms, malaise, or fatigue. Neurologic changes range from generalized headaches to altered mental status, seizures, and even coma. Generally, however, the mere presence of petechiae and thrombocytopenia are sufficient to lead to the diagnosis of TTP and consideration of treatment. The diagnosis is confirmed by the peripheral blood smear, which shows schistocytes, nucleated red blood cells, and basophilic stippling. Plasma exchange is the first-line therapy for TTP. The treatment consists of daily removal of a single volume of the patient's plasma, replaced with fresh, frozen plasma until thrombocytopenia, anemia, and associated symptoms are corrected. (See Schwartz 9th ed., p 1253-1254.)

7. Which of the following is a common indication for splenectomy in a patient with agnogenic myeloid metaplasia?
   A. Early satiety
   B. Thrombocytopenia
   C. Neutropenia
   D. Splenic rupture

Answer: A

The myeloproliferative disorders are characterized by an abnormal growth of cell lines in the bone marrow. They include chronic myeloid leukemia, acute myeloid leukemia, chronic myelomonocytic leukemia, essential thrombocythemia, polycythemia vera, and myelofibrosis, also known as *agnogenic myeloid metaplasia*. The common underlying problem leading to splenectomy in these disorders is symptomatic splenomegaly. Symptoms due to splenomegaly consist of early satiety, poor gastric emptying, heaviness or pain in the left upper quadrant, and even diarrhea. Hypersplenism, when it occurs in these conditions, usually is associated with splenomegaly. Splenectomy performed in the setting of the myeloproliferative disorders is generally for treatment of the pain, early satiety, and other symptoms of splenomegaly.

The term *myelofibrosis* may be used to describe either the generic condition of fibrosis of the bone marrow (which may be associated with a number of benign and malignant disorders) or a specific, chronic, malignant hematologic disease associated with splenomegaly, the presence of red blood cell and white blood cell progenitors in the bloodstream, marrow fibrosis, and extramedullary hematopoiesis, otherwise known as *agnogenic myeloid metaplasia (AMM)*. (See Schwartz 9th ed., p 1254.)

8. The treatment of choice in an otherwise healthy 22-year-old patient with a large, sepatated splenic abscess is
   A. Antibiotic therapy only
   B. Antibiotics + percutaneous drainage
   C. Antibiotics + partial splenectomy
   D. Antibiotics + splenectomy

Answer: D

Abscesses of the spleen are uncommon, with an incidence of 0.14 to 0.7% based on autopsy findings. They occur more frequently in tropical locations, where they are associated with thrombosed splenic vessels and infarction in patients with sickle cell anemia. Five distinct mechanisms of splenic abscess formation have been described: (a) hematogenous infection; (b) contiguous infection; (c) hemoglobinopathy; (d) immunosuppression, including HIV infection and chemotherapy; and (e) trauma. Presentation frequently is delayed, with most patients enduring symptoms for 16 to 22 days before diagnosis. Clinical manifestations include fever, left upper quadrant pain, leukocytosis, and splenomegaly in about one third of patients. The diagnosis is confirmed by ultrasound or CT scan, which has a 95% sensitivity and specificity. Upon discovery of a splenic abscess, broad-spectrum antibiotics should be started, with adjustment to more specific therapy based on culture results and continuation of treatment for 14 days. Splenectomy is the operation of choice, but percutaneous and open drainage are options for patients who cannot tolerate splenectomy. Percutaneous drainage is successful for patients with unilocular disease. (See Schwartz 9th ed., p 1255.)

9. Patients undergoing elective splenectomy should receive vaccinations against *Streptococcus pneumoniae, H. influenzae* type B, and meningococcus
   A. 2-4 weeks before surgery
   B. The day of surgery
   C. 1 week after surgery
   D. 1 month after surgery

Answer: A

Splenectomy imparts a small (<1 to 5%) but definite lifetime risk of fulminant, potentially life-threatening infection. Therefore, when elective splenectomy is planned, vaccinations against encapsulated bacteria should be given at least 2 weeks before surgery to protect against such infection. The most common bacteria to cause serious infections in asplenic hosts are *Streptococcus pneumoniae, H. influenzae* type B, and meningococcus. Vaccinations against these bacteria are available and should be given. If the spleen is removed emergently (e.g., for trauma), vaccinations should be given as soon as possible after surgery, with at least 1 to 2 days allowed for recovery. After splenectomy, annual influenza immunization is advisable. Splenectomized patients should be well educated regarding the potential consequences of overwhelming postsplenectomy infection and should be encouraged to maintain documentation of their own immunization status. (See Schwartz 9th ed., p 1256.)

10. The most common early complication after open splenectomy is
    A. Atelectasis
    B. Hemorrhage
    C. Subphrenic abscess
    D. Wound infection

Answer: A

Left lower lobe atelectasis is the most common complication after OS; pleural effusion and pneumonia also can occur. Hemorrhage can occur intraoperatively or postoperatively, presenting as subphrenic hematoma. Transfusions have become less common since the advent of LS, although the indication for operation influences the likelihood of transfusion as well. Subphrenic abscess and wound infection are among the perioperative infectious complications. (See Schwartz 9th ed., p 1260.)

CHAPTER 35

Abdominal Wall, Omentum, Mesentery, and Retroperitoneum

BASIC SCIENCE QUESTIONS

1. The inguinal ligament is the inferior-most part of which abdominal wall muscle?
   A. Transversalis
   B. Internal oblique
   C. External oblique
   D. Rectus abdominis

Answer: C

The *inguinal ligament* is the inferior-most edge of the external oblique aponeurosis, reflected posteriorly in the area between the anterior superior iliac spine and pubic tubercle. (See Schwartz 9th ed., p 1267.)

2. Which nerve root(s) supplies innervations to the skin of the umbilicus?
   A. C3, 4, and 5
   B. T1
   C. T4 and 5
   D. T10

Answer: D

Innervation of the anterior abdominal wall is segmentally related to specific spinal levels. The motor nerves to the rectus muscles, the internal oblique muscles, and the transversus abdominis muscles run from the anterior rami of spinal nerves at the T6 to T12 levels. The overlying skin is innervated by afferent branches of the T4 to L1 nerve roots, with the nerve roots of T10 subserving sensation of the skin around the umbilicus. (See Schwartz 9th ed., p 1269, and Fig. 35-1.)

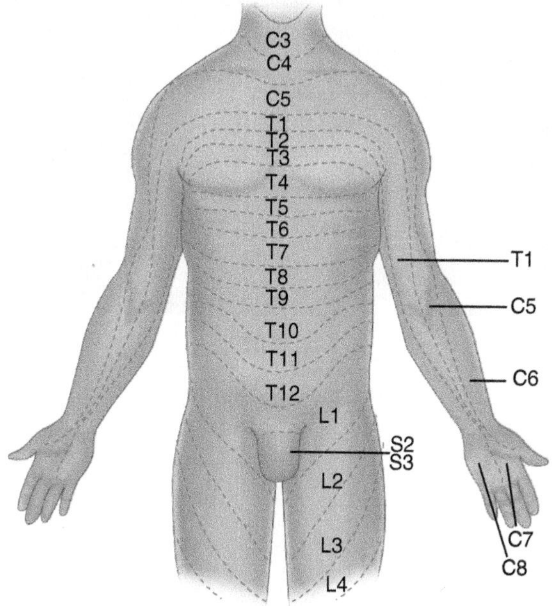

FIG. 35-1. Dermatomal sensory innervation of the abdominal wall. (Reproduced with permission from Moore KL, Dailey AF (eds): *Clinically Oriented Anatomy*, 4th ed. Philadelphia: Lippincott Williams & Wilkins, 1999, p 188.)

1. Which of the following (see Fig. 35-2) is a Rocky-Davis incision?

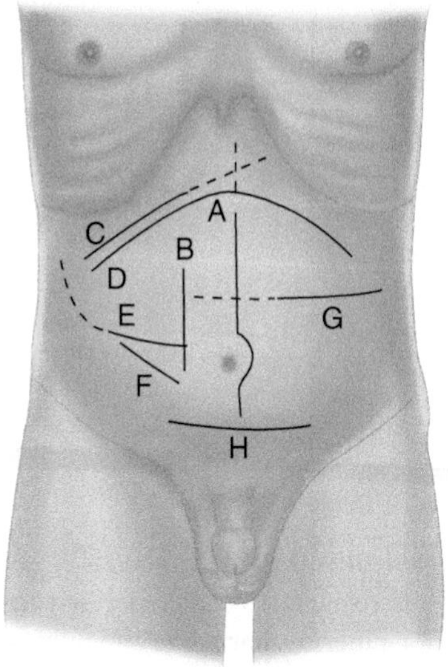

FIG. 35-2.

Answer: E
The incision labeled E is the Rocky-Davis muscle-splitting incision, most commonly used for open appendectomies. If exposure is not adequate, a Weir extension (dotted line) can be performed. (See Schwartz 9th ed., p 1270.)

2. The best treatment for the condition shown in Fig. 35-3 is
   A. Primary open repair
   B. Open repair using mesh
   C. Laparoscopic repair using mesh
   D. Observation

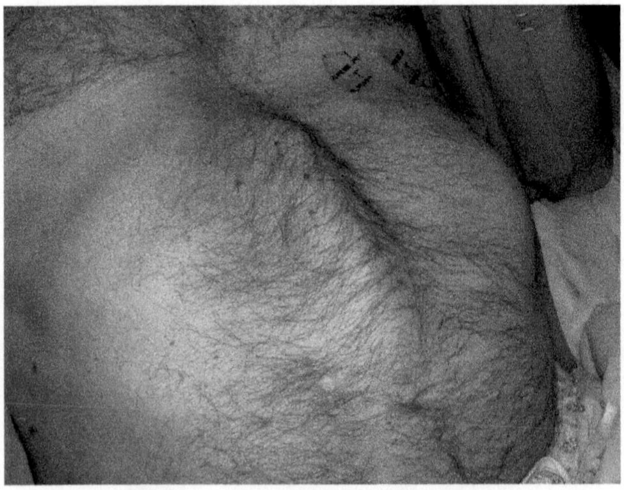

FIG. 35-3.

Answer: D
This is the typical, epigastric bulge of diastasis recti, which in the vast majority of patients needs no treatment. Rectus abdominis diastasis (or diastasis recti) is a clinically evident separation of the rectus abdominis muscle pillars. This results in a characteristic bulging of the abdominal wall in the epigastrium that is sometimes mistaken for a ventral hernia despite the fact that the midline aponeurosis is intact and no hernia defect is present. Diastasis may be congenital, as a result of a more lateral insertion of the rectus muscles to the ribs and costochondral junctions, but is more typically an acquired condition, occurring with advancing age, in obesity, or after pregnancy. In the postpartum setting, rectus diastasis tends to occur in women who are of advanced maternal age, who have a multiple or twin pregnancy, or who deliver a high-birth-weight infant. Diastasis is usually easily identified on physical examination. Computed tomographic (CT) scanning provides an accurate means of measuring the distance between the rectus pillars and can differentiate rectus diastasis from a true ventral hernia if clarification is required. Surgical correction of rectus diastasis by plication of the broad midline aponeurosis has been described for cosmetic indications and for alleviation of impaired abdominal wall muscular function. However, these approaches introduce the risk of an actual ventral hernia and are of questionable value in addressing pathology. (See Schwartz 9th ed., p 1271.)

3. A 48-year-old patient presents with sudden onset of bilateral lower abdominal pain after spasmodic coughing. On examination, there is an 8-cm, tender mass in the mid lower abdomen that remains unchanged with contraction of the rectus muscles. Which of the following is the most likely diagnosis?
   A. Ruptured aortic aneurysm
   B. Obturator hernia
   C. Spigelian hernia
   D. Rectus sheath hematoma

Answer: D

This patient has a typical history for rectus hematoma and a positive Fothergill's sign (a palpable abdominal mass that remains unchanged with contraction of the rectus muscles). Although rectus sheath hematomas are usually unilateral, if the hematoma is below the arcuate line, it may cross the midline. CT or MRI can be used to confirm the diagnosis. A spigelian hernia is herniation through the lateral rectus sheath, on the semilunar line. The oburator foramen is in the posterior pelvis, and obturator hernias usually present with bowel obstruction or medial thigh pain due to compression of the obturator nerve. A ruptured aortic aneurysm would usually present with back pain and a less prominent abdominal mass. (See Schwartz 9th ed., p 1272.)

4. The indications for surgery in a patient with a rectus sheath hematoma include
   A. Persistent pain after 24 hours
   B. Expanding hematoma after embolization
   C. Need for transfusion
   D. Need for ongoing anticoagulation

Answer: B

The primary indications for operating on a patient with a rectus sheath hematoma are hemodynamic instability and an expanding hematoma despite embolization. (See Schwartz 9th ed., p 1272, and Fig. 35-4.)

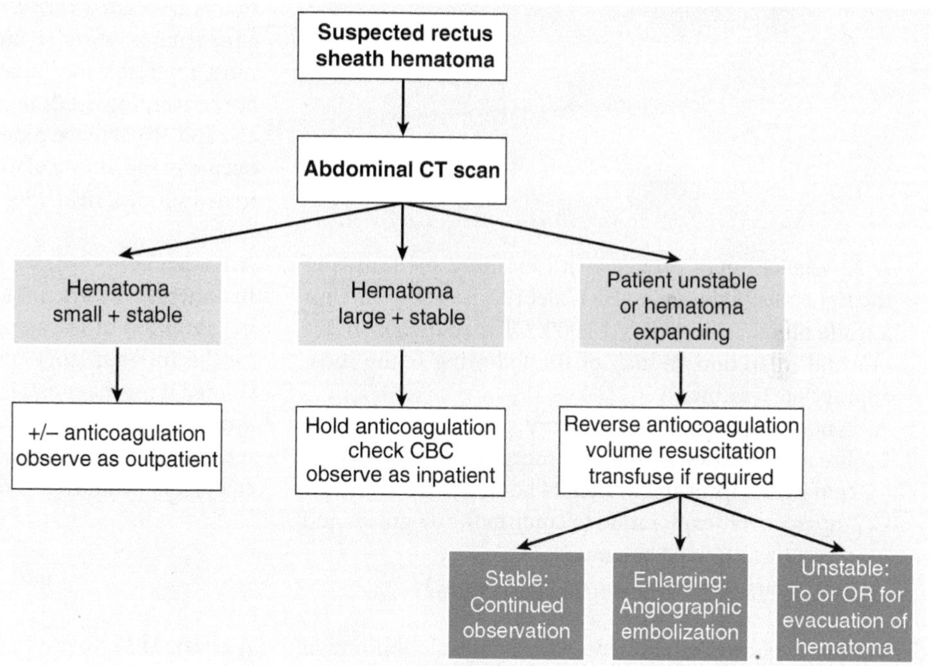

FIG. 35-4. Management algorithm for rectus sheath hematoma. Most patients present with a mass and/or pain and are managed without intervention. The potential for a rare catastrophic bleeding event must be recognized, however. Surgical evacuation is reserved for those circumstances in which clinical evidence of ongoing bleeding makes any other management option untenable. CBC = complete blood count; CT = computed tomography; OR = operating room.

5. Which of the following is the most important initial therapy for a patient with portal hypertension, ascites, and a tense umbilical hernia?
   A. Primary repair with concurrent placement of a peritoneal venous shunt
   B. Emergency primary repair to avoid hernia rupture
   C. Medical therapy to control the ascites
   D. Transjugular intrahepatic portocaval shunt followed by umbilical hernia repair

Answer: C

Treatment and control of the ascites with diuretics, dietary management, and paracentesis is the most appropriate initial therapy. Patients with refractory ascites may be candidates for transjugular intrahepatic portocaval shunting or eventual liver transplantation. Umbilical hernia repair should be deferred until after the ascites is controlled. (See Schwartz 9th ed., p 1273.)

6. In a patient with a permanent ileostomy and 4-cm infraumbilical midline incisional hernia, which of the following would be the most appropriate?
   A. Open primary closure
   B. Open mesh closure
   C. Component separation
   D. Observation

Answer: C

Although mesh repair would not be contraindicated in this patient, component separation has the advantage of no prosthetic material in a potentially contaminated wound.

Primary repair, even of small hernias (defects <3 cm), is associated with high reported hernia recurrence rates. In a randomized prospective study of open primary and open mesh incisional hernia repairs in 200 patients, investigators from the Netherlands found that after 3 years, recurrence rates were 43% and 24% for the two methods, respectively. Identified risk factors for recurrence were primary suture repair, postoperative wound infection, prostatism, and surgery for abdominal aortic aneurysm. These investigators concluded that mesh repair was superior to primary repair. In an effort to decrease the suture line tension associated with primary repair, Ramirez first described the components separation technique. Components separation entails the creation of large subcutaneous flaps lateral to the fascial defect followed by incision of the external oblique muscles and, if necessary, incision of the posterior rectus sheath bilaterally. These fascial releases allow for primary apposition of the fascia under far less tension than in simple primary repair. Components separation hernia repair is associated with a high wound infection risk (20%) and a recurrence rate of 18.2% at 1 year. Components separation is most applicable for the repair of incisional hernias when there are converging needs to (a) avoid the use of prosthetic materials, and (b) achieve a definitive repair. Most commonly this occurs in the setting of a contaminated or potentially contaminated surgical field. (See Schwartz 9th ed., p 1273.)

7. A 22-year-old man presents with localized peritonitis of the right lateral abdomen. He is afebrile, is eating, and has a white blood cell count of 12,000. CT scan demonstrates omental infarction. Which of the following is the most appropriate treatment?
   A. A nonsteroidal anti-inflammatory agent and observation
   B. Broad spectrum antibiotics, morphine with exploration if no improvement after 24 hours
   C. Laparoscopic exploration to confirm the diagnosis and resect the infarcted omentum
   D. Total omentectomy (open or laparoscopic)

Answer: A

In patients who are not toxic, supportive care will often result in resolution of the symptoms. Antibiotics are not indicated for this inflammatory condition. Laparoscopy should be considered if the diagnosis is not sure, or for progressive or severe symptoms. Resection of the infracted omentum leads to rapid resolution of the symptoms. A total omentectomy is not indicated. (See Schwartz 9th ed., p 1275.)

8. A 55-year-old woman presents with a palpable abdominal mass and abdominal pain. CT scan and exploration show scarring of the mesentery with shortening and retraction. The base of the mesentery is fibrotic and thickened. Following biopsy confirmation of your clinical diagnosis, which of the following is the best therapy for this patient?
   A. Surgical debulking of the tumor
   B. Chemotherapy
   C. Chemotherapy and radiation therapy
   D. Observation

Answer: D

This is the typical description of sclerosing mesenteritis. In most cases of sclerosing mesenteritis the process appears to be self-limited and may even demonstrate regression if followed with interval imaging studies. Clinical symptoms are very likely to improve without intervention, and therefore aggressive surgical treatments are generally not indicated. (See Schwartz 9th ed., p 1276.)

9. A 15-year-old girl presents with a mobile, 8-cm mid abdominal mass that moves freely from left to right but does not move superiorly or inferiorly. Which of the following is the most likely diagnosis?
   A. Omental cyst
   B. Mesenteric cyst
   C. Ovarian cyst
   D. Gastric duplication

Answer: B

Physical examination of a patient with a mesenteric cyst may reveal a mass lesion that is mobile only from the patient's right to left or left to right (Tillaux's sign), in contrast to the findings with omental cysts, which should be freely mobile in all directions. Although ovarian cysts are usually ballotable, they are rarely mobile. Gastric duplications are virtually never palpable. (See Schwartz 9th ed., p 1277.)

10. Which of the following drugs is associated with retroperitoneal fibrosis?
    A. Methysergide
    B. Omeprazole
    C. Prozac
    D. Dapsone

Answer: A

The strongest case for a causal relationship between medication and retroperitoneal fibrosis is made for methysergide, a semisynthetic ergot alkaloid used in the treatment of migraine headaches. Other medications that have been linked to retroperitoneal fibrosis include beta blockers, hydralazine, α-methyldopa, and entacapone, which inhibits catechol-*O*-methyltransferase and is used as an adjunct with levodopa in the treatment of Parkinson's disease. The retroperitoneal fibrosis regresses on discontinuation of these medications. Omeprazole, Prozac, and Dapsone have not been associated with retroperitoneal fibrosis. (See Schwartz 9th ed., p 1280.)

11. Which of the following is the most appropriate treatment for retroperitoneal fibrosis?
    A. Surgical débridement of potentially obstructing fibrosis
    B. Prevention of obstruction with anticoagulation (for IVC thrombosis) and ureteral stenting (for ureteral obstruction)
    C. High dose corticosteroids
    D. Observation

Answer: C

Corticosteroids, with or without surgery, are the mainstay of medical therapy. Surgical treatment consists primarily of ureterolysis or ureteral stenting and is required in patients who present with moderate or massive hydronephrosis. Laparoscopic ureterolysis has been shown to be as efficacious as open surgery in addressing this problem. Patients with iliocaval thrombosis require anticoagulation, although the required duration of this therapy is unclear. Prednisone is initially administered at a relatively high dose (60 mg every other day for 2 months) and then gradually tapered over the next 2 months. Therapeutic efficacy is assessed on the basis of patient symptoms and interval imaging studies. Cyclosporin, tamoxifen, and azathioprine also have been used to treat patients who respond poorly to corticosteroids. (See Schwartz 9th ed., p 1280.)

CHAPTER 36

Soft Tissue Sarcomas

BASIC SCIENCE QUESTIONS

1. Which of the following embryonic cell type is the most common origin of sarcomas?
   A. Ectoderm
   B. Mesoderm
   C. Endoderm
   D. Mesenchyme

Answer: B

Sarcomas are a heterogeneous group of tumors that arise predominantly from the embryonic mesoderm, but can also originate, as does the peripheral nervous system, from the ectoderm. (See Schwartz 9th ed., p 1284.)

2. Which of the following is an expected molecular event in an older patient with a sarcoma?
   A. Point mutation of an oncogene
   B. Translocation causing overexpression of an autocrine growth factor
   C. Oncogenic fusion transcription factor
   D. None of the above

Answer: D

Molecular genetics, cytogenetics, and expression profiling have been used to investigate sarcomas resulting in their classification into two main groups: those with defined diagnostic molecular events and those with variable histological and genetic changes. In general, the group of sarcoma patients with defined molecular events have been found to be younger with a defined histology suggesting a clear line of differentiation. The defined molecular events include point mutations, a translocation causing overexpression of an autocrine grow factor, or oncogenic fusion transcription factor. In contrast, sarcomas without currently identifiable genetic changes or expression profile signatures tend to occur in older patients exhibiting pleomorphoic cytology and p53 dysfunction. (See Schwartz 9th ed., p 1285.)

3. Which of the following mechanisms is felt to play the most significant role in the development of sarcomas?
   A. Activation of cancer suppressor genes
   B. Chromosomal translocation with activation of oncogenes
   C. Gene fusion with expression of oncoproteins
   D. Germ line mutation with suppression of oncogenes

Answer: C

Cytogenetic analysis of soft tissue tumors has identified distinct chromosomal translocations that seem to encode for oncogenes associated with certain sarcoma histologic subtypes. These specific genetic changes result in the in-frame fusion of genes and fused product codes for the expression of oncoproteins functioning as transcriptional activators or repressors. The best characterized gene rearrangements are found in Ewing's sarcoma (*EWS–FLI-1* fusion), clear-cell sarcoma (*EWS–ATF1* fusion), myxoid liposarcoma (*TLS–CHOP* fusion), alveolar rhabdomyosarcoma (*PAX3–FHKR* fusion), desmoplastic small round-cell tumor (*EWS–WT1* fusion), and synovial sarcoma (*SSX–SYT* fusion). It has been estimated that in aggregate, fusion gene-related sarcomas may account for up to 30% of all sarcomas. The oncogenic potential of many of these genes has been demonstrated *in vitro* and *in vivo*. These fusion genes provide not only specific diagnostic markers but encode chimeric proteins, both of which may be potential therapeutic targets. (See Schwartz 9th ed., p 1285.)

CLINICAL QUESTIONS

1. Which of the following is the most common soft tissue sarcoma in adults?
   A. Liposarcoma
   B. Leiomyosarcoma
   C. Synovial sarcoma
   D. Malignant fibrous histiocytoma

Answer: D

The most common histologic types of soft tissue sarcoma in adults (excluding Kaposi's sarcoma) are malignant fibrous histiocytoma (28%), leiomyosarcoma (12%), liposarcoma (15%), synovial sarcoma (10%), and malignant peripheral nerve sheath tumors (6%). (See Schwartz 9th ed., p 1284, and Table 36-1.)

TABLE 36-1 Relative frequency of histologic subtypes of soft tissue sarcoma

Histologic Subtypes	*n*	%
Malignant fibrous histiocytoma	349	28
Liposarcoma	188	15
Leiomyosarcoma	148	12
Unclassified sarcoma	140	11
Synovial sarcoma	125	10
Malignant peripheral nerve sheath tumor	72	6
Rhabdomyosarcoma	60	5
Fibrosarcoma	38	3
Ewing's sarcoma	25	2
Angiosarcoma	25	2
Osteosarcoma	14	1
Epithelioid sarcoma	14	1
Chondrosarcoma	13	1
Clear-cell sarcoma	12	1
Alveolar soft part sarcoma	7	1
Malignant hemangiopericytoma	5	0.4

Source: Data from Coindre JM, Terrier P, Guillou L, et al: Predictive value of grade for metastasis development in the main histologic types of adult soft tissue sarcomas: A study of 1240 patients from the French Federation of Cancer Centers Sarcoma Group. *Cancer* 91:1914, 2001.

2. Which of the following is the most common soft tissue sarcoma in children?
   A. Liposarcoma
   B. Leiomyosarcoma
   C. Rhabdomyosarcoma
   D. Chondrosarcoma

Answer: C

Associated with skeletal muscle, rhabdomyosarcomas are the most common soft tissue tumors among children younger than 15 years and can occur at any site that has striated muscle. These tumors generally present as a painless enlarging mass; about 24% in the genitourinary system, 20% in the extremities, 20% in the head and neck, 16% in the parameningeal region, and 22% in miscellaneous other sites. Regional lymphatic spread of tumor occurs frequently in extremity tumors and in paratesticular tumors. About 15 to 20% of cases have metastasis at presentation, most commonly (40 to 50%) involving the lungs, followed by bone marrow and bone. However, all patients are considered to have micrometastatic disease at presentation which is the rationale for universal chemotherapy. (See Schwartz 9th ed., p 1299.)

3. Malignant fibrous histiocytoma is most likely to metastasize to which of the following organs?
   A. Lung
   B. Liver
   C. Bone
   D. Lymph node

Answer: D

The dominant pattern of metastasis (of sarcomas) is hematogenous, primarily to the lungs. Lymph node metastases are rare (<5%) except for a few histologic subtypes such as epithelioid sarcoma, rhabdomyosarcoma, clear-cell sarcoma, synovial sarcoma, malignant fibrous histiocytoma, and angiosarcoma. (See Schwartz 9th ed., p 1284.)

4. Which of the following is a risk factor for developing a sarcoma?
   A. Hypaque (isotonic contrast)
   B. Trauma
   C. Chronic lymphedema
   D. Dental radiographs

Answer: C
In 1948, Stewart and Treves first described the association between chronic lymphedema after axillary dissection and subsequent lymphangiosarcoma. Lymphangiosarcoma has also been reported as occurring after filarial infections and in the lower extremities of patients with congenital or heritable lymphedema.

External radiation therapy is a rare but well-established risk factor for soft tissue sarcoma. An eightfold to 50-fold increase in the incidence of sarcomas has been reported among patients treated for cancer of the breast, cervix, ovary, testes, and lymphatic system. Dental radiographs would not expose the patient to enough radiation to increase the risk of sarcoma.

Thorotrast, which is a contrast material, has been implicated in carcinogenesis of sarcomas. There is no increased risk with exposure to Hypaque.

Although patients with sarcomas often report a history of trauma, no causal relationship has been established. More often, a minor injury calls attention to a preexisting tumor that may be accentuated by edema or hematoma. (See Schwartz 9th ed., p 1285.)

5. Which of the following syndromes is associated with an increased risk of developing a sarcoma?
   A. Familial adenomatous polyposis
   B. Ehlers-Danlos syndrome
   C. Down syndrome
   D. Turner syndrome

Answer: A
Sarcomas occur more commonly within several hereditary cancer syndromes including retinoblastoma, Li-Fraumeni syndrome, neurofibromatosis type I, and familial adenomatous polyposis. Germline mutations have been identified as causal in only a limited number of these disorders. Developments in the field of molecular biology have led to a better understanding of some of the basic cellular processes governed by oncogenes and tumor suppressor genes. (See Schwartz 9th ed., p 1285.)

6. Abdominal metastases are most likely to occur from which of the following tumors?
   A. Synovial sarcoma
   B. Rhabdomyosarcoma
   C. Leiomyosarcoma
   D. Myxoid liposarcoma

Answer: D
Computed tomography of the abdomen and pelvis should be done when histologic assessment of an extremity sarcoma reveals a myxoid liposarcoma, because this subtype is known to metastasize to the abdomen. (See Schwartz 9th ed., p 1286.)

7. The most appropriate initial method to biopsy a suspected 4-cm sarcoma of the lower leg is
   A. Core needle biopsy
   B. Suction biopsy
   C. Incisional biopsy
   D. Excisional biopsy

Answer: A
Core needle biopsy is a safe, accurate, and economical procedure for diagnosing sarcomas. The tissue sample obtained from a core needle biopsy is usually sufficient for several diagnostic tests such as electron microscopy, cytogenetic analysis, and flow cytometry. The reported complication rate for core needle biopsy is less than 1%.

Fine-needle aspiration is an acceptable method of diagnosing most soft tissue sarcomas, particularly when the results correlate closely with clinical and imaging findings. However, fine-needle aspiration biopsy is indicated for primary diagnosis of soft tissue sarcomas only at centers where cytopathologists have experience with these types of tumors. Incisional biopsy and excisional biopsy may change the outcome for patients by complicating staging. They are not considered the best initial diagnostic method for sarcomas >3 cm in diameter. (See Schwartz 9th ed., p 1287.)

8. In which of the following would an excisional biopsy of a suspected sarcoma be acceptable?
   A. 2-cm superficial flank mass
   B. 1.5-cm lesion of the dorsum of the hand
   C. 2-cm lesion over the calcaneus
   D. 4-cm superficial thigh mass

Answer: A
Excisional biopsy can be performed for easily accessible (superficial) extremity or truncal lesions smaller than 3 cm. Excisional biopsy should not be done for lesions involving the hands and feet, because definitive re-excision may not be possible after the biopsy. Excisional biopsy results have a 30 to 40% rate of recurrence when margins are positive or uncertain. Excisional biopsies rarely provide any benefit over other biopsy techniques and may cause postoperative complications that could ultimately delay definitive therapy. (See Schwartz 9th ed., p 1287.)

9. Which of the following has a low risk of metastasis?
   A. Clear-cell sarcoma
   B. Leiomyosarcoma
   C. Dermatosarcoma protuberans
   D. Chondrosarcoma

Answer: C
Tumors with limited metastatic potential include desmoid, atypical lipomatous tumor (also called *well-differentiated liposarcoma*), dermatofibrosarcoma protuberans, and hemangiopericytoma. Tumors with an intermediate risk of metastatic spread usually have a large myxoid component and include myxoid liposarcoma and extraskeletal chondrosarcoma. Among the highly aggressive tumors that have substantial metastatic potential are angiosarcoma, clear-cell sarcoma, pleomorphic and dedifferentiated liposarcoma, leiomyosarcoma, rhabdomyosarcoma, and synovial sarcoma. (See Schwartz 9th ed., p 1287.)

10. Which of the following is the most important determinant of prognosis for a patient with a sarcoma?
    A. Depth of invasion
    B. Cell type
    C. Histologic grade
    D. Tumor size

Answer: C
Histologic grade remains the most important prognostic factor for patients with sarcomas. For an accurate determination of tumor grade, an adequate tissue sample must be appropriately fixed, stained, and reviewed by an experienced sarcoma pathologist. The features that define grade are cellularity, differentiation, pleomorphism, necrosis, and the number of mitoses. Tumor grade has been shown to predict the development of metastases and overall survival. The metastatic potentials have been estimated at 5 to 10% for low-grade lesions, 25 to 30% for intermediate-grade lesions, and 50 to 60% for high-grade tumors. (See Schwartz 9th ed., p 1288.)

11. Which of the following is appropriate treatment following wide local excision of a 4-cm leiomyoma of the calf with negative margins and no metastases?
    A. Radiation therapy
    B. Systemic chemotherapy
    C. Isolated limb perfusion of chemotherapy
    D. Radiation therapy and chemotherapy

Answer: A
Small (<5 cm) primary tumors with no evidence of distant metastatic disease are managed with local therapy consisting of surgery, alone or in combination with radiation therapy, when wide pathologic margins are limited because of anatomic constraints. (See Schwartz 9th ed., p 1289, and Fig. 36-1.)

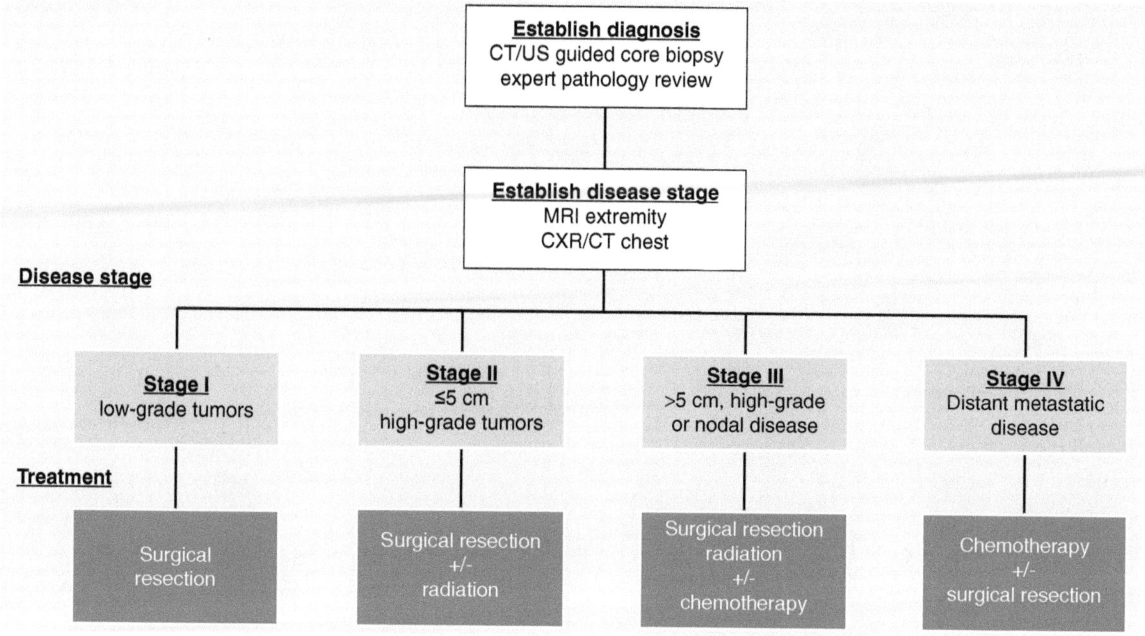

FIG. 36-1. Treatment algorithm of extremity soft tissue sarcoma. CT = computed tomography; CXR = chest x-ray; MRI = magnetic resonance imaging; US = ultrasound.

12. Which of the following sarcomas is most responsive to chemotherapy?
    A. Leiomyosarcoma
    B. Chondrosarcoma
    C. Liposarcoma
    D. Synovial sarcoma

Answer: D
As a group, sarcomas include histologic subtypes that are responsive to cytotoxic chemotherapy and subtypes that are universally resistant to current agents. A spectrum of chemosensitivity has been demonstrated for various histologic subtypes. In particular, synovial sarcoma and fibrosarcoma have been noted to be highly sensitive to chemotherapy. Liposarcoma and myxofibrosarcoma as having intermediate sensitivity to chemotherapy; and gastrointestinal stromal tumors and chondrosarcoma as being highly resistant to chemotherapy. (See Schwartz 9th ed., p 1293.)

13. The most common presenting symptom of a retroperitoneal sarcoma is
    A. A large abdominal mass
    B. Ureteral obstruction
    C. Rectal obstruction
    D. Lower extremity swelling from venous congestion

Answer: A
In contrast to extremity sarcomas, many retroperitoneal sarcomas present as large tumor masses abutting or involving vital structures, making margin-free resection difficult. As a result, locoregional recurrence is common (72% at 5 years) and prognosis for patients with retroperitoneal sarcoma is poor with 5-year survival estimated at 36 to 58%. (See Schwartz 9th ed., p 1295.)

14. The most appropriate surgical treatment for a 2-cm leiomyosarcoma of the greater curvature of the stomach is
    A. Local resection with 3-cm margin of normal tissue
    B. Subtotal gastrectomy
    C. Total gastrectomy
    D. Total gastrectomy and lymphadenectomy

Answer: A
Lymphatic spread is not the primary route of metastasis for gastrointestinal sarcomas. Consequently, lymphadenectomy is not routinely performed as part of resection. Based on published data and the primary pattern of distant (versus local) failure, the general recommendation is to perform a margin-negative resection with a 2- to 4-cm margin of normal tissue. (See Schwartz 9th ed., p 1297.)

15. Which of the following is used in the treatment of gastrointestinal stromal tumors?
    A. Doxirubicin
    B. Imatinib
    C. Bleomycin
    D. Methotrexate

Answer: B
Until recently, systemic treatment options for patient with unresectable or metastatic GIST were of little therapeutic benefit. Treatment with imatinib (Gleevec, ST1571), a selective c-Kit inhibitor, has resulted in impressive clinical responses in a large percentage of patients with unresectable or metastatic GISTs. (See Schwartz 9th ed., p 1298.)

CHAPTER 37

Inguinal Hernia

BASIC SCIENCE QUESTIONS

1. Poupart's ligament is composed of fibers from which muscle aponeurosis?
   A. Rectus abdominis
   B. Transversalis
   C. Internal oblique
   D. External oblique

Answer: D

The inguinal ligament is also known as *Poupart's ligament* and is comprised of the inferior fibers of the external oblique aponeurosis. The ligament stretches from the anterior superior iliac spine to the pubic tubercle. The ligament serves an important purpose as a readily identifiable boundary of the inguinal canal, as well as a sturdy structure used in various hernia repairs. (See Schwartz 9th ed., p 1308, and Fig. 37-1.)

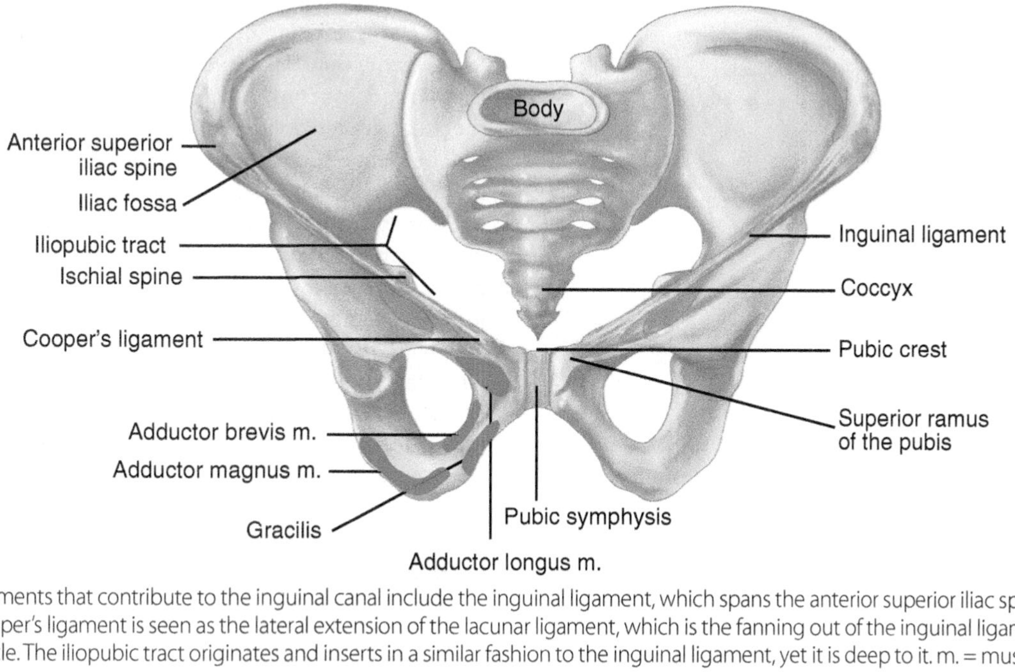

FIG. 37-1. Ligaments that contribute to the inguinal canal include the inguinal ligament, which spans the anterior superior iliac spine to the pubic bone. Cooper's ligament is seen as the lateral extension of the lacunar ligament, which is the fanning out of the inguinal ligament as it joins the pubic tubercle. The iliopubic tract originates and inserts in a similar fashion to the inguinal ligament, yet it is deep to it. m. = muscle.

2. The iliopubic tract
   A. Makes up the anterior border of the femoral canal
   B. Makes up the posterior border of the femoral canal
   C. Makes up the lateral border of the external inguinal ring
   D. Makes up the medial border of the external inguinal ring

Answer: A

The iliopubic tract is an aponeurotic band that begins at the anterior superior iliac spine and inserts into Cooper's ligament from above. It often is confused with the inguinal ligament secondary to common origin and insertion points. However, the iliopubic tract forms on the deep side of the inferior margin of the transverses abdominus and transversalis fascia. The inguinal ligament is on the superficial side of the musculoaponeurotic layer of these structures. The shelving edge of the inguinal ligament is a structure that more or less connects the iliopubic tract to the inguinal ligament. The iliopubic tract helps form the inferior margin of the internal inguinal ring as it courses medially, where it continues as the anterior and medial border of the femoral canal. (See Schwartz 9th ed., p 1308.)

3. Which nerve travels with the spermatic cord, entering the inguinal canal at the internal ring, and exiting at the external ring?
   A. Iliohypogastric nerve
   B. Ilioinguinal nerve
   C. Genitofemoral nerve
   D. Lateral femoral cutaneous nerve

Answer: B

The ilioinguinal nerve emerges from the lateral border of the psoas major and passes obliquely across the quadratus lumborum. At a point just medial to the anterior superior iliac spine, it crosses the internal oblique muscle to enter the inguinal canal between the internal and external oblique muscles and exits through the superficial inguinal ring. The nerve supplies the skin of the upper and medial thigh. In males, it also supplies the penis and upper scrotum, while supplying the mons pubis and labium majus in females.

The iliohypogastric nerve arises from T12–L1 and follows the ilioinguinal nerve. After the iliohypogastric nerve pierces the deep abdominal wall in its downward course, it courses between the internal oblique and transversus abdominis, supplying both. It then branches into a lateral cutaneous branch and an anterior cutaneous branch, which pierces the internal oblique and then external oblique aponeurosis above the superficial inguinal ring. A common variant is for the iliohypogastric and ilioinguinal nerves to exit around the superficial inguinal ring as a single entity.

The genitofemoral nerve arises from L1–L2, courses along the retroperitoneum, and emerges on the anterior aspect of the psoas. It then divides into the genital and femoral branches. The genital branch remains ventral to the iliac vessels and iliopubic tract as it enters the inguinal canal just lateral to the inferior epigastric vessels. In males, it travels through the superficial inguinal ring and supplies the scrotum and cremaster muscle. In females, it supplies the mons pubis and labia majora. The femoral branch courses along the femoral sheath, supplying the skin anterior to the upper part of the femoral triangle.

The lateral femoral cutaneous nerve arises from L2–L3, but emerges from the lateral border of the psoas muscle at the level of L4. It crosses the iliacus muscle obliquely toward the anterior superior iliac spine. It then passes inferior to the inguinal ligament where it divides to supply the lateral aspect of the thigh. (See Schwartz 9th ed., p 1310, and Fig. 37-2.)

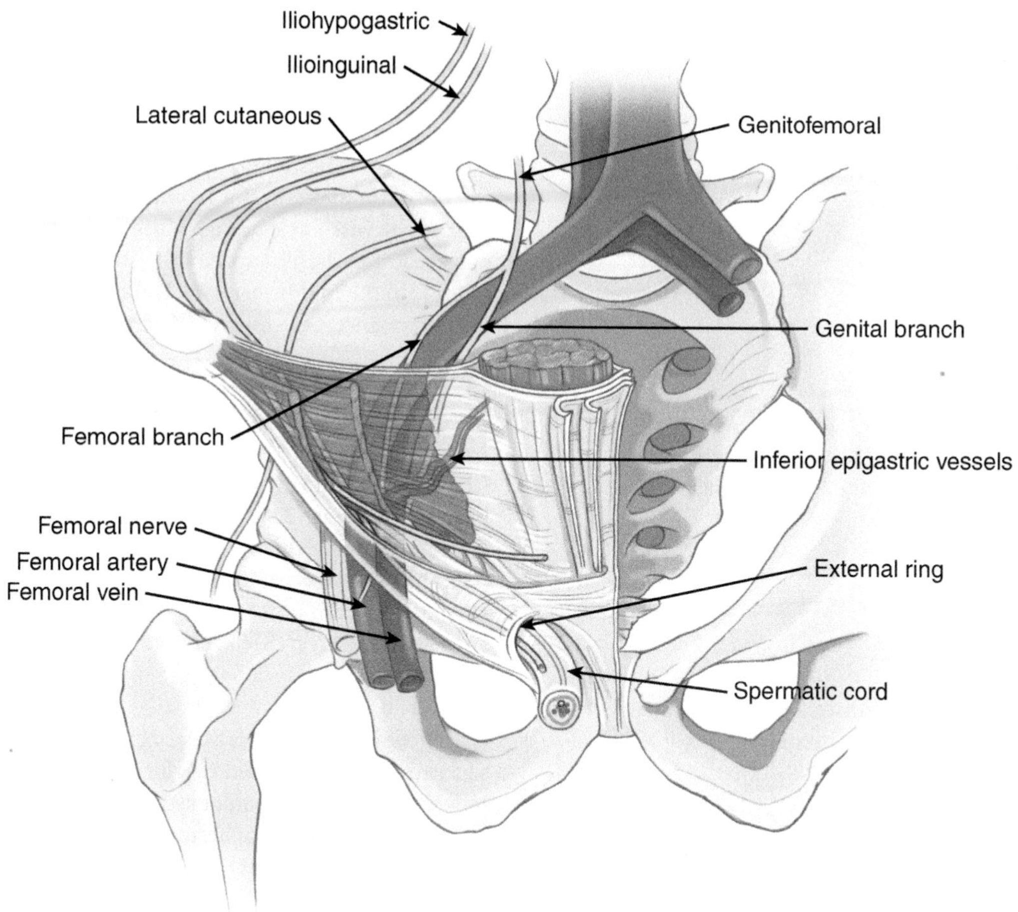
Iliohypogastric
Ilioinguinal
Lateral cutaneous
Genitofemoral
Genital branch
Femoral branch
Inferior epigastric vessels
Femoral nerve
Femoral artery
Femoral vein
External ring
Spermatic cord

FIG. 37-2. Anterior view of the five major nerves of the inguinal region.

4. Which of the following is one of the three borders of Hesselbach's triangle?
   A. Superior epigastric artery
   B. Edge of the transversalis muscle
   C. Inguinal ligament
   D. Internal inguinal ring

Answer: C

Direct hernias, on the contrary, are protrusions medial to the inferior epigastric vessels, in Hesselbach's triangle. The borders of the triangle are as such: the inguinal ligament forms the inferior margin, the edge of rectus abdominis is the medial border, and the inferior epigastric vessels are the superior or lateral border. (See Schwartz 9th ed., p 1312.)

5. Which of the following makes up one of the borders of the femoral ring?
   A. Medial edge of the rectus muscle
   B. Femoral artery
   C. Iliopubic tract
   D. Septum femorale

Answer: C

The femoral ring is bordered by sturdy structures that lend to its inflexibility. The posterior boundary consists of the iliacus fascia and Cooper's ligament, and the anterior boundary is the iliopubic tract and inguinal ligament, internally and externally, respectively. Medially, the border is made up of the aponeurosis of transverses abdominis and the transversalis fascia and laterally, the canal is bordered by the femoral vein and its connective tissue. Normal contents of the femoral canal include areolar preperitoneal tissue and fat and lymph nodes, most notably the node of Cloquet at its upper end. The distal end of the canal is closed by fatty tissue called the *septum femorale*. Once the integrity of this septum is lost, femoral herniation occurs. (See Schwartz 9th ed., p 1312.)

6. In performing a laparoscopic hernia repair, which of the following potential spaces is entered?
   A. Prussak's space
   B. Bogros's space
   C. Space of Disse
   D. Space of Traube

Answer: B

Two potential spaces exist deep to the peritoneum, and these are encountered once the peritoneal flap is created. Between the peritoneum and the posterior lamina of the transversalis fascia is Bogros's space. This area contains preperitoneal fat and areolar tissue. A less prominent space exists between the posterior and anterior laminae of the transversalis fascia termed the *vascular space*, as this is the location of the inferior epigastric vessels. The space of Disse is in the liver, Prussak's space is in the middle ear, and Traube's space is in the left upper abdomen. (See Schwartz 9th ed., p 1313.)

CLINICAL QUESTIONS

1. What percentage of adult patients with a unilateral inguinal hernia will have an unrecognized contralateral hernia?
   A. 7%
   B. 14%
   C. 22%
   D. 39%

Answer: C

In a study examining only patients with primary unilateral inguinal hernias, 22% were found to have an occult contralateral hernia during laparoscopic inguinal hernia repair. Although asymptomatic at time of diagnosis, these hernias have the potential to become clinically significant as the patient ages. (See Schwartz 9th ed., p 1306.)

2. Which of the following disorders is associated with an increased incidence of groin hernias?
   A. Down syndrome
   B. Osteogenesis imperfecta
   C. VACTERL association
   D. Biliary atresia

Answer: B

Osteogenesis imperfecta is a connective tissue disorder and is associated with an increased risk for groin hernias. Collagen disorders such as Ehlers-Danlos syndrome also are associated with an increased incidence of hernia formation (Table 37-1). Tissue analysis has revealed that there is a relationship between the aneurysmal component and hernias, owing to a pathologic extracellular matrix metabolism. (See Schwartz 9th ed., p 1308.)

TABLE 37-1 Connective tissue disorders associated with groin herniation
Osteogenesis imperfecta
Cutis laxa (congenital elastolysis)
Ehlers-Danlos syndrome
Hurler-Hunter syndrome
Marfan syndrome
Congenital hip dislocation in children
Polycystic kidney disease
Alpha$_1$-antitrypsin deficiency
Williams syndrome
Androgen insensitivity syndrome
Robinow's syndrome
Serpentine fibula syndrome
Alport's syndrome
Tel Hashomer camptodactyly syndrome
Leriche's syndrome
Testicular feminization syndrome
Rokitansky-Mayer-Küster syndrome
Goldenhar's syndrome
Morris syndrome
Gerhardt's syndrome
Menkes' syndrome
Kawasaki disease
Pfannenstiel syndrome
Beckwith-Wiedemann syndrome
Rubinstein-Taybi syndrome
Alopecia-photophobia syndrome

3. In the setting of an equivocal examination, which of the following has the greatest sensitivity in diagnosing an inguinal hernia?
   A. Repeat examination by a second surgeon
   B. Ultrasound
   C. CT scan
   D. MRI

Answer: D

Although CT scan is useful in ambiguous clinical presentations, little data exist to support its routine use in diagnosis. The use of MRI in assessing groin hernias was examined in a group of 41 patients scheduled to undergo laparoscopic inguinal hernia repair. Preoperatively, all patients underwent US and MRI. Laparoscopic confirmation of the presence of inguinal hernia was deemed the gold standard. Physical examination was found to be the least sensitive, whereas MRI was found to be the most sensitive. False positives were low on physical examination and MRI (one finding), but higher with US (four findings). With further refinement of technology, radiologic techniques will continue to improve the sensitivity and specificity rates of diagnosis, thereby serving a supplementary role in cases of uncertain diagnosis. (See Schwartz 9th ed., p 1318.)

4. A four-layer, suture repair of an inguinal hernia is a
   A. Pott's repair
   B. Shouldice repair
   C. McVay repair
   D. Lichtenstein repair

Answer: B

Shouldice repair: With the posterior inguinal floor exposed, an incision in the transversalis fascia is performed between the pubic tubercle and internal ring. Care is taken to avoid injury to any preperitoneal structures, and these are bluntly dissected to mobilize the upper and lower fascial flaps. The first layer of repair begins at the pubic tubercle where the iliopubic tract is sutured to the lateral edge of the rectus sheath, then progressing laterally. The inferior flap of the transversalis fascia, which includes the iliopubic tract, is sutured continuously to the posterior aspect of the superior flap of the transversalis fascia until the internal ring is encountered. At this point, the internal ring has been reconstituted. The suture is not tied here, but rather is continued back upon itself in the medial direction. At the internal ring, the second layer is the reapproximation of the superior edge of the transversalis fascia to the inferior fascial margin and the shelving edge of the inguinal ligament. The suture is then tied to the tail of the original stitch. A third suture is started at the tightened inguinal ring, joining the internal oblique and transversus abdominis aponeuroses to external oblique aponeurotic fibers just superficial to the inguinal ligament. This layer is continued to the pubic tubercle where it reverses upon itself to create a fourth suture line, which is similar and superficial to the third layer.

Pott's repair: high ligation of the sac only, with no repair of the inguinal canal—used for indirect hernias only.

McVay repair: Once the cord has been isolated, a transverse incision is performed through the transversalis fascia, thereby entering the preperitoneal space. A small amount of dissection of the posterior aspect of the fascia is performed to allow mobilization of the upper margin of the transversalis fascia. The floor of the inguinal canal is then reconstructed to restore its strength. Cooper's ligament is identified medially, and it is bluntly dissected to expose its surface. The upper margin of the transversalis fascia is then sutured to Cooper's ligament. The repair is continued laterally along Cooper's ligament, occluding the femoral canal.

Lichtenstein repair: Initial exposure and mobilization of cord structures is identical to other open approaches. Particular attention must be paid to blunt dissection of the inguinal canal to expose the shelving edge of the inguinal ligament and pubic tubercle, as well as provide a large area for mesh placement. Unlike the tissue-based repairs, the Lichtenstein repair does not include routine division of the transversalis fascia, thereby preventing the identification of a latent femoral hernia.... Instead, the floor and internal ring are reinforced through the application of the mesh. (See Schwartz 9th ed., p 1321, and Fig. 37-3.)

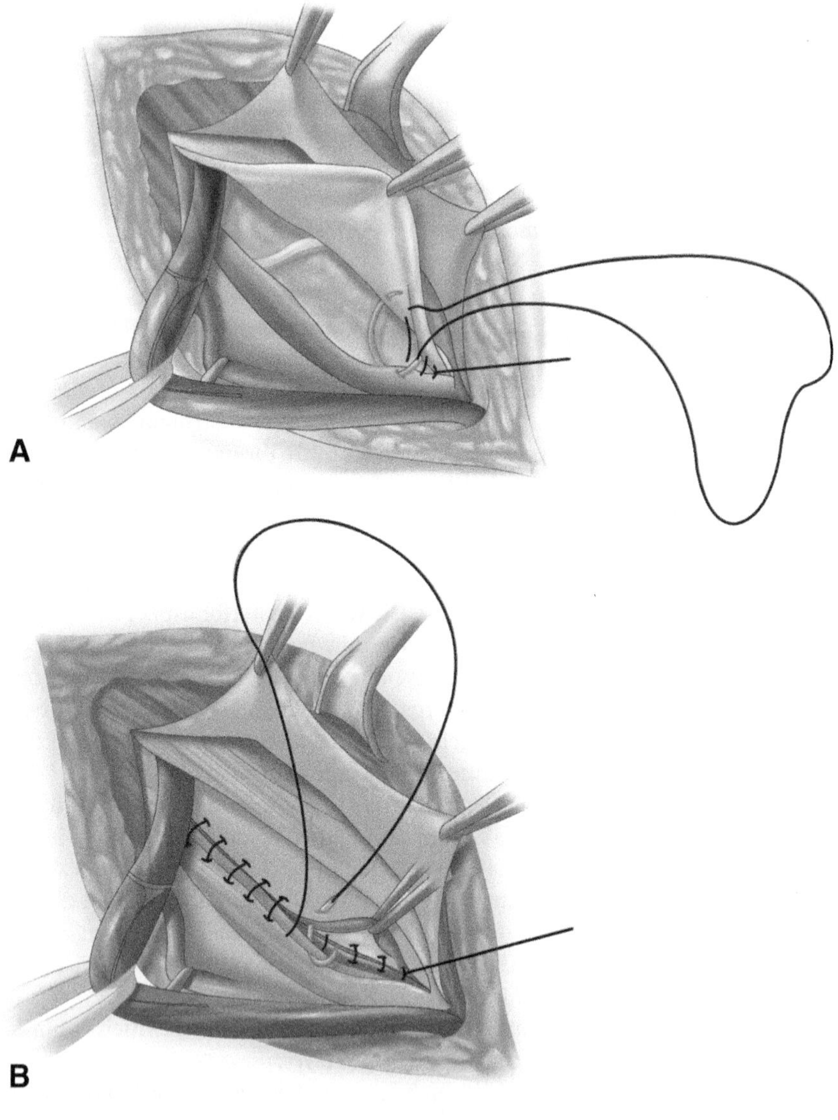

FIG. 37-3. The Shouldice repair. A. The iliopubic tract is sutured to the medial flap, which is made up of the transversalis fascia and the internal oblique and transverse abdominis muscles. B. This is the second of the four suture lines. After the stump of the cremaster muscle is picked up, the suture is reversed back toward the pubic tubercle approximating the internal oblique and transversus muscles to the inguinal ligament. Two more suture lines will eventually be created suturing the internal oblique and transversus muscles medially to an artificially created "pseudo" inguinal ligament developed from superficial fibers of the inferior flap of the external oblique aponeurosis parallel to the true ligament.

5. Contraindications for a transperitoneal laparoscopic inguinal hernia repair include
   A. Inability to tolerate general anesthesia
   B. Previous gastric surgery
   C. Morbid obesity
   D. Diabetes

Answer: A

There are several contraindications to the transperitoneal laparoscopic technique that must be taken into consideration. Because laparoscopy must be performed using general anesthesia, the patient must be able to hemodynamically tolerate both general anesthesia and the effects of pneumoperitoneum. As well, previous lower abdominal surgery, such as prostatectomy, or lower midline incisions for other abdominal procedures, are a relative contraindication to a laparoscopic approach secondary to the presence of scarred tissue in the preperitoneal space. (See Schwartz 9th ed., p 1332.)

6. Which of the following has the lowest recurrence rate after open inguinal hernia repair?
   A. Basini repair
   B. Shouldice repair
   C. McVay repair
   D. Marcy repair

Answer: B

Recurrence rates of tissue-based repairs vary according to procedure; however, large-scale analyses continue to confirm the Shouldice repair as the most superior. Surgeons who perform a large volume of the Shouldice repair are able to demonstrate recurrence rates around 1%. In less experienced hands, such low recurrence rates are not demonstrated, yet overall, recurrence rates for the Shouldice repair are consistently lower than those of the Bassini or McVay repair. The Marcy repair is a Bassini with narrowing of a widened internal ring. (See Schwartz 9th ed., p 1334.)

7. Ischemic orchitis is best treated with
   A. Re-exploration to relax tension at the internal ring
   B. Re-exploration for orchiectomy
   C. Nonsteroidal anti-inflammatory agents
   D. Nothing (no treatment is necessary)

Answer: C

Ischemic orchitis usually presents within the first week following inguinal hernia repair. The patient may present with a low-grade fever, but more commonly with an enlarged, indurated, and painful testicle. This complication occurs in <1% of all herniorrhaphies, but increases in the reoperations for recurrent inguinal hernias. Ischemic orchitis is likely caused by injury to the pampiniform plexus, not the testicular artery. Densely adherent or large hernia sacs that require extensive dissection may lead to injury of the pampiniform plexus. Reassurance, NSAIDs, and comfort measures are enacted to allow self-limited resolution of this complication. Long-term effects of ischemic orchitis are rare. (See Schwartz 9th ed., p 1337.)

8. A "sports hernia" is best described as
   A. A direct inguinal hernia in an athlete
   B. A stress-related groin hernia in an athlete
   C. A small tear or weakness in the posterior inguinal canal
   D. Pubis osteitis

Answer: C

Despite a classical presentation, the absence of clinical findings makes the diagnosis of a hernia more dubious. Occult hernias such as these may, in fact, be a sports hernia, otherwise known as a *sportsman's hernia* or *athletic pubalgia*. They are commonly seen in athletes that perform repetitive kicking, twisting, or turning, as in hockey, soccer, and football, which results in a weakness or tearing of the posterior inguinal wall. A similar abrupt motion in a nonathlete also may lead to this condition. The hernia often is not identified until the time of surgical exploration, where a number of different anomalies may be visualized. These include tearing of the transversalis fascia or conjoined tendon, tearing of the internal oblique or avulsion of the internal oblique at the pubic tubercle, or tear of the external oblique aponeurosis or widened external ring. The lack of standardization in the literature makes analysis difficult because oftentimes groin pain of other origins is included in the discussion of sports hernias. (See Schwartz 9th ed., p 1340.)

CHAPTER 38

Thyroid, Parathyroid, and Adrenal

BASIC SCIENCE QUESTIONS

1. The most common position of the RIGHT recurrent laryngeal nerve is
   A. Anterior to the inferior thyroid artery
   B. Posterior to the inferior thyroid artery
   C. Between the branches of the inferior thyroid artery
   D. Absent (nonrecurrent laryngeal nerve)

Answer: B

The left RLN arises from the vagus nerve where it crosses the aortic arch, loops around the ligamentum arteriosum, and ascends medially in the neck within the tracheoesophageal groove. The right RLN arises from the vagus at its crossing with the right subclavian artery. The nerve usually passes posterior to the artery before ascending in the neck, its course being more oblique than the left RLN. Along their course in the neck, the RLNs may branch, and pass anterior, posterior, or interdigitate with branches of the inferior thyroid artery (Fig. 38-1). The right RLN may be nonrecurrent in 0.5 to 1% of individuals and often is associated with a vascular anomaly. (See Schwartz 9th ed., p 1346.)

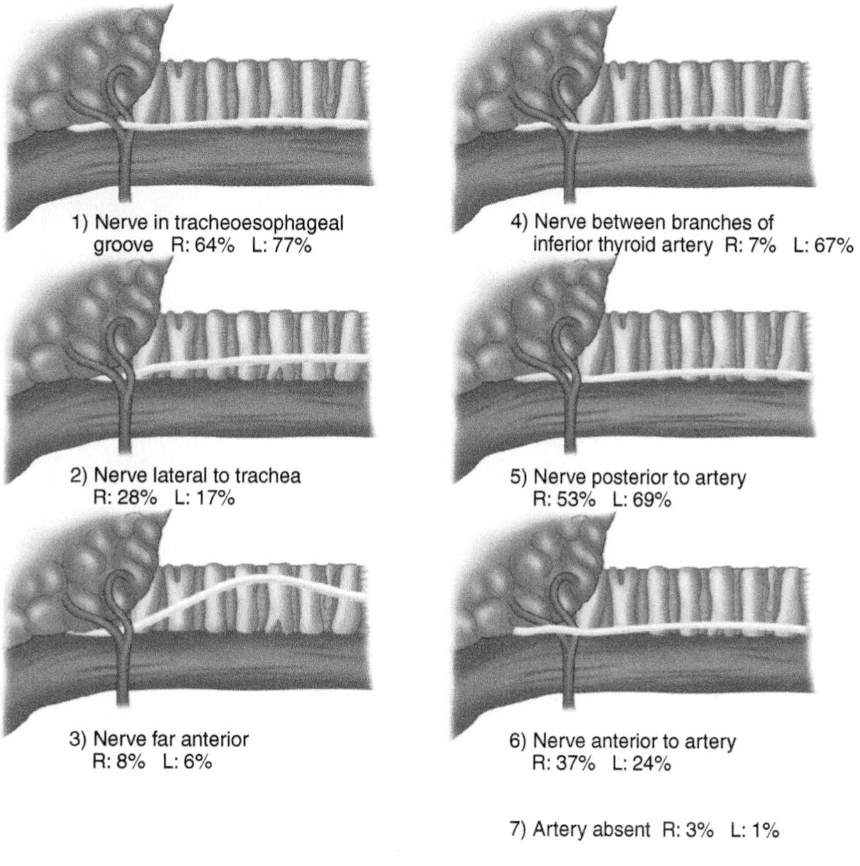

1) Nerve in tracheoesophageal groove R: 64% L: 77%
4) Nerve between branches of inferior thyroid artery R: 7% L: 67%
2) Nerve lateral to trachea R: 28% L: 17%
5) Nerve posterior to artery R: 53% L: 69%
3) Nerve far anterior R: 8% L: 6%
6) Nerve anterior to artery R: 37% L: 24%
7) Artery absent R: 3% L: 1%

FIG. 38-1. Relationship of recurrent laryngeal nerve to the inferior thyroid artery—the superior parathyroid is characteristically dorsal to the plane of the nerve, whereas the inferior gland is ventral to the nerve.

2. Thyroid hormone receptors
   A. Bind T_4
   B. Bind T_3
   C. Are present in the mitochondria
   D. Are present on the cell membrane

Answer: B
Free thyroid hormone enters the cell membrane by diffusion or by specific carriers and is carried to the nuclear membrane by binding to specific proteins. T_4 is deiodinated to T_3 and enters the nucleus via active transport, where it binds to the thyroid hormone receptor. The T_3 receptor is similar to the nuclear receptors for glucocorticoids, mineralocorticoids, estrogens, vitamin D, and retinoic acid. In humans, two types of T_3 receptor genes (α and β) are located on chromosomes 3 and 17. (See Schwartz 9th ed., p 1348.)

3. The inferior parathyroid glands are derived from the
   A. 1st branchial pouch
   B. 2nd branchial pouch
   C. 3rd branchial pouch
   D. 4th branchial pouch

Answer: C
In humans, the superior parathyroid glands are derived from the fourth branchial pouch, which also gives rise to the thyroid gland. The third branchial pouches give rise to the inferior parathyroid glands and the thymus. (See Schwartz 9th ed., p 1374.)

4. Parathormone secretion is stimulated by
   A. Hypermagnesemia
   B. Hypovitaminosis D
   C. Parasympathetic stimulation
   D. Severe hypokalemia

Answer: B
The parathyroid cells rely on a Gprotein coupled membrane receptor, designated the calcium-sensing receptor (CASR), to regulate PTH secretion by sensing extracellular calcium levels. PTH secretion also is stimulated by low levels of 1,25-dihydroxy vitamin D, catecholamines, and hypomagnesemia. (See Schwartz 9th ed., p 1376.)

5. Which of the following receptors has the greatest affinity for epinephrine?
   A. α adrenergic receptor
   B. β_1 adrenergic receptor
   C. β_2 adrenergic receptor
   D. γ adrenergic receptor

Answer: A
Adrenergic receptors are transmembrane-spanning molecules, which are coupled to G proteins. They may be subdivided into α and β subtypes, which are localized in different tissues, have varying affinity to various catecholamines, and mediate distinct biologic effects (Table 38-1). The receptor affinities for α receptors are—epinephrine > norepinephrine >> isoproterenol; β_1 receptors—isoproterenol > epinephrine = norepinephrine; and β_2 receptors—isoproterenol > epinephrine >> norepinephrine. There is no γ adrenergic receptor. (See Schwartz 9th ed., p 1392.)

TABLE 38-1 Catecholamine hormone receptors and effects they mediate

Receptor	Tissue	Function
α_1	Blood vessels	Contraction
	Gut	Decreased motility, increased sphincter tone
	Pancreas	Decreased insulin and glucagon release
	Liver	Glycogenolysis, gluconeogenesis
	Eyes	Pupil dilation
	Uterus	Contraction
	Skin	Sweating
α_2	Synapse (sympathetic)	Inhibits norepinephrine release
	Platelet	Aggregation
β_1	Heart	Chronotropic, inotropic
	Adipose tissue	Lipolysis
	Gut	Decreased motility, increased sphincter tone
	Pancreas	Increased insulin and glucagon release
β_2	Blood vessels	Vasodilation
	Bronchioles	Dilation
	Uterus	Relaxation

6. The left adrenal vein drains into the
   A. IVC
   B. Left renal vein
   C. Left gonadal vein
   D. Splenic vein

Answer: B

In contrast to the arterial supply, each adrenal usually is drained by a single, major adrenal vein. The right adrenal vein is usually short and drains into the IVC, whereas the left adrenal vein is longer and empties into the left renal vein after joining the inferior phrenic vein. (See Schwartz 9th ed., p 1389.)

7. Which of the following is an effect of thyroid hormones?
   A. Positive inotropic effect on the heart
   B. Maintenance of the normal hypoxic drive to breathe
   C. Increased protein turnover
   D. All of the above

Answer: D

Thyroid hormones affect almost every system in the body. They are important for fetal brain development and skeletal maturation. T_3 increases oxygen consumption, basal metabolic rate, and heat production by stimulation of Na^+/K^+ ATPase in various tissues. It also has positive inotropic and chronotropic effects on the heart by increasing transcription of the Ca^{2+} ATPase in the sarcoplasmic reticulum and increasing levels of beta-adrenergic receptors and concentration of G proteins. Myocardial alpha receptors are decreased and actions of catecholamines are amplified. Thyroid hormones are responsible for maintaining the normal hypoxic and hypercapnic drive in the respiratory center of the brain. They also increase GI motility, leading to diarrhea in hyperthyroidism and constipation in hypothyroidism. Thyroid hormones also increase bone and protein turnover and the speed of muscle contraction and relaxation. They also increase glycogenolysis, hepatic gluconeogenesis, intestinal glucose absorption, and cholesterol synthesis and degradation. (See Schwartz 9th ed., p 1349.)

8. The origin of the superior thyroid artery is
   A. Internal carotid artery
   B. External carotid artery
   C. Thyrocervical trunk
   D. Innominate artery

Answer: B

The superior thyroid arteries arise from the ipsilateral external carotid arteries and divide into anterior and posterior branches at the apices of the thyroid lobes. The inferior thyroid arteries arise from the thyrocervical trunk shortly after their origin from the subclavian arteries. The inferior thyroid arteries travel upward in the neck posterior to the carotid sheath to enter the thyroid lobes at their midpoint. A thyroidea ima artery arises directly from the aorta or innominate in 1 to 4% of individuals to enter the isthmus or replace a missing inferior thyroid artery. (See Schwartz 9th ed., p 1345, and Fig. 38-2.)

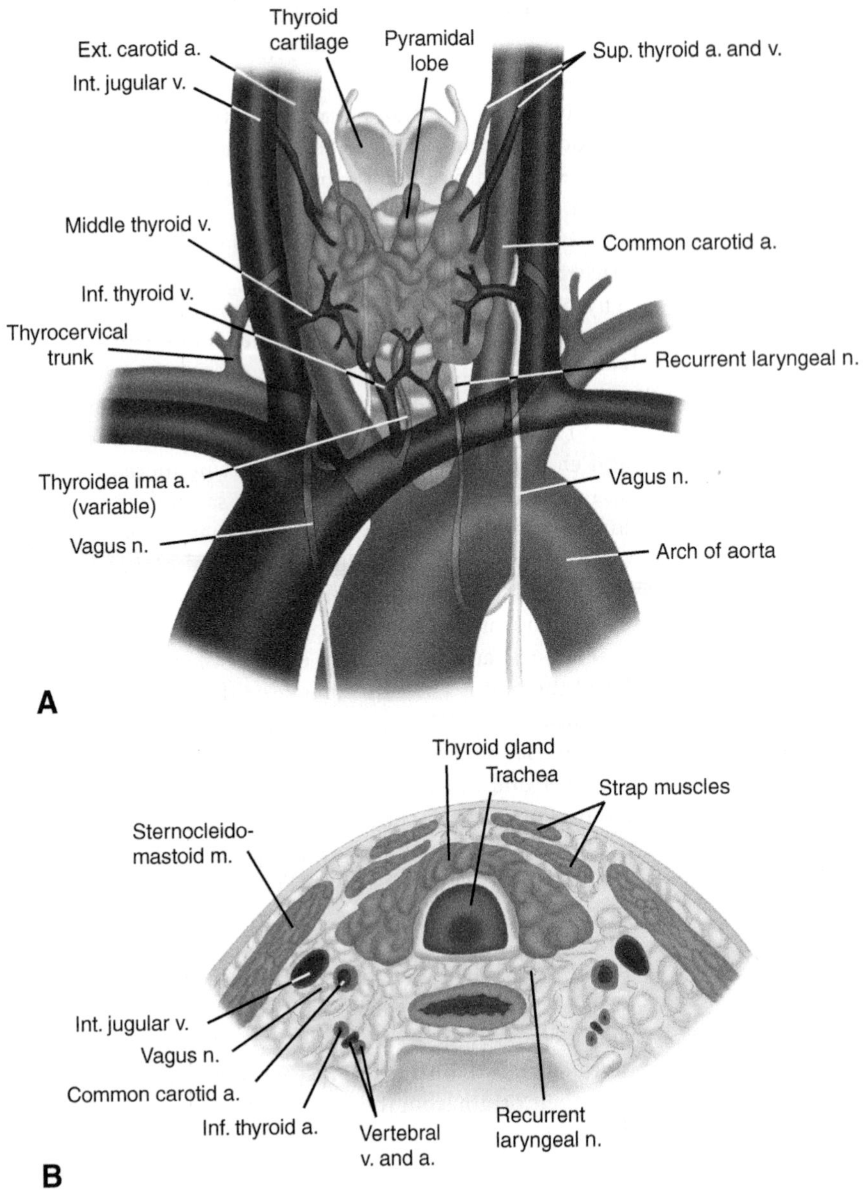
Thyroid cartilage
Pyramidal lobe
Ext. carotid a.
Int. jugular v.
Sup. thyroid a. and v.
Middle thyroid v.
Common carotid a.
Inf. thyroid v.
Thyrocervical trunk
Recurrent laryngeal n.
Thyroidea ima a. (variable)
Vagus n.
Vagus n.
Arch of aorta
A
Thyroid gland
Trachea
Strap muscles
Sternocleido-mastoid m.
Int. jugular v.
Vagus n.
Common carotid a.
Inf. thyroid a.
Vertebral v. and a.
Recurrent laryngeal n.
B

FIG. 38-2. Anatomy of the thyroid gland and surrounding structures, viewed anteriorly (A) and in cross-section (B). a. = artery; m. = muscle; n. = nerve; v. = vein.

9. The most common location of the superior parathyroid glands is
   A. Dorsal to the recurrent laryngeal nerve (RLN), within 1 cm of the junction of the RLN and inferior thyroid artery
   B. Ventral to the recurrent laryngeal nerve (RLN), within 1 cm of the junction of the RLN and inferior thyroid artery
   C. Dorsal to the recurrent laryngeal nerve (RLN), within 3 cm of the junction of the RLN and inferior thyroid artery
   D. Ventral to the recurrent laryngeal nerve (RLN), within 3 cm of the junction of the RLN and inferior thyroid artery

Answer: A

About 85% of individuals have four parathyroid glands that can be found within 1 cm of the junction of the inferior thyroid artery and the RLN. The superior glands are usually located dorsal to the RLN, whereas the inferior glands are usually found ventral to the RLN (Fig. 38-3). (See Schwartz 9th ed., p 1349.)

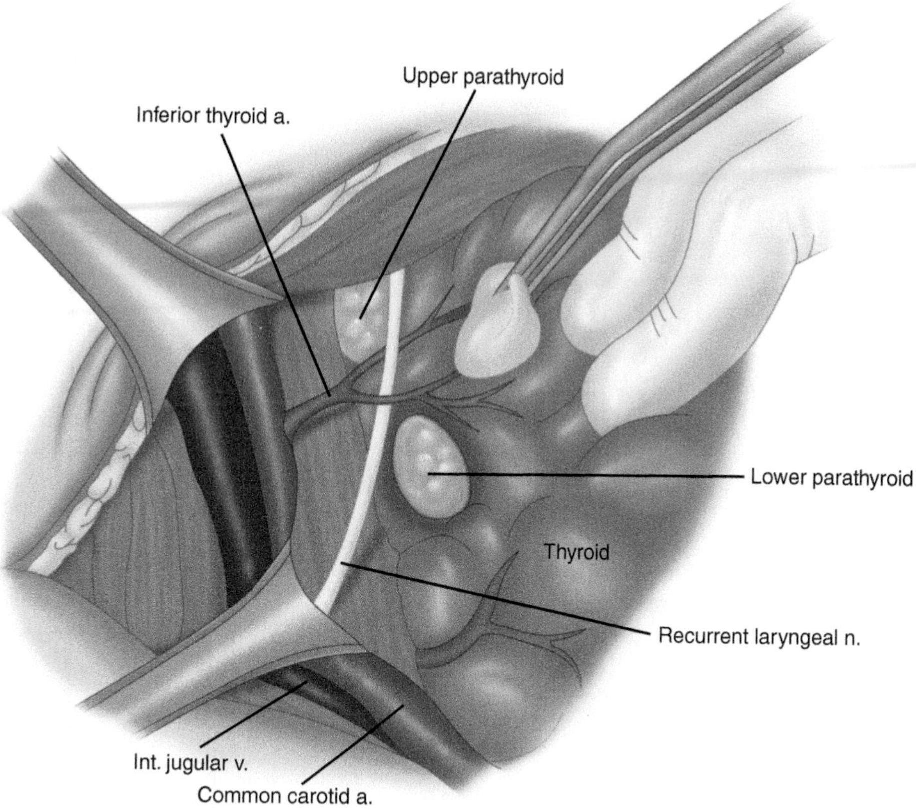

FIG. 38-3. Relationship of the parathyroids to the recurrent laryngeal nerve. a. = artery; v. = vein.

10. Secreted parathormone has a half-life of
    A. 2-4 minutes
    B. 45-60 minutes
    C. 3 hours
    D. 8 hours

Answer: A

Secreted PTH has a half-life of 2 to 4 minutes. In the liver, PTH is metabolized into the active N-terminal component and the relatively inactive C-terminal fraction. The C-terminal component is excreted by the kidneys and accumulates in chronic renal failure. (See Schwartz 9th ed., p 1376.)

11. Which of the following is the substrate for all catecholamines?
    A. Alanine
    B. Leucine
    C. Tryptophan
    D. Tyrosine

Answer: D

Catecholamine hormones (epinephrine, norepinephrine, and dopamine) are produced not only in the central and sympathetic nervous system but also in the adrenal medulla. The substrate, tyrosine, is converted to catecholamines via a series of steps shown in Fig. 38-4. (See Schwartz 9th ed., p 1392.)

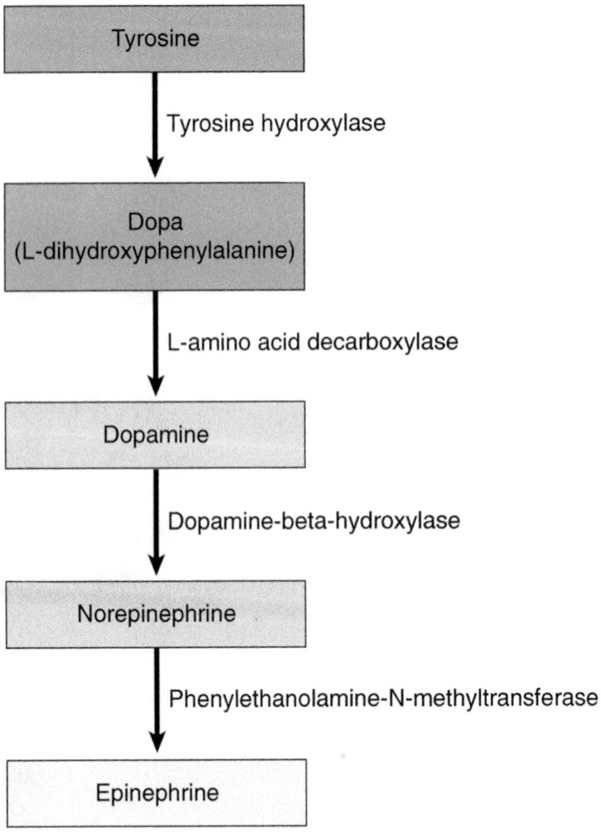

FIG. 38-4. Synthesis of catecholamines.

12. The adrenal cortex arises from
    A. Ectoderm
    B. Mesoderm
    C. Endoderm
    D. Neural crest

Answer: B

The cortex originates around the fifth week of gestation from mesodermal tissue near the gonads on the adrenogenital ridge. Therefore, ectopic adrenocortical tissue may be found in the ovaries, spermatic cord, and testes. The cortex differentiates further into a thin, definitive cortex and a thicker, inner fetal cortex. The latter is functional and produces fetal adrenal steroids by the eighth week of gestation, but undergoes involution after birth, resulting in a decrease in adrenal weight during the first three postpartum months. The definitive cortex persists after birth to form the adult cortex over the first 3 years of life. In contrast, the adrenal medulla is ectodermal in origin and arises from the neural crest. (See Schwartz 9th ed., p 1389.)

13. The inferior adrenal artery originates from the
    A. Phrenic artery
    B. Splenic artery
    C. Renal artery
    D. Aorta

Answer: C

Each adrenal gland is supplied by three groups of vessels—the superior adrenal arteries derived from the inferior phrenic artery, the middle adrenal arteries derived from the aorta, and the inferior adrenal arteries derived from the renal artery. Other vessels originating from the intercostal and gonadal vessels may also supply the adrenals. These arteries branch into about 50 arterioles to form a rich plexus beneath the glandular capsule and require careful dissection, ligation, and division during adrenalectomy. (See Schwartz 9th ed., p 1389.)

14. Which of the following is NOT an effect of glucocorticosteroids?
    A. Decreased muscle protein synthesis
    B. Decreased lipolysis
    C. Inhibition of bone formation
    D. Increased cardiac output

Answer: B

Glucocorticoids have important functions in intermediary metabolism but also affect connective tissue, bone, immune, cardiovascular, renal, and central nervous systems, as outlined in Table 38-2. (See Schwartz 9th ed., p 1391.)

TABLE 38-2 Functions of glucocorticoid hormones

Function/System	Effects
Glucose metabolism	Increased hepatic glycogen deposition, gluconeogenesis, decreased muscle glucose uptake and metabolism
Protein metabolism	Decreased muscle protein synthesis, increased catabolism
Fat metabolism	Increased lipolysis in adipose tissue
Connective tissue	Inhibition of fibroblasts, loss of collagen, thinning of skin, striae formation
Skeletal system	Inhibition of bone formation, increased osteoclast activity, potentiate the action of PTH
Immune system	Increases circulation of polymorphonuclear cells, decreases numbers of lymphocytes, monocytes, and eosinophils, reduces migration of inflammatory cells to sites of injury
Cardiovascular system	Increases cardiac output and peripheral vascular tone
Renal system	Sodium retention, hypokalemia, hypertension via mineralocorticoid effect, increased glomerular filtration via glucocorticoid effects
Endocrine system	Inhibits TSH synthesis and release, decreased TBG levels, decreased conversion of T_4 to T_3

PTH = parathyroid hormone; T_3 = 3,5',3-triiodothyronine; T_4 = thyroxine; TBG = thyroxine-binding globulin; TSH = thyroid-stimulating hormone.

15. The *RET* proto-oncogene is associated with
    A. Papillary thyroid cancer
    B. Hirschsprung's disease
    C. Pheochomocytoma
    D. All of the above

Answer: D

The *RET* proto-oncogene plays a significant role in the pathogenesis of thyroid cancers. It is located on chromosome 10 and encodes a receptor tyrosine kinase, which binds several growth factors such as glial-derived neurotrophic factor and neurturin. The *RET* protein is expressed in tissues derived from the embryonic nervous and excretory systems. Therefore, *RET* disruption can lead to developmental abnormalities in organs derived from these systems, such as the enteric nervous system (Hirschsprung's disease) and kidney. Germline mutations in the *RET* proto-oncogene are known to predispose to MEN2A, MEN2B, and familial MTCs, and somatic mutations have been demonstrated in tumors derived from the neural crest, such as MTCs (30%) and pheochromocytomas. (See Schwartz 9th ed., p 1361, and Table 38-3.)

TABLE 38-3 Oncogenes and tumor-suppressor genes implicated in thyroid tumorigenesis

Gene	Function	Tumor
Oncogenes		
RET	Membrane receptor with tyrosine kinase activity	Sporadic and familial MTC, PTC (RET/PTC rearrangements)
MET	Same	Overexpressed in PTC
TRK1	Same	Activated in some PTC
TSH-R	Linked to heterotrimeric G protein	Hyperfunctioning adenoma
Gsα (gsp)	Signal transduction molecule (GTP binding)	Hyperfunctioning adenoma, follicular adenoma
Ras	Signal transduction protein	Follicular adenoma and carcinoma, PTC
PAX8/PPARγ1	Oncoprotein	Follicular adenoma, follicular carcinoma
B-Raf (BRAF)	Signal transduction	PTC, tall cell and poorly differentiated, anaplastic
Tumor suppressors		
p53	Cell cycle regulator, arrests cells in G_1, induces apoptosis	De-differentiated PTC, FTC, anaplastic cancers
p16	Cell cycle regulator, inhibits cyclin dependent kinase	Thyroid cancer cell lines
PTEN	Protein tyrosine phosphatase	Follicular adenoma and carcinoma

FTC = follicular thyroid cancer; GTP = guanosine triphosphate; MTC = medullary thyroid cancer; PTC = papillary thyroid cancer.

16. Thyroxine (T_4) is composed of
    A. Two Diiodotyrosine (DIT) molecules
    B. One Diiodotyrosine (DIT) molecules and two mono-iodohyrosin (MIT) molecules
    C. Four monoiodohyrosin (MIT) molecules
    D. None of the above

Answer: A

The synthesis of thyroid hormone consists of several steps. The first, iodide trapping, involves active (ATP-dependent) transport of iodide across the basement membrane of the thyrocyte via an intrinsic membrane protein, the sodium/iodine (Na^+/I^-) symporter. Thyroglobulin (Tg) is a large (660 kDa) glycoprotein, which is present in thyroid follicles and has four tyrosyl residues. The second step in thyroid hormone synthesis involves oxidation of iodide to iodine and iodination of tyrosine residues on Tg, to form monoiodotyrosines (MIT) and diiodotyrosines (DIT). Both processes are catalyzed by thyroid peroxidase (TPO). A recently identified protein, pendrin, is thought to mediate iodine efflux at the apical membrane. The third step leads to coupling of two DIT molecules to form tetra-iodothyronine or thyroxine (T4), and one DIT molecule with one MIT molecule to form 3,5,3'-triiodothyronine (T3) or 3,3',5'–triiodothyronine reverse (rT_3). (See Schwartz 9th ed., p 1348.)

17. Which of the following is a function of aldosterone?
   A. Increased potassium absorption
   B. Increased hydrogen ion absorption
   C. Increased sodium absorption
   D. None of the above

Answer: C
Aldosterone functions mainly to increase sodium reabsorption and potassium and hydrogen ion excretion at the level of the renal distal convoluted tubule. Less commonly, aldosterone increases sodium absorption in salivary glands and GI mucosal surfaces. (See Schwartz 9th ed., p 1390.)

18. Glucocorticoids are produced in the
   A. Zona glomerulosa
   B. Zona fasciculate
   C. Zona reticularis
   D. Adrenal medulla

Answer: B
The adrenal cortex appears yellow due to its high lipid content and accounts for about 80 to 90% of the gland's volume. Histologically, the cortex is divided into three zones—the zona glomerulosa, zona fasciculata, and zona reticularis. The outer area of the zona glomerulosa consists of small cells and is the site of production of the mineralocorticoid hormone, aldosterone. The zona fasciculate is made up of larger cells, which often appear foamy due to multiple lipid inclusions, whereas the zona reticularis cells are smaller. These latter zones are the site of production of glucocorticoids and adrenal androgens. The adrenal medulla constitutes up to 10 to 20% of the gland's volume and is reddish brown in color. It produces the catecholamine hormones epinephrine and norepinephrine. (See Schwartz 9th ed., p 1389.)

19. The paired lateral thyroid anlages fuse with the median thyroid anlage in the 5th week of gestation. These paired lateral anlages originate from
   A. Ectoderm
   B. Mesoderm
   C. Endoderm
   D. Neural crest

Answer: C
The thyroid gland arises as an outpouching of the primitive foregut around the third week of gestation. It originates at the base of the tongue at the foramen cecum. Endoderm cells in the floor of the pharyngeal anlage thicken to form the medial thyroid anlage that descends in the neck anterior to structures that form the hyoid bone and larynx. During its descent, the anlage remains connected to the foramen cecum via an epithelial-lined tube known as the *Thyroglossal duct.* The epithelial cells making up the anlage give rise to the thyroid follicular cells. The paired lateral anlages originate from the fourth branchial pouch and fuse with the median anlage at approximately the fifth week of gestation. The lateral anlages are neuroectodermal in origin (ultimobranchial bodies) and provide the calcitonin producing parafollicular or C cells, which thus come to lie in the superoposterior region of the gland. (See Schwartz 9th ed., p 1344.)

20. Cholesterol is the precursor of all hormones produced in the adrenal gland. The first step in the synthesis of all adrenal hormones is to cleave cholesterol to produce
   A. Progesterone
   B. Pregnenolone
   C. 17α-hydroxypregnenolone
   D. 11-deoxy-corticosterone

Answer: B
Pregnenolone is produced by cleaving the cholesterol side chain and becomes the precursor to all adrenal hormones (Fig. 38-5). (See Schwartz 9th ed., p 1390.)

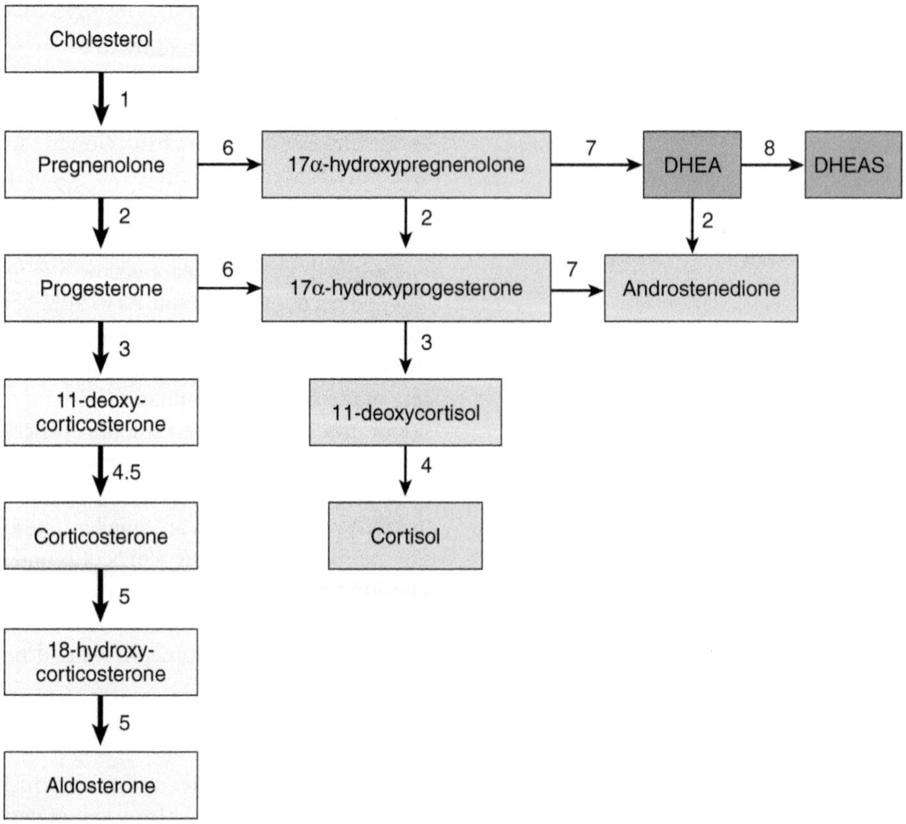

FIG. 38-5. Synthesis of adrenal steroids. The enzymes involved are (*1*) p450scc (cholesterol side chain cleavage), (*2*) 3*β*-hydroxysteroid dehydrogenase, (*3*) p450c21 (21 *β*-hydroxylase), (*4*) p450c11 (11 *β*-hydroxylase), (*5*) p450c11AS (aldosterone synthase), (*6*) p450c17 (17*α*-hydroxylase activity), (*7*) p450c17 (17, 20-lyase/desmolase activity), and (*8*) sulfokinase. DHEAS = dehydroepiandrosterone sulfate.

CLINICAL QUESTIONS

1. Propylthiouracil
   A. Can be given once a day in patients with hyperthyroidism
   B. Can cause agranulocytosis
   C. Does not affect the peripheral conversion of T_4 to T_3
   D. Does not cross the placenta

Answer: B

Antithyroid medications generally are administered in preparation for RAI ablation or surgery. The drugs commonly used are propylthiouracil (PTU, 100 to 300 mg three times daily) and methimazole (10 to 30 mg three times daily, then once daily). Methimazole has a longer half-life and can be dosed once daily. Both drugs reduce thyroid hormone production by inhibiting the organic binding of iodine and the coupling of iodotyrosines (mediated by TPO). In addition, PTU also inhibits the peripheral conversion of T_4 to T_3, making it useful for the treatment of thyroid storm. Both drugs can cross the placenta, inhibiting fetal thyroid function, and are excreted in breast milk, although PTU has a lower risk of transplacental transfer. Methimazole also has been associated with congenital aplasia; therefore, PTU is preferred in pregnant and breast-feeding women. Side effects of treatment include reversible granulocytopenia, skin rashes, fever, peripheral neuritis, polyarteritis, vasculitis, and, rarely, agranulocytosis and aplastic anemia. Patients should be monitored for these possible complications and should always be warned to stop PTU or methimazole immediately and seek medical advice should they develop a sore throat or fever. Treatment of agranulocytosis involves admission to the hospital, discontinuation of the drug, and broad-spectrum antibiotic therapy. Surgery should be postponed until the granulocyte count reaches 1000 cells/m^3. (See Schwartz 9th ed., p 1354.)

2. Which of the following is NOT commonly seen in patients with MEN1 syndrome?
   A. Gastrinoma
   B. Insulinoma
   C. Prolactinoma
   D. Pheochromocytoma

Answer: D

Pheochromocytomas are seen in patients with MEN2 syndrome. PHPT is the earliest and most common manifestation of MEN1[59] and develops in 80 to 100% of patients by age 40 years old. These patients also are prone to pancreatic neuroendocrine tumors and pituitary adenomas and, less commonly, to adrenocortical tumors, lipomas, skin angiomas, and carcinoid tumors of the bronchus, thymus, or stomach. About 50% of patients develop gastrinomas, which often are multiple and metastatic at diagnosis. Insulinomas develop in 10 to 15% of cases, whereas many patients have nonfunctional pancreatic endocrine tumors. Prolactinomas occur in 10 to 50% of MEN1 patients and constitute the most common pituitary lesion. (See Schwartz 9th ed., p 1377.)

3. Painful subacute thyroiditis
   A. Results in hypothyroidism in >80% of patients
   B. Occurs most commonly in women >70 years of age
   C. Is often preceded by an upper respiratory tract infection
   D. Requires thyroidectomy for relief of symptoms in >50% of patients

Answer: C

Painful thyroiditis most commonly occurs in 30- to 40-year-old women and is characterized by the sudden or gradual onset of neck pain, which may radiate toward the mandible or ear. History of a preceding upper respiratory tract infection often can be elicited. The gland is enlarged, exquisitely tender, and firm. The disorder classically progresses through four stages. An initial hyperthyroid phase, due to release of thyroid hormone, is followed by a second, euthyroid phase. The third phase, hypothyroidism, occurs in about 20 to 30% of patients and is followed by resolution and return to the euthyroid state in >90% of patients. A few patients develop recurrent disease.

Painful thyroiditis is self-limited, and therefore, treatment is primarily symptomatic. Aspirin and other NSAIDs are used for pain relief, but steroids may be indicated in more severe cases. Short-term thyroid replacement may be needed and may shorten the duration of symptoms. Thyroidectomy is reserved for the rare patient who has a prolonged course not responsive to medical measures or for recurrent disease. (See Schwartz 9th ed., p 1356.)

4. Which of the following tests has the highest sensitivity in localizing parathyroid adenomas?
   A. Ultrasound
   B. Fine cut CT scan
   C. PET scan
   D. Sestamibi scan

Answer: D

^{99m}Tc-labeled sestamibi is the most widely used and accurate modality with a sensitivity >80% for detection of parathyroid adenomas. Sestamibi (Cardiolite) initially was introduced for cardiac imaging and is concentrated in mitochondria-rich tissue. It was subsequently noted to be useful for parathyroid localization due to the delayed washout of the radionuclide from hypercellular parathyroid tissue compared to thyroid tissue. Sestamibi scans generally are complemented by neck ultrasound, which can identify adenomas with >75% sensitivity in experienced centers, and are most useful in identifying intrathyroidal parathyroids. Single-photon emission computed tomography, particularly when used with CT, has been shown to be superior to other nuclear medicine-based imaging. Specifically, single-photon emission computed tomography can indicate whether an adenoma is located in the anterior or posterior mediastinum (aortopulmonary window), thus enabling the surgeon to modify the operative approach accordingly. CT and MRI scans are less sensitive than sestamibi scans, but are helpful in localizing large paraesophageal and mediastinal glands. (See Schwartz 9th ed., p 1381.)

5. Which of the following drugs can cause thyroid storm in patients with hyperthyroidism?
   A. Amiodarone
   B. Labetalol
   C. Corticosteroids
   D. None of the above

Answer: A

Thyroid storm is a condition of hyperthyroidism accompanied by fever, central nervous system agitation or depression, cardiovascular dysfunction that may be precipitated by infection, surgery, or trauma. Occasionally, thyroid storm may result from amiodarone administration. This condition was previously associated with high mortality rates but can be appropriately managed in an intensive care unit setting. Beta blockers are given to reduce peripheral T_4 to T_3 conversion and decrease the hyperthyroid symptoms. Oxygen supplementation and hemodynamic support should be instituted. Non-aspirin compounds can be used to treat pyrexia and Lugol's iodine or sodium ipodate (intravenously) should be administered to decrease iodine uptake and thyroid hormone secretion. PTU therapy blocks the formation of new thyroid hormone and reduces peripheral conversion of T_4 to T_3. Corticosteroids often are helpful to prevent adrenal exhaustion and block hepatic thyroid hormone conversion. (See Schwartz 9th ed., p 1355.)

6. In patients with elevated thyroglobulin after total thyroidectomy for thyroid cancer, many physicians recommend a dose of 100 mCi of ^{131}I. Which of the following is a reported complication of this treatment?
   A. Sialadenitis
   B. Cerebral edema
   C. Bone marrow suppression
   D. Vocal cord paralysis

Answer: A

Sialadenitis, nausea, and vomiting are symptoms reported to occur with as little as 50 mCi of ^{131}I. (See Schwartz 9th ed., p 1367, and Table 38-4.)

TABLE 38-4 Complications of radioactive iodine therapy (^{131}I) and doses at which they are observed

Acute	Long-Term
Neck pain, swelling, and tenderness	Hematologic
Thyroiditis (if remnant present)	Bone marrow suppression (>500 mCi)
Sialadenitis (50–450 mCi), taste dysfunction	Leukemia (>1000 mCi)
Hemorrhage (brain metastases)	Fertility
Cerebral edema (brain metastases, 200 mCi)	Ovarian/testicular damage, infertility
Vocal cord paralysis	Increased spontaneous abortion rate
Nausea and vomiting (50–450 mCi)	Pulmonary fibrosis
Bone marrow suppression (200 mCi)	Chronic sialadenitis, nodules, taste dysfunction
	Increased risk of cancer
	Anaplastic thyroid cancer
	Gastric cancer
	Hepatocellular cancer
	Lung cancer
	Breast cancer (>1000 mCi)
	Bladder cancer
	Hypoparathyroidism

7. The most common cause of Cushing's syndrome is
   A. Adrenal adenoma
   B. Adrenal hyperplasia
   C. Ectopic ACTH production
   D. Pituitary adenoma

Answer: D

Although a bit confusing, the most common cause of Cushing's syndrome is Cushing's disease. *Cushing's syndrome* refers to a complex of symptoms and signs resulting from hypersecretion of cortisol regardless of etiology. In contrast, *Cushing's disease* refers to a pituitary tumor, usually an adenoma, which leads to bilateral adrenal hyperplasia and hypercortisolism. Cushing's syndrome (endogenous) is a rare disease, affecting 10 in 1 million individuals. It is more common in adults but may occur in children. Women are more commonly affected (male:female ratio 1:8). Although most individuals have sporadic disease, Cushing's syndrome may be found in MEN1 families and can result from ACTH-secreting pituitary tumors, primary adrenal neoplasms, or an ectopic ACTH-secreting carcinoid tumor (more common in men) or bronchial adenoma (more common in women).

Cushing's syndrome may be classified as ACTH-dependent or ACTH-independent (Table 38-5). The most common cause of hypercortisolism is exogenous administration of steroids. However, approximately 70% of cases of endogenous Cushing's syndrome are caused by an ACTH-producing pituitary tumor. Primary adrenal sources (adenoma, hyperplasia, and carcinoma) account for about 20% of cases and ectopic ACTH-secreting tumors account for <10% of cases. (See Schwartz 9th ed., p 1394.)

TABLE 38-5 Etiology of Cushing's syndrome

ACTH-dependent (70%)
- Pituitary adenoma or Cushing's disease (~70%)
- Ectopic ACTH production[a] (~10%)
- Ectopic CRH production (<1%)

ACTH-independent (20–30%)
- Adrenal adenoma (10–15%)
- Adrenal carcinoma (5–10%)
- Adrenal hyperplasia—pigmented micronodular cortical hyperplasia or gastric inhibitory peptide-sensitive macronodular hyperplasia (5%)

Other
- Pseudo-Cushing's syndrome
- Iatrogenic—exogenous administration of steroids

[a]From small cell lung tumors, pancreatic islet cell tumors, medullary thyroid cancers, pheochromocytomas, and carcinoid tumors of the lung, thymus, gut, pancreas, and ovary.
ACTH = adrenocorticotropic hormone; CTH = corticotrophin-releasing hormone.

8. Surgery is indicated in which of the following asymptomatic patients with primary hyperparathyroidism?
   A. Mildly elevated urinary calcium excretion (>100 mg/dl)
   B. Reduction in creatinine clearance by 10%
   C. Serum calcium >0.8 above the upper limits of normal
   D. Age <50 years

Answer: D

The guidelines for surgery in asymptomatic patients with primary hyperparathyroidism were recently reassessed at a second workshop on asymptomatic PHPT held at the National Institutes of Health in 2002 as shown in Table 38-6.... It now is recommended for patients with smaller elevations in serum calcium levels (>1 mg/dL above the upper limit of normal) and if BMD measured at any of three sites (radius, spine, or hip) is greater than 2.5 standard deviations below those of gender- and race-matched, not age-matched, controls (i.e., peak bone density or T score (rather than Z score) <2.5). The panel still recommends exercising caution in using neuropsychologic abnormalities, cardiovascular disease, GI symptoms, menopause, and elevated serum or urine indices of increased bone turnover as sole indications for parathyroidectomy. (See Schwartz 9th ed., p 1380.)

TABLE 38-6 Indications for parathyroidectomy in patients with asymptomatic primary HPT (2002 NIH consensus conference guidelines)

- Serum calcium >1 mg/dL above the upper limits of normal
- Life-threatening hypercalcemic episode
- Creatine clearance reduced by 30%
- Kidney stones on abdominal x-rays
- Markedly elevated 24-h urinary calcium excretion (≥400 mg/d)
- Substantially decreased bone mineral density at the lumbar spine, hip, or distal radius (>2.5 SD below peak bone mass, T score <–2.5
- Age <50 y
- Long-term medical surveillance not desired or possible

HPT = hyperparathyroidism; NIH = National Institutes of Health; SD = standard deviation.

9. A patient with a 1-cm medullary carcinoma of the right thyroid and no clinically significant adenopathy is best treated with
   A. Right thyroid lobectomy and isthmusectomy
   B. Right thyroid lobectomy and subtotal left thyroidectomy
   C. Total thyroidectomy
   D. Total thyroidectomy with central lymph node dissection

Answer: D
Total thyroidectomy is the treatment of choice for patients with MTC because of the high incidence of multicentricity, the more aggressive course, and the fact that ^{131}I therapy usually is not effective. Central compartment nodes frequently are involved early in the disease process, so that a bilateral central neck node dissection should be routinely performed. In patients with palpable cervical nodes or involved central neck nodes, ipsilateral or bilateral, modified radical neck dissection is recommended. (See Schwartz 9th ed., p 1368.)

10. The most common cause of primary hyperparathyroidism is
    A. Parathyroid adenoma
    B. Multiple parathyroid adenomas
    C. Parathyroid hyperplasia
    D. Parathyroid carcinoma

Answer: A
PHPT results from the enlargement of a single gland or parathyroid adenoma in approximately 80% of cases, multiple adenomas or hyperplasia in 15 to 20% of patients, and parathyroid carcinoma in 1% of patients. (See Schwartz 9th ed., p 1377.)

11. Which of the following can be seen in the ophthalmopathy of Graves' disease?
    A. Chemosis
    B. Proptosis
    C. Blindness
    D. All of the above

Answer: D
Approximately 50% of patients with Graves' disease develop clinically evident ophthalmopathy. Eye symptoms include lid lag (von Graefe's sign), spasm of the upper eyelid revealing the sclera above the corneoscleral limbus (Dalrymple's sign), and a prominent stare, due to catecholamine excess. True infiltrative eye disease results in periorbital edema, conjunctival swelling and congestion (chemosis), proptosis, limitation of upward and lateral gaze (from involvement of the inferior and medial rectus muscles, respectively), keratitis, and even blindness due to optic nerve involvement. The etiology of Graves' ophthalmopathy is not completely known; however, orbital fibroblasts and muscles are thought to share a common antigen, the TSHR. Ophthalmopathy is thought to result from inflammation caused by cytokines released from sensitized killer T lymphocytes and cytotoxic antibodies. (See Schwartz 9th ed., p 1353.)

12. Papillary cancer of the thyroid
    A. Is uncommon in children
    B. Is the most common thyroid cancer in patients with a history of external radiation
    C. Occurs more commonly in men
    D. All of the above

Answer: B
Papillary carcinoma accounts for 80% of all thyroid malignancies in iodine-sufficient areas and is the predominant thyroid cancer in children and individuals exposed to external radiation. Papillary carcinoma occurs more often in women, with a 2:1 female-to-male ratio, and the mean age at presentation is 30 to 40 years. (See Schwartz 9th ed., p 1362.)

13. There are 7 compartments of lymph nodes in the neck. Metastases from thyroid cancer are uncommon in
    A. Level I nodes
    B. Level III nodes
    C. Level V nodes
    D. Level VII nodes

Answer: A
The thyroid gland is endowed with an extensive network of lymphatics. Intraglandular lymphatic vessels connect both thyroid lobes through the isthmus and also drain to perithyroidal structures and lymph nodes. Regional lymph nodes include pretracheal, paratracheal, perithyroidal, RLN, superior mediastinal, retropharyngeal, esophageal, and upper, middle, and lower jugular chain nodes. These lymph nodes can be classified into seven levels as depicted in Fig. 38-6. The central compartment includes nodes located in the area between the two carotid sheaths, whereas nodes lateral to the vessels are present in the lateral compartment. Thyroid cancers may metastasize to any of these regions, although metastases to submaxillary nodes (level I) are rare (<1%). There also can be 'skip' metastases to nodes in the ipsilateral neck. (See Schwartz 9th ed., p 1347.)

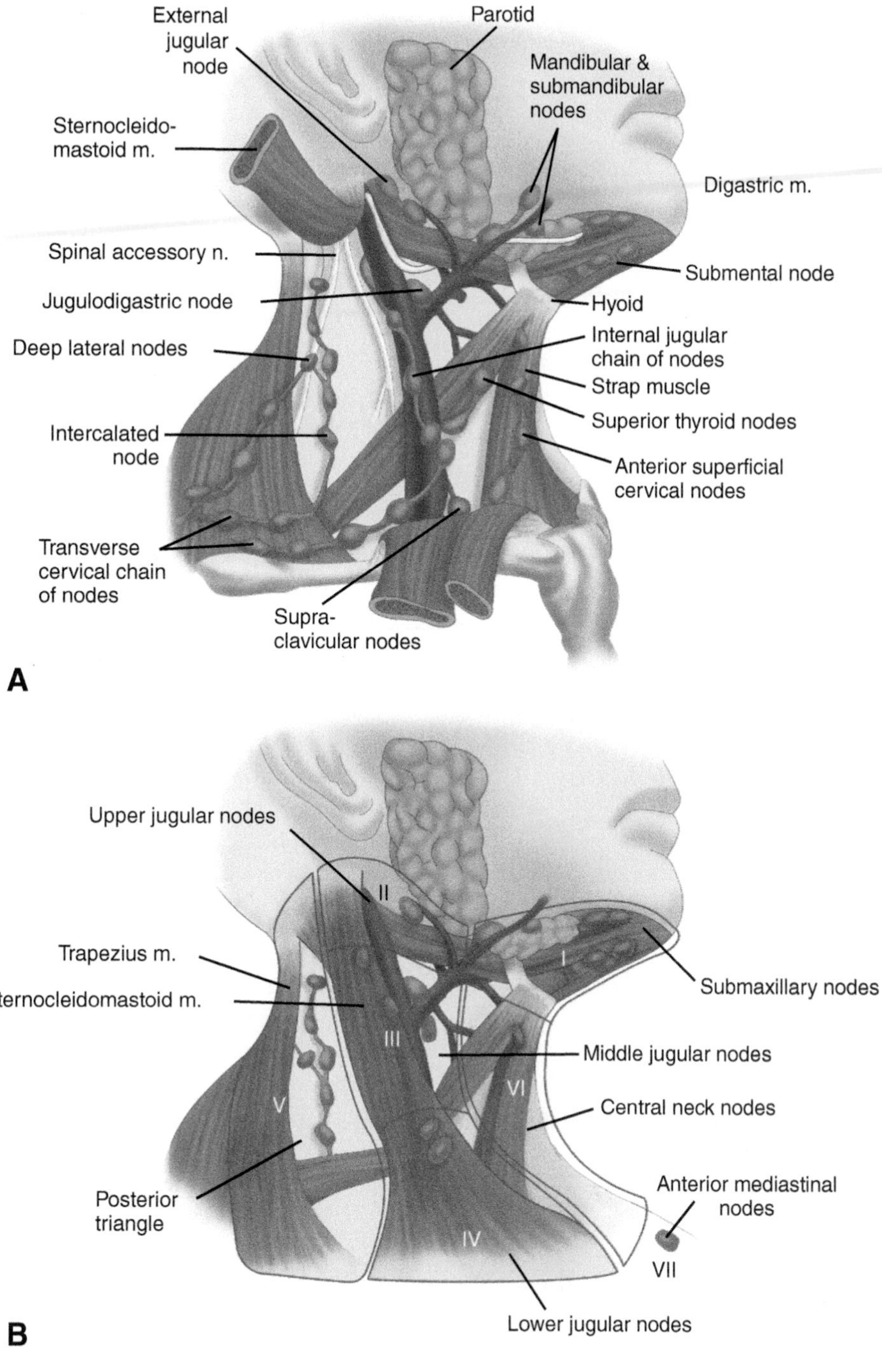

FIG. 38-6. A and B. Lymph nodes in the neck can be divided into six regions. Upper mediastinal nodes constitute level VII. m. = muscle; n. = nerve.

14. A patient with hypertension is diagnosed with hyperaldosteronism. A CT scan shows bilaterally enlarged adrenals without a mass. The most appropriate next intervention is
    A. Unilateral adrenalectomy
    B. Bilateral adrenalectomy
    C. Selective venous catheterization
    D. Medical management

Answer: C

If adrenal hyperplasia is suspected, the algorithm depicted in Fig. 38-7 is useful. Selective venous catheterization and adrenal vein sampling for aldosterone has been demonstrated to be 95% sensitive and 90% specific in localizing the aldosteronoma. Only 20 to 30% of patients with hyperaldosteronism secondary to bilateral adrenal hyperplasia benefit from surgery and, as described, selective venous catheterization is useful to predict which patients will respond. For the other patients, medical therapy with spironolactone, amiloride, or triamterene is the mainstay of management. (See Schwartz 9th ed., p 1394.)

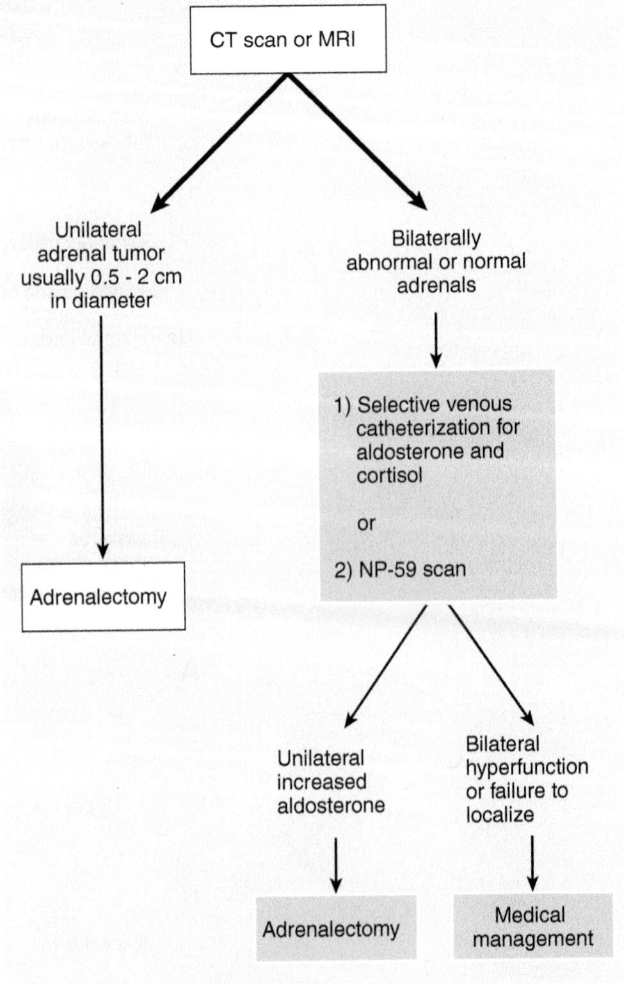

FIG. 38-7. Management of an adrenal aldosteronoma. CT = computed tomography; MRI = magnetic resonance imaging.

15. Papillary thyroid cancer of the clear cell variant is associated with
    A. Cowden's syndrome
    B. Familial adenomatous polyposis
    C. Werner's syndrome
    D. McCune-Albright syndrome

Answer: D

Nonmedullary thyroid cancers can occur in association with other known familial cancer syndromes such as Cowden's syndrome, Werner's (adult progeroid syndrome), and familial adenomatous polyposis (Table 38-7). (See Schwartz 9th ed., p 1360.)

TABLE 38-7 Familial cancer syndromes involving nonmedullary thyroid cancer

Syndrome	Gene	Manifestation	Thyroid Tumor
Cowden's syndrome	*PTEN*	Intestinal hamartomas, benign and malignant breast tumors	FTC, rarely PTC and Hürthle cell tumors
FAP	*APC*	Colon polyps and cancer, duodenal neoplasms, desmoids	PTC cribriform growth pattern
Werner's syndrome	*WRN*	Adult progeroid syndrome	PTC, FTC, anaplastic cancer
Carney complex type 1	*PRKAR1a*	Cutaneous and cardiac myxomas, breast and adrenal tumors	PTC, FTC
McCune-Albright syndrome	*GNAS1*	Polyostotic fibrous dysplasia, endocrine abnormalities, café-au-lait spots	PTC clear cell

FAP = familial adenomatous polyposis; FTC = follicular thyroid cancer; PTC = papillary thyroid cancer.

16. The initial treatment of choice for Riedel's thyroiditis is
    A. Observation
    B. Antibiotics
    C. Corticosteroids
    D. Surgery

Answer: D

Riedel's thyroiditis is a rare variant of thyroiditis also known as *Riedel's struma* or *invasive fibrous thyroiditis* that is characterized by the replacement of all or part of the thyroid parenchyma by fibrous tissue, which also invades into adjacent tissues.

Surgery is the mainstay of the treatment for Riedel's thyroiditis. The chief goal of operation is to decompress the trachea by wedge excision of the thyroid isthmus and to make a tissue diagnosis. More extensive resections are not advised due to the infiltrative nature of the fibrotic process that obscures usual landmarks and structures. Hypothyroid patients are treated with thyroid hormone replacement. Some patients who remain symptomatic have been reported to experience dramatic improvement after treatment with corticosteroids and tamoxifen. (See Schwartz 9th ed., p 1357.)

17. Which of the following should be the first drug to be started in a patient with a symptomatic pheochromocytoma?
    A. ACE inhibitor
    B. Alpha blocker
    C. Beta blocker
    D. Calcium channel blocker

Answer: B

Alpha blockers such as phenoxybenzamine are started 1 to 3 weeks before surgery at doses of 10 mg twice daily, which may be increased to 300 to 400 mg/d with rehydration. Patients should be warned about orthostatic hypotension. Other alpha blockers such as prazosin and other classes of drugs such as ACE inhibitors and calcium channel blockers are also useful. Beta blockers such as propranolol at doses of 10 to 40 mg every 6 to 8 hours often need to be added preoperatively in patients who have persistent tachycardia and arrhythmias. Beta blockers should only be instituted after adequate alpha blockade and hydration to avoid the effects of unopposed alpha stimulation, (i.e., hypertensive crisis and congestive heart failure). Patients also should be volume repleted preoperatively to avoid postoperative hypotension, which ensues with the loss of vasoconstriction after tumor removal. (See Schwartz 9th ed., p 1399.)

18. Following a total thyroidectomy for differentiated thyroid cancer, radioactive iodine ablation would be offered for all of the following patients EXCEPT
    A. Stage III disease
    B. Stage II disease <45 years of age
    C. Stage 1 disease with multifocal disease
    D. Stage 1 disease <45 years of age

Answer: D

RAI ablation currently is recommended for all patients with stage III or IV disease, all patients with stage II disease younger than 45 years old, most patients 45 years or older with stage II disease, and patients with stage I disease who have aggressive histologies, nodal metastases, multifocal disease, and extrathyroid or vascular invasion. (See Schwartz 9th ed., p 1365.)

19. Which of the following organisms is a common cause of acute (suppurative) thyroiditis?
    A. *Escherichia coli*
    B. *Pseudomonas aeruginous*
    C. *Streptococcus species*
    D. *Staphylococcus aureus*

Answer: C

The thyroid gland is inherently resistant to infection due to its extensive blood and lymphatic supply, high iodide content, and fibrous capsule. However, infectious agents can seed it (a) via the hematogenous or lymphatic route, (b) via direct spread from persistent pyriform sinus fistulae or thyroglossal duct cysts, (c) as a result of penetrating trauma to the thyroid gland, or (d) due to immunosuppression. *Streptococcus* and anaerobes account for about 70% of cases; however, other species also have been cultured. Acute suppurative thyroiditis is more common in children and often is preceded by an upper respiratory tract infection or otitis media. It is characterized by severe neck pain radiating to the jaws or ear, fever, chills, odynophagia, and dysphonia. Complications such as systemic sepsis, tracheal or esophageal rupture, jugular vein thrombosis, laryngeal chondritis, and perichondritis or sympathetic trunk paralysis may also occur. (See Schwartz 9th ed., p 1356.)

20. Thyroidectomy should be recommended for patients with Graves' disease who
    A. Are of the male gender
    B. Are >55 years of age
    C. Have large asymptomatic goiters
    D. Have a suspicious thyroid nodule

Answer: D

In North America, surgery is recommended when RAI is contraindicated as in patients who (a) have confirmed cancer or suspicious thyroid nodules, (b) are young, (c) are pregnant or desire to conceive soon after treatment, (d) have had severe reactions to antithyroid medications, (e) have large goiters causing compressive symptoms, and (f) are reluctant to undergo RAI therapy. Relative indications for thyroidectomy include patients, particularly smokers, with moderate to severe Graves' ophthalmopathy, those desiring rapid control of hyperthyroidism with a chance of being euthyroid, and those demonstrating poor compliance to antithyroid medications. (See Schwartz 9th ed., p 1355.)

21. Which of the following is an indication for surgery in patients with secondary hyperparathyroidism?
    A. Calciphylaxis
    B. PTH >250
    C. Progressive renal failure
    D. None of the above

Answer: A

Surgical treatment in secondary hyperparathyroidism was traditionally recommended for patients with bone pain, pruritus, and (a) a calcium-phosphate product ≥70, (b) calcium >11 mg/dL with markedly elevated PTH, (c) calciphylaxis, (d) progressive renal osteodystrophy, and (e) soft tissue calcification and tumoral calcinosis, despite maximal medical therapy. The role of parathyroidectomy in the era of calcimetics will require long-term studies; however, parathyroidectomy should be considered if PTH levels remain high despite optimal therapy. Calciphylaxis is a rare, limb- and life-threatening complication of secondary HPT characterized by painful (sometimes throbbing), violaceous, and mottled lesions usually on the extremities, which often become necrotic and progress to nonhealing ulcers, gangrene, sepsis, and death. These are critically ill, high-risk patients, but successful parathyroidectomy sometimes relieves symptoms. (See Schwartz 9th ed., p 1387.)

22. Thyroglossal duct cysts are most commonly located
    A. On the anterior border of the sternocleidomastoid muscle
    B. In the midline at the level of the hyoid
    C. Over the medial clavicular head
    D. In the midline just superior to the thyroid gland

Answer: B

Thyroglossal duct cysts are the most commonly encountered congenital cervical anomalies. During the fifth week of gestation, the thyroglossal duct lumen starts to obliterate, and the duct disappears by the eighth week of gestation. Rarely, the thyroglossal duct may persist in whole, or in part. Thyroglossal duct cysts may occur anywhere along the migratory path of the thyroid although 80% are found in juxtaposition to the hyoid bone.

The thyroid gland arises as an outpouching of the primitive foregut around the third week of gestation. It originates at the base of the tongue at the foramen cecum. Endoderm cells in the floor of the pharyngeal anlage thicken to form the medial thyroid anlage (Fig. 38-8) that descends in the neck anterior to structures that form the hyoid bone and larynx. During its descent, the anlage remains connected to the foramen cecum via an epithelial-lined tube known as the *thyroglossal duct*. (See Schwartz 9th ed., p 1344.)

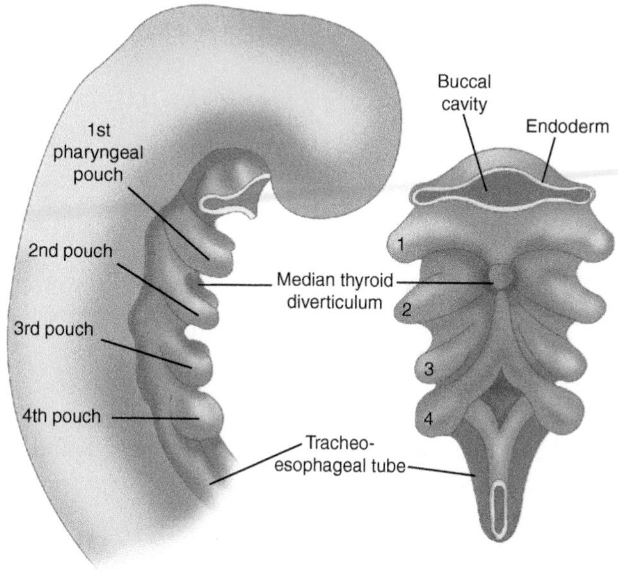

FIG. 38-8. Thyroid embryology—early development of the median thyroid anlage as a pharyngeal pouch. (Reproduced with permission from Embryology and developmental abnormalities, in Cady B, Rossi R (eds): *Surgery of the Thyroid and Parathyroid Glands.* Philadelphia: WB Saunders, 1991, p 6.)

23. Which of the following syndromes is NOT typically associated with an increased risk of pheochromocytoma?
  A. Familial adenomatous polyposis syndrome
  B. Carney's syndrome
  C. von Hippel-Lindau syndrome
  D. Sturge-Weber syndrome

Answer: A

Pheochromocytomas occur in families with MEN2A and MEN2B, in approximately 50% of patients. Both syndromes are inherited in an autosomal dominant fashion and are caused by germline mutations in the *RET* proto-oncogene. Another syndrome with an increased risk of pheochromocytomas is von Hippel-Lindau (VHL) disease, which also is inherited in an autosomal dominant manner. This syndrome also includes retinal angioma, hemangioblastomas of the central nervous system, renal cysts and carcinomas, pancreatic cysts, and epididymal cystadenomas. The incidence of pheochromocytomas in the syndrome is approximately 14%. The gene causing VHL has been mapped to chromosome 3p and is a tumor-suppressor gene. Pheochromocytomas also are included within the tumor spectrum of neurofibromatosis type 1 (NF1 gene) and other neuroectodermal disorders (Sturge-Weber syndrome and tuberous sclerosis), Carney's syndrome (gastric epithelioid leiomyosarcoma, pulmonary chondroma, and extra-adrenal paraganglioma), MEN1 syndrome, and the familial paraganglioma and pheochromocytoma syndrome caused by mutations in the succinyl dehydrogenase family of genes (SDHB, SDHC, and SDHD). (See Schwartz 9th ed., p 1399.)

24. The most common cause of hyperthyroidism is
  A. Graves' disease
  B. Toxic multinodular goiter
  C. Plummer's disease
  D. Thyroiditis

Answer: A

Graves' disease is by far the most common cause of hyperthyroidism in North America, accounting for 60 to 80% of cases. It is an autoimmune disease with a strong familial predisposition, female preponderance (5:1), and peak incidence between the ages of 40 and 60 years. Graves' disease is characterized by thyrotoxicosis, diffuse goiter, and extrathyroidal conditions including ophthalmopathy, dermopathy (pretibial myxedema), thyroid acropachy, gynecomastia, and other manifestations. (See Schwartz 9th ed., p 1353, and Table 38-8.)

TABLE 38-8 Differential diagnosis of hyperthyroidism

Increased Hormone Synthesis (Increased RAIU)	Release of Preformed Hormone (Decreased RAIU)
Graves' disease (diffuse toxic goiter)	Thyroiditis—acute phase of Hashimoto's thyroiditis, subacute thyroiditis
Toxic multinodular goiter	Factitious (iatrogenic) thyrotoxicosis
Plummer's disease (toxic adenoma)	"Hamburger thyrotoxicosis"
Drug induced—amiodarone, iodine	
Thyroid cancer	
Struma ovarii	
Hydatidiform mole	
TSH-secreting pituitary adenoma	

RAIU = radioactive iodine uptake; TSH = thyroid-stimulating hormone.

25. The most common adrenal mass incidentally found on CT scan (adrenal incidentaloma) is
    A. Adrenal cyst
    B. Adrenal hemorrhage
    C. Cortical adenoma
    D. Myelolipoma

Answer: C

The differential diagnosis of adrenal incidentalomas is shown in Table 38-9. Nonfunctional cortical adenomas account for the majority (36 to 94%) of adrenal incidentalomas in patients without a history of cancer. (See Schwartz 9th ed., p 1401.)

TABLE 38-9 Differential diagnosis of adrenal incidentaloma

Functioning Lesions	Nonfunctioning Lesions
Benign	Benign
Aldosteronoma	Cortical adenoma
Cortisol-producing adenoma	Myelolipoma
Sex-steroid–producing adenoma	Cyst
Pheochromocytoma	Ganglioneuroma
	Hemorrhage
Malignant	Malignant
Adrenocortical cancer	Metastasis
Malignant pheochromocytoma	Adrenocortical cancer

26. Which of the following would be the best initial treatment of a symptomatic lingual thyroid?
    A. Intravenous thyroxine
    B. Radioactive iodine ablation
    C. External beam radiation
    D. Local surgical excision

Answer: B

A lingual thyroid represents a failure of the median thyroid anlage to descend normally and may be the only thyroid tissue present. Intervention becomes necessary for obstructive symptoms such as choking, dysphagia, airway obstruction, or hemorrhage. Many of these patients develop hypothyroidism. Medical treatment options include administration of exogenous oral thyroid hormone to suppress thyroid-stimulating hormone (TSH) and radioactive iodine (RAI) ablation followed by hormone replacement. Surgical excision is rarely needed but, if required, should be preceded by an evaluation of normal thyroid tissue in the neck to avoid inadvertently rendering the patient hypothyroid. (See Schwartz 9th ed., p 1345.)

27. A patient is noted to have an adrenal mass on CT scan. Which of the following CT findings is most suggestive of adrenal cancer?
    A. Tumor heterogeneity
    B. Adjacent lymphadenopathy
    C. Size >6 cm
    D. Lesion enhancement

Answer: C

The size of the adrenal mass on imaging studies is the single most important criterion to help diagnose malignancy. In the series reported by Copeland, 92% of adrenal cancers were >6 cm in diameter. The sensitivity, specificity, and likelihood ratio of tumor size in predicting malignancy (based on Surveillance; Epidemiology, and End Results program data) was recently reported as 96%, 51%, and 2 for tumors ≥4 cm; and 90%, 78%, and 4.1 for tumors ≥6 cm. Other CT imaging characteristics suggesting malignancy include tumor heterogeneity, irregular margins, and the presence of hemorrhage and adjacent lymphadenopathy or liver metastases. Moderately bright signal intensity on T_2-weighted images (adrenal mass to liver ratio 1.2:2.8), significant lesion enhancement, and slow washout after injection of gadolinium contrast also indicate malignancy, as does evidence of local invasion into adjacent structures such as the liver, blood vessels (IVC), and distant metastases. (See Schwartz 9th ed., p 1397.)

28. The most sensitive test to diagnose a pheochromocytoma is
    A. Plasma vanillylmandellic acid (VMA)
    B. Urinary vanillylmandellic acid (VMA)
    C. Plasma metanephrines
    D. Urinary metanephrines

Answer: C

Recent studies have shown that plasma metanephrines are the most reliable tests to identify pheochromocytomas, with sensitivity approaching 100%.

Urinary metanephrines are 98% sensitive and also are highly specific for pheochromocytomas, whereas VMA measurements are slightly less sensitive and specific. False-positive VMA tests may result from ingestion of caffeine, raw fruits, or medications (α-methyldopa). Fractionated urinary catecholamines (norepinephrine, epinephrine, and dopamine) also are very sensitive but less specific for pheochromocytomas. (See Schwartz 9th ed., p 1399.)

29. Thyroid hormone production is inhibited by
    A. Epinephrine
    B. Glucocorticoids
    C. Human chorionic gonadotrophin
    D. Alphafetoprotein

Answer: B

Epinephrine and human chorionic gonadotrophin hormones stimulate thyroid hormone production. Thus, elevated thyroid hormone levels are found in pregnancy and gynecologic malignancies such as hydatidiform mole. In contrast, glucocorticoids inhibit thyroid hormone production. In severely ill patients, peripheral thyroid hormones may be reduced, without a compensatory increase in TSH levels, giving rise to the euthyroid sick syndrome. (See Schwartz 9th ed., p 1348.)

30. Which of the following should be the first diagnostic test ordered in a patient with a solitary thyroid nodule?
    A. Radioactive iodine scan
    B. CT or MRI
    C. Fine needle aspiration
    D. Core needle biopsy

Answer: C

FNAB has become the single most important test in the evaluation of thyroid masses and can be performed with or without ultrasound guidance. (See Schwartz 9th ed., p 1360, and Fig. 38-9.)

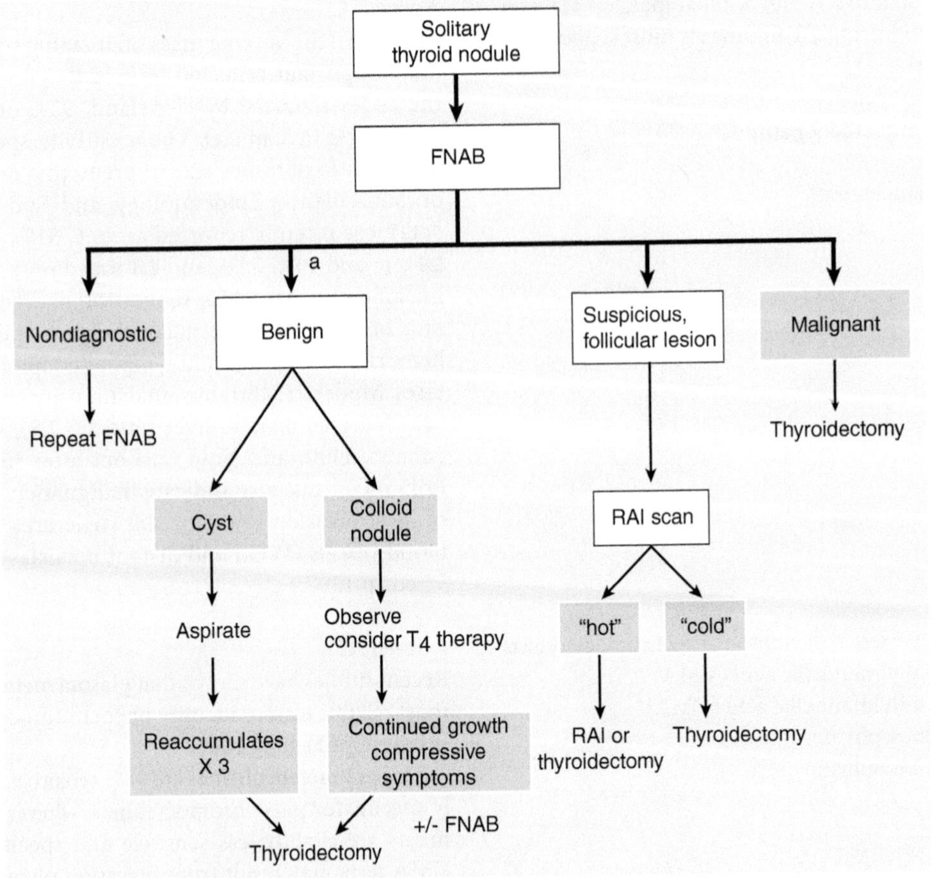

FIG. 38-9. Management of a solitary thyroid nodule. a = except in patients with a history of external radiation exposure or a family history of thyroid cancer; FNAB = fine-needle aspiration biopsy; RAI = radioactive iodine; T_4 = thyroxine.

31. Which of the following cancers does NOT occur in thyroglossal duct cysts?
    A. Papillary thyroid cancer
    B. Follicular thyroid cancer
    C. Medullary thyroid cancer
    D. Hürthle cell cancer

Answer: C

Approximately 1% of thyroglossal duct cysts are found to contain cancer, which is usually papillary (85%). The role of total thyroidectomy in this setting is controversial, but is advised in older patients with large tumors, particularly if there are additional thyroid nodules and evidence of cyst wall invasion or lymph node metastases. Squamous, Hürthle cell, and anaplastic cancers also have been reported but are rare. Medullary thyroid cancers (MTCs) are, however, not found in thyroglossal duct cysts. (See Schwartz 9th ed., p 1344.)

CHAPTER 39

Pediatric Surgery

BASIC SCIENCE QUESTIONS

1. Total body water in a full-term infant is approximately
   A. 60 mL/kg
   B. 80 mL/kg
   C. 100 mL/kg
   D. 120 mL/kg

Answer: B

At 12 weeks' gestation, the total body water of a fetus is approximately 94 mL/kg. By the time the fetus reaches full term, the total body water has decreased to approximately 80 mL/kg. Total body water drops an additional 5% within the first week of life, and by 1 year of life, total body water approaches adult levels, 60 to 65 mL/kg. (See Schwartz 9th ed., p 1412.)

2. Approximately how many calories per day are required to support growth in a newborn infant?
   A. 110 kcal/kg/day
   B. 90 kcal/kg/day
   C. 70 kcal/kg/day
   D. 55 kcal/kg/day

Answer: A

The protein and caloric requirements for the surgical neonate are shown in Table 39-1. (See Schwartz 9th ed., p 1413.)

TABLE 39-1 Nutritional requirements for the pediatric surgical patient

Age	Calories (kcal/kg per day)	Protein (g/kg per day)
0–6 mo	100–120	2
6 mo–1 y	100	1.5
1–3 y	100	1.2
4–6 y	90	1
7–10 y	70	1
11–14 y	55	1
15–18 y	45	1

3. Mutation in which of the following genes has been associated with Hirschsprung's disease?
   A. Glial cell line-derived neurotrophic factor (GDNF)
   B. "Rearranged during transfection" (RET)
   C. GDNF family receptor alphañ1 (Gfra-1)
   D. All of the above

Answer: D

Recent studies have shed light on the molecular basis for Hirschsprung's disease. Patients with Hirschsprung's disease have an increased frequency of mutations in several genes, including *GDNF*, its receptor *Ret*, and its coreceptor *Gfra-1*. Moreover, mutations in these genes also lead to aganglionic megacolon in mice, which provides the opportunity to study the function of the encoded proteins. Initial investigations indicate that *GDNF* promotes the survival, proliferation, and migration of mixed populations of neural crest cells in culture. Other studies have revealed that *GDNF* is expressed in the gut in advance of migrating neural crest cells and is chemoattractive for neural crest cells in culture. These findings raise the possibility that mutations in the *GDNF* or *Ret* genes could lead to impaired neural crest migration in utero and the development of Hirschsprung's disease. (See Schwartz 9th ed., p 1436.)

4. The glomerular filtration rate of a newborn is approximately
   A. 30% less than a normal adult
   B. 60% less than a normal adult
   C. 30% more than a normal adult
   D. 60% more than a normal adult

Answer: B

Precise management of a neonate's fluid status requires an understanding of changes in the glomerular filtration rate (GFR) and tubular function of the kidney. The full-term newborn's GFR is approximately 21 mL/min per square meter compared with 70 mL/min per square meter in an adult. Within the first year GFR increases steadily to the point that it essentially reaches adult levels by the end of the first year of life. The capacity to concentrate urine is very limited in preterm and term infants. In comparison with an adult who can concentrate urine to 1200 mOsm/kg, infants can concentrate urine at best to 600 mOsm/kg. Although infants are capable of secreting antidiuretic hormone, the aquaporin water channelñmediated osmotic water permeability of the infant's collecting tubules is severely limited compared with that of an adult, which leads to insensitivity to antidiuretic hormone. (See Schwartz 9th ed., p 1412.)

5. Third branchial cleft anomalies are located
   A. Anterior to the carotid artery
   B. Posterior to the carotid artery
   C. Lateral to the carotid artery
   D. Between the branches of the external and internal carotid arteries

Answer: B

Paired branchial clefts and arches develop early in the fourth gestational week. The first cleft and the first, second, third, and fourth pouches give rise to adult organs. The embryologic communication between the pharynx and the external surface may persist as a fistula. A fistula is seen most commonly with the second branchial cleft, which normally disappears, and extends from the anterior border of the sternocleidomastoid muscle superiorly, passes inward through the bifurcation of the carotid artery, and enters the posterolateral pharynx just below the tonsillar fossa. In contrast, a third branchial cleft fistula passes posterior to the carotid bifurcation. (See Schwartz 9th ed., p 1414.)

6. The blood volume of a 3-kg newborn infant is approximately
   A. 150 mL
   B. 240 mL
   C. 300 mL
   D. 450 mL

Answer: B

A useful guideline for estimating blood volume for the newborn infant is approximately 80 mL/kg of body weight. (See Schwartz 9th ed., p 1412.)

7. Approximately how many calories are in 1 ounce (30 mL) of breast milk?
   A. 20 kcal
   B. 30 kcal
   C. 42 kcal
   D. 50 kcal

Answer: A

There are approximately 0.67 kcal/cc in one mL of breast milk. Therefore, there are about 20 kcals in 1 ounce (30 mL) of breast milk. (See Schwartz 9th ed., p 1413, and Table 39-2.)

TABLE 39-2 Formulas for pediatric surgical neonates

Formula	Calories (kcal/mL)	Protein (g/mL)	Fat (g/mL)	Carbohydrate (g/mL)
Human milk	0.67	0.011	0.04	0.07
Milk based				
Enfamil 20	0.67	0.015	0.038	0.069
Similac 20	0.67	0.015	0.036	0.072
Soy based				
ProSobee LIPIL	0.67	0.02	0.036	0.07
Isomil	0.67	0.018	0.037	0.068
Special				
Pregestimil LIPIL	0.67	0.019	0.028	0.091
Alimentum	0.67	0.019	0.038	0.068
Preterm				
Enfamil	0.80	0.024	0.041	0.089
Premature LIPIL				
Neocate	0.71	0.023	0.035	0.081

1. Thyroglossal ducts are usually diagnosed at
   A. Birth
   B. 6-9 months of age
   C. 2-4 years of age
   D. 5-8 years of age

Answer: C

Thyroglossal duct cysts are most commonly appreciated in the 2- to 4-year-old child when the baby fat disappears and irregularities in the neck become more readily apparent. Usually the cyst is encountered in the midline at or below the level of the hyoid bone and moves up and down with swallowing or with protrusion of the tongue. Occasionally it presents as an intrathyroidal mass. Most thyroglossal duct cysts are asymptomatic. (See Schwartz 9th ed., p 1414.)

2. Malignant tumors are uncommon in children with sacrococcygeal teratomas. When they are present, however, the most common tumor is
   A. Rhabdomyosarcoma
   B. Neuroblastoma
   C. Yolk sac tumor
   D. Malignant teratoma

Answer D

Sacrococcygeal teratoma usually presents as a large mass extending from the sacrum in the newborn period. Diagnosis may be established by prenatal ultrasonography. In fetuses with evidence of hydrops and a large sacrococcygeal teratoma, prognosis is poor; thus prenatal intervention has been advocated in such patients. The mass may be as small as a few centimeters in diameter or as massive as the size of the infant (Fig. 39-1). The tumor has been classified based on the location and degree of intrapelvic extension. Lesions that grow predominantly into the presacral space often present later in childhood. The differential diagnosis consists of neural tumors, lipoma, and myelomeningoceles. Most tumors are identified at birth and are benign. Malignant yolk sac tumor histology occurs in a minority of these tumors. (See Schwartz 9th ed., p 1451.)

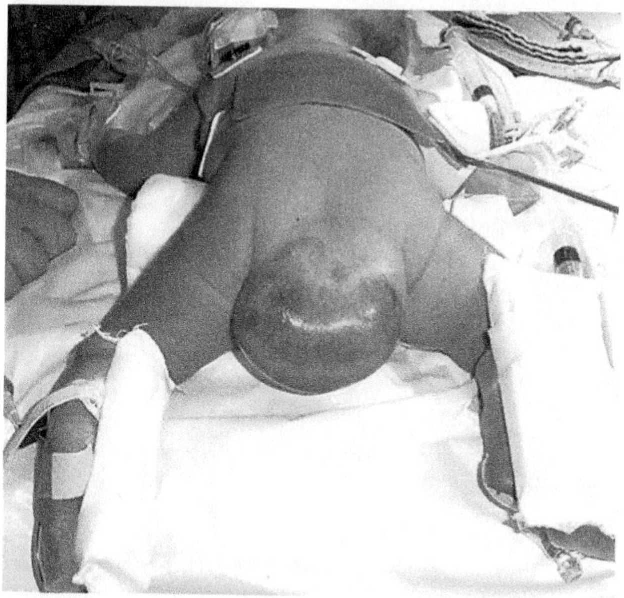

FIG. 39-1. Sacrococcygeal teratoma in a 2-day-old boy.

3. In children, hernias are most common
   A. In boys, on the left side
   B. In boys, on the right side
   C. In girls, on the left side
   D. In girls, on the right side

Answer: B

Inguinal hernias occur more commonly in males than in females (10:1) and are more common on the right side than the left. (See Schwartz 9th ed., p 1444.)

4. The mortality rate for congenital diaphragmatic hernia is approximately
   A. 15%
   B. 35%
   C. 50%
   D. 70%

Answer: C

The vast majority of infants with CDH develop immediate respiratory distress, which is due to the combined effects of three factors. First, the air-filled bowel in the chest compresses the mobile mediastinum, which shifts to the opposite side of the chest, so that air exchange in the contralateral lung is compromised. Second, pulmonary hypertension develops. This phenomenon results in persistent fetal circulation, with resultant decreased pulmonary perfusion, and impaired gas exchange. Finally, the lung on the affected side is often markedly hypoplastic, so that it is essentially nonfunctional. Varying degrees of pulmonary hypoplasia on the opposite side may compound these effects. As a result, neonates with CDH are extremely sick, and the overall mortality in most series is approximately 50%. (See Schwartz 9th ed., p 1416.)

5. A 5-week-old infant presents to the emergency room with bilious vomiting, lethargy, and poor urine output. Following resuscitation, based on the film in Fig. 39-2, the next intervention should be
   A. NG decompression and observation
   B. Upper GI series
   C. Contrast enema
   D. Laparotomy

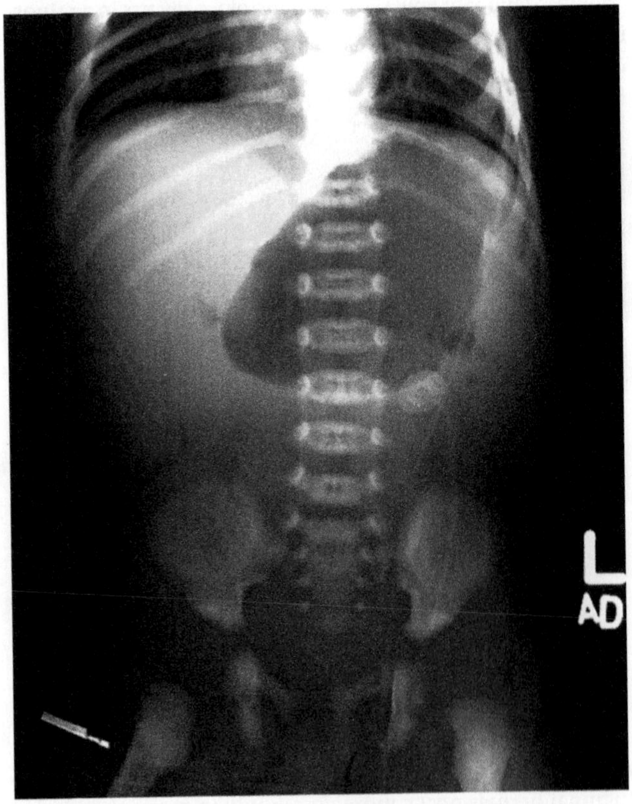

FIG. 39-2

Answer: D

Midgut volvulus can occur at any age, although it is seen most often in the first few weeks of life. Bilious vomiting is usually the first sign of volvulus, and all infants with bilious vomiting must be evaluated rapidly to ensure that they do not have intestinal malrotation with volvulus. This diagnosis should be suspected in a child with irritability and bilious emesis. If the condition is left untreated, vascular compromise of the midgut initially causes bloody stools but eventually results in circulatory collapse. Additional clues to the presence of advanced ischemia of the intestine include erythema and edema of the abdominal wall, which progresses to shock and death. It must be re-emphasized that the index of suspicion for this condition must be high, because abdominal signs are minimal in the early stages. Abdominal films show a paucity of gas throughout the intestine with a few scattered air-fluid levels (Fig. 39-2). When these findings are present, the patient should undergo immediate fluid resuscitation to ensure adequate perfusion and urine output, followed by prompt exploratory laparotomy. (See Schwartz 9th ed., p 1428.)

6. Which of the following is NOT part of the VACTERL complex?
   A. Vertebral anomalies
   B. Imperforate anus
   C. Congenital diaphragmatic hernia
   D. Renal anomalies

Answer: C
VACTERL syndrome is associated with *v*ertebral anomalies (absent vertebrae or hemivertebrae), *a*norectal anomalies (imperforate anus), *c*ardiac defects, *t*racheo*e*sophageal fistula, *r*enal anomalies (renal agenesis, renal anomalies), and *r*adial *l*imb anomalies (most often radial dysplasia). (See Schwartz 9th ed., p 1421.)

7. Intestinal duplications are most commonly located in the
   A. Duodenum
   B. Jejunum
   C. Ileum
   D. Colon

Answer: C
Intestinal duplications are mucosa-lined structures that are in continuity with the GI tract. Although they can occur at any level in the GI tract, duplications are found most commonly in the ileum within the leaves of the mesentery. Duplications may be long and tubular, but usually are cystic masses. In all cases, they share a common wall with the intestine. Symptoms associated with enteric duplication cysts include recurrent abdominal pain, emesis from intestinal obstruction, and hematochezia. Such bleeding typically results from ulceration in the duplication or in the adjacent intestine if the duplication contains ectopic gastric mucosa. (See Schwartz 9th ed., p 1435.)

8. A 2-week-old with mild respiratory distress is seen in the emergency room. Based on the chest radiograph obtained (see Fig. 39-3), the most likely diagnosis is
   A. Respiratory syncticial virus infection
   B. Spontaneous pneumothorax
   C. Congenital lobar emphysema
   D. Congenital pulmonary airway malformation

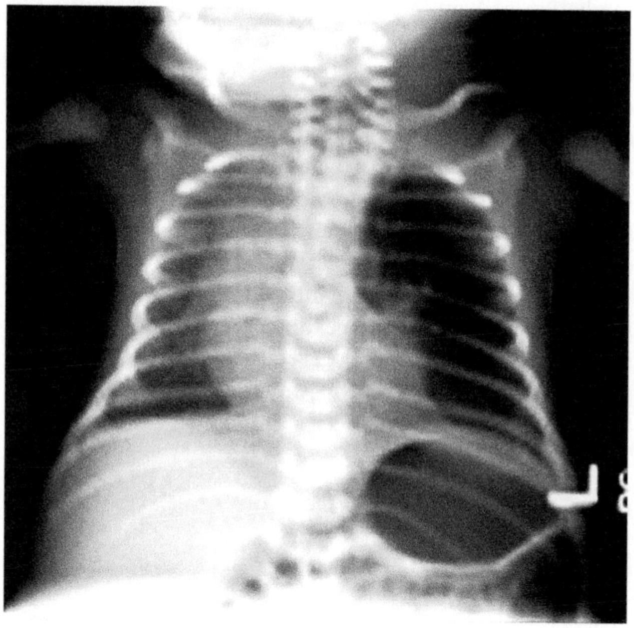

FIG. 39-3

Answer: C
Congenital lobar emphysema (CLE) is a condition manifested during the first few months of life as a progressive hyperexpansion of one or more lobes of the lung. It can be life-threatening in the newborn period, but in the older infant it causes less respiratory distress. Air entering during inspiration is trapped in the lobe. On expiration, the lobe cannot deflate and progressively overexpands, which causes atelectasis of the adjacent lobe or lobes. This hyperexpansion eventually shifts the mediastinum to the opposite side and compromises the other lung. CLE usually occurs in the upper lobes of the lung (left more often than right), followed next in frequency by the right middle lobe; however, it can occur in the lower lobes as well. It is caused by intrinsic bronchial obstruction from poor bronchial cartilage development or extrinsic compression.

Congenital pulmonary airway malformation (CPAM) consists of cystic proliferation of the terminal airway, which produces cysts lined by mucus-producing respiratory epithelium and elastic tissue in the cyst walls without cartilage formation. There may be a single cyst with a wall of connective tissue containing smooth muscle. Formerly known as *congenital cystic adenomatoid malformation*, CPAM may consist of a single large cyst or multiple cysts (type I), may be characterized by smaller and more numerous cysts (type II), or may resemble fetal lung without macroscopic cysts (type III). CPAMs frequently occur in the left lower lobe. However, this lesion can occur in any lobe or may occur in both lungs simultaneously. (See Schwartz 9th ed., p 1418.)

Spontaneous pneumothorax is rare in infants. Loculated airtrapping, like that seen on the chest radiograph in Fig. 39-3, is not usually seen with RSV infection.

9. The defect in gastroschisis is usually
   A. In the midline, superior to the umbilicus
   B. In the midline, inferior to the umbilicus
   C. To the right of the umbilicus
   D. To the left of the umbilicus

Answer: C

Gastroschisis is a congenital anomaly characterized by a defect in the anterior abdominal wall through which the intestinal contents freely protrude. Unlike with omphalocele, there is no overlying sac and the size of the defect is much smaller (<4 cm). The abdominal wall defect is located at the junction of the umbilicus and normal skin and is almost always to the right of the umbilicus. (See Schwartz 9th ed., p 1443.)

10. The most common type of choledochal cyst is
    A. Type I
    B. Type II
    C. Type III
    D. Type IV

Answer: A

Based on the classification system proposed by Alonso-Lej, five types of choledochal cyst are described. Type I cysts are characterized by fusiform dilatation of the bile duct. This type is the most common and is found in 80 to 90% of cases. Type II choledochal cysts appear as an isolated diverticulum protruding from the wall of the common bile duct. The cyst may be joined to the common bile duct by a narrow stalk. Type III choledochal cysts arise from the intraduodenal portion of the common bile duct and are also known as *choledochoceles*. Type IVA cysts consist of multiple dilatations of the intrahepatic and extrahepatic bile ducts. Type IVB choledochal cysts are multiple dilatations involving only the extrahepatic bile ducts. Type V cysts (Caroli's disease) consist of multiple dilatations limited to the intrahepatic bile ducts. (See Schwartz 9th ed., p 1440.)

11. A premature infant with bloody stools, bilious emesis, and the following KUB (see Fig. 39-4) should be treated with
    A. NG decompression and antibiotics
    B. Percutaneous abdominal drainage with peritoneal irrigation
    C. Exploratory laparotomy, resection of the involved bowel, and primary anastomosis
    D. Exploratory laparotomy, resection of the involved bowel, and end ostomies

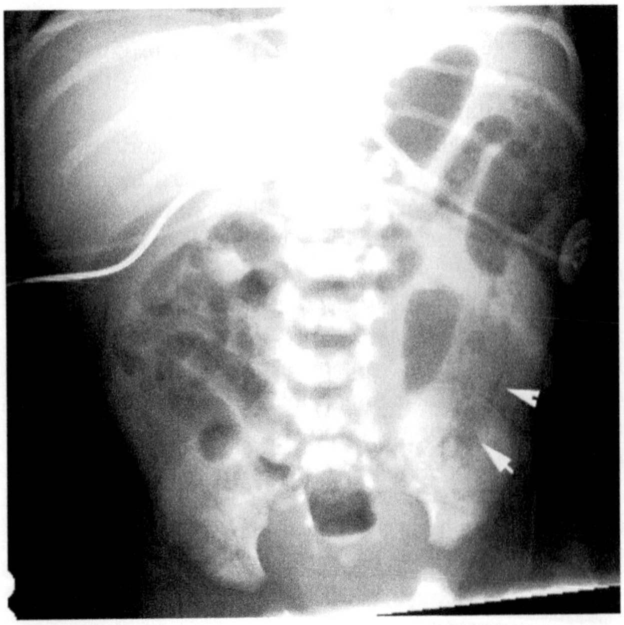

FIG. 39-4

Answer: A

In all infants suspected of having NEC, feedings are discontinued, a nasogastric tube is placed, and broad-spectrum parenteral antibiotics are given. The infant is resuscitated, and inotropes are administered to maintain perfusion as needed. Intubation and mechanical ventilation may be required to maintain oxygenation. TPN is started. Subsequent treatment may be influenced by the particular stage of NEC that is present. Patients with Bell stage I disease are closely monitored and generally remain on nil per os (NPO) status and are given IV antibiotics for 7 to 10 days before enteral nutrition is resumed. After this time, provided the infant fully recovers, feedings may be reinitiated. Patients with Bell II disease merit close observation. Serial physical examinations are performed to look for the development of diffuse peritonitis, a fixed mass, progressive abdominal wall cellulitis, or systemic sepsis. If the infant fails to improve after several days of treatment, consideration should be given to exploratory laparotomy. (See Schwartz 9th ed., p 1432.)

12. The most common type of tracheoesophageal anomaly is
    A. Pure esophageal atresia (without fistula)
    B. Esophageal atresia with distal fistula
    C. Esophageal atresia with proximal fistula
    D. Tracheoesophageal fistula (without atresia)

Answer: B

The five major varieties of EA and TEF are shown in Fig. 39-5. The most commonly seen variety is EA with distal TEF (type C), which occurs in approximately 85% of the cases in most series. The next most frequent is pure EA (type A), occurring in 8 to 10% of patients, followed by TEF without EA (type E). The latter occurs in 8% of cases and is also referred to as an *H-type fistula*, based on the anatomic similarity to that letter. EA with fistula between both the proximal and distal ends of the esophagus and trachea (type D) is seen in approximately 2% of cases, and type B, EA with TEF between the proximal esophagus and trachea, is seen in approximately 1% of cases. (See Schwartz 9th ed., p 1421, and Fig. 39-5.)

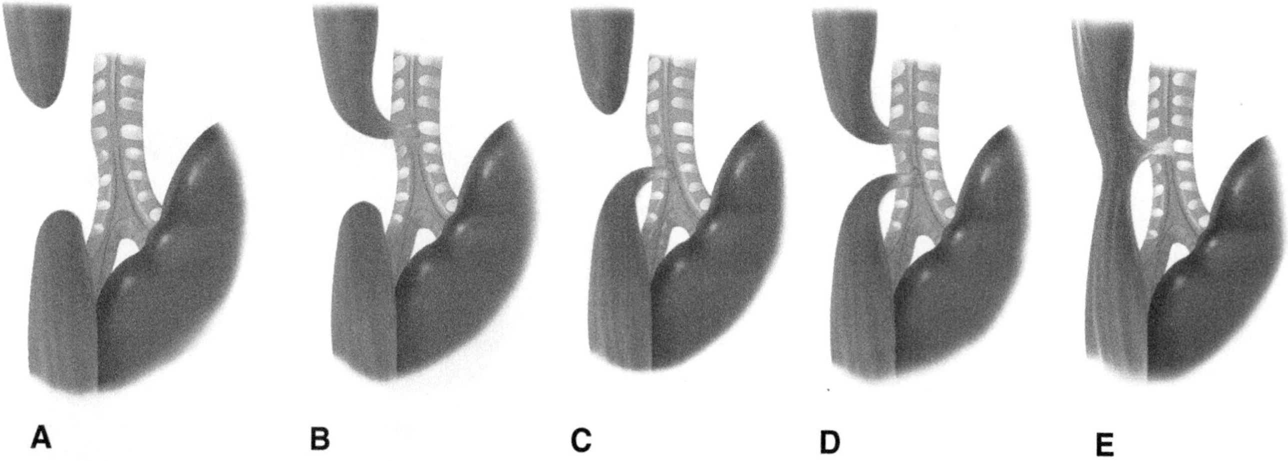

FIG. 39-5. The five varieties of esophageal atresia (EA) and tracheoesophageal fistula (TEF). **A.** Isolated EA. **B.** EA with TEF between the proximal segment of the esophagus and the trachea. **C.** EA with TEF between the distal esophagus and the trachea **D.** EA with fistula between both the proximal and distal ends of the esophagus and the trachea. **E.** TEF without EA (H-type fistula).

13. The expected survival for a patient with Stage IV Wilms' tumor is approximately
    A. 5%
    B. 33%
    C. 50%
    D. 80%

Answer: D

Wilms' tumor is the most common primary malignant tumor of the kidney in children. Approximately 500 new cases are seen annually in the United States, and most are diagnosed in children between 1 and 5 years of age with the peak incidence at age 3. Advances in the care of patients with Wilms' tumor have resulted in an overall cure rate of roughly 90%, even in the presence of metastatic spread.

Essentially, patients who have disease confined to one kidney that is completely excised surgically receive a short course of chemotherapy, and for this group a 97% 4-year survival is expected, with tumor relapse rare after that time. Patients who have more advanced disease or tumors with unfavorable histologic features receive more intensive chemotherapy and radiation therapy. Even in patients with stage IV disease, cure rates of 80% are achieved. (See Schwartz 9th ed., p 1449.)

14. The most common cause of serious head injury in toddlers is
    A. Motor vehicle accidents
    B. Fall from a height
    C. Autopedestrian accident
    D. Nonaccidental trauma

Answer: D

The central nervous system (CNS) is the most commonly injured system, and CNS trauma is the leading cause of death among injured children. In the toddler age group, nonaccidental trauma is the most common cause of serious head injury. Findings suggestive of abuse include the presence of retinal hemorrhage on funduscopic evaluation and intracranial hemorrhage without evidence of external trauma (indicative of a shaking injury) as well as fractures at different stages of healing on skeletal survey. (See Schwartz 9th ed., p 1452.)

15. Which of the following procedures is the procedure of choice to correct biliary atresia?
    A. Choledochojejunostomy
    B. Cholecystojejunostomy
    C. Hepatoportoenterostomy
    D. None of the above

Answer: C
Currently, first-line therapy for the treatment of biliary atresia consists of creation of a hepatoportoenterostomy, as described by Kasai. The purpose of this procedure is to promote bile flow into the intestine. The procedure is based on Kasai's observation that the fibrous tissue at the porta hepatis invests microscopically patent biliary ductules that, in turn, communicate with the intrahepatic ductal system. Transecting this fibrous tissue at the portal plate, which is invariably encountered cephalad to the bifurcating portal vein, opens these channels and establishes bile flow into a surgically constructed intestinal conduit, usually a Roux-en-Y limb of jejunum (Fig. 39-6). (See Schwartz 9th ed., p 1439.)

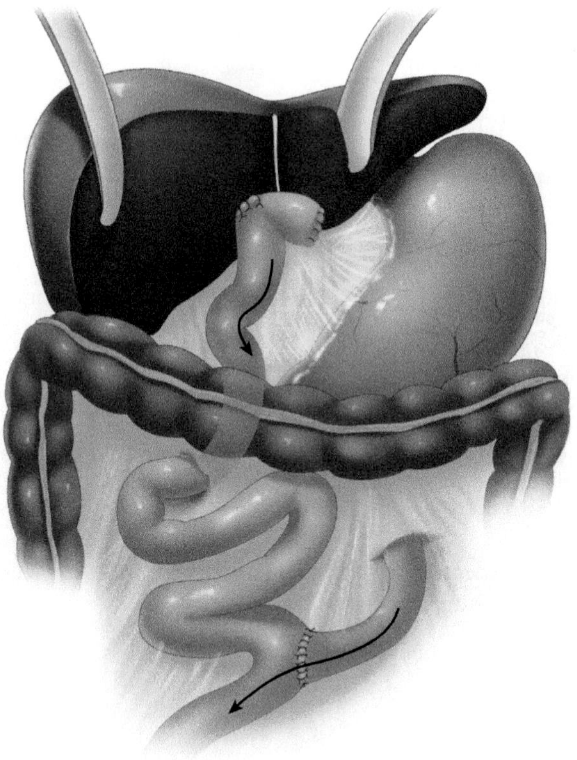

FIG. 39-6. Schematic illustration of the Kasai portoenterostomy for biliary atresia. An isolated limb of jejunum is brought to the porta hepatis and anastomosed to the transected ducts at the liver plate.

16. The diagnosis of Hirschsprung's is made by
    A. The clinical finding of inability to pass meconium
    B. The presence of a transition zone on contrast enema
    C. Genetic analysis
    D. Rectal biopsy

Answer: D
The definitive diagnosis of Hirschsprung's disease is made by rectal biopsy. Samples of mucosa and submucosa are obtained at 1 cm, 2 cm, and 3 cm from the dentate line. In the neonatal period this biopsy can be performed at the bedside without anesthesia, because samples are taken in bowel that does not have somatic innervation and thus the procedure is not painful to the child. (See Schwartz 9th ed., p 1436.)

17. Which of the following is a common site for a cystic hygroma?
    A. Anterior mediastinum
    B. Retroperitoneum
    C. Anterior triangle of the neck
    D. Axilla

Answer: D
Cystic hygroma (lymphangioma), occurring as a result of sequestration or obstruction of developing lymph vessels, occurs in approximately 1 in 12,000 births. Although the lesion can occur anywhere, the most common sites are in the posterior triangle of the neck, axilla, groin, and mediastinum. (See Schwartz 9th ed., p 1415.)

18. Which of the following is NOT typically associated with prune-belly syndrome?
 A. Lax abdominal wall
 B. Respiratory insufficiency
 C. Dilated ureters
 D. Bilateral undescended testes

Answer: B

Prune-belly syndrome is a disorder that is characterized by a constellation of symptoms including extremely lax lower abdominal musculature, dilated urinary tract including the bladder, and bilateral undescended testes (Fig. 39-7). (See Schwartz 9th ed., p 1443.)

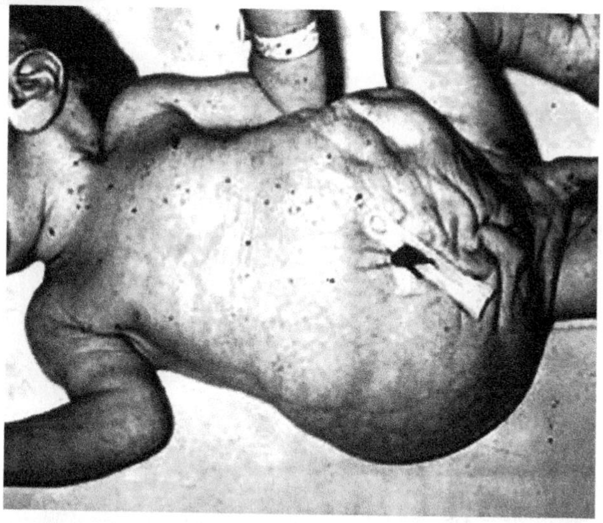

FIG. 39-7. Prune-belly (Eagle-Barrett) syndrome. Notice the flaccid abdomen.

19. Which of the following approaches is used for the repair of a type E (H-type) tracheoesophageal fistula?
 A. Right thoracotomy
 B. Left thoracotomy
 C. Cervical incision
 D. Median sternotomy

Answer: C

Patients with type E TEFs (commonly referred to as *H-type*) present beyond the newborn period. Presenting symptoms include recurrent chest infections, bronchospasm, and failure to thrive. The diagnosis can be suspected from the results of barium esophagography and confirmed by endoscopic visualization of the fistula. Surgical correction is generally possible through a cervical approach after placement of a balloon catheter across the fistula and requires mobilization and division of the fistula. Outcome is usually excellent. (See Schwartz 9th ed., p 1424.)

20. The most common associated anomaly in a boy with a high imperforate anus is
 A. Congenital heart defect
 B. Vertebral anomalies
 C. Posterior urethral valves
 D. Rectourethral fistula

Answer: D

In patients with imperforate anus, the rectum fails to descend through the external sphincter complex. Instead, the rectal pouch ends blindly in the pelvis, above or below the levator ani muscle. In most cases, the blind rectal pouch communicates more distally with the genitourinary system or with the perineum through a fistulous tract. Traditionally, the anatomic description of imperforate anus has characterized it as either 'high' or 'low' depending on whether the rectum ends above the levator ani muscle complex or partially descends through this muscle. Based on this classification system, in male patients with high imperforate anus the rectum usually ends as a fistula into the membranous urethra. In females, high imperforate anus often occurs in the context of a persistent cloaca. In both males and females, low lesions are associated with a fistula to the perineum. In males, the fistula connects with the median raphe of the scrotum or penis. In females, the fistula may end within the vestibule of the vagina, which is located immediately outside the hymen, or at the perineum. (See Schwartz 9th ed., p 1437.)

Congenital heart disease, vertebral anomalies, and posterior valves can all be seen in infants with imperforate anus and the VACTERL complex but these anomalies are not as common as the rectourethral fistula.

21. A newborn is evaluated for abdominal distention and bilious vomiting. Based on the KUB in Fig. 39-8, the initial intervention for this child should be a
   A. Contrast enema
   B. Upper gastrointestinal series
   C. Rectal biopsy
   D. Laparotomy

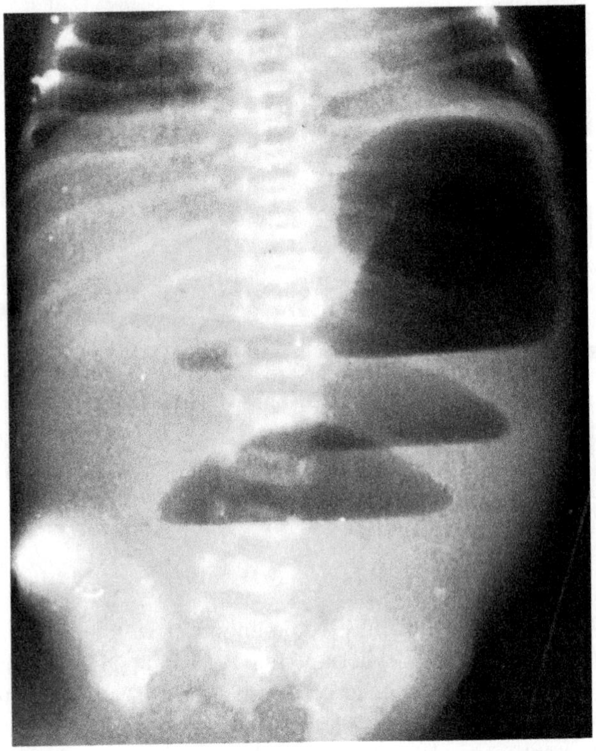

FIG. 39-8

Answer: D

In cases in which the diagnosis of complete intestinal obstruction is determined based on the clinical picture and the presence of staggered air-fluid levels on plain abdominal films, the child can be brought to the operating room after appropriate resuscitation. In these circumstances, there is little extra information to be gained by performing a barium enema study. In contrast, when diagnostic uncertainty exists, or when distal intestinal obstruction is apparent, a barium enema study is useful to establish whether a microcolon is present and to diagnose the presence of meconium plugs, small left colon syndrome, Hirschsprung's disease, or meconium ileus. (See Schwartz 9th ed., p 1427.)

22. The most appropriate intervention for a 3-month-old asymptomatic infant with a 1-cm firm mass in the center of the sternocleidomastoid muscle is
   A. Fine-needle aspiration
   B. Trucut needle biopsy
   C. Surgical excision
   D. Physical therapy

Answer: D

The presence of a lateral neck mass in infancy in association with rotation of the head toward the opposite side of the mass indicates the presence of congenital torticollis. This lesion results from fibrosis of the sternocleidomastoid muscle. The mass may be palpated in the affected muscle in approximately two thirds of cases. Histologically, the lesion is characterized by the deposition of collagen and fibroblasts around atrophied muscle cells. In the overwhelming majority of cases, physical therapy based on passive stretching of the affected muscle is of benefit. Rarely, surgical transection of the sternocleidomastoid muscle may be indicated. (See Schwartz 9th ed., p 1416.)

23. Orchidopexy (for an undescended testes)
   A. Improves fertility
   B. Decreases cancer risk
   C. Increases the risk of trauma to the testes
   D. Increases the risk of torsion of the testes

Answer: A

It is now established that cryptorchid testes show an increased predisposition to malignant degeneration. In addition, fertility is decreased when the testicle is not in the scrotum. For these reasons, surgical placement of the testicle in the scrotum (orchidopexy) is indicated. This procedure does improve the fertility potential, although it is never normal. Similarly, the testicle is still at risk of malignant change, although its location in the scrotum facilitates potentially earlier detection of a testicular malignancy. Other reasons to consider orchidopexy include the risk of trauma to a testicle located at the pubic tubercle, increased incidence of torsion, and the psychologic impact of an empty scrotum in a developing male. The reason for malignant degeneration has not been established, but the evidence points to an inherent abnormality of the testicle that predisposes it to incomplete descent and malignancy rather than malignancy as a result of an abnormal environment. (See Schwartz 9th ed., p 1446.)

24. The initial treatment of an infant with complete bowel obstruction from uncomplicated meconium ileus is
    A. NG decompression
    B. Contrast enemas
    C. Laparotomy and irrigation of the bowel lumen with *N*-acetylcysteine (purse-string enterotomy)
    D. Laparotomy with resection of the distended distal ileum and creation of an ileostomy

Answer: B

The treatment strategy for infants with meconium ileus depends on whether the patient has complicated or uncomplicated meconium ileus. Patients with uncomplicated meconium ileus can be treated nonoperatively. A dilute water-soluble contrast agent is advanced through the colon under fluoroscopic control into the dilated portion of the ileum. The enema may be repeated at 12-hour intervals over several days until all the meconium is evacuated. If surgical intervention is required because of failure of contrast enemas to relieve obstruction, operative irrigation with dilute contrast agent, *N*-acetylcysteine (Mucomyst), or saline through a purse-string suture may be successful. Alternatively, resection of the distended terminal ileum is performed, and the meconium pellets are flushed from the distal small bowel. At this point, ileostomy and mucus fistula may be created from the proximal and distal ends, respectively. Alternatively, a Bishop-Koop anastomosis or an end-to-end anastomosis may be performed. (See Schwartz 9th ed., p 1429.)

25. What is the approximate success rate for air enema reduction of intussusceptions in children?
    A. <10%
    B. 25%
    C. 50%
    D. 75%

Answer: D

In the patient [with an intussusceptions who is] in stable condition, the air enema is both diagnostic and often curative. It constitutes the preferred method of diagnosis and nonoperative treatment of intussusception. Air is introduced with a manometer and the pressure that is administered is carefully monitored. Under most instances, this should not exceed 120 mmHg. Successful reduction is marked by free reflux of air into multiple loops of small bowel and symptomatic improvement as the infant suddenly becomes pain free. Unless both of these indications are observed, it cannot be assumed that the intussusception is reduced. If reduction is unsuccessful and the infant's condition remains stable, the infant should be brought back to the radiology suite for a repeat attempt at reduction after a few hours. This strategy has improved the success rate of nonoperative reduction in many centers. In addition, hydrostatic reduction with barium may be useful if pneumatic reduction is unsuccessful. The overall success rate of radiographic reduction varies based on the experience of the center but is typically between 60 and 90%. (See Schwartz 9th ed., p 1433.)

26. The most common ovarian neoplasm in children is
    A. Teratoma
    B. Dysgerminoma
    C. Granulosa-theca cell tumors
    D. Epithelial tumors

Answer: A

Neoplastic lesions are categorized based on the three primordia that contribute to the ovary: mesenchymal components of the urogenital ridge, germinal epithelium overlying the urogenital ridge, and germ cells migrating from the yolk sac. The most common variety is germ cell tumors. Germ cell tumors are classified based on the degree of differentiation and the cellular components involved. The least differentiated tumors are the dysgerminomas, which share features similar to those of seminomas in males. Although these are malignant tumors, they are extremely sensitive to radiation and chemotherapy. The most common lesions are the teratomas, which may be mature, immature, or malignant. The degree of differentiation of the neural elements of the tumor determines the degree of immaturity. The sex cord stromal tumors arise from the mesenchymal components of the urogenital ridge. These include granulosa-theca cell tumors and Sertoli-Leydig cell tumors. These tumors often produce hormones that result in precocious puberty or hirsutism, respectively. Epithelial tumors, although rare, do occur in children. These include serous and mucinous cystadenomas. (See Schwartz 9th ed., p 1446.)

27. The standard surgical procedure for a patient with confirmed Hirschsprung's disease is
    A. Transverse colostomy
    B. "Leveling" colostomy
    C. Primary pull-through in the newborn period
    D. Irrigations with primary pull-through at age 3-6 months

Answer: C
It is now well established that a primary pull-through procedure can be performed safely, even in the newborn period. This approach follows the same treatment principles as a staged procedure and saves the patient from an additional operation. Many surgeons perform the intra-abdominal dissection using the laparoscope. This approach is especially useful in the newborn period, because it provides excellent visualization of the pelvis. (See Schwartz 9th ed., p 1436.)

28. The most common location for a congenital diaphragmatic hernia is
    A. Left posterolateral
    B. Right posterolateral
    C. Left anteromedial
    D. Right anteromedial

Answer: A
The most common variant of a congenital diaphragmatic hernia (CDH) is a posterolateral defect, also known as a *Bochdalek's hernia.* This anomaly is encountered more commonly on the left (80 to 90% of cases). (See Schwartz 9th ed., p 1416.)

29. Which of the following indicates a poor prognosis in a patient with neuroblastoma?
    A. Hyperdiploid DNA
    B. Absence of *N-myc* amplification
    C. Age <1 year
    D. Age >13 years

Answer: D
A number of biologic variables have been studied in children with neuroblastoma. An open biopsy is often required to provide sufficient tissue for analysis. The presence of hyperdiploid tumor DNA is associated with a favorable prognosis, whereas *N-myc* amplification is associated with a poor prognosis regardless of patient age. The Shimada classification describes tumors as having either favorable or unfavorable histologic features based on the degree of differentiation, the mitosis-karyorrhexis index, and the presence or absence of schwannian stroma. In general, children of any age with localized neuroblastoma and infants <1 year of age with advanced disease and favorable disease characteristics have a high likelihood of disease free survival. By contrast, older children with advanced disease have a significantly decreased chance for cure even with intensive therapy. For example, aggressive multiagent chemotherapy has resulted in a 2-year survival rate of approximately 20% in older children with stage IV disease. Neuroblastoma in the adolescent has a worse long-term prognosis regardless of stage or site and, in many cases, a more prolonged course. (See Schwartz 9th ed., p 1450.)

30. Appropriate management of a stable child with a grade IV splenic injury is
    A. Observation
    B. Embolization
    C. Splenorrhaphy
    D. Splenectomy

Answer: A
The spleen is injured relatively commonly in blunt abdominal trauma in children. The extent of injury to the spleen is graded (Table 39-3), and management is governed by the injury grade. Current treatment involves a nonoperative approach in most cases, even for grade IV injuries, assuming the patient is hemodynamically stable. This approach avoids surgery in most cases. All patients should be placed in a monitored unit, and

type-specific blood should be available for transfusion. When nonoperative management is successful, as it is in most cases, an extended period of bedrest is prescribed. This optimizes the chance for healing and minimizes the likelihood of reinjury. A typical guideline is to keep the child on extremely restricted activity for 2 weeks longer than the grade of spleen injury (i.e., a child with a grade IV spleen injury is prescribed 6 weeks of restricted activity). (See Schwartz 9th ed., p 1453, and Table 39-3.)

TABLE 39-3	Grading of splenic injuries
Grade I	Subcapsular hematoma, <10% surface area capsular tear, <1 cm in depth
Grade II	Subcapsular hematoma, nonexpanding, 10–50% surface area; intraparenchymal hematoma, nonexpanding, <2 cm in diameter; capsular tear, active bleeding, 1–3 cm, does not involve trabecular vessel
Grade III	Subcapsular hematoma, >50% surface area or expanding; intraparenchymal hematoma, >2 cm or expanding; laceration >3 cm in depth or involving trabecular vessels
Grade IV	Ruptured intraparenchymal hematoma with active bleeding; laceration involving segmental or hilar vessels producing major devascularization (>25% of spleen)
Grade V	Shattered spleen; hilar vascular injury that devascularizes spleen

31. Approximately what percentage of patients who have undergone a Kasai procedure for biliary atresia will be alive with their native liver 10 years after the procedure?
   A. 10%
   B. 25%
   C. 33%
   D. 50%

Answer: D
A recent review of the data of the Japanese Biliary Atresia Registry, which includes the results for 1381 patients, showed that the 10-year survival rate was 53% without transplantation and 66.7% with transplantation. (See Schwartz 9th ed., p 1440.)

32. Which of the following is NOT part of Cantrell's pentalogy?
   A. Omphalocele
   B. Ectopia cordis
   C. Posterolateral diaphragmatic hernia
   D. Cardiac anomalies

Answer: C
Omphalocele has an incidence of approximately 1 in 5000 live births and occurs in association with special syndromes such as exstrophy of the cloaca (vesicointestinal fissure), the Beckwith-Wiedemann constellation of anomalies (macroglossia, macrosomia, hypoglycemia, visceromegaly, and omphalocele) and the Cantrell pentalogy (lower thoracic wall malformations such as cleft sternum, ectopia cordis, epigastric omphalocele, anterior midline diaphragmatic hernia, and cardiac anomalies). (See Schwartz 9th ed., p 1442.)

33. The optimal time for reduction and repair of a congenital diaphragmatic hernia is
   A. At birth, after initial stabilization of the baby
   B. Within the first 24 hours of life
   C. Within the first 72 hours of life
   D. None of the above

Answer: D
In the past, correction of the hernia was felt to be a surgical emergency, and these patients underwent surgery shortly after birth. It is now accepted that the presence of persistent pulmonary hypertension which results in right-to-left shunting across the open foramen ovale or the ductus arteriosus and pulmonary hypoplasia are the leading causes of cardiorespiratory insufficiency. Current management therefore is directed toward preventing or reversing the pulmonary hypertension and minimizing barotrauma while optimizing oxygen delivery. In patients who are not placed on ECMO, repair should be performed once the hemodynamic status has been optimized. (See Schwartz 9th ed., p 1417.)

34. Which of the following would be expected in a baby with delayed diagnosis of pyloric stenosis?
A. Hyperchloremia, low urine pH
B. Hyperchloremia, high urine pH
C. Hypochloremia, low urine pH
D. Hypochloremia, high urine pH

Answer: C
Infants with HPS develop a hypochloremic, hypokalemic metabolic alkalosis. The urine pH is high initially but eventually drops because hydrogen ions are preferentially exchanged for sodium ions in the distal tubule of the kidney as the hypochloremia becomes severe. (See Schwartz 9th ed., p 1426.)

35. Which of the following is associated with duodenal atresia?
A. Trisomy 13
B. Trisomy 16
C. Trisomy 18
D. Trisomy 21

Answer: D
Approximately one third of newborns with duodenal atresia have associated Down syndrome (trisomy 21). These patients should be evaluated for associated cardiac anomalies. (See Schwartz 9th ed., p 1427.)

36. The blood supply of a pulmonary sequestration is from the
A. Pulmonary artery
B. Bronchial artery
C. Innominate artery
D. Aorta

Answer: D
In pulmonary sequestration, a mass of lung tissue, usually in the left lower chest, lacks the usual connections to the pulmonary artery or tracheobronchial tree and its blood supply is derived directly from the aorta. There are two kinds of sequestration. In extralobar sequestration a small area of nonaerated lung is separated from the main lung mass, has a systemic blood supply, and usually is located immediately above the left diaphragm. It is commonly found in cases of CDH. Intralobar sequestration more commonly occurs within the parenchyma of the left lower lobe but also can occur on the right. (See Schwartz 9th ed., p 1418, and Fig. 39-9.)

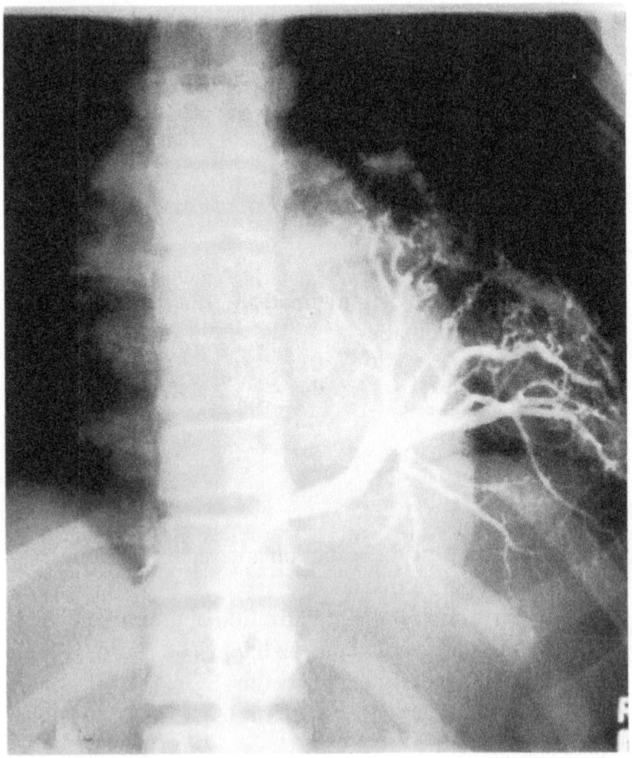

FIG. 39-9. Arteriogram showing large systemic artery supply to an intralobar sequestration of the left lower lobe.

CHAPTER 40

Urology

BASIC SCIENCE QUESTIONS

1. The blood supply of the distal ureter is provided by branches of the
   A. Aorta
   B. Renal arteries
   C. Lumbar arteries
   D. Iliac arteries

Answer: D

The blood supply of the proximal ureter derives from the aorta and renal artery and comes mainly from the medial direction. However, once it crosses the iliac vessels at the pelvic brim near where the iliac vessels bifurcate, it derives its blood supply laterally from branches from the iliac arteries. The blood supply has implications for managing ureteral injuries. Mobilizing the distal ureter for anastomosis requires releasing its lateral attachments, which results in ischemia, so for this reason, distal ureteral injuries are typically managed by bringing the proximal ureter to the bladder. (See Schwartz 9th ed., p 1460.)

2. Which of the following does NOT supply arterial blood to the testes?
   A. Testicular artery
   B. Deferential artery
   C. Scrotal artery
   D. Cremasteric artery

Answer: C

The blood supply enters the testis at the superior pole by way of the spermatic cord. In addition to the vas deferens, the cord carries three separate sources of arterial blood flow—the testicular artery that branches from the aorta below the renal artery, the cremasteric artery, and the deferential artery. Interruption of one of the arteries during vasectomy or inguinal surgery will not result in ischemia to the testis.

The cremasteric artery is a branch of the inferior epigastric artery, and the deferential artery is a branch of the superior vesicular artery. There is no scrotal artery. (See Schwartz 9th ed., p 1461.)

3. Which portion of the bladder is intraperitoneal?
   A. Dome only
   B. Dome and body
   C. Dome, body, and neck
   D. None of the above

Answer: D

The urinary bladder is situated in the retropubic space in an extraperitoneal position. A portion of the bladder dome is adjacent to the peritoneum, so ruptures at this point can result in intraperitoneal urine leakage. (See Schwartz 9th ed., p 1460.)

4. Hydroceles form between
   A. The external spermatic and cremasteric fascia
   B. The cremasteric and internal spermatic fascia
   C. The internal spermatic fascia and the parietal layer of the tunica vaginalis
   D. The visceral and parietal layers of the tunica vaginalis

Answer: D

Beneath the skin of the scrotum, from superficial to deep, are the dartos, external spermatic, cremasteric, and internal spermatic fascias. These layers are not always distinct. Beneath the internal fascia are the parietal and visceral layers of the tunica vaginalis, between which hydroceles form. The visceral layer of the tunica vaginalis is adherent to the testis. (See Schwartz 9th ed., p 1461.)

5. The left spermatic vein drains into the
   A. Left iliac vein
   B. Left inferior epigastric vein
   C. Left side of the inferior vena cava
   D. Left renal vein

Answer: D

The right spermatic vein drains directly into the inferior vena cava. On the left, the spermatic vein drains into the left renal vein. (See Schwartz 9th ed., p 1461.)

CLINICAL QUESTIONS

1. Patients with bladder stones are at increased risk for which of the following bladder cancers?
   A. Adenocarcinoma
   B. Transitional cell carcinoma
   C. Squamous cell carcinoma
   D. Choriocarcinoma

Answer: C

The most common form of bladder cancer in the United States is transitional cell carcinoma (TCC). Tobacco use, followed by occupational exposure to various carcinogenic materials such as automobile exhaust or industrial solvents are the most frequent risk factors, though many with the disease have no identifiable risks. Other forms of bladder cancer, such as adenocarcinoma and squamous cell carcinoma, occur in distinct patient populations. Patients with chronic irritation from catheters, bladder stones, or schistosomiasis infection are at risk for the squamous cell variant while those with urachal remnants or bladder exstrophy have an increased risk of adenocarcinoma. (See Schwartz 9th ed., p 1461.)

2. Emphysematous pyelonephritis is most commonly caused by
   A. *Clostridia perfringens*
   B. *Escherichia coli*
   C. Group A *Streptococcus*
   D. *Bacteroides* species

Answer: B

Emphysematous pyelonephritis is a life-threatening infection that results from complicated pyelonephritis by gas-producing organisms. It is an acute necrotizing infection of the kidney that occurs predominantly in diabetic patients. Patients frequently present with sepsis and ketoacidosis. *Escherichia coli* appears to be the most frequent organism responsible for this infection. Patients require supportive care, IV antibiotics, and relief of any urinary tract obstruction. Emphysematous pyelonephritis can be subdivided based on extent of infection. Those with gas confined to the parenchyma frequently can be managed conservatively with placement of a nephrostomy tube to allow drainage of purulent material. Patients with extensive involvement of the perirenal tissue may not respond to conservative management, and strong consideration should be given to expeditious nephrectomy, particularly if the patient is displaying signs of sepsis. (See Schwartz 9th ed., p 1470.)

3. Expectant management may be considered for men with prostate cancer who
   A. Have a Gleason score >10
   B. Are <55 years of age
   C. Have low volume disease as determined by biopsy
   D. Have a PSA level <35

Answer: C

Expectant management may be a useful strategy in men with anticipated survival of <10 years, low Gleason score (≤6), early-stage disease (cT1c), and small volume disease as determined by biopsy. Patients should be watched closely with digital rectal exam, PSA testing, and repeat biopsy at 1 year to assess the possible progression of disease.

Prostate cancer is graded according to the Gleason scoring system. A primary and secondary score are assigned based on the most common and second most common histologic pattern. Grades run from 1 for the most differentiated to 5 for the least. The grades are added to give the Gleason score. In current practice, scores below 6 are almost never assigned. Gleason score, preoperative PSA level, and digital rectal exam are used to estimate the likelihood of whether the cancer is localized, locally advanced, or metastatic. Prostate cancer with high Gleason scores (8 to 10) or a high PSA level (>20) is much more likely to have spread, often at a micrometastatic level. (See Schwartz 9th ed., p 1465.)

4. A blunt injury to the kidney with a 2-cm, nonexpanding hematoma and a small amount of urinary extravasation is
   A. A grade 1 injury
   B. A grade 2 injury
   C. A grade 3 injury
   D. A grade 4 injury

Answer: D

Any injury that involves the collecting system (implied by the urinary leak) is a grade 4 injury. The AAST grading system is shown in Table 40-1. (See Schwartz 9th ed., p 1466.)

TABLE 40-1 American Association for the Surgery of Trauma renal injury scale

Grade	Injury Type	Description
1	Contusion	Microscopic or gross hematuria with normal imaging
	Hematoma	Subcapsular, nonexpanding without parenchymal laceration
2	Hematoma	Nonexpanding perirenal hematoma confined to renal retroperitoneum <1 cm in depth without urinary extravasation
3	Laceration	>1 cm in depth without collecting system rupture or urinary extravasation
4	Laceration	Parenchymal laceration through cortex, medulla, and collecting system
4	Vascular	Main renal artery or vein injury with contained hemorrhage
5	Laceration	Completely shattered kidney
5	Laceration	Avulsion of renal hilum leading to devascularized kidney

Source: Adapted with permission from Moore EE et al: Organ injury scaling. *Surg Clin North Am* 75:293, 1995. Copyright © Elsevier.

5. Injuries to the distal ureter should be treated with
   A. Primary repair
   B. End-to-end anastomosis after spatulation
   C. Uretero-ureterostomy (to the contralateral ureter)
   D. Ureteral reimplantation

Answer: D

Surgical repair depends on location and extent of injury. A suture in place briefly may be removed usually without consequence. Partial injuries can be primarily repaired, although all devitalized tissue must be débrided to avoid delayed tissue breakdown and urinoma formation. Ureteral stents should be placed in this situation to facilitate healing without stricture. Lower ureteral injuries (below the iliac vessels) are best treated with ureteral reimplant, as the blood supply can be tenuous, and strictures are more common with a distal uretero-ureterostomy. Midureteral level injuries can be treated with a uretero-ureterostomy if a spatulated, tension-free repair can be achieved. For longer defects, the bladder can be mobilized and brought up to the psoas muscle (psoas hitch). For additional length, a tubularized flap of bladder (Boari flap) can be created and anastomosed to the remaining ureter. Renal mobilization with nephropexy by anchoring to the psoas muscle can provide additional length. Autotransplantation, transuretero-ureterostomy, and ileal ureter are rarely needed during an acute setting. (See Schwartz 9th ed., p 1466.)

6. Elevated serum levels of alpha fetoprotein in a man with a firm testicular mass make which of the following diagnoses most likely?
   A. Seminomatous germ cell tumor
   B. Nonseminomatous germ cell tumor
   C. Leydig cell tumor
   D. Sertoli cell tumor

Answer: B

All solid testicular masses observed on physical examination and documented on ultrasound are malignant until proven otherwise, because the vast majority are cancerous. Initial studies must include tumor markers, including alpha-fetoprotein and beta human chorionic gonadotrophin. Elevated tumor markers are found almost exclusively in nonseminomatous germ cell tumor, though occasionally seminomas will cause a modest rise in beta human chorionic gonadotrophin.

Most testicular neoplasms arise from the germ cells, though nongerm cell tumors arise from Leydig's or Sertoli's cells. The nongerm cell tumors are rare and generally follow a more benign course. Germ cell cancers are categorically divided into seminomatous and nonseminomatous forms that follow different treatment algorithms. (See Schwartz 9th ed., p 1462.)

7. Which of the following types of renal calculi will NOT be seen on CT scan?
   A. Calcium oxalate
   B. Struvite (magnesium ammonium phosphate)
   C. Uric acid
   D. Crystalline excreted indinavir

Answer: D

Urolithiasis, or urinary calculus disease, may affect up to 10% of the population over the course of a lifetime. Calculi are crystalline aggregates of one or more components, most commonly calcium oxalate. They also may contain calcium phosphate, magnesium ammonium phosphate (struvite), uric acid, or cystine. Calcium and struvite-containing stones often are visible on plain radiographs, but CT scans will demonstrate all calculi except those composed of crystalline-excreted indinavir, an antiretroviral medication. (See Schwartz 9th ed., p 1472.)

8. A patient with renal cell carcinoma with extension into the IVC (tumor thrombus) is best treated with
   A. Radiotherapy
   B. Chemotherapy
   C. Thrombolytic therapy
   D. Surgery

Answer: D

Up to 10% of RCC invades the lumen of the renal vein or vena cava. The degree of venous extension directly impacts the surgical approach. Patients with thrombus below the level of the liver can be managed with cross-clamping above and below the thrombus and extraction from a cavotomy at the insertion of the renal vein (Fig. 40-1A). Usually, the thrombus is not adherent to the vessel wall. However, cross-clamping the vena cava above the hepatic veins can drastically reduce cardiac preload, and therefore, bypass techniques often are necessary. For thrombus above the hepatic veins, a multidisciplinary approach with either venovenous or cardiopulmonary bypass is necessary. In cases of invasion of the wall of the vena cava or atrium, deep hypothermic circulatory arrest may be used to give a completely bloodless field. Tumor thrombus embolization to the pulmonary artery is a rare but known complication during these cases and is associated with a high mortality (Fig. 40-1B). For cases of extensive tumor thrombus, intraoperative transesophageal echocardiography should be considered for monitoring and assessment of possible thrombus embolization. If a thrombus embolization occurs, a sternotomy/cardiopulmonary bypass with extraction of the thrombus may be life saving. (See Schwartz 9th ed., p 1464.)

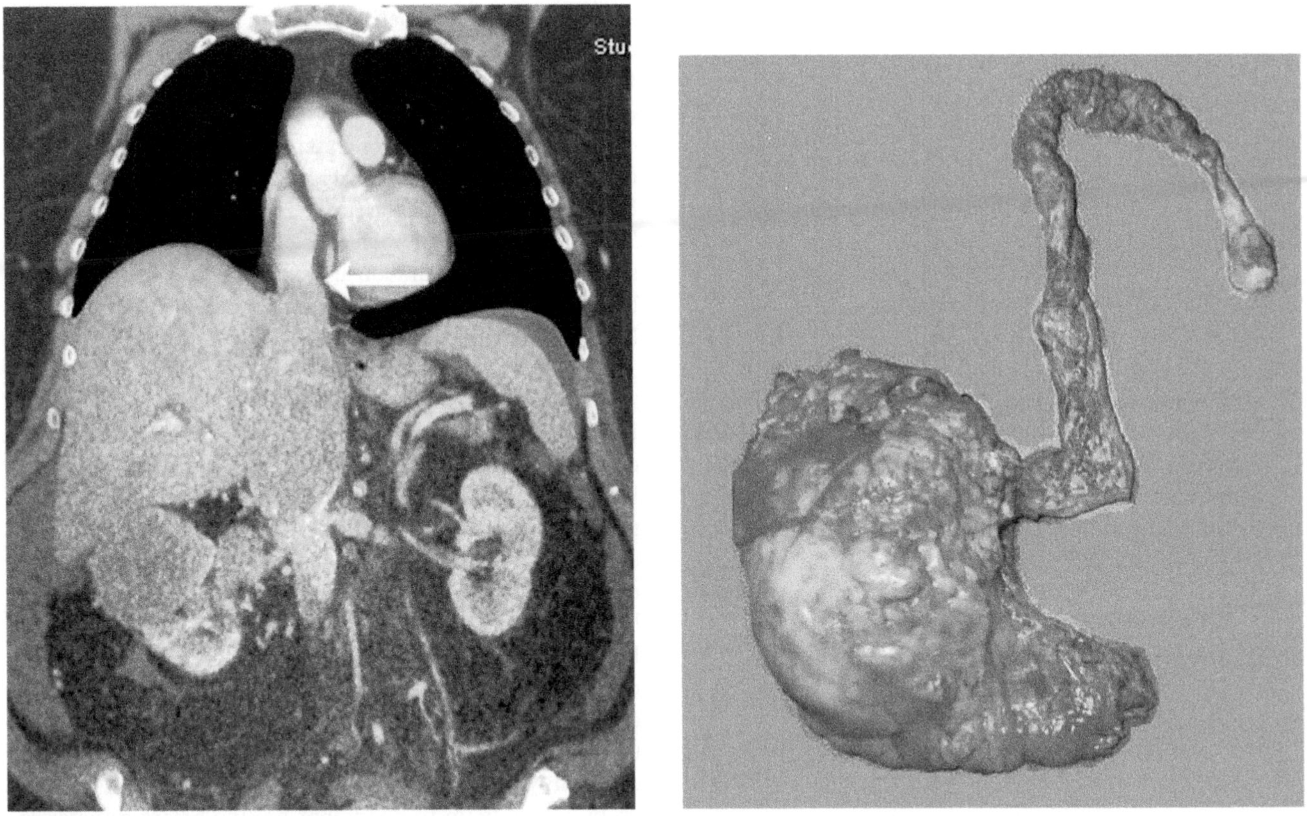

A B

FIG. 40-1. Inferior vena cava thrombus. A. A multidetector computed tomographic image displaying a tumor thrombus extending above the diaphragm (*arrow*) arising from a right renal mass. B. An en bloc removal of a different right renal mass with a tumor thrombus that extended to the pulmonary artery. This patient is alive 6 years after surgery.

9. The most common noncontinent urinary diversion procedure after cystectomy is
   A. Orthotopic neobladder (ileal pouch)
   B. Ileal conduit
   C. Appendiceal conduit
   D. Ureterostomy

Answer: B

Patients have multiple reconstructive options, including continent and noncontinent urinary diversions following cystectomy. The orthotopic neobladder has emerged as a popular urinary diversion for patients without urethral involvement. This diversion type involves the detubularization of a segment of bowel, typically distal ileum, which is then refashioned into a pouch that is anastomosed to the proximal urethral. Detubularization decreases intrapouch filling pressure, which improves urinary storage capacity. The external sphincter is still intact, and voiding is achieved through sphincteric relaxation and a Valsalva's maneuver. The most common noncontinent diversion is the ileal conduit, whereby a segment of distal ileum is isolated with one end brought out through the abdominal wall as a urostomy. Ileal conduits are preferred for renal insufficiency because urine is not 'stored' and therefore has less time in contact with the absorptive surface of the ileal segment. Conduits are also used when the bladder is unresectable, but urinary diversion is necessary due to intractable bleeding or severe voiding pain. Each segment of bowel that is used offers its own advantages and inherent complications. (See Schwartz 9th ed., p 1461.)

10. Initial management of a patient with priapism includes
    A. Bed rest, narcotics, and hydration
    B. Administration of beta blockers
    C. Placement of an 18-g IV catheter into the corpus cavernosum
    D. Surgical exploration

Answer: C

The management of priapism is rapid detumescence with the goal of preservation of future erectile function. The ability to achieve normal erections is directly related to length of the episode of priapism. Low-flow priapism can be confirmed with a penile blood gas of the cavernosal bodies demonstrating hypoxic, acidotic blood. Initial management can include oral agents such as pseudoephedrine or baclofen, but more aggressive measures usually are necessary to achieve rapid detumescence. Insertion of a large gauge needle (18 gauge) into the lateral aspect of one corporal body allows thorough aspiration and irrigation of both corporal bodies because of widely communicating channels. Injection of phenylephrine (up to 200 mg in 20 mL normal saline) into the corporal bodies may be required. For those with sickle cell disease, hydration and oxygen administration should be performed first, as that is sometimes successful in this group. (See Schwartz 9th ed., p 1470.)

11. A patient with a complex pelvic fracture is scheduled for open reduction and fixation of the fractures in the operating room. He also has an extraperitoneal bladder injury with a contained area of extravasation. The best treatment for the bladder injury is
    A. Leaving a Foley catheter in place for 7-10 days
    B. Percutaneous drainage of the extravasation and Foley catheter drainage of the bladder
    C. Transurethral repair of the bladder injury
    D. Open repair of the bladder injury

Answer: D
Extraperitoneal bladder injuries can typically be managed with catheter drainage for 7 to 10 days. If intraoperative exploration is to occur for other injuries, repair can be performed at that time. For patients with pelvic injuries that require an open operation with placement of metal hardware, repair of the bladder rupture should be performed if possible. Intraperitoneal bladder injuries should be explored immediately and repaired. However, for cases of a missed intraperitoneal injury, patients often do well with catheter drainage only. For large ruptures after repair, a suprapubic tube is recommended, but a large urethral catheter is sufficient for smaller injuries. All injuries, especially those managed nonoperatively, should be followed up by a cystogram to document healing before catheter removal. (See Schwartz 9th ed., p 1467.)

12. Paraphimosis refers to
    A. Inability to retract the foreskin
    B. Inability to reduce the foreskin after it has been retracted
    C. Infection of the foreskin
    D. Excessive length of foreskin

Answer: B
Paraphimosis is a common problem that represents a true medical emergency. When foreskin is retracted for prolonged periods, constriction of the glans penis may ensue. This is particularly likely in hospitalized patients who are confined to bed or who have altered mentation. Edema often forms in the genitals of supine patients due to the dependent position of that area. Patients with diminished consciousness will not be aware of the penile pain from paraphimosis, which may delay recognition of the problem until too late. Delay can be catastrophic as penile necrosis may occur due to ischemia. (See Schwartz 9th ed., p 1470.)

13. Which of the following is an absolute indication for surgical exploration of an injured kidney?
    A. Grade V injury
    B. Large urinoma from a collecting duct injury
    C. Contained hematoma >5 cm in diameter
    D. Renovascular hypertension

Answer: A
The absolute and relative indications for surgical exploration of an injured kidney are listed in Table 40-2. (See Schwartz 9th ed., p 1465, 66.)

TABLE 40-2 Indications for surgical intervention for renal trauma

Absolute indications
1. Persistent, life-threatening hemorrhage from probable renal injury
2. Renal pedicle avulsion (grade V injury)
3. Expanding, pulsatile, or uncontained retroperitoneal hematoma
Relative indications
1. Large laceration of the renal pelvis or avulsion of the ureteropelvic junction
2. Coexisting bowel or pancreatic injuries
3. Persistent urinary leakage, postinjury urinoma, or perinephric abscess with failed percutaneous or endoscopic management
4. Abnormal intraoperative one-shot IV urogram
5. Devitalized parenchymal segment with associated urine leak
6. Complete renal artery thrombosis of both kidneys or of a solitary kidney when renal perfusion appears preserved
7. Renal vascular injuries after failed angiographic management
8. Renovascular hypertension

Source: Adapted with permission from Santucci RA, Wessells H, Bartsch G, et al: Evaluation and management of renal injuries: Consensus statement of the renal trauma subcommittee. *BJU Int* 93:937, 2004.

14. A patient with a complete anterior urethral injury after a high speed motor vehicle accident is best initially managed by
    A. Placement of a Foley catheter for 8-10 days
    B. Placement of a Foley catheter for 1 month
    C. Placement of a suprapubic catheter
    D. Immediate repair

Answer: C

Blunt anterior urethral injury can be managed in multiple ways and only small series are available in the literature to compare methods. Immediate surgical repair is not recommended in the acute setting with the exception of low velocity penetrating injuries. If the patient is stable with minimal hematoma formation, repair should be considered. In this setting of a 1- to 2-cm defect, the urethra can be débrided, spatulated, and anastomosed in an end-to-end, watertight fashion. Large defects should have treatment deferred, as grafts or flaps may be required for repair and the success may diminish with infections. For most cases, catheter drainage is recommended. Many advocate avoiding a placement of a urethral catheter, as it may convert a partial tear to a complete dissection. However, a single gentle passage performed by a urologist is safe. For a complete disruption, the placement of a suprapubic tube is recommended; however, a stricture at the site of injury may ensue. (See Schwartz 9th ed., p 1467.)

15. Following documentation of a firm mass in the testes by ultrasound in a 32-year-old male, tissue should be obtained for diagnosis by
    A. Fine-needle aspiration
    B. Core-needle biopsy
    C. Open biopsy
    D. Orchiectomy

Answer: D

There is no role for percutaneous biopsy of testicular masses due to the risk of seeding the scrotal wall and changing the natural retroperitoneal lymphatic drainage of the testicle, because the testes have a remarkably predictable pattern of lymphatic drainage. In cases where metastatic disease to the testicle is suspected, an open testicular biopsy by delivery of the testicle through the inguinal canal is recommended. Lymphoma may involve one or both testes, but evidence of the disease usually is present elsewhere in the body, although relapses may be isolated to the testes. (See Schwartz 9th ed., p 1462.)

16. Following transurethral resection of a superficial (noninvasive) transitional cell carcinoma, which of the following is instilled in the bladder to decrease the risk of recurrence?
    A. Cyclophosphamide
    B. Cis-platinum
    C. Methotrexate
    D. BCG (bacille Calmette-Guérin)

Answer: D
Patients with nonmuscle invasive TCC (confined to the bladder mucosa or submucosa) can be managed with transurethral resection alone. However, patients are at risk for recurrence and progression to muscle-invasive disease. Tumor grade is extremely important in assessing the risk of disease progression. Those patients with high-grade disease or recurrent tumors can be treated with intravesical agents such as bacille Calmette-Guérin or mitomycin C. These agents decrease risk of progression and recurrence, by induction of an effective immunologic antitumor response in the case of bacilli Calmette-Guérin and through direct cytotoxicity for mitomycin C. (See Schwartz 9th ed., p 1461.)

Adriamycin is actually used on occasion to prevent recurrences, whereasile cyclophosphamide is never used.

17. Which one of the following syndromes is associated with an increased risk of renal cell carcinoma?
    A. Down syndrome
    B. Von Hippel-Lindau syndrome
    C. Neurofibromatosis type 1
    D. Osteogenesis imperfecta

Answer: B
Most cases of RCC are sporadic, but many hereditary forms have been described. These syndromes frequently involve a germline mutation in a tumor-suppressor gene. Von Hippel-Lindau disease is associated with multiple tumors including clear-cell RCC. The involved gene, *vhl*, also frequently is mutated or hypermethylated in sporadic RCC. Other rare forms include Birt-Hogg-Dubé syndrome, where patients get oncocytomas or chromophobe tumors. Patients with hereditary papillary RCC and hereditary leiomyomatosis develop papillary RCC. (See Schwartz 9th ed., p 1463.)

18. Which of the following classes of medication is the most common initial treatment of men with symptomatic benign prostatic hypertrophy (BPH)?
    A. Alpha agonist
    B. Alpha blocker
    C. Beta agonist
    D. Beta blocker

Answer: B
Medical treatment of BPH is usually the first step. Alpha blockers act on alpha receptors in the smooth muscle of the prostate and decrease its tone. 5α-Reductase inhibitors, which block the conversion of testosterone to the more potent dihydrotestosterone, shrink the prostate over several months. (See Schwartz 9th ed., p 1471.)

'Blockers' and 'antagonists' are the same thing. '*Agonists*' areis better becausesince they do exist but are not used for BPH.

19. In a patient with extensive Fournier's gangrene involving the scrotum, the testes
    A. Are usually involved and must be resected
    B. Are usually involved but can be watched for 24-48 hours before deciding to perform an orchiectomy
    C. Are usually not involved but should be removed due to the potential for post-operative pain
    D. Are usually not involved and can be transposed to the soft tissue of the thigh

Answer: D
Prompt débridement of nonviable tissue and broad-spectrum antibiotics is necessary to prevent further spread [of infection in patients with Fournier's gangrene] (Fig. 40-2A and B). If there is damage to the external sphincter, patients may require a colostomy. As the testes have a separate blood supply, they are usually not threatened and do not need to be removed. They may be tucked subcutaneously into the thigh ('thigh pouch') to ease postoperative management.

The testes are occasionally left exposed but wrapped in wet-to-dry dressings if there is a plan to do skin grafting in the immediate post-débridement time frame. They may be tucked subcutaneously into the thigh or left exposed wrapped in wet to dry dressings if early skin grafting is possible. (See Schwartz 9th ed., p 1469.)

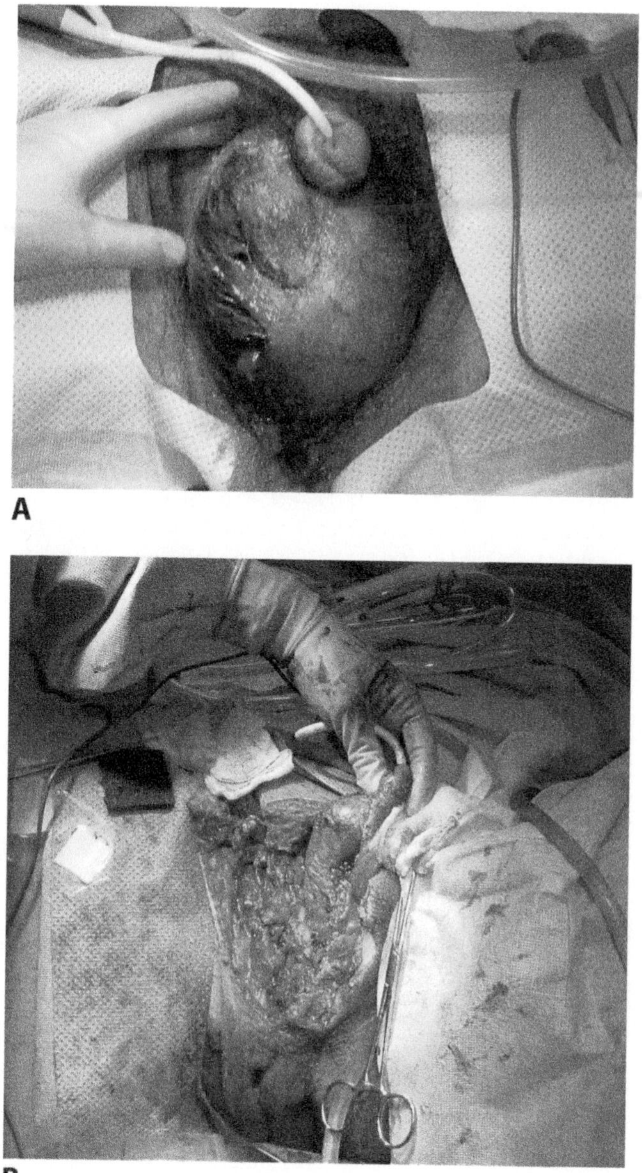

A

B

FIG. 40-2. Fournier's gangrene. A. Necrotic scrotal skin from Fournier's gangrene. B. Débridement of gangrenous tissue. Note the extensive débridement, which is commonly required. The right testicle required removal in this case (the left is wrapped in gauze), but typically the testes are not involved with the necrotic process.

20. Which of the following types of renal carcinoma has the worst prognosis?
    A. Clear cell
    B. Papillary
    C. Chromophobe
    D. Collecting duct

Answer: D

Various histologic subtypes of renal carcinoma include clear-cell, papillary (types I and II), chromophobe, collecting duct, and unclassified forms. Collecting duct and unclassified forms have dismal prognosis and very little response to systemic therapy. (See Schwartz 9th ed., p 1462.)

CHAPTER 41

Gynecology

BASIC SCIENCE QUESTIONS

1. The round ligament leaves the abdomen through the internal inguinal ring to attach to the mons pubis. Its proximal origin is
   A. The broad ligament
   B. The uterosacral ligament
   C. The uterine cervical junction
   D. The cornu of the uterus

Answer: D

Emanating from the uterine cornu and traveling through the inguinal canal are the round ligaments, eventually attaching to the subcutaneous tissue of the mons pubis. (See Schwartz 9th ed., p 1479, and Fig. 41-1.)

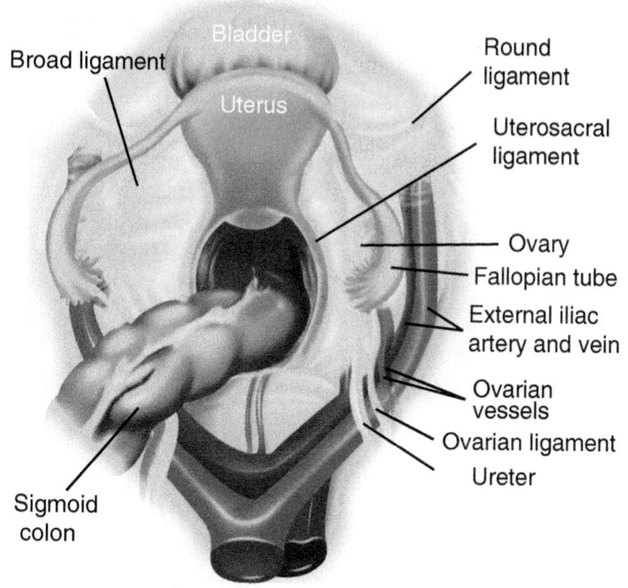

FIG. 41-1. Internal pelvic anatomy, from above.

2. Which of the following physiologic changes occurs during pregnancy?
   A. Increased systemic vascular resistance
   B. Decreased minute ventilation
   C. Decreased gastric motility
   D. Decreased fibrinogen

Answer: C

Table 41-1 summarizes the physiologic changes due to pregnancy. Gastric motility is decreased. Systemic vascular resistance, minute ventilation, and fibrinogen are all increased. (See Schwartz 9th ed., p 1487.)

TABLE 41-1 Physiologic changes due to pregnancy
Cardiovascular changes
Increased cardiac output
Increased blood volume
Decreased systemic vascular resistance
Decreased venous return from lower extremities
Respiratory changes
Increased minute ventilation
Decreased functional residual capacity
GI changes
Decreased gastric motility
Delayed gastric emptying
Coagulation changes
Increased clotting factors (II, V, VII, VIII, IX, X, and XII)
Increased fibrinogen
Increased risk for venous thromboembolism
Renal changes
Increased renal plasma flow and glomerular filtration rate
Ureteral dilation
Initial increased bladder capacity

Source: Adapted with permission from Gabbe S, Niebyl J, Simpson J: *Obstetrics: Normal and Problem Pregnancies*, 4th ed. Philadelphia: Churchill Livingstone, 2001, Chap. 19, p 608. Copyright © Elsevier.

CLINICAL QUESTIONS

1. Which of the following groups of women should receive an annual cervical cytologic examination (Pap smear)?
   A. Starting at age 18, regardless ofn onset of intercourse, and yearly thereafter
   B. Starting after 5 years of onset of sexual intercourse and yearly thereafter
   C. Starting after first sexual intercourse at any age
   D. All women starting after 3 years of onset of sexual intercourse or by age 21 and until 30 years of age

Answer: D

The present guidelines for cervical cytology recommend annual evaluation for all sexually active women up to the age of 30 years old. After age 30, cervical cytology may be extended to every 2 to 3 years if cytology has remained negative and/or testing for human papillomavirus (HPV) high-risk types has been negative. This can be achieved with either liquid techniques or the older smear technique, recognizing that the accepted approach is moving to liquid techniques as they allow for reflex testing of HPV high-risk subtypes as appropriate. (See Schwartz 9th ed., p 1481.)

2. The most common cause of vaginitis is
   A. Human papillomavirus
   B. Anaerobic bacteria
   C. Candida albicans
   D. Trichomonas vaginalis

Answer: B

BV (bacterial vaginitis) is the most common cause of vaginal discharge, accounting for 50% of cases. It results from reduction in concentration of the normally dominant lactobacilli and increase in concentration of anaerobic organisms like *Gardnerella vaginalis*, *Mycoplasma hominis*, *Bacteroides* spp, and others. Diagnosis is made by microscopy and involves recognition of clue cells, which are epithelial cells studded with adherent bacteria causing their margins to be obliterated. The discharge typically produces a fishy odor upon addition of KOH (amine or Whiff test).

Candida and trichomonas are also common causes of vaginitis. HPV is associated with cervical aplasia and does not cause vaginitis. (See Schwartz 9th ed., p 1484, and Table 41-2.)

TABLE 41-2 Features of common causes of vaginitis

	Bacterial Vaginosis	Vulvovaginal Candidiasis	Trichomoniasis
Pathogen	Anaerobic organisms	*Candida albicans*	*Trichomonas vaginalis*
% of Vaginitis	40	30	20
pH	>4.5	<4.5	>4.5
Signs and symptoms	Malodorous, adherent discharge	White discharge, vulvar erythema, pruritus, dyspareunia	Malodorous purulent discharge, vulvovaginal erythema, dyspareunia
Wet mount	Clue cells	Pseudohyphae or budding yeasts in 40% of cases	Motile trichomonads
KOH mount		Pseudohyphae or budding yeasts in 70% of cases	
Amine test	+	–	–
Treatment	Metronidazole 500 mg bid × 7 d or 2 g single dose, metronidazole or clindamycin vaginal cream	Oral fluconazole 150 mg single dose, vaginal antifungal preparations	Metronidazole 2 g single dose and treatment of partner

+ = positive; – = negative; KOH = potassium hydroxide.

3. A patient presents with a single genital ulcer. Of the following, the most likely cause is:
   A. Herpes
   B. Chancroid
   C. Lymphgranuloma venereum
   D. Granuloma inguinale

Answer: C

Lymphogranuloma venereum usually presents with a single ulcer. Herpes and chancroid most commonly have multiple lesions. Granuloma inguinale is variable in its presentation. The other infection that commonly presents with a single ulcer (chancre) is the primary stage of syphilis. (See Schwartz 9th ed., p 1485.)

4. With no treatment, what percent of patients with primary syphilis eventually progresses to tertiary disease?
   A. 10%
   B. 30%
   C. 50%
   D. 70%

Answer: B

The primary stage [of syphilis] is marked by the appearance of a single ulcer (chancre). The chancre usually is firm, round, painless, may be accompanied by regional adenopathy, and develops at the site of entry of the bacterium. It lasts 3 to 6 weeks, and it heals without treatment. However, without treatment, the primary infection progresses to secondary syphilis and eventually to tertiary disease in 30% of cases, after a variable latent phase that usually lasts for years. During pregnancy, syphilis can be transmitted to the fetus and may result in the varied manifestations of congenital syphilis syndrome, which may results in fetal hydrops and intrauterine fetal demise. The diagnosis of syphilis is typically made by examination and serologic testing. Nonspecific nontreponemal tests such as rapid plasma reagin and Venereal Disease Research Laboratories are used for screening, and specific treponemal tests such as fluorescent-labeled treponema antibody absorption and microhemagglutination assay for antibodies to *T. pallidum* are used for confirmation. (See Schwartz 9th ed., p 1485.)

5. Appropriate antibiotic treatment for chancroid is
   A. Penicillin
   B. Acyclovir
   C. Azithromycin
   D. Doxycycline

Answer: C

There are four antibiotics that can be used to treat chancroid (see Table 41-3): azithromycin, ceftriaxone, ciprofloxacin, and erythromycin.

Chancroid is a contagious sexually transmitted ulcerative disease of the vulva caused by *Haemophilus ducreyi*, small gram-negative rods that exhibit parallel alignment on Gram's staining ("school of fish"). After a short incubation period, the patient usually develops multiple painful soft ulcers on the vulva, mainly on the labia majora and, less commonly, on the labia minora or involving the perineal area. The chancroid ulcer has ragged, irregular borders and a base that bleeds easily and is covered with grayish exudates. Approximately half the patients will develop painful inguinal lymphadenitis within 2 weeks of an untreated infection, which may undergo liquefaction and presents as buboes. These may rupture and discharge pus. Diagnosis is made by Gram's stain and, less commonly, by culture. (See Schwartz 9th ed., p 1485.)

TABLE 41-3 Clinical features of genital ulcer syndromes

	Herpes	Syphilis	Chancroid	Lymphogranuloma Venereum	Granuloma Inguinale (Donovanosis)
Pathogen	HSV type II and, less commonly, HSV type I	*Treponema palladium*	*Haemophilus ducreyi*	*Chlamydia trachomatis* L1–L3	*Calymmatobacterium granulomatis*
Incubation period	2–7 d	Typically 2–4 wk (can range from 1–12 wk)	1–14 d	3 d–6 wk	1–4 wk (up to 6 mo)
Primary lesion	Vesicle	Papule	Papule or pustule	Papule, pustule, or vesicle	Papule
Number of lesions	Multiple, may coalesce	Usually one	Usually multiple, may coalesce	Usually one	Variable
Diameter (mm)	1–2	5–15	2–20	2–10	Variable
Edges	Erythematous	Sharply demarcated, elevated, round, or oval	Undermined, ragged, irregular	Elevated, round, or oval	Elevated, irregular
Depth	Superficial	Superficial or deep	Excavated	Superficial or deep	Elevated
Base	Serous, erythematous	Smooth, nonpurulent	Purulent	Variable	Red and rough ("beefy")
Induration	None	Firm	Soft	Occasionally firm	Firm
Pain	Common	Unusual	Usually very tender	Variable	Uncommon
Lymphadenopathy	Firm, tender, often bilateral	Firm, nontender, bilateral	Tender, may suppurate, usually unilateral	Tender, may suppurate, loculated, usually unilateral	Pseudoadenopathy
Treatment	Acyclovir 400 mg PO tid × 7–10 d for primary infection and 400 mg PO tid × 5 d for episodic management	Primary, secondary, and early latent (<1 y): benzathine PCN-G 2.4 million U IM × 1 Late latent (>1 y) and latent of unknown duration: benzathine PCN-G 2.4 million units IM qwk × 3	Azithromycin 1 g PO or ceftriaxone 250 mg IM × 1 *or* Ciprofloxacin 500 mg PO bid × 3 d *or* Erythromycin base 500 mg PO tid × 7 d	Doxycycline 100 mg PO bid × 21 d *or* Erythromycin base 500 mg PO qid × 21 d	Doxycycline 100 mg PO bid × 3 wk until all lesions have healed
Suppression	Acyclovir 400 mg PO bid for those with frequent outbreak	—	—	—	—

HSV = herpes simplex virus; PCN-G = penicillin.
Data from Stenchever M, Droegemueller W, Herbst A, et al: *Comprehensive Gynecology*, 4th ed. St Louis: Mosby, 2001.

6. A 32-year-old woman presents with a swollen, red, tender 3-cm mass in the posterior aspect of the right labia majora at the vaginal orifice. In addition to antibiotics, the appropriate treatment for this lesion is
   A. Observation
   B. Aspiration and cytologic evaluation
   C. Resection of the mass
   D. Incision, drainage, and Word catheter

Answer: D

Bartholin's glands (great vestibular glands) are located at the vaginal orifice at the 4 and 8 o'clock positions and they are rarely palpable in normal patients. They are lined with cuboidal epithelium and secrete mucoid material to keep the vulva moist. Their ducts are lined with transitional epithelium and their obstruction secondary to inflammation may lead to the development of a Bartholin's cyst or abscess. Bartholin's cysts range in size from 1 to 3 cm, and are detected on examination or recognized by the patient. They occasionally result in discomfort and dyspareunia and require treatment. Cysts and ducts can become infected and form abscesses. Infections are often polymicrobial; however, sexually transmitted *Neisseria gonorrhea* and *C. trachomatis* are sometimes implicated. Abscesses usually present as acutely inflamed, exquisitely tender masses. Treatment consists of incision and drainage and placement of a Word catheter, a small catheter with a balloon tip, for 2 to 3 weeks to allow for formation and epithelialization of a new duct. Appropriate antibiotic therapy should be instituted and modified based upon culture results. Recurrent cysts or abscesses are usually marsupialized, but on occasion necessitate excision of the whole gland. Marsupialization is done by incising the cyst or abscess wall and securing its lining to the skin edges with interrupted sutures. Cysts or abscesses that fail to resolve after drainage and those occurring in patients >40 years of age should be biopsied to exclude malignancy. (See Schwartz 9th ed., p 1485.)

7. A young female presents with fever, nausea and vomiting, abdominal pain, and a pelvic mass. While in the ED she was given IV fluids and started on IV antibiotics. However, within an hour of presentation she rapidly progressed to septic shock. She was taken to surgery where a ruptured tubo-ovarian abscess was identified. In addition to appropriate antibiotic therapy, the surgical treatment of choice in this unstable patient is
   A. Washout with planned re-exploration in 24-48 hours
   B. Pelvic drainage
   C. Resection of the involved Fallopian tube
   D. Total abdominal hysterectomy and bilateral salpingo-oophorectomy

Answer: D

Surgical intervention becomes necessary if medical therapy of a tubo-ovarian abscess fails or if the abscess ruptures. Rupture of a tubo-ovarian abscess is a surgical emergency with a high mortality rate if not recognized and managed promptly. In addition to management of the septic shock state, total abdominal hysterectomy and bilateral salpingo-oophorectomy is the procedure of choice; however, conservative surgery must be considered in young patients desiring of future fertility. The abdomen should be explored for metastatic abscesses, and special attention must be paid to bowel, bladder, and ureteral safety due to the friability of the infected tissue and the adhesions commonly encountered at the time of surgery. Placement of an intraperitoneal drain and mass closure of the peritoneum, muscle, and fascia with delayed-absorbable or permanent sutures is advised. (See Schwartz 9th ed., p 1486.)

8. In a nulliparous young female with contraindications to methotrexate therapy, a nonruptured ectopic pregnancy should be treated by
   A. Observation if the patient is hemodynamically stable and the Hb is >12 gm/dL
   B. Removal of the products of conception by milking to distal end of the Fallopian tube
   C. Antimesenteric salpingotomy and removal of products of conception
   D. Unilateral salpingectomy

Answer: C

Early ectopic pregnancies can be managed with methotrexate. Advanced ectopic pregnancy or a patient with unstable vital signs is managed by laparoscopy or laparotomy. Linear salpingostomy along the antimesenteric border and removal of the products of conception is a reasonable option unless the oviduct has already ruptured and a large hemoperitoneum already exists, in which case removal of the tube should be performed. (See Schwartz 9th ed., p 1487.)

9. The material most commonly used for a urethral sling (for urinary incontinence) is
   A. Wire mesh bands
   B. Prolene suture in doublets
   C. Gortex mesh bands
   D. Autograft rectus fascia or allograft fascia lata.

Answer: D

A variety of organic and synthetic graft materials have been used to construct suburethral slings. Synthetic materials fell out of favor after a high incidence of postoperative urinary retention and urethral damage were found to be associated with their use. Currently, the most commonly used sling materials include autografts of rectus fascia and processed cadaveric allografts (fascia lata).

The procedure is performed by a combined abdominovaginal approach, using a small transverse suprapubic skin incision. The space of Retzius is entered using a blunt clamp or closed heavy Mayo scissors to penetrate the perineal membrane along the inferior aspect of the descending pubic ramus. A Bozeman clamp or long-angled ligature carrier is used to perforate the rectus fascia two fingerbreadths superior to the pubic bone just medial to the pubic tubercle, and the instrument is guided along the back of the pubic bone through the space of Retzius and into the vaginal incision to retrieve one arm of the sling. After bringing up the other side of the sling, and confirming the absence of urinary tract injury, the sling arms are tied.

Cure rates range from 75 to 95% for the many different types of sling procedures. Slings are associated with higher complication rates than most other incontinence procedures, most frequently involving voiding dysfunction, urinary retention, new-onset urge incontinence, and foreign-body erosion. (See Schwartz 9th ed., p 1490.)

10. Paget's disease of the vulva is associated with
    A. Invasive adenocarcinoma
    B. Papillary carcinoma of the thyroid
    C. Retroperitoneal fibrosis
    D. Melanoma

Answer: A

Paget's disease of the vulva is an intraepithelial disease of unknown etiology that affects mostly white postmenopausal women in their sixth decade of life. It causes chronic vulvar itching and is sometimes associated with an underlying invasive vulvar adenocarcinoma or invasive cancers of the breast, cervix, or GI tract. Grossly, the lesion is variable but usually confluent, raised, erythematous to violet, and waxy in appearance. Biopsy is required for diagnosis; the disease is intraepithelial and characterized by Paget's cells with large pale cytoplasm. Treatment is assessment for other potential concurrent adenocarcinomas and then surgical removal by wide local resection of the involved area with a 2-cm margin. Free margins are difficult to obtain because the disease usually extends beyond the clinically visible area. Intraoperative frozen section of the margins can be done to ensure complete resection. Unfortunately, Paget's vulvar lesions have a high likelihood of recurrence even after securing negative resection margins. (See Schwartz 9th ed., p 1491.)

11. Up to what percentage of cervical cancer in the United States could be prevented if girls were vaccinated against HPV prior to infection?
    A. 10%
    B. 30%
    C. 50%
    D. 70%

Answer: D

The oncogenes of high-risk HPV are both initiating and promoting for cervical cancer. Other correlates with disease include concurrent active HIV infection with immunosuppression, smoking, and probably other genetic factors. It is anticipated that early vaccination, before infection, will function as primary prevention for cervical cancer. It is expected to reduce both the risk and frequency of high-grade CIN, but also translate to marked reduction in actual invasive cancer, requiring 20 to 40 years to see full impact. However, not all high-risk HPV subtypes are covered in the two vaccines available in 2009. Thus, vaccination will likely prevent approximately 70% of cancers in the United States, depending on regional area distribution of oncogenic subtypes. Vaccines are approved for girls ages 9 to 26, but are recommended preferentially for the younger girls as there was a stronger immunologic response seen. (See Schwartz 9th ed., p 1494.)

12. At the time of laparoscopic cholecystectomy, extensive endometriosis is noted in the pelvis. The patient denies pelvic pain and has completed her family with no desire for future pregnancies. The best treatment is
    A. Follow clinically; no treatment is indicated
    B. Oral contraceptive pills (OCPs)
    C. Danazole
    D. Ablation of the lesions with electrocautery

Answer: A

Endometriosis is the finding of ectopic endometrial glands and stroma outside the uterus. It a common condition affecting 10% of the general population, and it is an incidental finding at the time of laparoscopy in >20% of asymptomatic women. It is especially prevalent in patients suffering from chronic pelvic pain (80%) and infertility (20 to 50%).

Expectant management is appropriate in asymptomatic patients. Those with mild symptoms can be managed successfully with cyclic or continuous OCPs combined with the as- needed use of analgesics such as NSAIDs. Moderate symptoms are treated with medroxyprogesterone acetate 10 to 20 mg orally daily or 150 mg IM injection every 3 months. Its use should be limited to 2 years or less because of its negative effects on bone density. Severe symptoms are treated with either danazol or gonadotropin-releasing hormone (GnRH) agonists to induce medical pseudomenopause. Danazol has been largely abandoned secondary to its marked androgenic side effects, such as acne and hirsutism. GnRH agonists act by suppressing the release of gonadotropins (luteinizing and follicle-stimulating hormones) from the pituitary gland and are available in injections or nasal spray preparations.

Conservative surgical therapy [for symptomatic patients] is a popular option because it can be done at the time of the diagnostic laparoscopy and usually involves lysis of adhesions, ablation of endometriotic implants using carbon dioxide laser or electrocautery, and/or resection of deep endometriotic implants. (See Schwartz 9th ed., p 1497.)

13. Which of the following is a contraindication to uterine artery embolization for treatment of a symptomatic leiomyoma?
    A. Solitary lesion 6 cm in diameter
    B. Plans for future pregnancies
    C. Submucosal location
    D. Intramural location

Answer: B

Management options of leiomyomas are tailored to the individual patient, depending on her age and desire for fertility and the size, location, and symptoms of the myomas. Conservative management options include OCPs, medroxyprogesterone acetate, GnRH agonists, uterine artery embolization, and myomectomy. Uterine artery embolization is contraindicated in patients planning future pregnancy and frequently results in acute degeneration of myomas requiring hospitalization for pain control. Myomectomy is indicated in patients with infertility and those who wish to preserve their reproductive capabilities and can be done by laparoscopy, hysteroscopy, or laparotomy. (See Schwartz 9th ed., p 1498, and Fig. 41-2.)

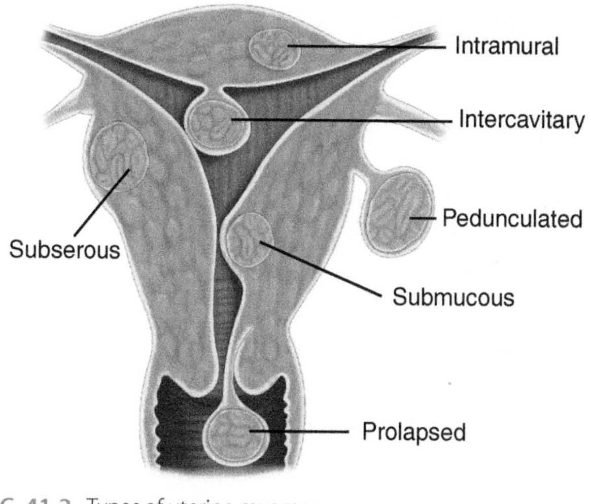

FIG. 41-2. Types of uterine myomas.

14. A 38-year-old patient with a family history of colon and endometrial cancer in multiple first- and second -degree relatives is diagnosed with endometrial cancer herself. She should be offered :
    A. MRI of the brain
    B. Colonoscopy and genetic testing
    C. Bone marrow biopsy
    D. Ultrasound of the thyroid

Answer: B

Hereditary nonpolyposis coli cancer, a cancer family syndrome, also known as Lynch II syndrome, is an autosomal dominant inherited predisposition to develop colorectal carcinoma and other extracolonic cancers, predominantly including tumors of the uterus and ovaries, with rare but defined inclusion of breast cancer. The risk of colorectal carcinoma is as high as 75% by age 75 years old. Affected female patients have a 40% and 10% lifetime risk of developing uterine and ovarian cancers, respectively. Surveillance has not been proven to identify disease in early stage for these patients but is (informally) recommended and should include annual cervical cytology, mammography, transvaginal ultrasound (TVUS), CA measurements, and an endometrial biopsy. (See Schwartz 9th ed., p 1499.)

15. The average distance from the umbilicus to the aorta in a woman of normal weight is
    A. 6 cm
    B. 9 cm
    C. 12 cm
    D. 15 cm

Answer: A

The aorta is only approximately 6 cm from the umbilicus. The distance is even less if the abdominal wall is compressed towards the spine. This is critically important to recognize when placing Varess needles for induction of laparoscopic pneumoperitoneum. (See Schwartz 9th ed., p 1506, and Fig. 41-3).

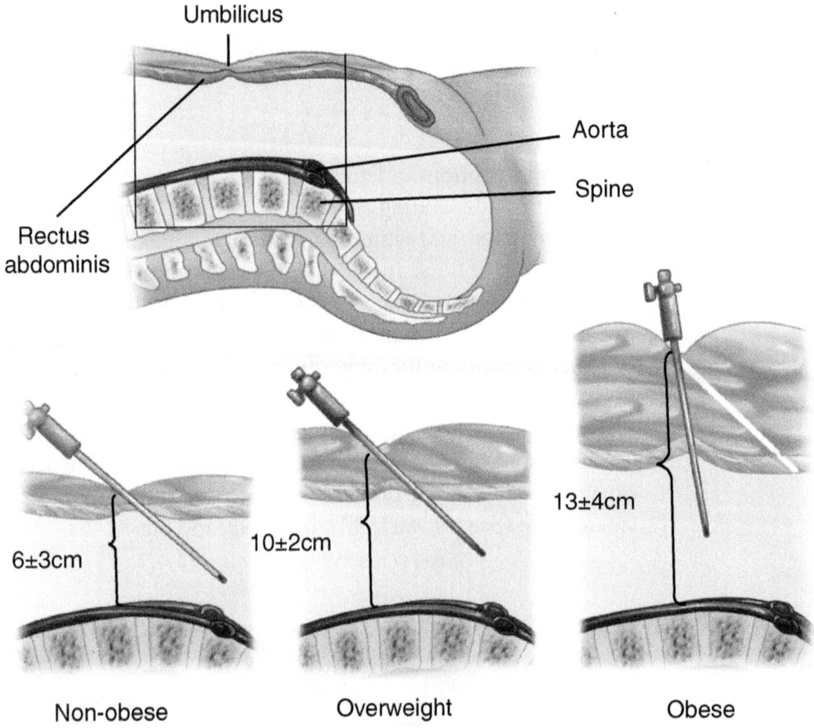

FIG. 41-3. Changes in the anterior abdominal wall anatomy with weight.

16. Which of the following is considered a risk factor for epithelial ovarian cancer?
    A. Pregnancy
    B. Tubal ligation
    C. OCP use for >5 years
    D. Endometriosis

Answer: D

Patients with endometriosis are at increased risk for epithelial ovarian cancer. Pregnancy, tubal ligation, and oral contraceptive (OCP) use for >5 years decrease the risk of developing epithelial ovarian cancer.

Ovarian endometriosis can mimic ovarian/tubal cancer symptoms and also can be associated with an increase in CA 125. It has been associated with an increased risk of malignant ovarian disease of endometrioid and clear-cell histology with reported relative risks in the range of 1.4. (See Schwartz 9th ed., p 1508, and Table 41-4.)

TABLE 41-4 Risk and protective factors for epithelial ovarian and fallopian tube cancers

Protective Factors	Risks
Oral contraceptive use, especially >5 y	Primary and secondary infertility
Tubal ligation	Nulliparity
Lactation	*BRCA1/2* mutation and HNPCC syndrome
Pregnancy	Family history without genetic risk
Oophorectomy, salpingectomy	Endometriosis
	Personal history of breast cancer or first-degree relative with breast cancer
	? Hormone replacement therapy

HNPCC = hereditary nonpolyposis colorectal cancer.

17. Which of the following is one of the variables included in the ovarian cancer symptom index?
   A. Constipation
   B. Dysuria
   C. Early satiety
   D. Menstrual irregularity

Answer: C

Common symptoms for either benign or malignant ovarian tumors include pelvic discomfort, cramping, pain, fullness, headache, backache, and others. These are all symptoms that can be attributed to a variety of pathology from infection to pregnancy to irritable bowel syndrome to cancer. Recent work has identified an ovarian cancer symptom index (Table 41-5), now adopted/supported by the Ovarian Cancer National Alliance, the Gynecologic Cancer Foundation, the Society of Gynecologic Oncologists, and the American Cancer Society. It is based on a 2007 publication by Goff and colleagues, and describes symptoms of bloating, pelvic or abdominal pain, difficulty eating or feeling full quickly, and urinary symptoms of urgency or frequency. These are symptoms that women with ovarian cancer report as newly developed and persistent, or representing a distinct change from their personal norm. The consensus statement says that if the symptom(s) persist for more than a few weeks, the woman should seek medical care. This medical attention should include an evaluation specifically targeted for identification of gynecologic malignancy. (See Schwartz 9th ed., p 1508.)

TABLE 41-5 Ovarian cancer symptom index (2007) and ACOG guidelines for patient referral to gynecologic oncology

Ovarian Cancer Symptom Index	ACOG Guidelines for Referral of Premenopausal Women with Mass Suspicious for Ovarian Cancer	ACOG Guidelines for Referral of Postmenopausal Women with Mass Suspicious for Ovarian Cancer
Development of, change in, and/or persistence in:	One or more of:	One or more of:
Bloating	CA 125 > 200 U/mL	Elevated CA 125
Pelvic or abdominal pain	Ascites	Ascites
Difficulty eating or feeling full quickly	Evidence of abdominal or distant metastasis	Nodular or fixed pelvic mass
Urinary symptoms of urgency or frequency	Family history of one or more first-degree relatives with ovarian or breast cancer	Evidence of abdominal or distant metastasis
		Family history of one or more first-degree relatives with ovarian or breast cancer

ACOG = American College of Obstetricians and Gynecologists.

18. At the time of laparoscopic appendectomy in a 26-year-old nulliparous female, an isolated 4-cm right ovarian mass was identified. A right salpingo-oophorectomy was performed. The abdominal and pelvic surveys were negative and the contralateral ovary was normal. Pathologic examination revealed a mucinous borderline tumor confined to the ovary. The most appropriate management is
   A. Clinical follow-up
   B. Contralateral oophorectomy
   C. Total abdominal hysterectomy
   D. Total abdominal hysterectomy + chemotherapy

Answer: A

LMP [low malignant potential] tumor, also known as *borderline tumor*, is histologically different from true malignancy. It is seen in the ovary with case reports of occurrences in fallopian tubes and accounts for approximately 15% of ovarian neoplasms. The World Health Organization defines LMP tumors as characterized by epithelial proliferation greater than seen in benign tumors and lack of destructive (ovarian) stromal invasion. This entity has an earlier median age of onset, up to two decades earlier than epithelial malignant tumors. Presentation is predominantly stage I and II, and histology includes all subtypes identified for frank malignancy: papillary serous, mucinous, clear-cell, endometrioid, and transitional or Brenner tumor. Surgical intervention is the recommendation of choice. Stages I and II LMP tumors have a 10-year survival of nearly 100%. (See Schwartz 9th ed., p 1509.)

CHAPTER 42

Neurosurgery

BASIC SCIENCE QUESTIONS

1. The motor strip of the cerebral cortex is located in the
   A. Frontal lobes
   B. Temporal lobes
   C. Parietal lobes
   D. Occipital lobes

Answer: A

The frontal areas are involved in executive function, decision making, and restraint of emotions. The motor strip, or precentral gyrus, is the most posterior component of the frontal lobes, and is arranged along a homunculus with the head inferior and lateral to the lower extremities superiorly and medially. The motor speech area (Broca's area) lies in the left posterior inferior frontal lobe in almost all right-handed people and in up to 90% of left-handed people. The parietal lobe lies between the central sulcus anteriorly and the occipital lobe posteriorly. The postcentral gyrus is the sensory strip, also arranged along a homunculus. (See Schwartz 9th ed., p 1516.)

2. The maximum level of intracranial pressure (ICP) that is considered normal is
   A. 6 mmHg
   B. 10 mmHg
   C. 14 mmHg
   D. 18 mmHg

Answer: C

ICP normally varies between 4 and 14 mmHg. Sustained ICP levels above 20 mmHg can injure the brain. The Monro-Kellie doctrine states that the cranial vault is a rigid structure, and therefore, the total volume of the contents determines ICP. The three normal contents of the cranial vault are brain tissue, blood, and CSF. The brain's contents can expand due to swelling from traumatic brain injury (TBI), stroke, or reactive edema. Blood volume can increase by extravasation to form a hematoma, or by reactive vasodilation in a hypoventilating, hypercarbic patient. CSF volume increases in the setting of hydrocephalus. Addition of a fourth element, such as a tumor or abscess, also will increase ICP. (See Schwartz 9th ed., p 1520.)

3. The sympathetic nervous system arises from
   A. Cranial nerves III, VII, IX, and X
   B. Cranial nerves II, IV, V, and VII
   C. The thoracolumbar spinal segments
   D. Spinal segments S_2, S_3, and S_4

Answer: C

The ANS is divided into the sympathetic, parasympathetic, and enteric systems. The sympathetic system drives the 'fight or flight' response, using epinephrine to increase heart rate, blood pressure, blood glucose, and temperature, as well as to dilate the pupils. It arises from the thoracolumbar spinal segments. The parasympathetic system promotes the 'rest and digest' state, and uses acetylcholine to maintain basal metabolic function under nonstressful circumstances. It arises from cranial nerves III, VII, IX, and X, and from the second to fourth sacral segments. The enteric nervous system controls the complex synchronization of the digestive tract, especially the pancreas, gallbladder, and small and large bowels. It can run autonomously but is regulated by the sympathetic and parasympathetic systems. (See Schwartz 9th ed., p 1518.)

4. Motor information is carried from the brain in the
   A. Corticospinal tract
   B. Medial lemnicus tracts
   C. Spinothalamic tracts
   D. Mesencephalic tracts

Answer: A
The brain stem consists of the midbrain (mesencephalon), pons (metencephalon), and medulla (myelencephalon). Longitudinal fibers run through the brain stem, carrying motor and sensory information between the cerebral hemispheres and the spinal cord. The corticospinal tract is the major motor tract, while the medial lemniscus and the spinothalamic tracts are the major sensory tracts. The nuclei of cranial nerves III through XII are also located within the brain stem. These nerves relay the motor, sensory, and special sense functions of the eye, face, mouth, and throat.

The principal motor tract is the corticospinal tract. It is a two-neuron path, with an upper motor neuron and a lower motor neuron. The upper motor neuron cell body is located within the motor strip of the cerebral cortex. The axon travels through the internal capsule to the brain stem, decussates at the brain stem–spinal cord junction, and travels down the contralateral corticospinal tract to the lower motor neuron in the anterior horn at the appropriate level. The lower motor neuron axon then travels via peripheral nerves to its target muscle. Damage to upper motor neurons results in hyperreflexia and mild atrophy. Damage to lower motor neurons results in flaccidity and significant atrophy. (See Schwartz 9th ed., p 1517.)

CLINICAL QUESTIONS

1. The standard treatment for an asymptomatic 2-cm chronic subdural hematoma is
   A. Observation and serial CT scan
   B. Placement of bedside ventriculostomy
   C. Burr hole drainage
   D. Crainiotomy

Answer: C
A chronic SDH >1 cm or any symptomatic SDH should be surgically drained. Unlike acute SDH, which consists of a thick, congealed clot, chronic SDH typically consists of a viscous fluid, with a texture and the dark brown color reminiscent of motor oil. A simple burr hole can effectively drain most chronic SDHs. However, the optimal treatment of chronic SDH remains controversial. Most authorities agree that burr hole drainage should be attempted first to obviate the risks of formal craniotomy. A single burr hole placed over the dependent edge of the collection can be made, and the space copiously irrigated until the fluid is clear. A second, more anterior burr hole can then be placed if the collection does not drain satisfactorily due to containment by membranes. The procedure is converted to open craniotomy if the SDH is too congealed for irrigation drainage, the complex of membranes prevents effective drainage, or persistent hemorrhage occurs that cannot be reached with bipolar cautery through the burr hole. (See Schwartz 9th ed., p 1526.)

2. The most common malignant tumor of the brain in children is
   A. Ganglioneuroma
   B. Neuroblastoma
   C. Medulloblastoma
   D. Glioblastoma multiforme

Answer: C
Neural and mixed tumors are a diverse group that includes tumors variously containing normal or abnormal neurons and/or normal or abnormal glial cells. Primitive neuroectodermal tumors arise from bipotential cells, capable of differentiating into neurons or glial cells.

Primitive neuroectodermal tumor is the most common type of medulloblastoma. Most occur in the first decade of life, but there is a second peak around age 30. Medulloblastoma is the most common malignant pediatric brain tumor. (See Schwartz 9th ed., p 1540.)

3. Which of the following spinal fractures should be suspected in a patient wearing a lap belt at the time of a head-on collision?
   A. Jefferson fracture
   B. Hangman's fracture
   C. Chance fracture
   D. Burst fracture

Answer: C

Chance fracture is a flexion-distraction injury causing failure of the middle and posterior columns, sometimes with anterior wedging. Typical injury is from a lap seat-belt hyperflexion with associated abdominal injury. It often is unstable and associated with neurologic deficit.

Jefferson fracture is a bursting fracture of the ring of C1 (the atlas) due to compression forces.

Traditionally considered a hyperextension/distraction injury from placement of the noose under the angle of the jaw, hangman's fractures also may occur with hyperextension/compression, as with diving accidents, or hyperflexion.

Burst fracture is a pure axial compression injury causing failure of the anterior and middle columns. (See Schwartz 9th ed., p 1528.)

4. Invasive monitors of intracerebral pressure are usually placed in the
   A. Right frontal lobe
   B. Left frontal lobe
   C. Right parietal lobe
   D. Left parietal lobe

Answer: A

There are several methods of monitoring intracranial physiology. The three described here are bedside intensive care unit (ICU) procedures and allow continuous monitoring. All three involve making a small hole in the skull with a hand-held drill. They generally are placed in the right frontal region to minimize the neurologic impact of possible complications such as hemorrhage. The most reliable monitor, *always*, is an alert patient with a reliable neurologic examination. If a reliable neurologic examination is not possible due to the presence of brain injury, sedatives, or paralytics, and if there is active and unstable intracranial pathology, then invasive monitoring is required. (See Schwartz 9th ed., p 1519.)

5. Following a closed head injury, clear fluid is seen draining from a patient's nose. Which of the following tests is most sensitive in determining if the fluid is cerebrospinal fluid (CSF)?
   A. Glucose level
   B. Halo test
   C. Fluid:serum LDH ratio
   D. Beta-transferrin

Answer: D

Copious clear drainage from the nose or ear makes the diagnosis of CSF leakage obvious. Often, however, the drainage may be discolored with blood or small in volume if some drains into the throat. The halo test can help differentiate. Allow a drop of the fluid to fall on an absorbent surface such as a facial tissue. If blood is mixed with CSF, the drop will form a double ring, with a darker center spot containing blood components surrounded by a light halo of CSF. If this test is indeterminate, the fluid can be sent for beta-transferrin testing, which will only be positive if CSF is present. (See Schwartz 9th ed., p 1523.)

6. Which of the following is NOT part of Cushing's triad?
   A. Hypertension
   B. Pinpoint pupils
   C. Irregular respirations
   D. Bradycardia

Answer: B

Patients with increased ICP, also called intracranial hypertension (ICH), often will present with headache, nausea, vomiting, and progressive mental status decline. Cushing's triad is the classic presentation of ICH: hypertension, bradycardia, and irregular respirations. This triad is usually a late manifestation. (See Schwartz 9th ed., p 1521.)

7. The most common tumor of peripheral nerves is
   A. Nerve sheath sarcoma
   B. Schwannoma
   C. Neurofibroma
   D. Neuroepithelioma

Answer: B

Schwannomas are the most common peripheral nerve tumors, also referred to as *neurilemomas* or *neurinomas*. Most occur in the third decade of life. These benign tumors arise from Schwann cells, which form myelin in peripheral nerves. The most characteristic presentation is a mass lesion with point tenderness and shooting pains on direct palpation.

Neurofibromas arise within the nerve and tend to be fusiform masses, unlike schwannomas, which tend to grow out of the nerve. Neurofibromas often present as a mass that is tender to palpation. They usually lack the shooting pains characteristic of schwannomas.

Malignant nerve sheath tumors include solitary sarcomas, degenerated neurofibromas, and neuroepitheliomas. Patients with malignant peripheral nerve tumors typically complain of constant pain, rather than pain only on palpation, and are more likely to have motor and sensory deficits in the distribution of the parent nerve. (See Schwartz 9th ed., p 1549.)

8. Clinical findings which can be seen in a patient who is brain dead include
   A. Minimally reactive pupil unilaterally
   B. No spontaneous breathing with a $PaCO_2$ of 50 mmHg
   C. Minimal, unilateral decorticate posturing to painful stimulus
   D. Positive triple flexion reflex of the leg

Answer: D

A neurologist, neurosurgeon, or intensivist generally performs the clinical brain death examination. Two examinations consistent with brain death 12 hours apart, or one examination consistent with brain death followed by a consistent confirmatory study generally is sufficient to declare brain death (see below). Hospital regulations and local laws regarding documentation should be followed closely.

Establish the absence of complicating conditions before beginning the examination. The patient must be normotensive, euthermic, and oxygenating well. The patient may not be under the effects of any sedating or paralytic drugs.

Documentation of no brain stem function requires the following: nonreactive pupils; lack of corneal blink, oculocephalic (doll's eyes), oculovestibular (cold calorics) reflexes; and loss of drive to breathe (apnea test). The apnea test demonstrates no spontaneous breathing even when $PaCO_2$ is allowed to rise above 60 mmHg.

Deep central painful stimuli are provided by bilateral forceful twisting pinch of the supraclavicular skin and pressure to the medial canthal notch. Pathologic responses such as flexor or extensor posturing are *not* compatible with brain death. Spinal reflexes to peripheral pain, such as triple flexion of the lower extremities, are compatible with brain death. (See Schwartz 9th ed., p 1527.)

9. Following a gunshot wound to the spine, a patient has loss of motor control on one side of his body. The most likely diagnosis is
   A. Crush injury to the spinal cord
   B. Brown-Sequard syndrome
   C. Central cord syndrome
   D. Anterior cord syndrome

Answer: B

Penetrating, compressive, or ischemic cord injury can lead to several characteristic presentations based on the anatomy of injury. The neurologic deficits may be deduced from the anatomy of the long sensory and motor tracts and understanding of their decussations. Four patterns are discussed.

First, injury to the entire cord at a given level results in anatomic or functional cord transaction with total loss of motor and sensory function below the level of the lesion. The typical mechanism is severe traumatic vertebral subluxation reducing spinal canal diameter and crushing the cord.

Second, injury to half the cord at a given level results in Brown-Sequard syndrome, with loss of motor control and proprioception ipsilaterally and loss of nociception and thermoception contralaterally. The typical mechanism is a stab or gunshot wound.

Third, injury to the interior gray matter of the cord in the cervical spine results in a central cord syndrome, with upper extremity worse than lower extremity weakness and varying degrees of numbness. The typical mechanism is transient compression of the cervical cord by the ligamentum flavum buckling during traumatic neck hyperextension. This syndrome occurs in patients with pre-existing cervical stenosis. Fourth, injury to the ventral half of the cord results in the anterior cord syndrome, with paralysis and loss of nociception and thermoception bilaterally. The typical mechanism is an acute disc herniation or ischemia from anterior spinal artery occlusion. (See Schwartz 9th ed., p 1529, and Fig. 42-1.)

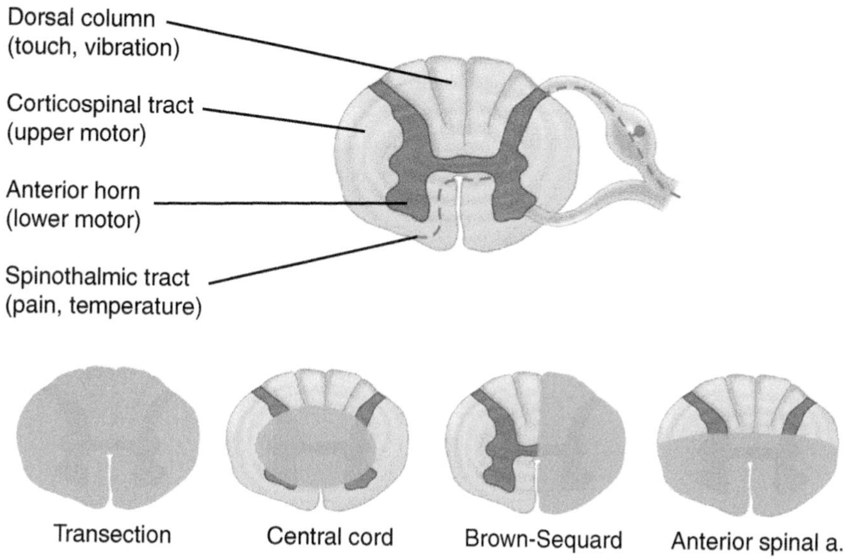
Dorsal column
(touch, vibration)
Corticospinal tract
(upper motor)
Anterior horn
(lower motor)
Spinothalmic tract
(pain, temperature)
Transection
Central cord
Brown-Sequard
Anterior spinal a.

FIG. 42-1. Spinal cord injury patterns. a. = artery. (Adapted with permission from Hoff J, Boland M: Neurosurgery, from *Principles of Surgery*, 7th ed. New York: McGraw-Hill, 1999, p 1837.)

10. Which of the following is a criterion that must be met for the nonoperative management of an epidural hematoma?
    A. Clot volume <30 cm^3
    B. Maximum thickness <2.5 cm
    C. GCS >12
    D. No previous history of systemic hypertension

Answer: A

Open craniotomy for evacuation of the congealed clot and hemostasis generally is indicated for EDH. Patients who meet all of the following criteria may be managed conservatively: clot volume <30 cm^3, maximum thickness <1.5 cm, and GCS score >8.10. (See Schwartz 9th ed., p 1525.)

11. The most common origin for metastatic tumors to the brain is
    A. Breast
    B. Lung
    C. Colon
    D. Kidney

Answer: B

The sources of most cerebral metastases are (in decreasing frequency): lung, breast, kidney, GI tract, and melanoma. Lung and breast cancers account for more than half of cerebral metastases. Metastatic cells usually travel to the brain hematogenously and frequently seed the gray-white junction. Other common locations are the cerebellum and the meninges. Meningeal involvement may result in carcinomatous meningitis, also known as *leptomeningeal carcinomatosis*. (See Schwartz 9th ed., p 1537.)

12. Temporal lesions most commonly cause which of the following forms of brain herniation?
    A. Subfalcine herniation
    B. Uncal herniation
    C. Central transtentorial herniation
    D. Tonsillar herniation

Answer: B

Temporal lesions push the uncus medially and compress the midbrain. This phenomenon is known as *uncal herniation*. The posterior cerebral artery (PCA) passes between the uncus and midbrain and may be occluded, leading to occipital infarct. Masses higher up in the hemisphere can push the cingulate gyrus under the falx cerebri. This process is known as *subfalcine herniation*. The anterior cerebral artery (ACA) branches run along the medial surface of the cingulate gyrus and may be occluded, leading to medial frontal and parietal infarcts. Diffuse increases in pressure in the cerebral hemispheres can lead to central, or transtentorial, herniation. Increased pressure in the posterior fossa can lead to upward central herniation or downward tonsillar herniation through the foramen magnum. Uncal, transtentorial, and tonsillar herniation can cause direct damage to the very delicate brain stem. Figure 42-2 diagrams patterns of herniation. (See Schwartz 9th ed., p 1521.)

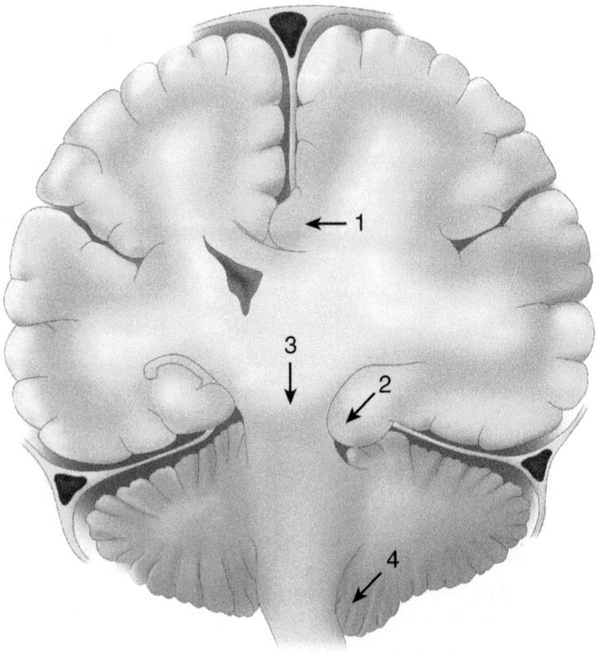

FIG. 42-2. Schematic drawing of brain herniation patterns. *1.* Subfalcine herniation. The cingulate gyrus shifts across midline under the falx cerebri. *2.* Uncal herniation. The uncus (medial temporal lobe gyrus) shifts medially and compresses the midbrain and cerebral peduncle. *3.* Central transtentorial herniation. The diencephalon and midbrain shift caudally through the tentorial incisura. *4.* Tonsillar herniation. The cerebellar tonsil shifts caudally through the foramen magnum. (Reproduced with permission from Cohen DS, Quest DO: Increased intracranial pressure, brain herniation and their control, in Wilkins RH, Rengachary SS (eds): *Neurosurgery*, 2nd ed. New York: McGraw Hill, 1996, p 349.)

13. The initial dose of methylprednisolone that should be given to a patient with an acute spinal cord injury is
    A. 5 mg/kg
    B. 15 mg/kg
    C. 30 mg/kg
    D. 50 mg/kg

Answer: C

The National Acute Spinal Cord Injury studies (NASCIS I and II) provide the basis for the common practice of administering high-dose steroids to patients with acute SCI. A 30-mg/kg IV bolus of methylprednisolone is given over 15 minutes, followed by a 5.4-mg/kg per hour infusion begun 45 minutes later. The infusion is continued for 23 hours if the bolus is given within 3 hours of injury, or for 47 hours if the bolus is given within 8 hours of injury. The papers indicate greater motor and sensory recovery at 6 weeks, 6 months, and 1 year after acute SCI in patients who received methylprednisolone. However, the NASCIS trial data have been extensively criticized, as many argue that the selection criteria and study design were flawed, making the results ambiguous. Patients who receive such a large corticosteroid dose have increased rates of medical and ICU complications, such as pneumonias, which have a deleterious effect on outcome. A clear consensus on the use of spinal-dose steroids does not exist. A decision to use or not use spinal-dose steroids may be dictated by local or regional practice patterns, especially given the legal liability issues surrounding SCI. Patients with gunshot or nerve root (cauda equina) injuries or those who are pregnant, <14 years old, or on chronic steroids were excluded from the NASCIS studies and should not receive spinal dose steroids. (See Schwartz 9th ed., p 1531.)

14. Which of the following is the most common mechanism of spinal cord injury following a dive into shallow water?
    A. Compression
    B. Flexion
    C. Extension
    D. Rotation

Answer: C

Arching the neck and back extends the spine. Extension loads the spine posteriorly and distracts the spine anteriorly. High extension forces occur during rear-end motor vehicle collisions (especially if there is no headrest), frontward falls when the head strikes first, or diving into shallow water.

Bending the head and body forward into a fetal position flexes the spine. Flexion loads the spine anteriorly (the vertebral bodies) and distracts the spine posteriorly (the spinous process and interspinous ligaments). High flexion forces occur during front-end motor vehicle collisions, and backward falls when the head strikes first.

Force applied along the spinal axis (axial loading) compresses the spine. Compression loads the spine anteriorly and posteriorly. High compression forces occur when a falling object strikes the head or shoulders, or when landing on the feet, buttocks, or head after a fall from height. A pulling force in line with the spinal axis distracts the spine. Distraction unloads the spine anteriorly and posteriorly. Distraction forces occur during a hanging, when the chin or occiput strikes an object first during a fall, or when a passenger submarines under a loose seat belt during a front-end motor vehicle collision.

Force applied tangential to the spinal axis rotates the spine. Rotation depends on the range of motion of intervertebral facet joints. High rotational forces occur during off-center impacts to the body or head or during glancing automobile accidents. (See Schwartz 9th ed., p 1527.)

15. Findings in an anterior cerebral artery stroke include
    A. Language deficits
    B. Contralateral leg weakness
    C. Contralateral homonymous hemianopsia
    D. Horner's syndrome

Answer: B

The anterior cerebral artery (ACA) supplies the medial frontal and parietal lobes, including the motor strip, as it courses into the interhemispheric fissure. ACA stroke results in contralateral leg weakness.

The middle cerebral artery (MCA) supplies the lateral frontal and parietal lobes and the temporal lobe. MCA stroke results in contralateral face and arm weakness. Dominant-hemisphere MCA stroke causes language deficits.

The posterior cerebellar artery (PCA) supplies the occipital lobe. PCA stroke results in a contralateral homonymous hemianopsia.

The posterior inferior cerebellar artery (PICA) supplies the lateral medulla and the inferior half of the cerebellar hemispheres. PICA stroke results in nausea, vomiting, nystagmus, dysphagia, ipsilateral Horner's syndrome, and ipsilateral limb ataxia. The constellation of symptoms resulting from PICA occlusion is referred to as the *lateral medullary* or *Wallenberg's syndrome*. (See Schwartz 9th ed., p 1533.)

16. In decorticate posturing, the patient's extremities
   A. Withdraw to pain
   B. Extend in response to pain
   C. Flex in response to pain
   D. None of the above

Answer: C
Characteristic motor reactions to pain in patients with depressed mental status include withdrawal from stimulus, localization to stimulus, flexor (decorticate) posturing, extensor (decerebrate) posturing, or no reaction (in order of worsening pathology). (See Schwartz 9th ed., p 1518.)

17. The most common intramedullary spinal tumor in adults is
   A. Hemangioma
   B. Ependymoma
   C. Astocytoma
   D. Osteoblastoma

Answer: B
Ependymomas are the most common intramedullary tumors in adults. There are several histologic variants. The myxopapillary type occurs in the conus medullaris or the filum terminale in the lumbar region and has the best prognosis after resection. The cellular type occurs more frequently in the cervical cord.

Astrocytomas are the most common intramedullary tumors in children, although they also occur in adults. They may occur at all levels, although more often in the cervical cord. The tumor may interfere with the CSF-containing central canal of the spinal cord, leading to a dilated central canal, referred to as *syringomyelia* (*syrinx*).

Hemangiomas and osteoblastomas are extramedullary tumors. (See Schwartz 9th ed., p 1543.)

18. A patient who localizes to pain, is confused, and opens his eyes to pain has a Glasgow Coma Scale score of
   A. 9
   B. 10
   C. 11
   D. 12

Answer: C
The GCS is determined by adding the scores of the best responses of the patient in each of three categories. The motor score ranges from 1 to 6, verbal from 1 to 5, and eyes from 1 to 4. The GCS therefore ranges from 3 to 15, as detailed in Table 42-1. (See Schwartz 9th ed., p 1522.)

TABLE 42-1 The Glasgow Coma Scale score[a]

Motor Response		Verbal Response		Eye-Opening Response	
Obeys commands	6	Oriented	5	Opens spontaneously	4
Localizes to pain	5	Confused	4	Opens to speech	3
Withdraws from pain	4	Inappropriate words	3	Opens to pain	2
Flexor posturing	3	Unintelligible sounds	2	No eye opening	1
Extensor posturing	2	No sounds	1		
No movement	1				

[a]Add the three scores to obtain the Glasgow Coma Scale (GCS) score, which can range from 3 to 15. Add "T" after the GCS if intubated and no verbal score is possible. For these patients, the GCS can range from 3T to 10T.

19. Patients with symptoms from a Chiari I malformation may complain of
   A. Seizures
   B. Extremity weakness
   C. Eye pain
   D. Ataxia

Answer: B
Chiari I malformation is the caudal displacement of the cerebellar tonsils below the foramen magnum. It may be seen as an incidental finding on MRI scans in asymptomatic patients. Symptomatic patients usually present with headache, neck pain, or symptoms of myelopathy, including numbness or weakness in the extremities. A syrinx may be associated, but the brain stem and lower cranial nerves are normal in Chiari I malformations. Chiari II malformations are more severe and involve caudal displacement of the lower brain stem and stretching of the lower cranial nerves. Symptomatic patients may be treated with suboccipital craniectomy to remove the posterior arch of the foramen magnum, along with removal of the posterior ring of C1. Removal of these bony structures relieves the compression of the cerebellar tonsils and cervicomedullary junction, and may allow reestablishment of normal CSF flow patterns. (See Schwartz 9th ed., p 1554, and Fig. 42-3.)

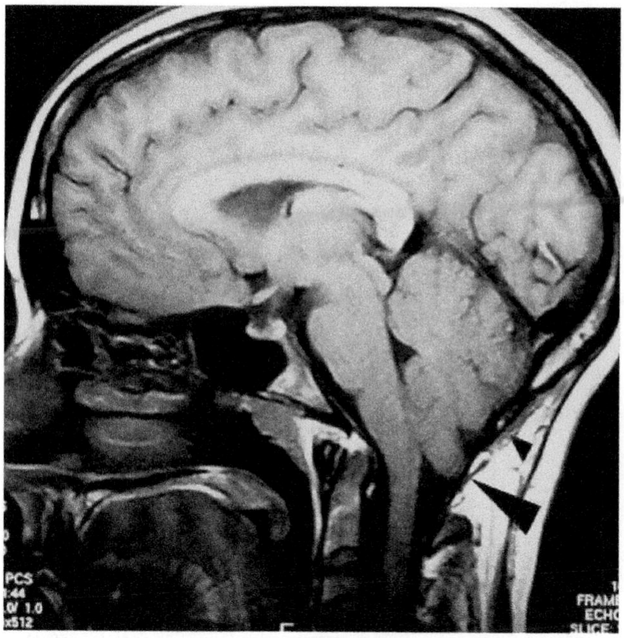

FIG. 42-3. T1-weighted sagittal magnetic resonance imaging of a patient with a Chiari I malformation. The *large arrowhead* points to the cerebellar tonsils. The *small arrowhead* points to the posterior arch of the foramen magnum.

20. Unilateral loss of visual acuity and pulsatile proptosis is suggestive of
    A. Retinal artery aneurysm
    B. Carotid-cavernous fistula
    C. Hypertensive crisis
    D. Carotid artery dissection

Answer: B

Traumatic vessel wall injury to the portion of the carotid artery running through the cavernous sinus may result in a carotid-cavernous fistula (CCF). This creates a high-pressure, high-flow pathophysiologic blood flow pattern. CCFs classically present with pulsatile proptosis (the globe pulses outward with arterial pulsation), retro-orbital pain, and decreased visual acuity or loss of normal eye movement (due to damage to cranial nerves III, IV, and VI as they pass through the cavernous sinus). Symptomatic CCFs should be treated to preserve eye function. Fistulae may be closed by balloon occlusion using interventional neuroradiology techniques. Fistulae with wide necks are difficult to treat and may require total occlusion of the parent carotid artery. (See Schwartz 9th ed., p 1527.)

21. Hemorrhagic strokes most commonly involve the
    A. Cerebellum
    B. Basal ganglia
    C. Pons
    D. Brain stem

Answer: B

Hemorrhagic stroke typically occurs within the basal ganglia or cerebellum [Table 42-2]. The patient is usually hypertensive on admission and has a history of poorly controlled hypertension. Such patients are more likely to present with lethargy or obtundation, compared to those who suffer an ischemic stroke. Depressed mental status results from brain shift and herniation secondary to mass effect from the hematoma in deep structures. Ischemic stroke does not cause mass effect acutely; and therefore, patients are more likely to present with normal consciousness and a focal neurologic deficit. Hemorrhagic strokes tend to present with a relatively gradual decline in neurologic function as the hematoma expands, rather than the immediately maximal symptoms caused by ischemic stroke. (See Schwartz 9th ed., p 1534.)

TABLE 42-2	Anatomic distribution of intracranial hemorrhages and correlated symptoms	
% of Intracranial Hemorrhages	**Location**	**Classic Symptoms**
50	Basal ganglia (putamen, globus pallidus), internal capsule	Contralateral hemiparesis
15	Thalamus	Contralateral hemisensory loss
10–20	Cerebral white matter (lobar)	Depends on location (weakness, numbness, partial loss of visual field)
10–15	Pons	Hemiparesis; may be devastating
10	Cerebellum	Lethargy or coma due to brain stem compression and/or hydrocephalus
1–6	Brain stem (excluding pons)	Often devastating

22. The most common primary malignant tumor of the brain is
    A. Oligodendoglioma
    B. Ependymoma
    C. Astrocytoma
    D. Ganglioglioma

Answer: C

Astrocytoma is the most common primary CNS neoplasm. The term *glioma* often is used to refer to astrocytomas specifically, excluding other glial tumors. Astrocytomas are graded from I to IV. Grades I and II are referred to as low-grade astrocytoma, grade III as anaplastic astrocytoma, and grade IV as glioblastoma multiforme (GBM).

Oligodendroglioma accounts for approximately 10% of gliomas. They often present with seizures. Calcifications and hemorrhage on CT or MRI suggest the diagnosis.

The lining of the ventricular system consists of cuboidal/columnar ependymal cells from which ependymomas may arise. Although most pediatric ependymomas are supratentorial, two thirds of adult ependymomas are infratentorial.

Ganglioglioma is a mixed tumor in which both neurons and glial cells are neoplastic. They occur in the first three decades of life, often in the medial temporal lobe, as circumscribed masses that may contain cysts or calcium and may enhance. (See Schwartz 9th ed., p 1540.)

23. Eccymosis behind the ear ("Battle sign") is indicative of which of the following?
    A. Parietal skull fracture
    B. Temporal skull fracture
    C. Basilar skull fracture
    D. Occipital skull fracture

Answer: C

Fractures of the skull base are common in head-injured patients, and they indicate significant impact. They are generally apparent on routine head CT, but should be evaluated with dedicated fine-slice coronal-section CT scan to document and delineate the extent of the fracture and involved structures. If asymptomatic, they require no treatment. Symptoms from skull base fractures include cranial nerve deficits and CSF leaks. A fracture of the temporal bone, for instance, can damage the facial or vestibulocochlear nerve, resulting in vertigo, ipsilateral deafness, or facial paralysis. A communication may be formed between the subarachnoid space and the middle ear, allowing CSF drainage into the pharynx via the eustachian tube or from the ear (otorrhea). Extravasation of blood results in ecchymosis behind the ear, known as *Battle's sign*. A fracture of the anterior skull base can result in anosmia (loss of smell from damage to the olfactory nerve), CSF drainage from the nose (rhinorrhea), or periorbital ecchymoses, known as *raccoon eyes*. (See Schwartz 9th ed., p 1523.)

24. Which of the following is standard treatment for a significant posttraumatic CSF leak?
    A. Placement of a lumbar drain
    B. Lumbar blood patch
    C. Endoscopic sinus exploration with mucosal repair
    D. Craniotomy and closure of the dural tear

Answer: A

Many CSF leaks will heal with elevation of the head of the bed for several days. A lumbar drain can augment this method. A lumbar drain is a catheter placed in the lumbar CSF cistern to decompress the cranial vault and allow the defect to heal by eliminating normal hydrostatic pressure. There is no proven efficacy of antibiotic coverage for preventing meningitis in patients with CSF leaks. (See Schwartz 9th ed., p 1523.)

25. A patient presents to the ER with a sudden, severe headache. Based on the CT scan in Fig. 42-4, what is the most likely diagnosis?
    A. Subarachnoid hemorrhage
    B. Subdural hematoma
    C. Diffuse axonal injury
    D. Epidural hematoma

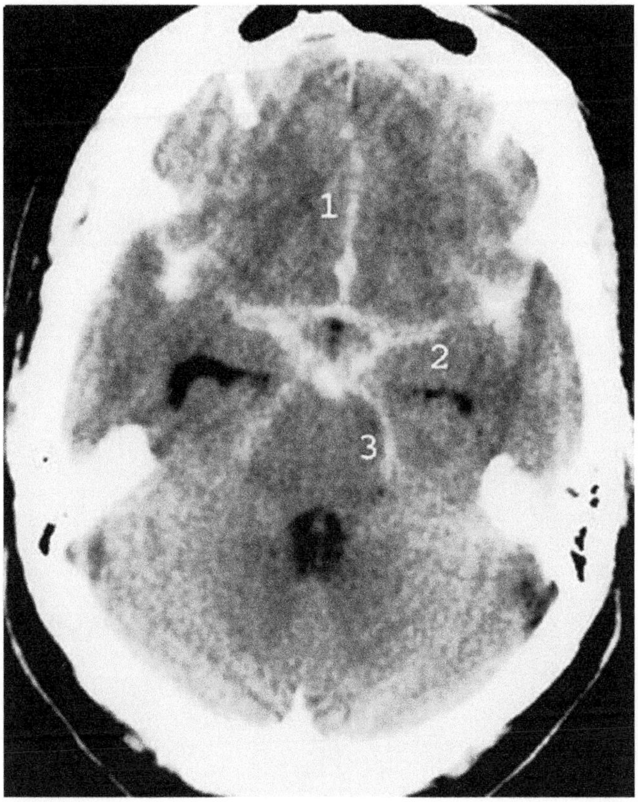

FIG. 42-4.

Answer: A

The image shown is a computed tomography scan of a patient who experienced a sudden, severe headache. Subarachnoid hemorrhage is visible as hyperdense signal in the interhemispheric fissure (*1*), bilateral sylvian fissures (*2* shows the left fissure), and in the ambient cisterns around the midbrain (*3*). This gives the classic five-pointed-star appearance of a subarachnoid hemorrhage. Visible temporal tips of the lateral ventricles indicate hydrocephalus. (See Schwartz 9th ed., p 1536.)

26. A patient with a crush injury to the arm has motor and sensory deficits that indicate a radial nerve injury. The most appropriate management is
    A. Immediate operative exploration and repair
    B. EMG 5-7 days after injury; surgical exploration if nerve conduction is decreased
    C. EMG 3-4 weeks after injury; surgical exploration if nerve conduction is decreased
    D. Surgical exploration if there is no functional improvement after 3 months

Answer: D

The sensory and motor deficits [in a patient with a peripheral nerve injury] should be accurately documented. Deficits are usually immediate. Progressive deficit suggests a process such as an expanding hematoma and may warrant early surgical exploration. Clean, sharp injuries may also benefit from early exploration and reanastomosis. Most other peripheral nerve injuries should be observed. EMG/NCS studies should be done 3 to 4 weeks postinjury if deficits persist. Axon segments distal to the site of injury will conduct action potentials normally until Wallerian degeneration occurs, rendering EMG/NCS before 3 weeks uninformative. Continued observation is indicated if function improves. Surgical exploration of the nerve may be undertaken if no functional improvement occurs over

3 months. If intraoperative electrical testing reveals conduction across the injury, continue observation. In the absence of conduction, the injured segment should be resected and end-to-end primary anastomosis attempted. However, anastomoses under tension will not heal. A nerve graft may be needed to bridge the gap between the proximal and distal nerve ends. The sural nerve often is harvested, as it carries only sensory fibers and leaves a minor deficit when resected. The connective tissue structures of the nerve graft may provide a pathway for effective axonal regrowth across the injury. (See Schwartz 9th ed., p 1532.)

27. The motor scoring system is a 5-point scale to assess motor strength. A patient who is able to move only against gravity (but not against resistance) would have a motor score of
    A. 2
    B. 3
    C. 4
    D. 5

Answer: B
(See Schwartz 9th ed., p 1518, and Table 42-3.)

TABLE 42-3 Motor scoring system

Grade	Description
0	No muscle contraction
1	Visible muscle contraction without movement across the joint
2	Movement in the horizontal plane, unable to overcome gravity
3	Movement against gravity
4	Movement against some resistance
5	Normal strength

CHAPTER 43

Orthopedic Surgery

BASIC SCIENCE QUESTIONS

1. The location marked (see Fig. 43-1) is which segment of a long bone?
   A. Growth plate
   B. Epiphysis
   C. Metaphysis
   D. Diaphysis

Answer: D

Much of an orthopedic surgeon's practice concerns treatment of the "long bones." Long bones generally consist of an epiphysis (the portion of the bone on either end which usually contains an articular surface). The epiphysis is formed from an epiphyseal ossification center at either end of most long bones separated from the metaphysis of the long bone by the growth plate (Fig. 43-1). After skeletal maturity, the ends of bones continue to be referred to as the epiphyseal region. The metaphysis of a long bone is the region immediately below the growth plate or its remnant. The metaphysis tapers to become the shaft or diaphysis of the long bone. (See Schwartz 9th ed., p 1559.)

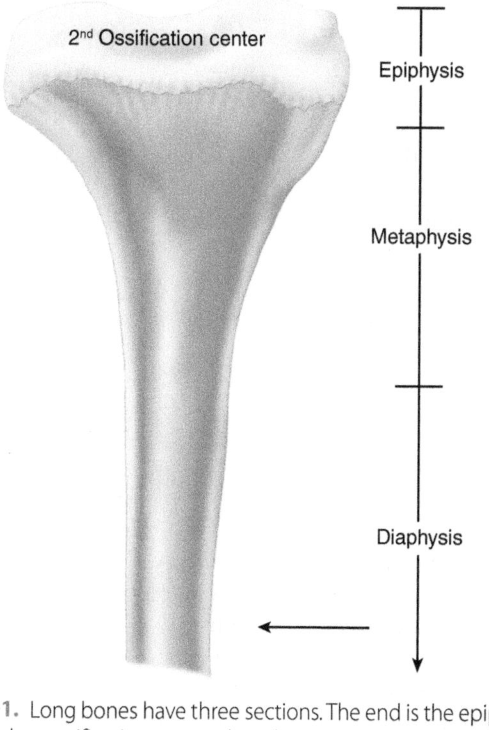

FIG. 43-1. Long bones have three sections. The end is the epiphysis or secondary ossification center, the adjacent area is the metaphysis, and the middle of the bone is the diaphysis. The metaphysis is broader than the diaphysis, has a thin cortex, and is composed of primarily cancellous bone.

2. Turn over of cortical bone is
   A. 2 times faster than trabecular bone
   B. 8 times faster than trabecular bone
   C. 2 times slower than trabecular bone
   D. 8 times slower than trabecular bone

Answer: D

It is important to know that all bone is subject to turnover with resorption and new bone formation, occurring in both the trabecular bone and the cortex. Cortical bone does turn over considerably slower than trabecular bone, however, by a factor of approximately seven or eight (Fig. 43-2). (See Schwartz 9th ed., p 1559, 60.)

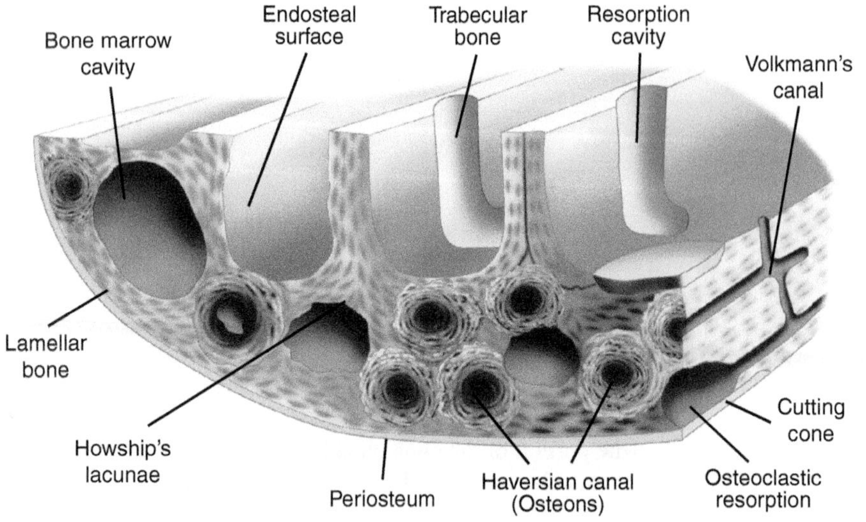

FIG. 43-2. The cellular and structural organization of bone.

3. Which of the following bone tumors is characterized by a 11:22 translocation?
   A. Giant cell tumor of the bone
   B. Chordoma
   C. Chondroblastoma
   D. Ewing's sarcoma

Answer: D

Ewing's sarcoma of bone, or Ewing's tumor, is a small, round cell sarcoma most common in children and younger adults. Ewing's sarcoma is most common in the long bones, especially the metaphyseal regions of the femur, tibia, and humerus. Patients present with complaints of local pain, interestingly, often accompanied by fever. Ewing's sarcoma is an undifferentiated tumor occurring in children and primarily involves the diaphysis of long bones.... These tumors have a characteristic 11:22 translocation that can be very helpful in making the correct diagnosis. (See Schwartz 9th ed., p 1559.)

4. Which of the following is NOT one of the three stages of fracture repair?
   A. Hormonal
   B. Circulatory
   C. Metabolic
   D. Mechanical

Answer: A

The biologic and histologic events in fracture repair can be divided into three general stages. The duration and classification of each stage is variable based on age, general health, and other factors. Additionally, these stages can overlap, as there are no definitive features to suggest progression of one stage to another. The three stages are (a) circulatory, which includes closure of any wound and primary callus formation, (b) metabolic, the stage where the primary callus is reinforced leading to clinical union, and (c) mechanical, the stage in which the united bone is remodeled along the lines of stress. (See Schwartz 9th ed., p 1561.)

5. Which of the following stimulates differentiation of mesenchymal cells into osteoblasts in response to a fracture?
   A. Bone morphogenic protein
   B. Platelet-derived growth factor
   C. Insulin-like growth factor
   D. Transforming growth factor beta

Answer: A

Bone morphogenic protein is a low molecular weight protein that can influence the differentiation of mesenchymal cells into mature osteoblasts. Other protein factors that can affect fracture healing include insulin-like growth factor, transforming growth factor beta, and platelet-derived growth factor (PDGF). Insulin-like growth factor stimulates bone cell proliferation and the production of cartilage matrix. Transforming growth factor beta induces the synthesis of cartilage, proteoglycans, and type II collagen. PDGF stimulates proliferation of osteoblasts and increases the rate of synthesis of type I collagen. PDGF is also known to be a chemotactic agent and induces the migration of inflammatory cells into the callus. (See Schwartz 9th ed., p 1562.)

6. The cell of origin of a chordoma is
   A. Notochordal
   B. Synovial
   C. Periosteal
   D. Plasma cell

Answer: A
Chordomas are slow-growing malignancies derived from embryonic notochord cells. Chordomas nearly always arise in the axial skeleton and most commonly involve the occiput or the sacrum. They can be found in the vertebrae. Chordomas are not found in the extremities. About one third of these tumors arise intracranially (skull base), and about half are found in the sacrum, with the rest in the spine. (See Schwartz 9th ed., p 1595.)

7. Lateral stability of the ankle is provided by
   A. The tarsal navicular
   B. The medial meniscus
   C. The deltoid ligament
   D. The fibula

Answer: C
The ankle joint is comprised of the talus, tibia, and fibula. The talus normally fits immediately beneath the distal tibia and is restrained medially by the buttress that the medial malleolus provides. Laterally, the talus is restrained by the articular surface of the fibula which, in precise alignment with the distal tibia, allows for flexion and extension of the ankle. Ligamentous stability of the medial ankle is provided by the 'deltoid' ligament that attaches to the medial malleolus of the tibia and talus. Stability of the talofibular joint is provided by the anterior talofibular ligament (a common site for sprains of the ankle), the calcaneal-fibular ligament, and the posterior talofibular ligaments. (See Schwartz 9th ed., p 1565.)

CLINICAL QUESTIONS

1. Which of the following orthopedic screws are most commonly used to secure a distal bone fragment to a more proximal fragment?
   A. Cortical screws
   B. Cancellous screws
   C. Lag screws
   D. Thompson screws

Answer: C
A *cortical screw* is a screw with a large inner diameter and shallow screw threads. This screw is designed to have a high breaking strength for its total diameter, and the screws threads are intended to engage cortical bone. Purchase of shallow screw threads in cortical bone can be excellent. *Cancellous screws* have a deeper thread pattern and a smaller inner shaft diameter. They are designed to obtain fixation in less dense cancellous bone. *Lag screws* also are commonly used. These are screws in which only the distal portion of the screw length is threaded. These screws penetrate one bone fragment without thread fixation. When a second fracture fragment is engaged by the threaded portion of the screw, turning the screw head tight down to the cortex of the first bony fragment will pull or 'lag' the distal fragment toward the screw head. Compression of the fractured bones is the result. (See Schwartz 9th ed., p 1563.)

2. The most appropriate treatment for posterior dislocation of the medial clavicle (at the sternoclavicular joint) is
   A. Analgesics only
   B. Ipsilateral sling to immobilize the shoulder
   C. Closed reduction
   D. Open reduction and internal fixation

Answer: C
Fractures of the medial third of the clavicle are rare. Often what appears to be a fracture of the medial clavicle is actually a dislocation of the sternoclavicular joint. When anteriorly displaced, this injury, while painful, requires only symptomatic treatment. In contrast, posterior dislocation of the sternoclavicular joint can impinge the great vessels and may be managed by closed reduction. With general anesthesia, the arm is abducted and a lateral force is applied, and a towel, clip, or bone holding clamp can be used to apply anterior forces on the clavicle that can relocate this joint. These maneuvers should be undertaken only when a surgeon is available for any associated great vessel injury. Fortunately, such injuries are rare. (See Schwartz 9th ed., p 1574.)

3. Which of the following statements is true about pilon fractures?
   A. Closed reduction and casting is successful in the majority of patients
   B. Skin complications are rare
   C. Delayed open reduction and internal fixation is the treatment of choice
   D. Posttraumatic arthritis is rare

Answer: C

High-energy fractures of the distal tibia and fibula that involve both the distal shaft of the tibia and the weightbearing surface are called *tibial plafond fractures* or, more commonly, *pilon fractures*. Due to the subcutaneous nature of these high energy fractures, skin complications, compartment syndromes, wound healing problems, and nonunions frequently complicate the care of patients with pilon fractures, which represent one of the most difficult challenges in the entire field of orthopedic trauma (Fig. 43-3). Pilon fractures almost always are displaced and are almost universally associated with significant soft tissue damage. Treatment nearly always involves open reduction and internal fixation of the bone fragments with as meticulous reconstruction of the ankle joint as possible. Immediate reconstructive surgery rarely is undertaken, however, because of the extremely high incidence of soft tissue complications. In most cases, the lower limb is stabilized by external fixation often with limited open reduction and internal fixation of the fibula to help establish and maintain anatomic length. A definitive reconstruction procedure on the tibia often is postponed until the acute swelling has resolved. This approach has been shown to lessen the incidence of soft tissue complications. With or without appropriate stabilization and timing, wound complications are common. Wound breakdown is seen in >10% of such injuries. The incidence of wound infection is high as are nonunion of the distal fragments. Posttraumatic arthritic joints are distressingly common. (See Schwartz 9th ed., p 1567.)

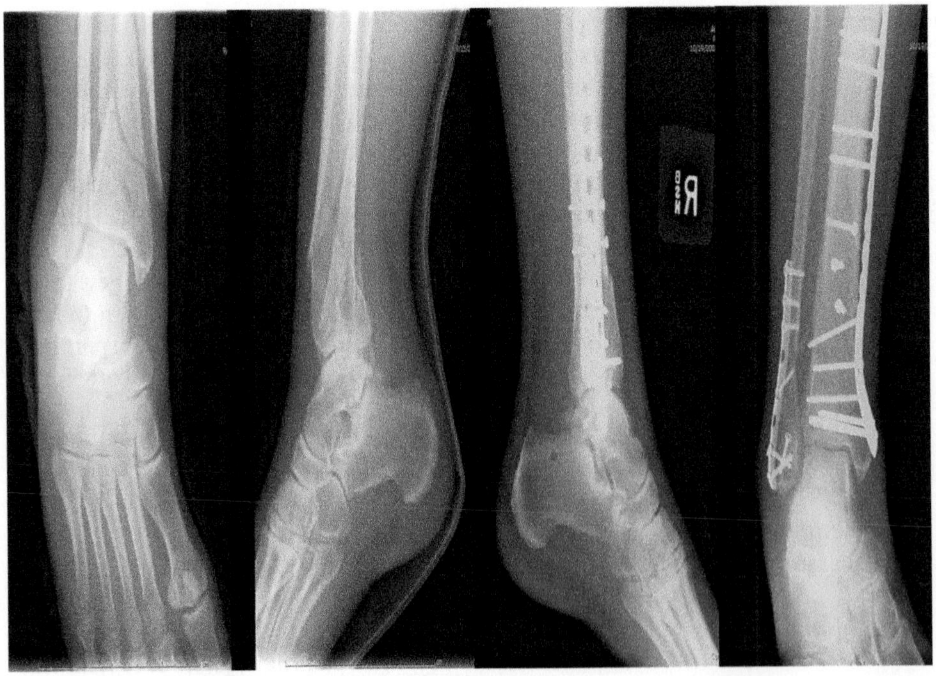

FIG. 43-3. Radiographs of a severe fracture of the distal tibia and fibula, before and after open reduction and internal fixation. High-energy trauma to the distal leg can frequently lead to neurovascular injury, compartment syndrome, and wound healing problems.

4. The most common bone malignancy in children is
   A. Periosteal sarcoma
   B. Ewing's sarcoma
   C. Osteosarcoma
   D. Rhabdomyosarcoma

Answer: C

High-grade *osteogenic sarcomas* generally take origin from within the medullary cavity of the bone and are the most common type of osteogenic sarcoma. It is the most common bone malignancy in children and is especially common in the distal femur, proximal tibia, and proximal humerus. (See Schwartz 9th ed., p 1592.)

5. Pubic ramus fractures are most often associated with
   A. Injuries to the urethra
   B. Injuries to a hollow viscus
   C. Sacral fractures
   D. Acetabular fractures

Answer: C

Pubic ramus fractures are frequently associated with concurrent sacral fractures. Vertical fractures through the sacral ala often involving multiple sacral foramina frequently occur with this injury. Interestingly, the sacral fractures are often quite nondisplaced and may be difficult or impossible to see on plain x-ray images. Nondisplaced fractures of the sacrum and minimally displaced fractures of the pelvic rami usually are managed with analgesics and mobilization. These injuries are compatible with full weightbearing. (See Schwartz 9th ed., p 1572.)

6. A 6-year-old presents with a tibial fracture of the metaphysis extending across the growth plate. This would be a
   A. Salter-Harris type 1 fracture
   B. Salter-Harris type 2 fracture
   C. Salter-Harris type 3 fracture
   D. Salter-Harris type 4 fracture

Answer: B

Classification of growth plate injuries has important implications as doctors communicate about the treatment of a patient. The exact type of physeal injury is important for the prognosis and treatment of the fracture. Salter and Harris described a very useful classification of growth plate injuries. A type I injury is a simple transverse failure of the physis without involvement of the ossified epiphysis or metaphysis. A Salter-Harris type II fracture contains a component of fracture through the growth plate in continuity with a fracture of the metaphysis. Salter-Harris type III fracture occurs partially through the epiphysis and partially through the growth plate. These fractures are essentially always intra-articular. A Salter-Harris type IV injury is one which has a fracture line extending through the physis extending from the metaphysis through into the epiphysis. Finally, a Salter-Harris type V injury is a subtle injury where the physis itself is injured but not displaced. (See Schwartz 9th ed., p 1602.)

7. Which of the following is most diagnostic for a compartment syndrome?
   A. Compartment pressure >25 mmHg
   B. Compartment pressure 20 mmHg higher than diastolic pressure
   C. Tense extremity on palpation
   D. Disproportionate pain and painful passive stretch of the compartment muscles

Answer: D

The diagnosis of a compartment syndrome is a clinical one, based on complaints of local pain out of proportion to the apparent injury, in association with pain, on passive stretch of the involved muscles. This situation can arise after a period of ischemia, after local blunt trauma, and, frequently, in the presence of an acute fracture. Measurement of compartment pressures, using one of a number of commercially available devices, involves inserting a needle into the suspected muscle compartments to measure pressure. Pressure measurements alone are not reliable to absolutely rule in or rule out the diagnosis, but they can be a useful adjunct to clinical assessment, particularly valuable in obtunded or unconscious patients. Pressure measurements that are greater than 30 mmHg or within 30 mmHg of the diastolic blood pressure are consistent, but not absolutely diagnostic with the presence of a compartment syndrome. The diagnosis is a clinical one. (See Schwartz 9th ed., p 1563.)

8. Which of the following is associated with fractures of the calcaneus?
   A. Ligamentous injury to the knee
   B. Dislocation of the hip
   C. Fracture of the femur
   D. Spinal fracture

Answer: D

Fractures of the calcaneus are common and frequently are associated with falls from a height. In assessing patients presenting with a fractured calcaneus, the orthopedist should always consider a possible concurrent fracture of the spine, as these injuries frequently occur together. (See Schwartz 9th ed., p 1563.)

9. Which of the following is the preferred treatment for a Monteggia fracture dislocation of the proximal forearm?
   A. Closed reduction of both ulna and radius
   B. Closed reduction of ulna, open reduction and fixation of radius
   C. Open reduction and fixation of the ulna, closed reduction of the radius
   D. Open reduction and fixation of the ulna and radius

Answer: C

This particular injury pattern is relatively common, and unfortunately, the dislocation of the radial head sometimes is unrecognized. In almost every case, an internal fixation of the ulna is indicated with closed reduction of the radial head. The treating surgeon must be alert to possible neurovascular injury and compartment syndrome. Late complications to this injury can include heterotopic ossification and redislocation of the radial head. (See Schwartz 9th ed., p 1576.)

10. Which of the following is the first radiographic finding of osteomyelitis?
    A. Localized osteoporosis
    B. Periosteal thickening
    C. Patchy sclerosis
    D. Lytic area

Answer: A

In patients with acute osteomyelitis, the radiologic features do not appear until 1 to 14 days after the onset of symptoms. The initial x-ray appearance is a vague, localized osteoporosis as a result of the removal of the dead trabecular bone and initial stages of endosteal resorption. This transforms to a mottled appearance on the plain film as more bone is resorbed, with the end result of a lytic area with or without a sequestrum. As the infection progresses, the radiologic and morphologic features transform as the inflammation becomes chronic. The marrow gradually is replaced by fibrous tissue, and the inflammatory cells are composed of mononuclear cells (i.e., lymphocytes and plasma cells). Radiologically, this appears as patchy sclerosis in the intramedullary space. A sinus tract may be appreciated especially on CT and magnetic resonance imaging (MRI). The periosteal reaction becomes more compact and often can appear lamellated. (See Schwartz 9th ed., p 1577.)

11. A 4-year-old presents with a fracture of the femur (mid shaft) with 20% of anterior angulation. Which of the following is the best treatment for this child?
    A. Traction and bed rest
    B. Closed reduction and application of a spica cast
    C. Open reduction and internal fixation (plate)
    D. Open reduction and intramedullary fixation

Answer: B

In children, femur fractures are usually low-energy injuries in contrast to adult femur fractures. Fractures of the femoral shaft in pediatric patients <6 years old may be managed with a spica cast. Minor degrees of angular deformity are acceptable and will remodel. More major degrees of angular deformities (up to 30° in the sagittal plane) may be acceptable because of the growth potential in these very young patients. Fractures in patients >6 years of age can be managed by limited internal fixation. Flexible intramedullary nails are popular in the treatment of this injury. A patient who is approaching skeletal maturity (14 years or older) may be managed by a rigid intramedullary reamed nail, much as would be used in an adult. (See Schwartz 9th ed., p 1602.)

12. Which of the following injuries is associated with forced dorsiflexion of the foot?
    A. Fracture of the talus
    B. Fracture of the navicular
    C. Fracture of the cuneiform
    D. Fracture of the cuboid

Answer: A

Fractures of the talus are common and frequently the result of forced dorsal flexion of the foot and ankle.

The tarsal bones (the navicular, the cuboid, and the three cuneiform bones) link the hind foot to the metatarsals. The precise arrangements of these bones provide mechanical stability to the arch of the foot. The large articular surfaces of these bones, however, also make avascular necrosis a potential complication with any fracture. Isolated fractures of the tarsal bones are uncommon. The force needed to fracture these bones is usually quite high. Such injuries are associated with trauma to adjacent structures, frequently including dislocations of the tarsometatarsal joints. (See Schwartz 9th ed., p 1564.)

13. Which of the following femur fractures is rarely associated with significant blood loss?
    A. Femoral neck fracture
    B. Intertrochanteric fracture
    C. Distal femoral metaphysis fracture
    D. Femoral shaft fracture

Answer: A

Fractures of the femoral neck comprise approximately one half of all fractures of the proximal femur. They are most common in elderly patients. The anatomy of the hip joint is an important consideration in the management of this fracture. The hip joint capsule extends from the rim of the acetabulum to the base of the neck of the femur. Fractures of the femoral neck are, therefore, entirely intrascapular. (See Schwartz 9th ed., p 1570.)

14. A large acute tear in the medial meniscus in a young athlete is best treated by
    A. Immobilization and anti-inflammatory agents
    B. Repair of the meniscus
    C. Resection of the meniscus
    D. Resection of the meniscus and replacement with allograft

Answer: B

Options for treatment of a meniscal tear include resection and reshaping of the torn area, generally preferred for small tears (Fig. 43-4). Very large tears in young active patients usually are treated by primary meniscal repair, generally using arthroscopic technique (Fig. 43-5). Complete excision of a torn meniscus, once quite popular, is now recommended only rarely because of loss of the meniscal load distributing function that can accelerate osteoarthritic change in the knee. On some occasions, badly injured menisci in young active patients can be successfully treated by allograft replacement of the meniscus from a cadaver source. The long-term results of this approach are not yet clear. (See Schwartz 9th ed., p 1579, 80, 81.)

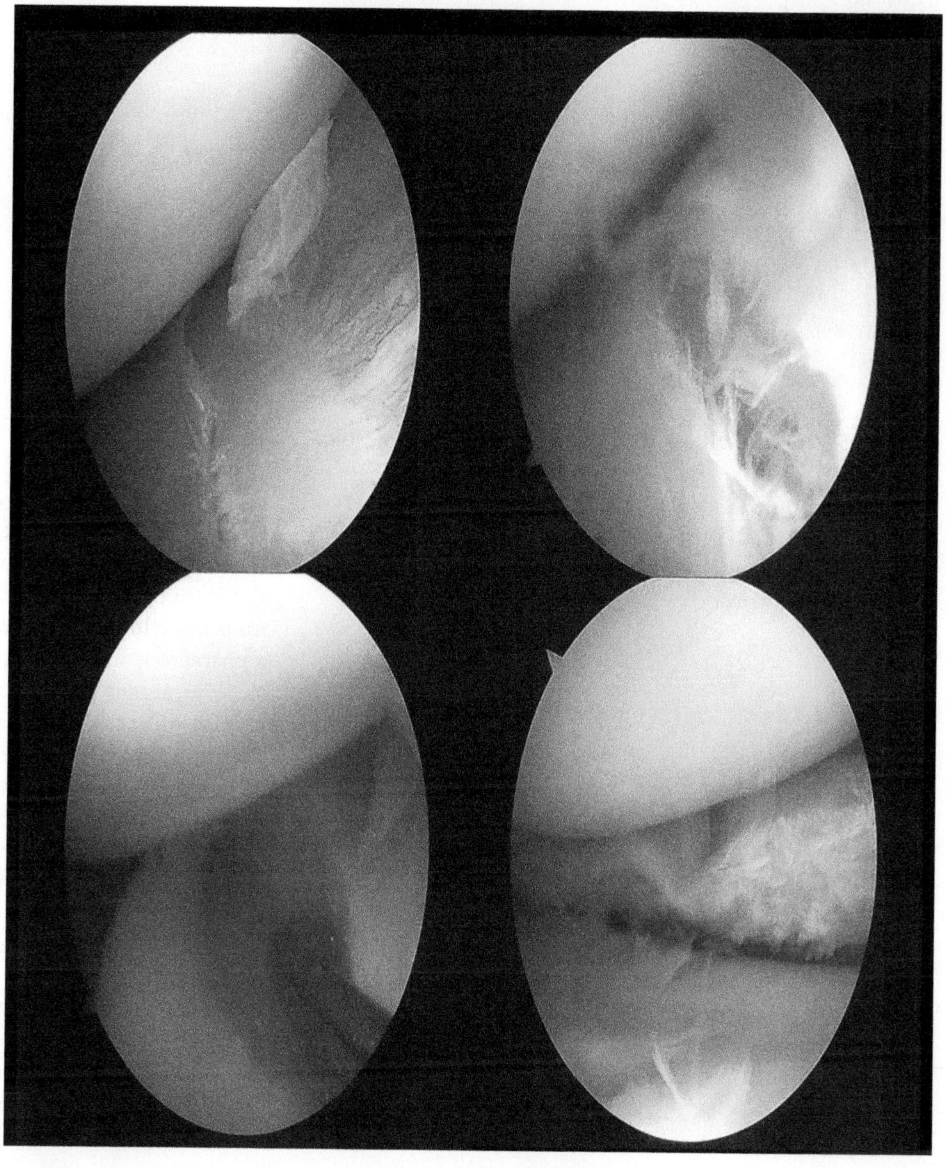

FIG. 43-4. Arthroscopic images of a tear of the medial meniscus of the knee before (*top*) and after (*bottom*) arthroscopic débridement. (*Courtesy of Dr. David Green.*)

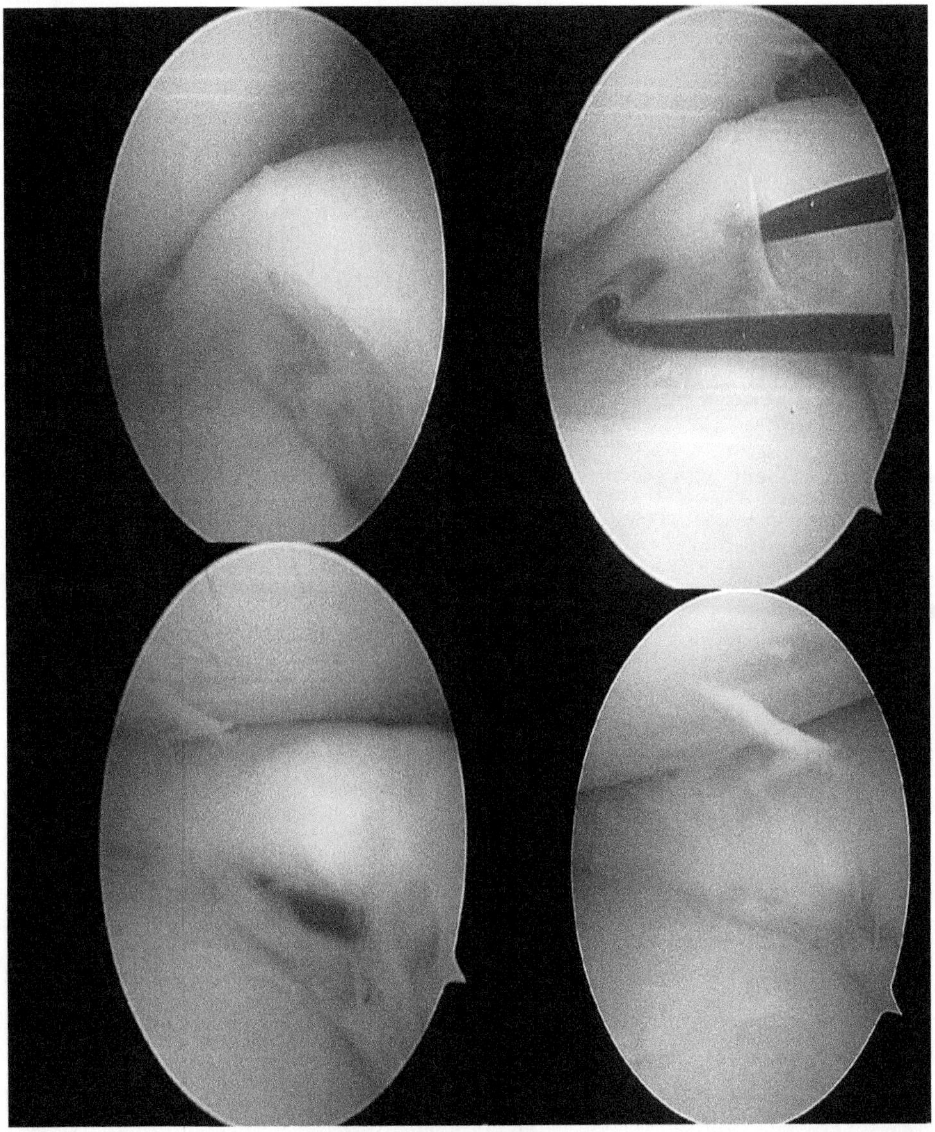

FIG. 43-5. Arthroscopic images of a vertical tear of the medial meniscus. The tear is repaired using a buried suture" technique. (*Courtesy of Dr. David Green.*)

15. A 15-year-old athlete with knee pain and severe point tenderness at the tibial tubercle most likely has
    A. Osgood-Schlatter disease
    B. Legg-Calvé-Perthes disease
    C. Slipped capital femoral epiphysis (SCFE)
    D. Tibial torsion

Answer: A

Osgood-Schlatter disease is a very common problem most often seen in athletically active adolescents. This disorder is characterized by ossification in the distal patellar tendon at the point of its insertion onto the tibial apophysis. This disorder is thought to result from mechanical stress on the tendinous insertional area. X-ray views of the involved knee show a characteristic irregularity in the insertional area and often show separately discrete ossicles within the tendon itself. The disease will present with severe local pain and exquisite tenderness in the area of the tibial tubercle. Effective treatment for the disease can be obtained by activity restriction, which is generally quite unwelcomed by the patient. If the symptoms are improved, athletic participation can be reasonable. In almost every case, symptoms do regress after skeletal maturity or the discontinuance of active athletic participation. In rare cases, persistive symptoms into adulthood can occur. Moderate success can be obtained by surgical excision of ossicles within the tendon of adults.

Legg-Calvé-Perthes disease, also known as *coxa plana*, is a condition of the pediatric hip characterized by a flattened, misshapen femoral head. The etiology of the problem is related to osteonecrosis of the proximal femoral epiphysis and is thought to result from vascular compromise. Legg-Calvé-Perthes disease generally presents in children, usually males, between the ages of 4 and 8 years old. Presenting symptoms generally include groin or knee pain, decreased hip range of motion, and a limp.

A *slipped capital femoral epiphysis* (SCFE) is an acquired disorder of the epiphysis thought to be associated with weakness in the perichondrial ring of the growth plate. Children within the ages of 10 to 16 years old are noted to have the displacement of the epiphysis on the femoral neck. In most cases, there is no identifiable trauma history. It is not known whether this is acquired insidiously or acutely. It is associated with African American heritage and obesity and is somewhat more common in boys than in girls. Twenty-five percent of cases are bilateral.

Tibial torsion is the most common cause of an intoeing gait. This is most frequently noted in 1- and 2-year-old children. This is often bilateral. Although occasionally intoeing can be marked, pediatric tibial torsion will completely resolve without treatment in almost every case. (See Schwartz 9th ed., p 1606.)

16. Which of the following is the most common cervical fracture seen after a diving accident?
    A. Dens (odontoid) fracture (C1)
    B. Hangman fracture (C2)
    C. Compression fracture (C3-7)
    D. Burst fracture (C3-6)

Answer: D

Burst fractures of the cervical spine arise as a result of failure under axial loads. Unrestrained motor vehicle occupants striking a windshield and diving accidents are common injury mechanisms. The burst fracture is distinct from the compression fracture, however, in that the posterior cortex of the vertebral body is fractured. This frequently results in displacement (retropulsion) of bony fragments into the canal, which can cause neurologic injury and dysfunction.

The Jefferson fracture is a fracture of the C1 ring. The C1 vertebra does not have a true anterior body as do all of the rest of the vertebrae. The rather thin anterior and posterior rings are subject to fracture, particularly with axial load injuries. The Jefferson fracture results in a lateral spread of the lateral masses of C1, which are visible on an AP (through the mouth) x-ray image of the upper cervical spine. This injury actually results in an increase in the size of the spinal canal, and thus, rarely is associated with neurologic injury.

Hangman's fractures or traumatic spondylolisthesis of C2 are fractures that occur through the pars interarticularis of C2 (the segment of the posterior elements between the superior and inferior facets of C2). This fracture results from sudden extension forces on the neck causing a fracture through this area of C2, which is one of the thinner portions of the posterior elements of this vertebra.

Compression fractures of the cervical spine refer to an axial load injury with failure of the end plate, but preservation of the posterior cortex of the vertebral body. This will occur in the vertebrae of C3 to C7 and may or may not be associated with a fracture of the anterior cortex. In either case, with the posterior cortex of the vertebral body intact, no compromise of the neural elements results. (See Schwartz 9th ed., p 1583, 85 and Fig. 43-6.)

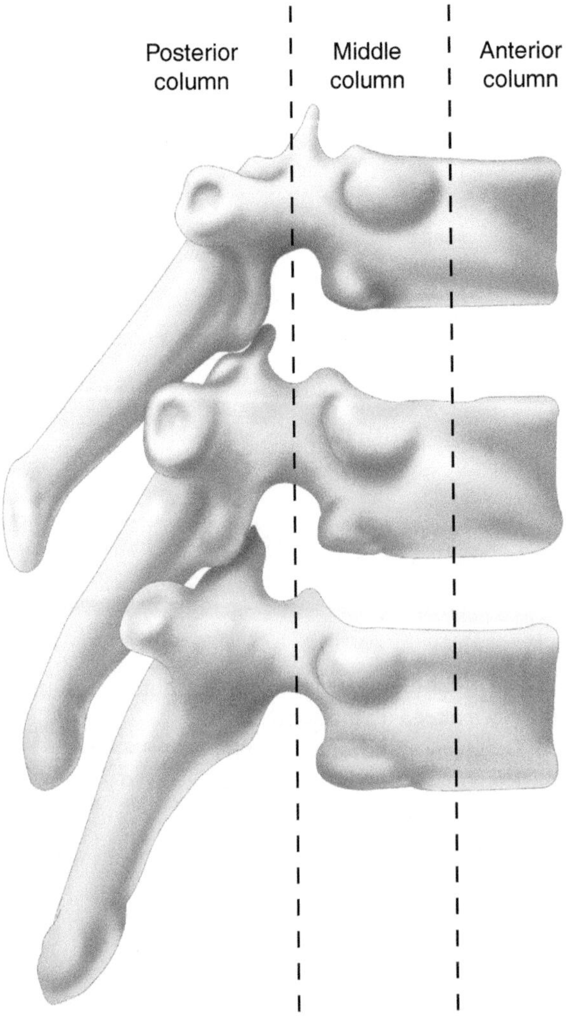

FIG. 43-6. The spine can be thought of as three columns. Two of three can maintain stability.

17. Following attempts at closed reduction, a lateral malleolus fracture has a 2-mm displacement. Which of the following is the best treatment?
    A. No weight bearing for 2 weeks
    B. Splinting
    C. Casting
    D. Open reduction and internal fixation

Answer: D

An isolated distal fibula fracture, often referred to as a *lateral malleolus fracture*, should be anatomically reduced whenever possible. This often can be accomplished by closed reduction and casting (Figs. 43-7 and 43-8). If closed reduction maneuvers do not result in an anatomic or near-anatomic restoration of the anatomy of the ankle, precise open reduction and internal fixation is indicated. Even a disruption of as little as 1 mm in the position of the lateral malleolus can result in a lateral shift of the talus and a decreased contact area between the tibia and talus of almost 50% and can markedly accelerate degenerative arthritis. Surgical exposure of the distal fibula is by a lateral incision. Fracture fragments are precisely aligned and fixed in place generally using a screw and plate device. With accurate reduction and internal fixation, excellent function can result. (See Schwartz 9th ed., p 1566.)

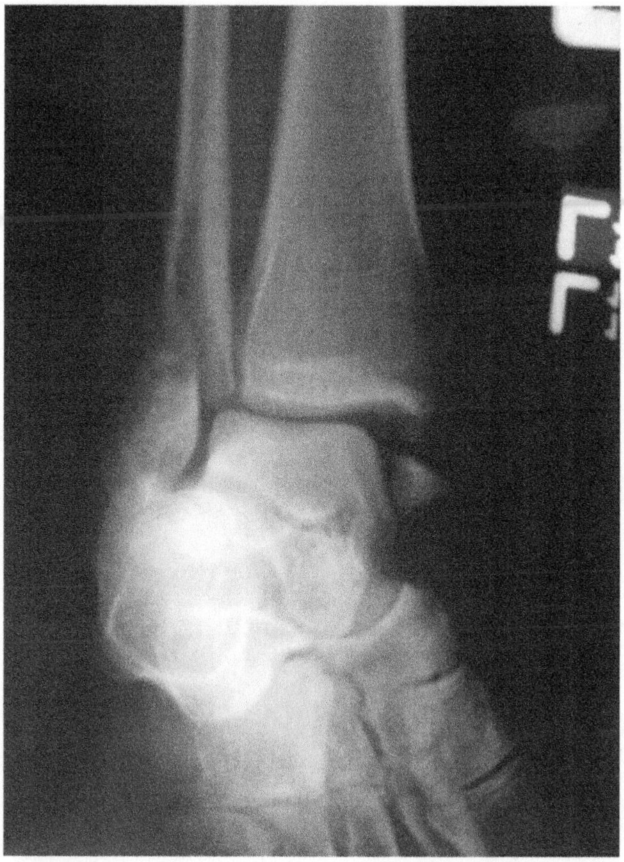

FIG. 43-7. Anteroposterior radiograph of a patient with a bimalleolar fracture.

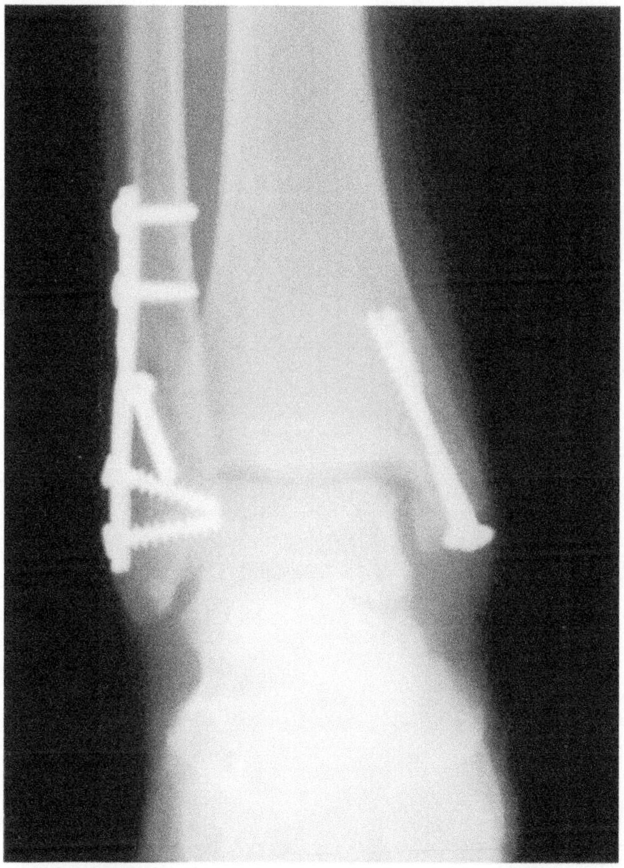

FIG. 43-8. Anteroposterior radiograph of a patient who has an open reduction and internal fixation of the bimalleolar ankle fracture.

18. The most appropriate initial treatment for a symptomatic osteoid osteoma of the distal tibia is
    A. Oral anti-inflammatory medication (aspirin or NSAID)
    B. Radiofrequency ablation
    C. Local resection
    D. Amputation

Answer: A

Osteoid osteoma is a benign bone-forming lesion of uncertain etiology that presents with a central radiolucent nidus (<1.5 cm) and dense surrounding sclerosis. This lesion occurs in patients under the age of 20 years old (usually under the age of 12) but can occasionally occur in older patients. They are predominantly intracortical in location except when they occur in the small bones of the hands and feet where they are intramedullary. Radiologically, they are noted to be a dense cortical sclerosis on plain film. The nidus can be difficult to observe, and CT often is helpful in this regard. Histologically, the nidus is a dense fibrovascular proliferation with abundant new bone formation and active osteoblastic and osteoclastic activity. The surrounding sclerosis is very dense and approaches that seen in the normal cortex. The pain produced by this tumor can be quite intense. Interestingly, this pain is predictably dramatically responsive to aspirin or NSAID medication. Indeed, regular medication with anti-inflammatories often can present definitive treatment for these lesions which in a significant proportion of cases spontaneously regress, usually after a period of 1 to 7 years. Should more aggressive treatment be contemplated, an accessible lesion can be treated by percutaneous radiofrequency ablation (heat administered through high frequency alternating currents). On other occasions, it can be treated by surgical excision. (See Schwartz 9th ed., p 1590.)

CHAPTER 44

Surgery of the Hand and Wrist

BASIC SCIENCE QUESTIONS

1. There are eight pulleys on the flexor surface of each finger. The two pulleys that are the most important to prevent bowstringing of the flexor tendons are
   A. A2 and A4
   B. A1 and A3
   C. A2 and C2
   D. A1 and C1

Answer: A

In the hand, the pulleys maintain the long flexor tendons in close apposition to the fingers and thumb. There are no extensor pulleys within the hand. Each finger has five annular and three cruciate pulleys (Fig. 44-1). The second and fourth (A2 and A4) pulleys are the critical structures that prevent bowstringing of the finger. The remaining pulleys can be divided as needed for surgical exposure or to relieve a stricture area. (See Schwartz 9th ed., p 1614.)

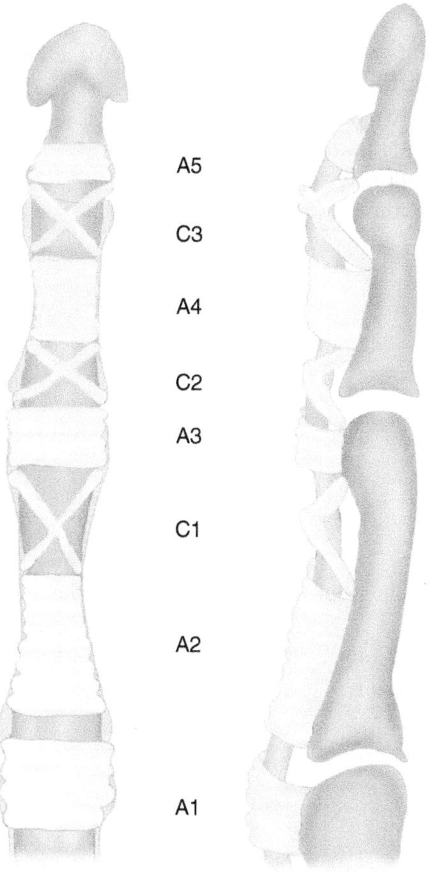
A5
C3
A4
C2
A3
C1
A2
A1

FIG. 44-1. Drawing of anteroposterior and lateral view of the pulley system.

2. In the proximal forearm, the radial artery travels deep to which of the following muscles?
   A. Flexor carpi radialis
   B. Brachioradialis
   C. Palmaris longus
   D. Flexor digitorum superficialis

Answer: B

The radial artery travels under the brachioradialis muscle in the forearm. At the junction of the middle and distal thirds of the forearm, the artery becomes superficial and palpable, passing just radial to the FCR tendon. At the wrist level, the artery splits into two branches. The smaller, superficial branch passes volarly into the palm to contribute to the superficial palmar arch. The larger branch passes dorsally over the scaphoid bone, under the EPL and EPB tendons (known as the *anatomic snuffbox*), and back volarly between the proximal thumb and index finger metacarpals to form the superficial palmar arch. (See Schwartz 9th ed., p 1614.)

3. Initial therapy for a patient with a functionally significant Duputryren's contracture is
   A. Physical therapy
   B. Steroid injection
   C. Splinting
   D. Surgery

Answer: D

Most nonoperative management techniques will not delay the progression of disease. Corticosteroid injections may soften nodules and decrease discomfort associated with them, but are ineffective against cords. Splinting similarly has been shown not to retard disease progression. Injectable clostridial collagenase has shown promise in clinical trials but has not yet been reported in large or long-term series. It also is not yet commercially available. For patients with advanced disease, including contractures of the digits that limit function, surgery is the mainstay of therapy. Although rate of progression should weigh heavily in the decision of whether or not to perform surgery, general guidelines are MP contracture of 30° or more and/or PIP contracture of 20° or more. (See Schwartz 9th ed., p 1630.)

4. In patients with severe arthritis of the MP joint unresponsive to medication, arthrodesis will
   A. Relieve pain
   B. Maintain extension
   C. Maintain flexion
   D. All of the above

Answer: A

When conservative measures fail, two principal surgical options exist: arthrodesis and arthroplasty. The surgeon and patient must decide together as to whether conservative measures have failed. Surgery for arthritis, whether arthrodesis or arthroplasty, is performed for the purpose of relieving pain. Arthrodesis, fusion of a joint, provides excellent relief of pain and is durable over time. However, it comes at the price of total loss of motion. Silicone implant arthroplasty has been available for over 40 years. Rather than a true replacement of the joint, the silicone implant acts as a spacer between the two bones adjacent to the joint. This allows for motion without bony contact that would produce pain. Long-term studies have shown that all implants fracture over time, but usually continue to preserve motion and pain relief. (See Schwartz 9th ed., p 1629.)

5. The movement of the fingers away from the middle finger is called
   A. Abduction
   B. Adduction
   C. Supination
   D. Pronation

Answer: A

The hand is highly mobile in space to allow maximum flexibility in function. As such, a number of directions particular to the hand are necessary to properly describe position, motion, etc. *Palmar* (or volar) refers to the anterior surface of the hand in the anatomic position; *dorsal* refers to the posterior surface in the anatomic position. The hand can rotate at the wrist level; rotation to bring the palm down is called *pronation*, to bring the palm up is called *supination*. Because the hand can rotate in space, the terms medial and lateral are avoided. Radial and ulnar are used instead as these terms do not vary with respect to the rotational position of the hand. Abduction and adduction, when used on the hand, refer to movement of the digits away from and toward the middle finger, respectively (Fig. 44-2). (See Schwartz 9th ed., p 1610-1612.)

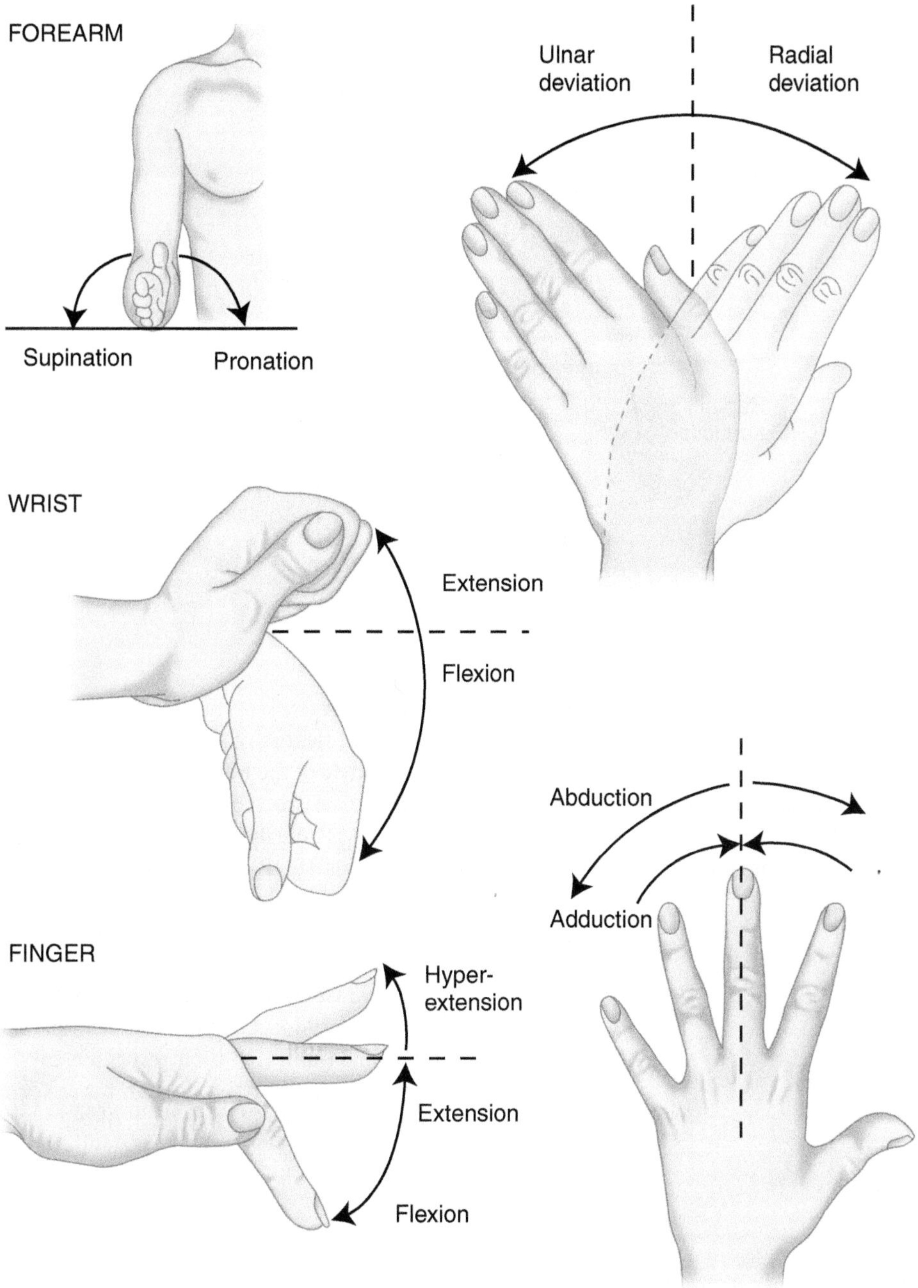

FIG. 44-2. Terminology of common hand motions. (Reproduced with permission from American Society for Surgery of the Hand (ed): *The Hand: Examination and Diagnosis*, 3rd ed. Copyright © Elsevier, 1990.) (*continued*)

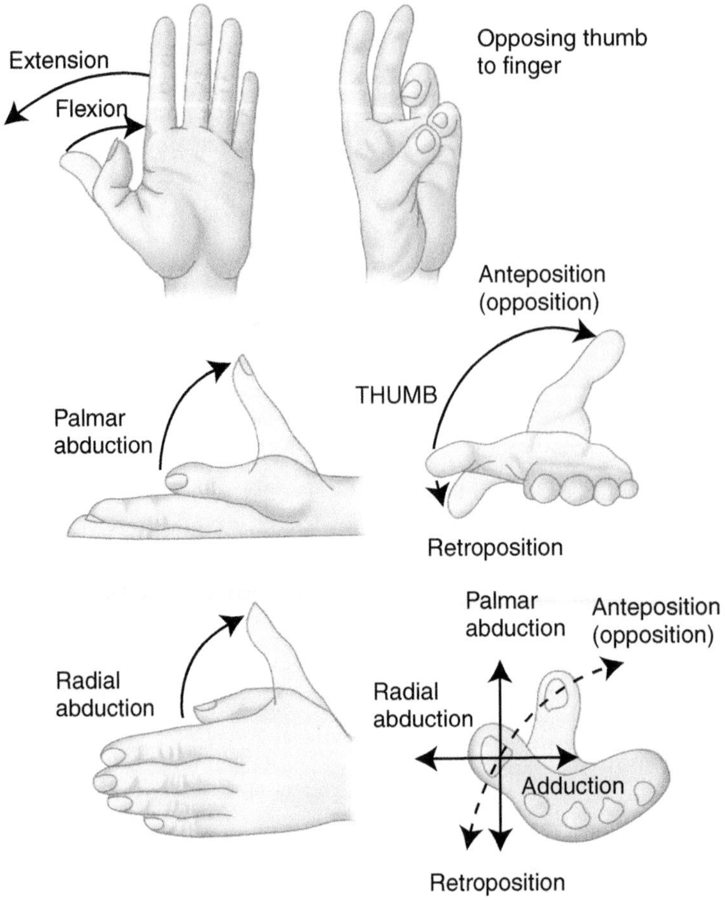

FIG. 44-2. (*continued*)

6. All of the muscles that flex the interphalangeal joints of the fingers originate from
   A. The medial condyle of the humerus
   B. The lateral condyle of the humerus
   C. The distal shaft of the humerus
   D. The deltoid tuberosity of the humerus

Answer: A

The long flexors of the fingers all originate from the medial epicondyle of the humerus. The flexor digitorum superficialis (FDS) inserts on the base of the middle phalanx of each finger and primarily flexes the PIP joint. The flexor digitorum profundus (FDP) inserts on the base of the distal phalanx and primarily flexes the DIP joint. The flexor pollicis longus (FPL) originates more distally, from the ulna, radius, and interosseous membrane between them in the forearm. It inserts on the base of the distal phalanx of the thumb and primarily flexes the IP joint. All of these tendons can also flex the more proximal joint(s) in their respective rays. All of these muscles are innervated by the median nerve (or its branches) except the FDP to the ring and small finger, which are innervated by the ulnar nerve. (See Schwartz 9th ed., p 1610;1613.)

CLINICAL QUESTIONS

1. Appropriate management of a paronychia includes
   A. Needle puncture of the nail
   B. Incision and drainage through the lateral nail plate
   C. Elevation of the nail fold from the nail plate
   D. None of the above

Answer: C

Early treatment of a paronychia is warm compresses or soaks and an antistaphylococcal antibiotic. First-generation cephalosporins have traditionally been used, but the increasing prevalence of methicillin-resistant *S. aureus* has led the authors to begin empiric treatment with vancomycin. Fluctuant swelling or visible pus should be drained with a Freer elevator or the bevel of an 18-gauge needle inserted between the nail and nail fold (Fig. 44-3). If the abscess resides under the eponychial fold, then a proximally based flap of eponychium can be reflected up to allow for better drainage. An abscess that extends below the nail necessitates partial removal of the nail plate. A thin gauze wick should be inserted for 24 to 48 hours to maintain patency of the drainage tract. (See Schwartz 9th ed., p 1634.)

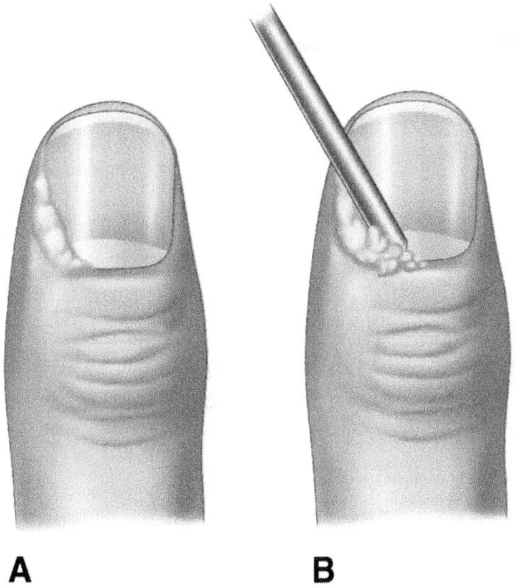

FIG. 44-3. Paronychia. A. Fluctuance in the nail fold is the hallmark of this infection. B. Technique of drainage between the nail plate and nail fold.

2. The Jahss maneuver is used to reduced fractures of the
   A. Scaphoid
   B. Lunate
   C. 5th metacarpal
   D. 2nd metacarpal

Answer: C

Angulated fractures of the small finger MC ('boxer's fracture') are another common injury seen in the ER. Typical history is that the patient struck another individual or rigid object with a hook punch. These often are stable after reduction using the Jahss maneuver (Fig. 44-4). (See Schwartz 9th ed., p 1620.)

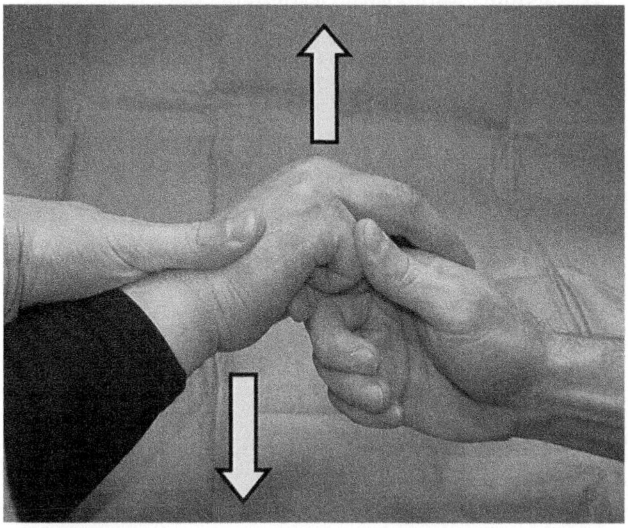

FIG. 44-4. The Jahss maneuver. The surgeon fully flexes the patient's small finger into the palm and secures it in his distal hand. The proximal hand controls the wrist and places the thumb on the patients fracture apex (the most prominent dorsal point). The examiner distracts the fracture, pushes dorsally with the distal hand (*up arrow*) and resists dorsal motion with the proximal hand (*down arrow*).

3. Phalen's test is used in the diagnosis of
   A. Postoperative neuroma
   B. Scaphoid nonunion
   C. Carpal tunnel syndrome
   D. Trigger finger

Answer: C

Physical examination of a patient with suspected carpal tunnel syndrome should begin with inspection. Look for evidence of wasting of the thenar muscles. Tinel's sign should be tested over the median nerve from the volar wrist flexion crease to the proximal palm. Phalen's test (maximal flexion of the wrist for 1 minute) and reverse Phalen's (maximal extension) are tested. Applying pressure over the carpal tunnel while flexing the wrist has been shown in one series to have the highest sensitivity as compared to Phalen's and Tinel's signs. Strength of the thumb in opposition also should be tested. (See Schwartz 9th ed., p 1627.)

4. In a young, healthy patient, the most appropriate treatment for a nondisplaced scaphoid wrist fracture is
   A. Immobilization in a thumb spica cast for 4 weeks
   B. Immobilization in a wrist cock-up cast for 6 weeks
   C. Percutaneous screw fixation
   D. Open reduction and plate fixation

Answer: C

In general terms, most nondisplaced fractures do not require surgical treatment. The scaphoid bone of the wrist is a notable exception to this rule. Due to peculiarities in its vascular supply, particularly vulnerable at its proximal end, nondisplaced scaphoid fractures can fail to unite in up to 20% of patients, even with appropriate immobilization. Recent developments in hardware and surgical technique have allowed stabilization of the fracture with minimal surgical exposure. One prospective randomized series of scaphoid wrist fractures demonstrated shortening of time to union by up to 6 weeks in the surgically treated group, but no difference in rate of union. Surgical treatment for nondisplaced scaphoid fractures is not indicated for all patients, but may be useful in the younger, more active patient who would benefit from an earlier return to full activity. (See Schwartz 9th ed., p 1619.)

5. A chemical burn to the hand with hydrofluoric acid should be treated with
   A. Sodium bicarbonate irrigation
   B. Calcium gluconate gel
   C. Early tangential excision
   D. Dilute sodium hypochlorite irrigation

Answer: B

Chemical burns of the hands are continuously flushed with water until the pain significantly decreases or stops. Acid burns may require 20 minutes of irrigation while alkali burns may require several hours of irrigation. Hydrofluoric acid burns are a special consideration. This type of burn is marked by slow onset of severe pain as the compound reaches deeper tissues. Hydrofluoric acid avidly binds tissue and circulating calcium, resulting in hypocalcemia that can lead to cardiac arrhythmia and arrest. Following water irrigation, a mixture of calcium gluconate in an aqueous jelly is placed into a surgical glove, which is then used to cover the burned hand. Effectiveness of treatment is assessed by relief of pain. If topical therapy does not relieve pain, then locally injected intra-arterial calcium may be necessary. (See Schwartz 9th ed., p 1641.)

6. An injury to a finger flexor tendon at the level of the web space is a
   A. Zone I injury
   B. Zone II injury
   C. Zone III injury
   D. Zone IV injury

Answer: B

Flexor tendon injuries are described based on zones (Fig. 44-5). Up until 40 years ago, zone 2 injuries were always reconstructed and never repaired primarily due to concern that the bulk of repair within the flexor sheath would prevent tendon glide. The work of Dr. Kleinert and colleagues at the University of Louisville changed this 'axiom' and established the principle of primary repair and early controlled mobilization postoperatively. Flexor tendon injuries should always be repaired in the OR. Although they do not need to be repaired on the day of injury, the closer to the day of injury they are repaired, the easier it will be to retrieve the retracted proximal end. (See Schwartz 9th ed., p 1621.)

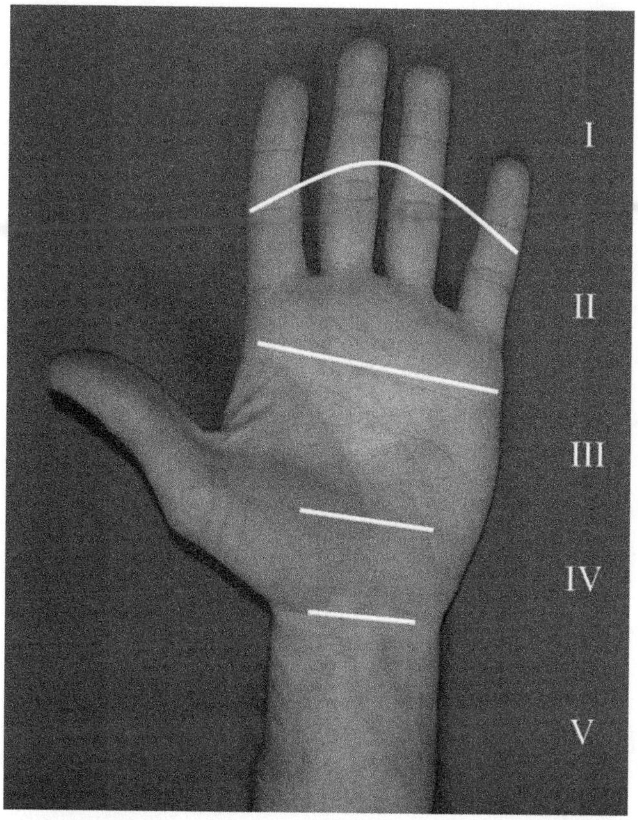

FIG. 44-5. The zones of flexor tendon injury: *I.* Flexor digitorum superficialis insertion to the flexor digitorum profundus insertion. *II.* Start of the A1 pulley to the flexor digitorum superficialis insertion. *III.* End of the carpal tunnel to the start of the A1 pulley. *IV.* Within the carpal tunnel. *V.* Proximal to the carpal tunnel.

7. The most common location for a ganglion cyst is
   A. The dorsal wrist
   B. The volar wrist
   C. Flexor tendon sheath
   D. Dorsal DIP joint

Answer: A

Ganglion cysts are the most common soft tissue tumors in the hand. These lesions can be painful and usually are found on the dorsal wrist, followed by the volar wrist, flexor tendon sheath, and the dorsal DIP joint (the mucous cyst). These non-neoplastic, mucinous, fluid-filled pseudocysts arise from synovial linings of irritated and inflamed joints, ligaments, and tendon sheaths. As they have no epithelial lining, the focus of treatment is the site of production or leakage of the synovial fluid, rather than the cyst itself. (See Schwartz 9th ed., p 1638.)

8. The most common congenital anomaly of the hand is
   A. Polydactyly
   B. Syndactyly
   C. Constriction band syndrome
   D. Radial club hand

Answer: B

Syndactyly, in which two or more fingers are fused together, is the most common congenital hand deformity. Syndactyly occurs in seven out of every 10,000 live births. There is a familial tendency to develop this deformity. This deformity often involves both hands, and males are more often affected than females. (See Schwartz 9th ed., p 1642.)

9. The incision to treat a felon is placed
   A. Laterally on each side of the finger
   B. Longitudinally, centered on the area of maximal fluctuence
   C. Between the nail fold and nail plate
   D. Transversely across the tip of the finger

Answer: B

The procedure to drain a felon is straightforward (Fig. 44-6). A digital block is performed. This is followed by a short skin incision. Only the skin is incised. Pus is evacuated using a blunt instrument to decrease the chance of severing a digital nerve or entering the tendon sheath. Gauze is loosely packed into the wound to prevent skin closure. A loose dressing and finger splint is applied. The hand is elevated and splinted. (See Schwartz 9th ed., p 1634.)

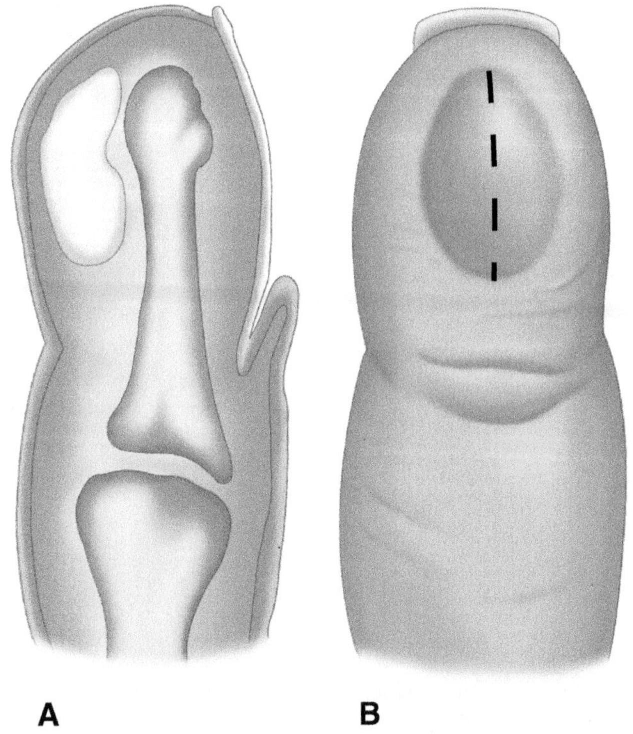

FIG. 44-6. A and B. The area of purulence in a felon is located in the pad of the distal phalanx as shown. B. A longitudinally oriented incision is made over the area of maximal fluctuance; this incision should not cross the distal interphalangeal joint crease. See text for additional details.

10. Which of the following is NOT one of Kanavel's signs of flexor tendon sheath infection?
    A. Finger held in slight flexion
    B. Fusiform swelling
    C. Tenderness along the flexor tendon sheath
    D. Pain with passive flexion of the finger

Answer: D

Patients with infectious flexor tenosynovitis (FTS) present with complaints of pain, redness, and fever. Physical examination reveals Kanavel's 'cardinal' signs of flexor tendon sheath infection, which are finger held in slight flexion, fusiform swelling, tenderness along the flexor tendon sheath, and pain over the flexor sheath with passive extension of the digit (Fig. 44-7A). (See Schwartz 9th ed., p 1636.)

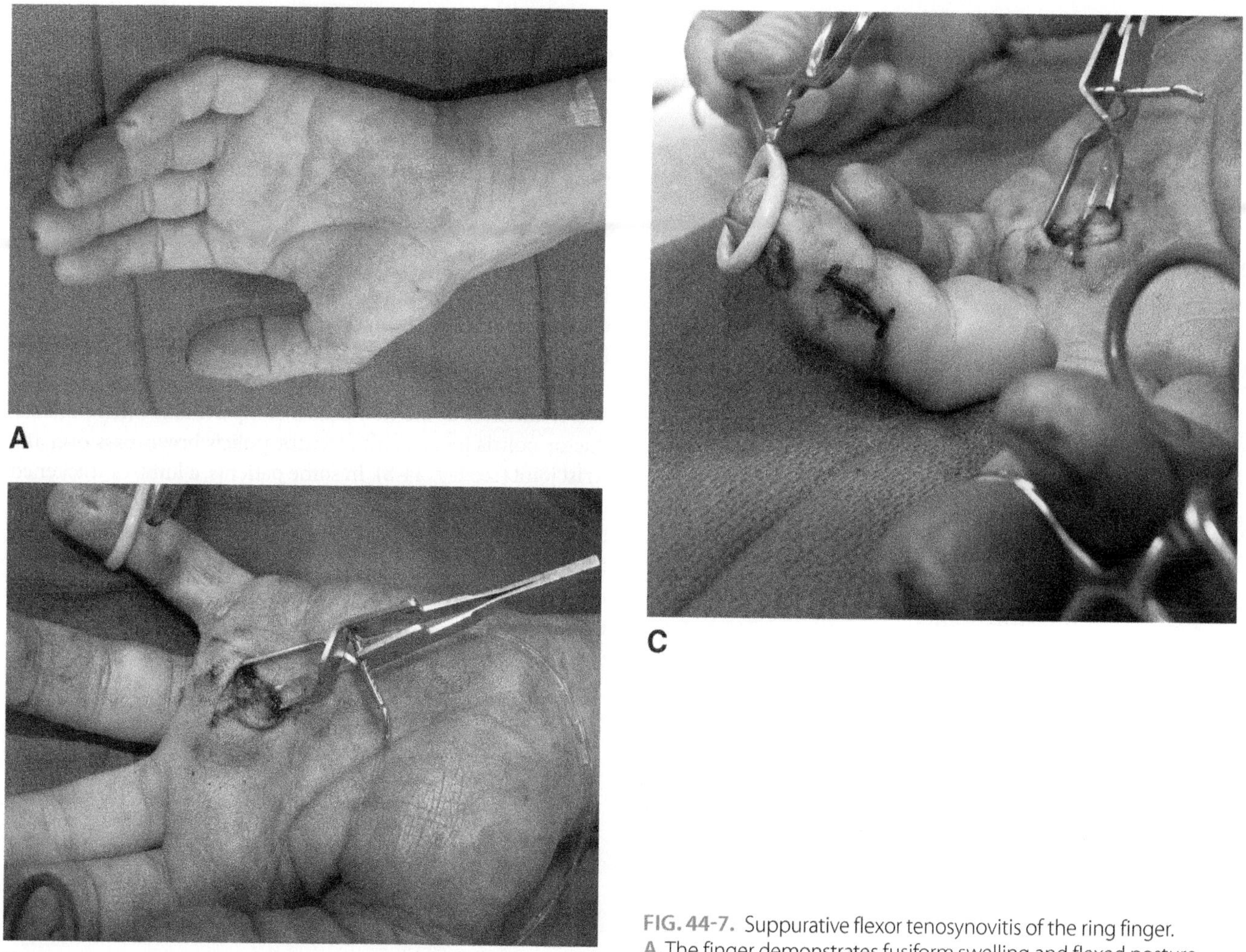

FIG. 44-7. Suppurative flexor tenosynovitis of the ring finger. A. The finger demonstrates fusiform swelling and flexed posture. B. Proximal exposure for drainage. C. Distal drainage incision.

11. The most important part of the initial management of a burn of the hand is
    A. Elevation
    B. Early range of motion exercise
    C. Early débridement
    D. Early grafting

Answer: A

Edema formation in burned hands hinders motion and may be a factor in later contracture formation. The hands must be elevated above the level of the heart to minimize edema formation. This is the most important initial step in the management of hand burns and can be done in any sized burn without hindering resuscitation, pulmonary, or other critical care management. (See Schwartz 9th ed., p 1640.)

12. The best initial treatment for "trigger finger" is
    A. Splinting for 4-6 weeks
    B. Physical therapy
    C. Steroid injection
    D. Surgery

Answer: C

Stenosing tenosynovitis of the flexor tendon sheath, also known as *trigger finger* (TF), is one of the most common upper limb problems to be encountered in hand surgery practice. The condition starts with discomfort in the palm during movements of the involved digits. Gradually, the flexor tendon causes painful popping or snapping as the patient flexes and extends the digit. The patient often will present with a digit locked in a flexed position, which may require gentle passive manipulation to regain full extension.

Nonoperative treatment includes limiting the activities that aggravate the condition. Splinting and/or oral anti-inflammatory medication may help. If symptoms continue, a corticosteroid injection into the tendon sheath at the pulley is often effective in relieving the trigger digit. The authors prefer triamcinolone acetonide (40 mg/mL) mixed with 0.5% plain bupivacaine.

The needle is inserted at the MC head, advanced until bone is encountered, and then withdrawn approximately 0.5 mm until resistance gives way, allowing the medication to be injected. Approximately 1 mL is deposited in the tendon sheath. The needle is withdrawn and pressure is applied. Fingers with irreducible flexion contractures should be treated with surgery, not steroid injection. (See Schwartz 9th ed., p 1631.)

13. The primary symptom in De Quervain's tenosynovitis is pain in the
    A. Radial wrist
    B. Ulnar wrist
    C. Dorsal wrist
    D. Volar wrist

Answer: A

Patients with De Quervain's tenosynovitis usually present with complaints of pain, several weeks to months in duration, along the radial aspect of the wrist aggravated by thumb motion. The most common symptoms are pain when grasping or pinching and tenderness at the first dorsal compartment, where the abductor policis longus and extensor policis brevis pass over the wrist joint (see Fig. 44-8). In some patients, a lump or thickened mass can be felt in the area 1 to 2 cm proximal to the radial styloid. Severe, sharp pain can be elicited by having the patient flex the thumb across the palm, make a fist, and then ulnarly deviate the wrist (Finkelstein's test) (Fig. 44-9). There should be no tenderness in the forearm proximal to the first dorsal compartment. (See Schwartz 9th ed., p 1632, image 44-8 on pg 1613.)

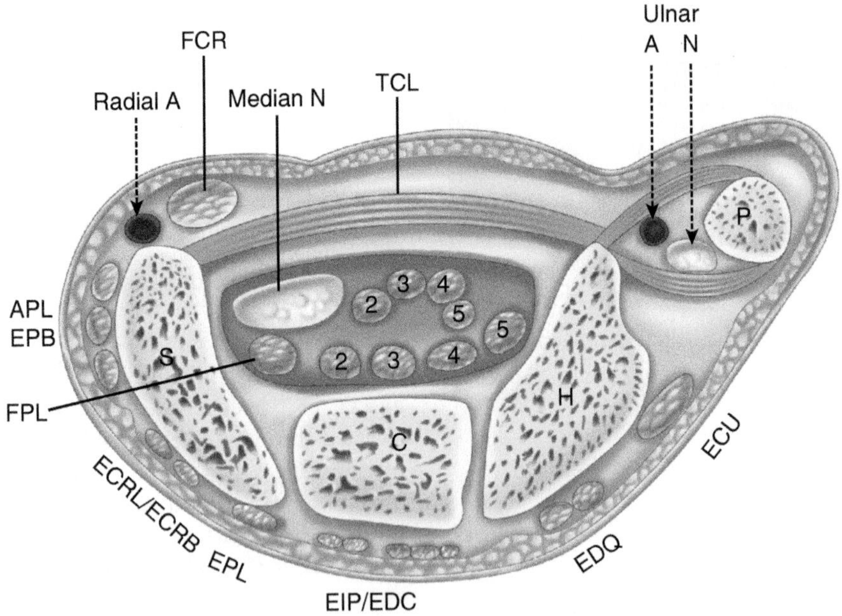

FIG. 44-8. Cross-section of the wrist at the midcarpal level. The relative geography of the neurologic and tendinous structures can be seen. The transverse carpal ligament (TCL) is the roof of the carpal tunnel, passing volar to the median nerve and long flexor tendons. The TCL is also the floor of the ulnar tunnel, or Guyon's canal, passing dorsal to the ulnar artery and nerve. The wrist and digital extensor tendons are also seen, distal to their compartments on the distal radius and ulna. Bones: C = capitate; H = hamate; P = pisiform; S = scaphoid. Tendons (flexor digitorum superficialis is volar to flexor digitorum profundus within the carpal tunnel): 2 = index finger; 3 = middle finger; 4 = ring finger; 5 = small finger. A = artery; APL = abductor pollicis longus; ECRB = extensor carpi radialis brevis; ECRL = extensor carpi radialis longus; ECU = extensor carpi ulnaris; EDC = extensor digitorum communis; EDQ = extensor digiti quinti; EIP = extensor indices proprius; EPB = extensor pollicis brevis; EPL = extensor pollicis longus; FCR = flexor carpi radialis; FPL = flexor pollicis longus; N = nerve.

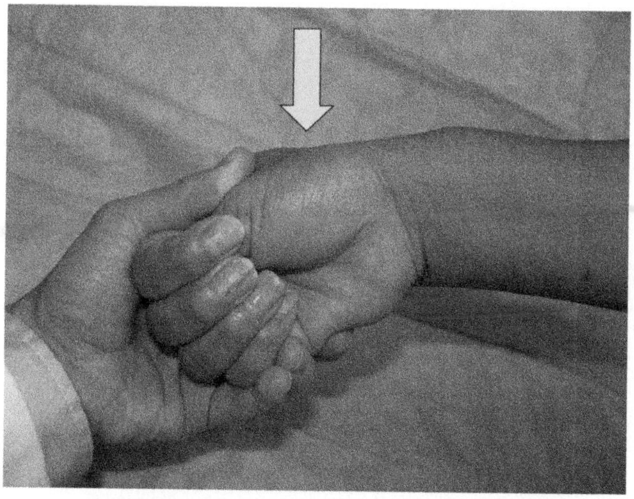

FIG. 44-9. Finkelstein's test. The patient places the thumb in the palm and makes a loose fist. The examiner then ulnarly deviates the patient's wrist (as indicated by the *arrow*). Pain at the first dorsal compartment with this maneuver is a positive response.

14. The most common benign bone tumor of the hand is
    A. Lipoma
    B. Fibroma
    C. Enchondroma
    D. Giant cell tumor of the tendon sheath

Answer: C

Enchondromas arise from cartilage and are the most common primary bone tumors of the hand. These lesions account for >90% of bone tumors seen in the hand. The proximal phalanges are the most common sites of occurrence, followed by the MC bones. On radiographs, an enchondroma usually is seen as a well-defined radiolucent lesion in the diaphysis or metaphysis and also may have a well-defined sclerotic rim. Although these tumors are benign, local bony destruction can lead to pathologic fracture. (See Schwartz 9th ed., p 1638.)

15. Which of the following is the most appropriate treatment for a crush injury to the fingertip with a laceration greater than 1 cm^2 with less than 50% of the nailbed remaining?
    A. Primary repair
    B. Débridement and wound care to allow healing by secondary intention
    C. Operative shortening of the bone for primary stump closure
    D. Volar V-Y flap closure of the laceration

Answer: C

For the common scenario, complex lacerations with minimally displaced fracture(s) and no loss of perfusion, the wound is cleansed, closed, and splinted in the ER. To properly assess the nail bed, the nail plate (hard part of the nail) should be removed. A Freer periosteal elevator is well suited for this purpose. Lacerations are repaired with 6-0 fast gut suture. Great care must be taken when suturing as excessive traction with the needle can further lacerate the tissue. After repair, the nail folds are splinted with the patient's own nail plate (if available) or with aluminum foil from the suture pack. This is done to prevent scarring from the nail folds down to the nail bed that would further compromise healing of the nail. In some situations, tissue may have been avulsed in the injury and be unavailable for repair. Choice of treatment options depends on the amount and location of tissue loss (Fig. 44-10). For wounds <1 cm^2 with no exposed bone, secondary intention will produce excellent functional and aesthetic results. For larger wounds or wounds with bone exposed, one must decide if the finger is worth preserving at the current length or if shortening to allow for primary closure is a better solution. A useful guideline is the amount of fingernail still present; if greater than 50% is present, local or regional flap coverage may be a good solution. (See Schwartz 9th ed., p 1622.)

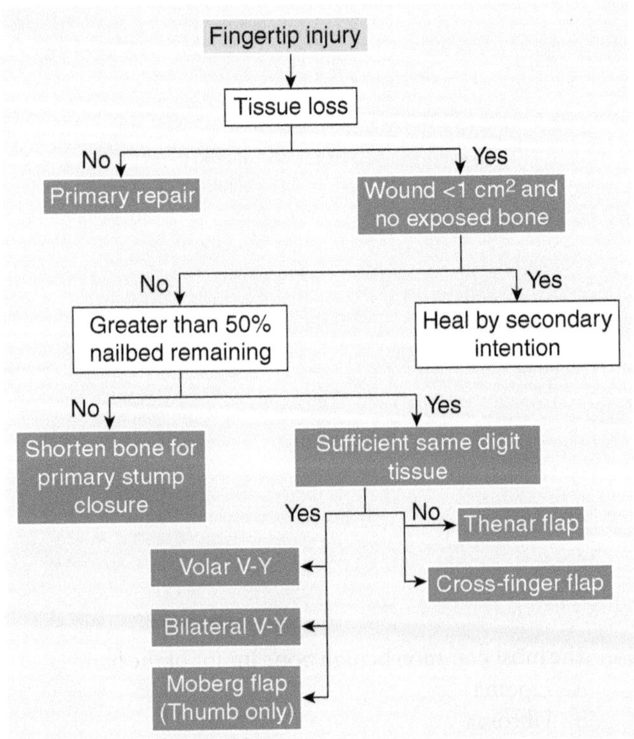

FIG. 44-10. Treatment algorithm for management of fingertip injuries. See text for description of flaps.

16. The primary treatment of herpetic whitlow is
    A. Dry dressings
    B. Wound débridement
    C. Intralesional acyclovir
    D. Intravenous acyclovir

Answer: A

Herpetic whitlow usually resolves spontaneously in 2 to 3 weeks. The main goals of treatment are to prevent both oral inoculation and spread of the infection, as well as to obtain symptomatic relief. The involved digit should be kept covered with a dry dressing. Some authors recommend treatment with oral acyclovir for 10 days if the diagnosis is made early in symptom onset, although acyclovir has not been demonstrated to shorten the course of this self-limited infection. Stronger evidence exists to recommend oral acyclovir for recurrent infections during the prodromal stage, as well as in immunocompromised patients. Infection can recur in 30 to 50% of patients, but the initial infection is typically the most severe. (See Schwartz 9th ed., p 1635.)

CHAPTER 45

Plastic and Reconstructive Surgery

BASIC SCIENCE QUESTIONS

1. The first stage of healing in a skin graft is
   A. Revascularization
   B. Inosculation
   C. Imbibition
   D. None of the above

Answer: C
Skin graft take occurs in three phases, imbibition, inosculation, and revascularization. Plasmatic imbibition refers to the first 24 to 48 hours after skin grafting, during which time a thin film of fibrin and plasma separates the graft from the underlying wound bed. It remains controversial whether this film provides nutrients and oxygen to the graft or merely a moist environment to maintain the ischemic cells temporarily until a vascular supply is re-established. After 48 hours a fine vascular network begins to form within the fibrin layer. These new capillary buds interface with the deep surface of the dermis and allow for transfer of some nutrients and oxygen. This phase, called *inosculation*, transitions into revascularization, the process by which new blood vessels either directly invade the graft or anastomose to open dermal vascular channels and restore the pink hue of skin. These phases are generally complete by 4 to 5 days after graft placement. During these initial few days the graft is most susceptible to deleterious factors such as infection, mechanical shear forces, and hematoma or seroma. (See Schwartz 9th ed., p 1650.)

2. The chance an offspring will have a cleft lip if one of the parents has a cleft lip is
   A. 4%
   B. 10%
   C. 25%
   D. 100%

Answer: A
Factors that likely increase the incidence of clefting include increased parental age, drug use and infections during pregnancy, smoking during pregnancy, and a family history of orofacial clefting. The increased chance of clefting when there is an affected parent is approximately 4%. (See Schwartz 9th ed., p 1658.)

3. The deepest layer of the scalp is
   A. Subcutaneous tissue
   B. Loose areolar tissue
   C. Pericranium
   D. Galea aponeurotica

Answer: C
The scalp is formed of five layers: *S*kin, sub*C*utaneous tissue, galea *A*poneurotica, *L*oose areolar tissue, and *P*ericranium (SCALP). (See Schwartz 9th ed., p 1675.)

CLINICAL QUESTIONS

1. The best incision to excise a lesion on the bridge of the nose is
   A. Vertical
   B. Horizontal
   C. Oblique
   D. Circular

Answer: B

Although the term *Langer's lines* often is used interchangeably with the term *relaxed skin tension lines*, the former lines describe skin tension vectors observed in the stretched integument of cadavers exhibiting rigor mortis, whereas the latter lines lay perpendicular to and more accurately reflect the action of underlying muscle. Kraissl's lines, which run along natural wrinkles and skin creases, tend also to follow the relaxed skin tension lines (Fig. 45-1). Relaxed skin tension lines may be exploited to create incisions and reconstructions that minimize anatomic distortion and improve cosmesis. (See Schwartz 9th ed., p 1648.)

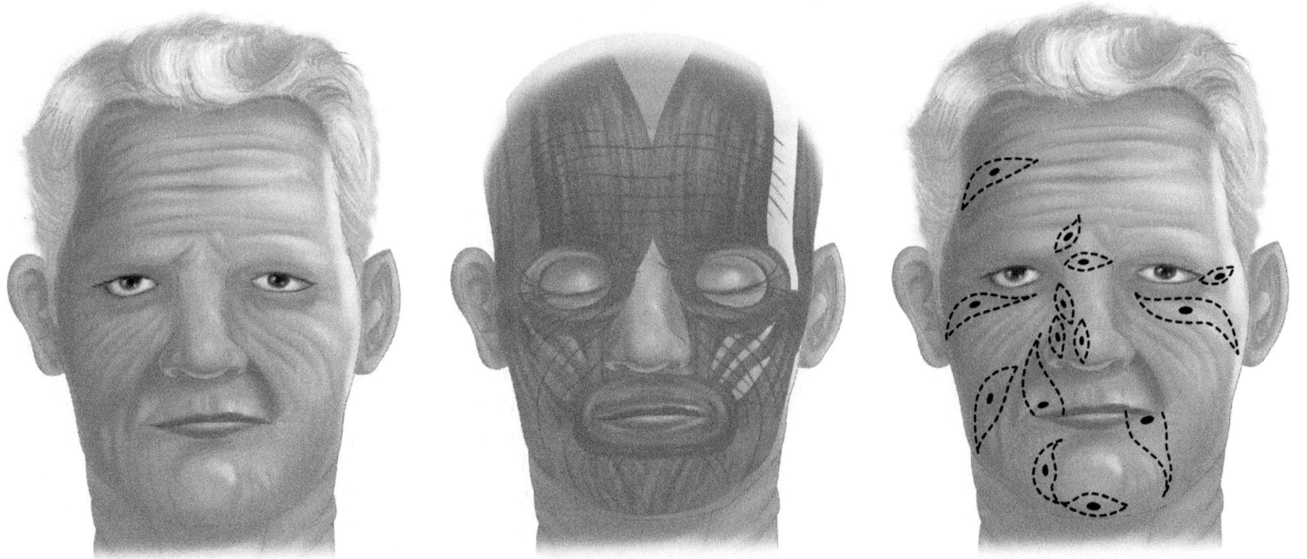

FIG. 45-1. Relaxed skin tension lines. (Reprinted with permission from Wilhelmi BJ, Blackwell SJ, Phillips LG: Langer's lines: To use or not to use. *Plast Reconstr Surg* 104:208, 1999.)

2. The first step in the treatment of a newborn with a complex cleft lip and palate is
   A. Nasoalveolar molding prosthetics in infancy, followed by staged repair
   B. Repair of the cleft lip at 3 months of age, followed by the palate repair
   C. Repair of the cleft palate at 6 months of age, followed by the lip repair
   D. Single stage repair (lip and palate) at 9-12 months of age

Answer: A

Attempts to lessen the deformity and set the stage for the surgical repair of the lip and nose begin with a process known as *presurgical infant orthopedics (PSIO)*, which includes procedures such as nasoalveolar molding (NAM). NAM repositions the neonatal alveolar segments, brings the lip elements into close approximation, stretches the deficient nasal components, and turns wide complete clefts into the morphology of narrow 'incomplete' clefts. After PSIO with NAM, the definitive single-stage cleft lip and nose repair is performed at 3 to 6 months of age. With this initial operation, the lip deformity is repaired and a primary nasoplasty reconstructs the cleft lip nasal deformity. If the family does not have access to PSIO or have the resources for this time-intensive therapy, a cleft lip adhesion can be performed as an initial stage in the repair. The preliminary cleft lip adhesion unites the upper lip and nasal sill, truly converting complete clefts into incomplete clefts. A cleft lip adhesion is performed in the first or second month of life, and the definitive cleft lip and nose repair follows at 4 to 6 months. After the definitive cleft lip and nose repair, the cleft palate is repaired in a single stage at 9 to 12 months of age. (See Schwartz 9th ed., p 1658.)

3. Which is the first fracture repaired in a patient with multiple facial fractures (panfacial fracture)?
   A. Mandibular
   B. Maxillary
   C. Nasomaxillary
   D. Zygomatic

Answer: D

Fractures of multiple bones in various locations fall into the category of panfacial fracture. These may involve frontal and maxillary sinus fractures, NOE fractures, orbital and ZMC fractures, palatal fractures, and complex mandible fractures. The difficulty in the repair of these injuries lies not in the technical aspects of fixation but in the re-establishment of normal relationships between facial features in the absence of all pretraumatic reference points. Without proper correction of bony fragment relationships, facial width is exaggerated and facial projection is lost. The key point in approaching the patient with a panfacial fracture is first to reduce and repair the zygomatic arches and frontal bar to establish the frame and width of the face. The nasomaxillary and zygomaticomaxillary buttresses may then be repaired within this correct frame. Next, the maxilla may be reduced to this framework, followed by palatal fixation if needed. Finally, now that the midface relationships have been corrected, maxillary-mandibular fixation can be applied with the mandible in correct occlusion followed by plating of any mandibular fractures. (See Schwartz 9th ed., p 1672.)

4. Involution of a hemangioma occurs in 50% of children by
   A. 6 months of age
   B. 1 year of age
   C. 2 years of age
   D. 5 years of age

Answer: D

Hemangioma growth frequently peaks before the first year, and then the lesions enter the *involuting phase* in which growth is commiserate with the child. The involuting phase is characterized by diminishing endothelial activity and luminal enlargement. The lesion begins to 'gray,' losing its intense reddish color and taking on a purple-gray shade with overlying 'crepe paper' skin. The involution phase continues until 5 to 10 years of age. Regression of the lesion is then complete. The *involuted phase* begins in 50% of children by 5 years of age and in 70% by 7 years. (See Schwartz 9th ed., p 1667.)

5. Conditioning of a transverse rectus abdominus myocutaneous (TRAM) flap can be achieved by
   A. Placing ice packs on the abdominal wall for 1 hour before surgery
   B. Placing ice packs on the abdominal wall for 1 hour × 7 days before surgery
   C. Dividing the inferior epigastric artery 2 weeks before surgery
   D. Dividing the superior epigastric artery 2 weeks before surgery

Answer: C

Conditioning refers to any procedure that increases the reliability of a flap. Invoking the delay phenomenon, for example, has improved the survival of flaps whose use is frequently complicated by unpredictable partial necrosis, such as the pedicled transverse rectus abdominis myocutaneous (TRAM) flap. The procedure can be particularly useful in patients at higher risk, such as those who are obese, smoke, or have received radiotherapy. One method of delay for the pedicled TRAM flap is to divide a major portion of its blood supply, the deep inferior epigastric artery on both sides, approximately 2 weeks before transfer. In response, blood from the anatomic angiosome of the superior epigastric artery appears to flow into that of the interrupted deep inferior epigastric artery via intervening choke vessels. As a result, the flap becomes conditioned to rely on the superior epigastric artery. The TRAM flap can then be transferred based on the superior epigastric artery with less risk of its distal portions becoming ischemic and possibly necrotic. (See Schwartz 9th ed., p 1654.)

6. Which of the following has the highest degree of secondary contraction?
   A. Thin split-thickness skin graft
   B. Thick split-thickness skin graft
   C. Meshed thick split-thickness skin graft
   D. Full-thickness skin graft

Answer: A

Many of the characteristics of a split-thickness graft are determined by the amount of dermis present. Less dermis translates into less primary contraction (the degree to which a graft shrinks in dimensions after harvesting and before grafting), more secondary contraction (the degree to which a graft contracts during healing), and better chance of graft survival. Thin split grafts have low primary contraction, high secondary contraction, and high reliability of graft take, often even in imperfect recipient beds. Thin grafts, however, tend to heal with abnormal pigmentation and poor durability compared with thick-split grafts and full-thickness grafts. Thick-split grafts have more primary contraction, show less secondary contraction, and may take less hardily. Split grafts may be meshed to expand the surface area that can be covered. This technique is particularly useful when a large area must be resurfaced, as in major burns. Meshed grafts usually also have enhanced reliability of engraftment, because the fenestrations allow for egress of wound fluid and excellent contour matching of the wound bed by the graft. (See Schwartz 9th ed., p 1651.)

7. The generally longest reliable length:width ratio for a random pattern flap is
   A. 1:1
   B. 2:1
   C. 3:1
   D. 4:1

Answer: C

Random pattern flaps have a blood supply based on small, unnamed blood vessels in the dermal-subdermal plexus, as opposed to the discrete, well-described, directional vessels of axial pattern flaps (Fig. 45-2). Random flaps are typically used to reconstruct relatively small, full-thickness defects that are not amenable to skin grafting. Unlike axial pattern flaps, random flaps are limited by their geometry. The generally accepted reliable length:width ratio for a random flap is 3:1. (See Schwartz 9th ed., p 1651.)

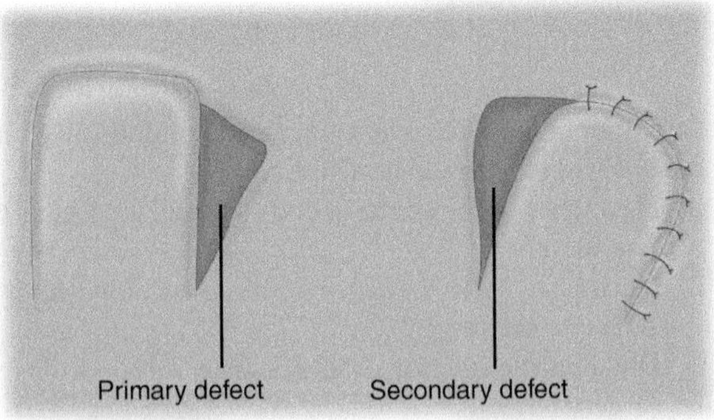

FIG. 45-2. Random pattern transposition flap.

8. Which of the following is a component of the Klippel-Trénaunay syndrome?
   A. Capillary malformations
   B. Venous malformations
   C. Lymphatic malformations
   D. All of the above

Answer: D

Vascular malformations are subclassified by vessel type, such as lymphatic, capillary, venous, or arterial, and by rheologic characteristics, such as slow flow and fast flow. Slow-flow lesions include capillary malformations (CMs) and telangiectasias, lymphatic malformations (LMs), and venous malformations (VMs). Fast-flow lesions include arterial malformations (AMs) and arteriovenous malformations (AVMs). In addition, there are combined malformations. One such combined lesion occurs in Klippel-Trénaunay syndrome in which CMs, LMs, and VMs are found and may be associated with soft tissue and skeletal hypertrophy in one or more of the limbs. (See Schwartz 9th ed., p 1667.)

9. The treatment of stage II pressure sores is
   A. Local wound care only
   B. Extensive débridement and local wound care
   C. Direct closure
   D. Skin grafting

Answer: A

Pressure ulcers are described by their stage, based on depth of tissue injury (Table 45-1). Stage I and II ulcers are treated conservatively with dressing changes and basic pressure ulcer prevention strategies as already discussed. Patients with stage III or IV ulcers should be evaluated for surgery. (See Schwartz 9th ed., p 1694.)

TABLE 45-1 National Pressure Ulcer Advisory Panel staging system

Classification	Description
Stage I	Intact skin with nonblanchable redness
Stage II	Partial-thickness loss of dermis; may present as blister
Stage III	Full-thickness loss of dermis with visible subcutaneous fat (no deeper structures exposed)
Stage IV	Full-thickness loss of dermis with exposed bone, tendon, or muscle
Unstageable	Full-thickness loss of dermis with ulcer base obscured by eschar

10. Which of the following is one of the most common locations for orbital fractures?
    A. Superior
    B. Laterosuperior
    C. Lateral
    D. Medial

Answer: D

Orbital fractures may involve the orbital roof, floor, or lateral or medial walls. The most common orbital fracture is the orbital floor blow-out fracture caused by direct pressure to the globe and sudden increase in intraorbital pressure. Because the medial floor and inferior medial wall are made of the thinnest bone, fractures occur most frequently at these locations. (See Schwartz 9th ed., p 1671.)

11. The most appropriate treatment of a septal hematoma following blunt trauma to the nose is
    A. Observation
    B. Aspiration
    C. Incision and drainage
    D. Operative repair of the fracture

Answer: C

The nose is the most common facial fracture site due to its prominent location, and such fracture can involve the cartilaginous nasal septum, the nasal bones, or both. It is important to perform an intranasal examination to determine whether a septal hematoma is present. If present, a septal hematoma must be incised, drained, and packed to prevent pressure necrosis of the nasal septum and long-term midvault collapse. (See Schwartz 9th ed., p 1672.)

12. What is the maximum defect (percent tissue lost) of the upper eyelid that can be repaired primarily?
    A. 5%
    B. 10%
    C. 25%
    D. 40%

Answer: C

Defects comprising <25% of the upper eyelid can generally be closed primarily in pentagonal approximating fashion. For defects involving 25 to 50% of the upper eyelid, lateral canthotomy (release of the lateral canthal tendon) and cantholysis (release of the superior limb of the lateral palpebral tendon) can be performed to allow advancement and are often combined with use of a lateral semicircular flap. Defects larger than 50% of the upper eyelid may be reconstructed with a Cutler-Beard full-thickness advancement flap or a modified Hughes tarsoconjunctival advancement flap. (See Schwartz 9th ed., p 1674.)

13. The maximum width (at the umbilicus) of a midline abdominal wound that can be closed by the component separation technique is
    A. 6 cm
    B. 12 cm
    C. 18 cm
    D. 24 cm

Answer: C

The separation-of-components procedure has enjoyed much success in closing large midline defects without resorting to mesh. This procedure involves advancement of bilateral myofascial flaps consisting of the anterior rectus fascia/rectus abdominis/internal oblique/transversus abdominis muscle complex. Mobility of this myofascial unit is created by release of the external oblique muscle at the semilunate line. Midline defects measuring up to 10 cm superiorly, 18 cm centrally, and 8 cm inferiorly can be closed using separation of components. This technique is less effective in closing lateral defects, for which regional muscle and fascial flaps are usually better suited (rectus abdominis flap, internal oblique flap, external oblique flap). (See Schwartz 9th ed., p 1690.)

14. Optimal time for repair of a facial nerve injured during a surgical procedure is
    A. Immediately
    B. 2 weeks after injury
    C. 4-6 weeks after injury
    D. 3 months after injury

Answer: A

Traumatic injuries to the facial nerve without segmental nerve loss are best treated with primary end-to-end neurorrhaphy of the facial nerve stumps. The success of this repair depends on accurate approximation of nerve ends and achievement of a tension-free epineural repair with fine sutures, usually 8-0 nylon or finer. In segmental facial nerve loss due to trauma or oncologic resection, interpositional nerve grafts lead to the most successful reconstruction and may approach the results of primary repair. Grafting ideally is performed at the time of the injury rather than in delayed fashion. Donor nerves include the cervical plexus, great auricular nerve, and sural nerve. (See Schwartz 9th ed., p 1681.)

15. The most likely diagnosis in the child shown in Fig. 45-3 is
    A. Craniosynostosis
    B. diGeorge syndrome
    C. Treacher Collins syndrome
    D. Pierre Robin syndrome

Answer: C

Treacher Collins syndrome, also known as *mandibulofacial dysostosis*, is a type of craniofacial clefting disorder representing bilateral 6-7-8 clefts. This autosomal dominant disorder with variable penetrance has the following manifestations: hypoplasia of the zygomas, asymmetry and hypoplasia of the mandible, ear anomalies, and colobomas of the lower eyelids. (See Schwartz 9th ed., p 1663.)

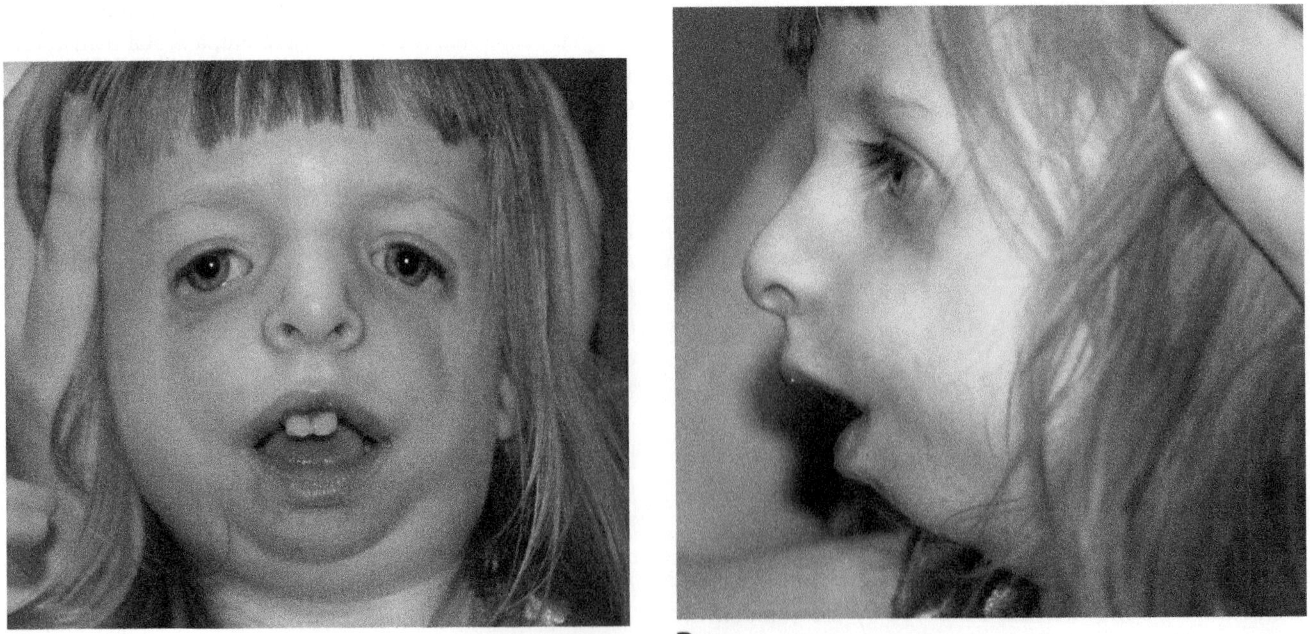

A B

FIG. 45-3.

16. The child shown in Fig. 45-4 is at increased risk for
    A. Brain aneurysm
    B. Hepatic hemangioma
    C. Leptomeningeal vascular anomalies
    D. Visceral aneurysm

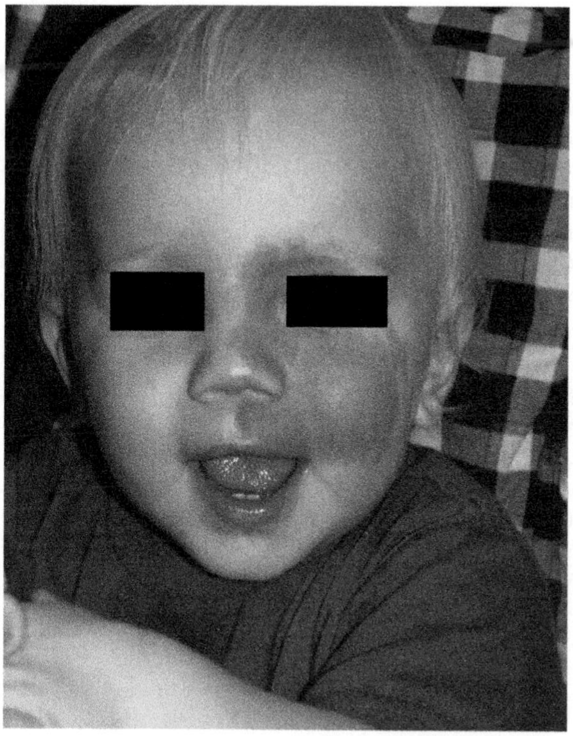

FIG. 45-4.

Answer: C

This is a child with Sturge-Weber syndrome. Capillary malformations (CMs) are pink-red macular vascular stains that are present at birth and persist throughout life. These lesions tend to become more verrucous and darker throughout life. CMs are effectively treated with a pulsed-dye laser, and the results often are better with treatment in infancy and young childhood. Laser therapy often is repetitive and prolonged. CMs of the head and neck, historically called *port-wine stains*, may be associated with Sturge-Weber syndrome, which includes vascular involvement of the leptomeninges and ocular pathology. (See Schwartz 9th ed., p 1667, 68.)

17. Immediate breast reconstruction (at the time of mastectomy) is associated with
    A. Delay in starting chemotherapy
    B. Decreased ability to detect an early recurrence
    C. Slightly increased mortality
    D. None of the above

Answer: D

A number of studies have shown that breast reconstruction, both immediate and delayed, does not impede standard oncologic treatment, does not delay detection of recurrent cancer, and does not change the overall mortality associated with the disease. (See Schwartz 9th ed., p 1682.)

18. Which of the following is a sign of venous occlusion in a free flap?
    A. Increasing warmth
    B. Increasing coolness
    C. Increasing paleness
    D. Increasing sluggishness of pinprick bleeding

Answer: A

Clinical flap monitoring continues after successful restoration of arterial inflow and venous outflow. The mainstay of postoperative free flap monitoring is clinical assessment (see Table 45-2), although supplementary instrument monitoring also can be helpful. (See Schwartz 9th ed., p 1657.)

TABLE 45-2 Clinical signs of arterial and venous compromise in a free flap[a]

Clinical Sign	Arterial Compromise	Venous Compromise
Color	Becoming paler	Increasingly reddish or purplish
Temperature	Becoming cooler	Becoming warmer
Tissue turgor	Reducing	Increasing
Capillary refill time	Becoming slower	Becoming faster
Pinprick bleeding	Increasingly sluggish	Quickening (and darkening)

[a]Note that venous and arterial compromise may coexist, and one may lead to the other.

19. A child with more than three cutaneous hemangiomas should undergo
    A. Abdominal ultrasound
    B. CT of the abdomen
    C. MRI of the brain
    D. MRA of the abdominal vasculature

Answer: A

Hemangiomas are solitary in 80% of cases and multiple in 20%. In children with multiple (more than three) cutaneous hemangiomas, abdominal ultrasound is suggested to rule out hemangiomatosis with visceral involvement. (See Schwartz 9th ed., p 1667.)

20. The flap illustrated in Fig. 45-5 is a
    A. Transposition flap
    B. Bipedicle flap
    C. Interpolation flap
    D. Rotational flap

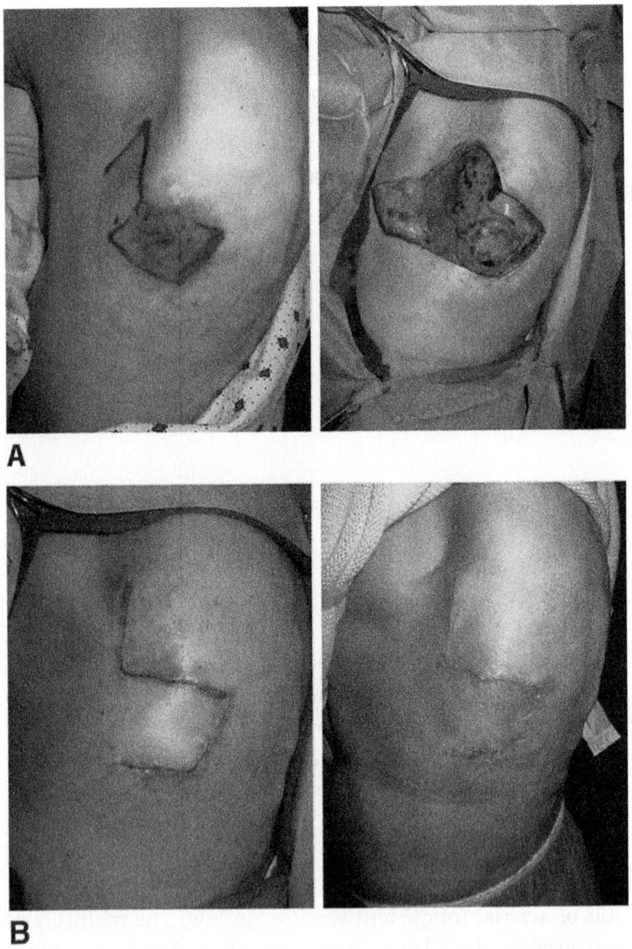

FIG. 45-5. (Photographs reproduced with permission from M. Gimbel.)

Answer: A

The flap illustrated is a rhomboid (Limberg) transposition flap. A *transposition flap* is rotated about a pivot point into an adjacent defect. A *Z-plasty* is a type of transposition flap in which two flaps are rotated, each into the donor site of the other, to achieve central limb lengthening. Another common transposition flap is the *rhomboid (Limberg) flap*. The *bipedicle flap* is comprised of two mirror-image transposition flaps that share their distal, undivided margin. *Rotational flaps* are similar to transpositional flaps but differ in that they are semicircular. *Advancement flaps* slide forward or backward along the flap's long axis. Two common variants include the rectangular advancement flap and the V-Y advancement flap. Like transposition flaps, *interpolation flaps* rotate about a pivot point. Unlike transposition flaps, they are inset into defects near, but not adjacent, to the donor site. An example of an interpolation flap is the thenar flap for fingertip reconstruction. (See Schwartz 9th ed., p 1651.)

CHAPTER 46

Surgical Considerations in the Elderly

BASIC SCIENCE QUESTIONS

1. For each decade of advanced age, cardiac output decreases by approximately
   A. 2%
   B. 5%
   C. 10%
   D. 14%

Answer: C
Cardiac complications are the leading cause of perioperative complications and death in surgical patients of all age groups, but particularly among the elderly. This is because they likely have existing cardiac dysfunction, combined with normal physiologic decline and poor functional reserve. The combined effect of depletion of intravascular volume, age-related impairment of response to catecholamines, and increased myocardial relaxation time adversely affects the functioning of an elderly patient under stress in the perioperative period. Aging has been demonstrated to cause a decrease in cardiac output by approximately 1% per year. Older individuals fail to augment heart rate to the same extent as younger individuals. More importantly, the ability to increase cardiac output with aging is dependent on ventricular dilatation, which is determined by preload. This is precisely the reason that careful attention must be paid to volume status in the perioperative period. Dehydration or poor resuscitation may occur in elderly surgical patients for a variety of reasons, and both are poorly tolerated. Over one half of all postoperative deaths in elderly patients and 11% of postoperative complications are a result of impaired cardiac function under physiologic stress. (See Schwartz 9th ed., p 1712.)

2. Maximal pulmonary capacity at age 70 is what percent of maximal pulmonary capacity at age 30?
   A. 90%
   B. 70%
   C. 50%
   D. 30%

Answer: C
The result of the changes that occur with the respiratory system with aging limits the maximal breathing capacity by age 70 to 50% of the capacity present at age 30. In addition, there is a decline in the forced expiratory volume in 1 second (FEV1) with advancing age. It is estimated that humans lose 35 mL of their FEV1 per year over the age of 35 years old. There is a slow decline between ages 35 and 65 years old followed by a much more progressive decline at approximately 75 years of age. (See Schwartz 9th ed., p 1712.)

3. Which one of the following changes occurs in the kidney with aging?
   A. Increased filtration area
   B. Increased creatinine clearance
   C. Decreased glomerular filtration rate
   D. Decreased sensitivity to many anesthetic agents

Answer: C
Renal size and volume decrease with age, accompanied by intrarenal vascular changes. There is a decrease in the number of glomeruli and nephron mass, resulting in decreased filtration area. Subsequently, serum creatinine concentration is an insensitive indicator of renal function in the elderly. The physiologic changes in renal function in elderly patients increase

susceptibility to renal ischemia as well as to nephrotoxic agents. Age-related changes in renal function result from progressive glomerulosclerosis and reduction in renal mass resulting in decreased creatinine clearance and glomerular filtration rate. This is worsened by a decline in cardiac output with increasing age and subsequent decrease in renal blood flow. It has been shown that patients with impaired glomerular filtration rate are more susceptible to volume changes that occur in the perioperative period. Furthermore, decreased drug elimination can potentiate the effects of nephrotoxic drugs and prolong the sedative effects of anesthetics and narcotic used for postoperative pain management. (See Schwartz 9th ed., p 1712.)

CLINICAL QUESTIONS

1. Which of the following is one of the physiologic changes of aging?
   A. Decreased fat mass
   B. Decreased pulmonary closing volume
   C. Decreased vascular baroreceptor sensitivity
   D. Decreased renal glucose threshold

Answer: C
(See Schwartz 9th ed., p 1711.)

2. The most common indication for surgery in the elderly is
   A. Obstructive vascular disease
   B. Thrombotic vascular disease
   C. Biliary tract disease
   D. Colorectal disease

Answer: C
Acute appendicitis and acute cholecystitis are examples of common acute surgical pathologies with which elderly patients present late or have delayed diagnosis or misdiagnosis. This often leads to higher rates of perforation and complications that adversely affect morbidity and mortality. In fact, biliary tract disease, including acute cholecystitis, is the most common indication for surgical intervention in the elderly. This is likely related to age-related changes within the biliary system, specifically increased lithogenicity of bile and increased prevalence of cholelithiasis. Delayed diagnosis may lead to complications such as ascending cholangitis and gallstone ileus. (See Schwartz 9th ed., p 1711.)

3. Which of the following tests of function in an elderly patient can be used to predict the time to recover after surgery?
   A. Hand grip strength
   B. Timed up and go test
   C. Functional reach test
   D. All of the above

Answer: D
It is important that a thorough preoperative evaluation include an accurate assessment of the functional status of surgical candidates as well as their cognitive level of functioning. This ensures that operative intervention will not significantly impair the quality of life of an elderly surgical candidate. The ability to withstand the stress of surgical interventions is dependent on functional reserve and ability to build an appropriate response to perioperative stress. The ability to perform activities of daily living (ADL) such as feeding, dressing, bathing, and toileting have been correlated with postoperative morbidity and mortality. Preoperative functional assessment can be measured by hand grip strength, timed up and go, and functional reach tests. All of these tests independently predicted better recovery and shorter time to recover ADL after major surgery. In addition, these tests provide an accurate assessment of a patientís muscle mass, nutritional status, coordination, gait speed, balance, and mobility. Proper functional assessment will accurately predict rehabilitation needs, estimate biologic reserve, and even signal complications. (See Schwartz 9th ed., p 1714.)

4. Protein energy malnutrition in an elderly surgical patient can result in
   A. Decreased range of motion of major joints
   B. Decreased glomerular filtration rate
   C. Decreased mucosal proliferation
   D. Decreased mental status

Answer: C

Protein energy malnutrition (PEM) also can result from keeping surgical patients who may already have inadequate nutritional reserve NPO. This may occur in a short period in the elderly, malnourished surgical patient in a hypermetabolic state induced by stress of illness and surgery. The physiologic consequences of PEM are multiple and include anorexia, hepatic dysfunction, decreased mucosal proliferation, and sarcopenia. A good marker of PEM is hypoalbuminemia, also shown to be an extremely accurate predictor of surgical outcomes. The incidence of postoperative complications was increased in patients with serum albumin levels <3.5 g/L. In fact, current recommendations indicate that if patients demonstrate compromise of nutritional status as defined by >10% weight loss and serum albumin level <2.5 g/dL, they should be considered for a minimum of 7 to 10 days of nutritional repletion prior to surgery. (See Schwartz 9th ed., p 1714.)

5. Which of the following is an independent predictor of mortality in elderly patients undergoing major cardiovascular surgery?
   A. Age >75
   B. ASA class 2 or greater
   C. Renal insufficiency
   D. Reactive airway disease

Answer: C

Interestingly, despite some degree of age bias in referral patterns for elderly patients to undergo major cardiac surgery, advanced age alone is not a predictor of poorer outcomes or increased mortality when compared to younger patients. It has been demonstrated that emergency operations, preoperative New York Heart Association (NYHA) functional class 3 or greater, and chronic renal failure were the main predictors of increased operative mortality. In one study, preoperative renal dysfunction, cerebrovascular disease, valve surgery, and catastrophic state were independent predictors of increased mortality in elderly patients. Elderly patients with nondialysis-dependent renal dysfunction had a 60% chance of death during a 5-year follow-up period compared to 25% in elderly patients without a history of renal dysfunction. Similarly, the presence of cerebrovascular disease resulted in a twofold increase in mortality among elderly patients. Even patients who were 80 years of age or more did not have any significant increase in surgical risk and within this population, the 4-year actuarial survival was 70.5% with an event-free survival of approximately 60.6%. (See Schwartz 9th ed., p 1716.)

6. The most common valvular abnormality requiring surgery in elderly patients is
   A. Aortic stenosis
   B. Aortic insufficiency
   C. Mitral stenosis
   D. Mitral insufficiency

Answer: A

There also is an increasing percentage of the geriatric population presenting with symptomatic valvular disease requiring intervention. The most common valvular abnormality present in elderly patients is calcific aortic stenosis, which can lead to angina and syncope. The operative mortality from aortic valve replacement is estimated to be between 3 and 10%, with an average of approximately 7.7%. If aortic stenosis is allowed to progress without operative intervention, CHF will ensue. The average survival of these patients is approximately 1.5 to 2 years. If a patient is a candidate for operative intervention, age should not be a deterrent, especially considering the potential to increase life expectancy. (See Schwartz 9th ed., p 1716.)

7. Renal transplantation in elderly patients
   A. Should be considered only if predicted life expectancy is >5 years
   B. Requires greater immunosuppression than in younger recipients
   C. May be accomplished by transplanting two kidneys from "extended criteria donors"
   D. Results in worse graft function than in younger recipients

Answer: C

In the last decade, there has been a shift favoring the transplantation of kidneys from older donors as well as transplantation of donor grafts to older recipients. A new strategy is the use of "extended criteria donors" (ECDs) for elderly recipients, using dual kidney transplantation to increase the net total nephron mass, resulting in favorable outcomes. The increased nephron mass achieved with dual kidney transplantation compensated for the possible decreased renal function with advancing age. The net result is that recipients demonstrate similar postoperative graft function when compared to single kidney transplantation. Elderly recipients of ECD kidneys demonstrated a 25% decrease in risk of mortality compared to waitlisted patients on hemodialysis.

Successful kidney transplantation is preferred treatment for ESRD and long-term patient survival is higher in elderly patients who have been transplanted compared to those that remain on hemodialysis. The projected life span for patients currently on the transplant waiting list who are age 60 to 74 years old is approximately 6 years. This increases to 10 years posttransplantation. For comparison, the expected life span of a 70-year-old patient in the general population is 13.4 years. Among dialysis patients ages 70 years and older, renal transplantation was associated with a 41% lower risk of death compared to age matched wait-listed patients. A clear survival advantage also has been demonstrated in carefully selected patients 75 years and older. A benefit is observed among patients whose life expectancy is expected to exceed 1.8 years.

Elderly patients have better graft function, with decreased incidence of delayed graft function and fewer episodes of acute rejection, than do younger patients. This may be the result of decreased immune competence with aging. (See Schwartz 9th ed., p 1717.)

8. What percent of breast cancers in the United States are diagnosed after 75 years of age?
   A. 5%
   B. 15%
   C. 25%
   D. 35%

Answer: C

It is projected that there will be a 72% increase in the number of elderly women diagnosed with breast cancer in the United States by 2025. Furthermore, 50% of breast cancers occur after the age of 65 years old and 25% after the age of 75 years old. The estimated risk for development of new breast cancer is one in 24 women aged 60 to 79 years old compared to one in 24 in women aged 40 to 59 years old. (See Schwartz 9th ed., p 1719.)

9. Which one of the following lung cancers is more common in elderly patients than younger patients?
   A. Small cell
   B. Squamous cell
   C. Adenocarcinoma
   D. Large cell

Answer: B

Non–small cell lung cancer accounts for roughly 80% of all lung cancer cases, and >50% of these patients are >65 years of age. Interestingly, approximately 30% of these patients are 70 years or older at diagnosis. Lung cancer is highly prevalent among elderly patients, so much so that a 2-cm, asymptomatic, solitary pulmonary nodule in a 70-year-old male smoker has a >70% chance of being an occult lung cancer. Squamous cell carcinomas are more common among elderly patients than among younger patients, and these tumors are associated with a higher incidence of local disease, tend to have lower recurrence rates, and have longer survival times than non-squamous cancers. In cases of resectable primary lung cancer, surgery remains the treatment of choice independent of age. (See Schwartz 9th ed., p 1720.)

10. Thyroid cancer in the elderly, when compared to younger patients
   A. Has a lower mortality rate
   B. Has a lower risk of metastases
   C. Is more likely to have vascular invasion
   D. Is proportionally less likely to be follicular carcinoma

Answer: C

Papillary carcinoma in elderly patients tends to be sporadic with a bell-shaped distribution of age at presentation, occurring primarily in patients aged 30 to 59 years old. The incidence of papillary carcinoma decreases in patients >60 years of age. However, patients >60 years of age have increased risk of local recurrence and for the development of distant metastases. Metastatic disease may be more common in this population secondary to delayed referral for surgical intervention because of the misconception that the surgeon will be unwilling to operate on an elderly patient with thyroid disease. Age is also a prognostic indicator for patients with follicular carcinoma. There is a 2.2 times increased risk of mortality from follicular carcinoma per 20 years of increasing age. Therefore, prognosis for elderly patients with differentiated thyroid carcinomas is worse when compared to younger counterparts. The higher prevalence of vascular invasion and extracapsular extension among older patients is, in part, responsible for the poorer prognosis in geriatric patients. (See Schwartz 9th ed., p 1723.)

11. Indications for surgical treatment of primary hyperparathyroidism in elderly patients include
   A. 10% decrease in creatinine clearance
   B. Urinary calcium excretion >100 mg
   C. Serum calcium >12.0
   D. Altered mental status

Answer: D

Approximately 2% of the geriatric population, including 3% of women 75 years of age or older, will develop primary hyperparathyroidism. Specific indications for operative intervention regardless of age include a 30% decrease in creatinine clearance, 24-hour urinary calcium excretion >400 mg, and decreased bone density. Elderly patients are especially prone to developing mental manifestations of hyperparathyroidism that may be severe enough to produce a dementia-like state. There often is a significant improvement in mental status after parathyroidectomy. (See Schwartz 9th ed., p 1724.)

CHAPTER 47

Anesthesia of the Surgical Patient

BASIC SCIENCE QUESTIONS

1. The therapeutic index is the
   A. ratio of the sensitivity and efficacy of a drug
   B. ratio of the lethal dose and effective dose of a drug
   C. ratio of the efficacy and potency of a drug
   D. ratio of the sensitivity and potency of a drug

Answer: B

The *lethal dose* (LD_{50}) of a drug produces death in 50% of animals to which it is given. The average sensitivity to a particular drug can be expressed through the calculation of the effective dose; ED_{50} would have the desired effect in 50% of the general population. The ratio of the lethal dose and effective dose, LD_{50}/ED_{50}, is the *therapeutic index.* A drug with a high therapeutic index is safer than a drug with a low or narrow therapeutic index.

The *potency* of a drug is the dose required to produce a given effect, such as pain relief or a change in heart rate. The *efficacy* of any therapeutic agent is its power to produce a desired effect. (See Schwartz 9th ed., p 1734.)

2. Local anesthetics block nerve conduction by their effect on the
   A. Calcium channel
   B. Sodium channel
   C. Potassium channel
   D. None of the above

Answer: B

The common characteristic of all local anesthetics is a reversible block of the transmission of neural impulses when placed on or near a nerve membrane. Local anesthetics block nerve conduction by stabilizing sodium channels in their closed state, preventing action potentials from propagating along the nerve. The individual local anesthetic agents have different recovery times based on lipid solubility and tissue binding, but return of neural function is spontaneous as the drug is metabolized or removed from the nerve by the vascular system. (See Schwartz 9th ed., p 1736.)

3. Which of the following induction agents does NOT work by its effect on the γ-aminobutyric acid (GABA) receptor?
   A. Ketamine
   B. Propofol
   C. Etomidate
   D. Thiopental

Answer: A

Ketamine differs from the above IV agents in that it produces analgesia as well as amnesia. Its principal action is on the *N*-methyl-D-aspartate receptor; it has no action on the GABA receptor. Propofol is an alkylated phenol that inhibits synaptic transmission through its effects at the GABA receptor.

Etomidate is an imidazole derivative used for IV induction. Its rapid and almost complete hydrolysis to inactive metabolites results in rapid awakening. Like the above IV agents, etomidate acts on the GABA receptor.

The most common barbiturates are thiopental, thiamylal, and methohexital. The mechanism of action is at the γ-GABA receptor, where they inhibit excitatory synaptic transmission. (See Schwartz 9th ed., p 1737.)

4. Reversal of a neuromuscular blockade is accomplished by
   A. Direct antagonism of the agent
   B. Increase in acetylcholine
   C. Increasing breakdown of the neuromuscular blocking agent
   D. None of the above

Answer: B
Reversal agents raise the concentration of the neurotransmitter acetylcholine to a higher level than that of the neuromuscular blocking agent. This is accomplished by the use of anticholinesterase agents, which reduce the breakdown of acetylcholine. The most commonly used agents are neostigmine, pyridostigmine, and edrophonium. (See Schwartz 9th ed., p 1749.)

5. Which of the following local anesthetic agents is an ester?
   A. Lidocaine
   B. Mepivacaine
   C. Prilocaine
   D. Benzocaine

Answer: D
Local anesthetics are divided into two groups based on their chemical structure: the amides and the esters. In general, the amides are metabolized in the liver and the esters are metabolized by plasma cholinesterases, which yield metabolites with slightly higher allergic potential than the amides.

Lidocaine, bupivacaine, mepivacaine, prilocaine, and ropivacaine have in common an amide linkage between a benzene ring and a hydrocarbon chain that, in turn, is attached to a tertiary amine. The benzene ring confers lipid solubility for penetration of nerve membranes, and the tertiary amine attached to the hydrocarbon chain makes these local anesthetics water soluble.

Cocaine, procaine, chloroprocaine, tetracaine, and benzocaine have an ester linkage in place of the amide linkage mentioned above in the Amides section. (See Schwartz 9th ed., p 1736.)

CLINICAL QUESTIONS

1. Which of the following anesthetic agents has the longest duration?
   A. Prilocaine
   B. Etidocaine
   C. Procaine
   D. Mepivacaine

Answer: B
Etidocaine is the longest acting local anesthetic. (See Schwartz 9th ed., p 1736, and Table 47-1.)

TABLE 47-1 Biologic properties of commonly used local anesthetics

Agent	Equianesthetic Concentration (%)	Approximate Anesthetic Duration (min)	Site of Metabolism
Esters			
Procaine	2	50	Plasma
Chloroprocaine	2	45	Plasma
Tetracaine	0.25	175	Plasma
Amides			
Prilocaine	1	100	Liver/lung
Lidocaine	1	100	Liver
Mepivacaine	1	100	Liver
Bupivacaine	0.25	175	Liver
Ropivacaine	0.3	150	Liver
Etidocaine	0.25	200	Liver

Source: Reproduced with permission from Mather LE, Tucker GT: Properties, absorption, and disposition of local anesthetic agents, in Cousins MJ, Bridenbaugh PO (eds): *Cousins and Bridenbaugh's Neural Blockade in Clinical Anesthesia and Pain Medicine*, 4th ed. Philadelphia: Lippincott Williams & Wilkins, 2009, p 49.

2. What is the maximum number of cc's of 1% lidocaine that can be used for local anesthesia in a 20-kg child?
   A. 5 ml
   B. 10 ml
   C. 20 ml
   D. 50 ml

Answer: B
The toxic dose of lidocaine is approximately 5 mg/kg; that of bupivacaine is approximately 3 mg/kg. Calculation of the toxic dose before injection is imperative. It is helpful to remember that for any drug or solution, 1% = 10 mg/mL.

For a 50-kg person, the toxic dose of bupivacaine would be approximately 3 mg/kg = 150 mg. A 0.5% solution of bupivacaine is 5 mg/mL, so 150 mL/5 mg/mL = 30 mL as the upper limit for infiltration. For lidocaine in the same patient, the calculation is 50 kg × 5 mg/mL = 250 mg toxic dose. If a 1% solution is used, the allowed amount would be 250 mg/10 mg/mL = 25 mL. (See Schwartz 9th ed., p 1736.)

3. Succinylcholine should NOT be used for induction in a patient with
   A. An open femur fracture
   B. A crush injury to the lower extremity
   C. Atherosclerotic occlusion of the femoral artery
   D. A burn to the foot

Answer: B

Although the rapid onset (<60 seconds) and rapid offset (5 to 8 minutes) make succinylcholine ideal for management of the airway in certain situations, total body muscle fasciculations can cause postoperative aches and pains, an elevation in serum potassium levels, and an increase in intraocular and intragastric pressure. Its use in patients with burns or traumatic tissue injuries may result in a high enough rise in serum potassium levels to produce arrhythmias and cardiac arrest. (See Schwartz 9th ed., p 1738.)

4. Which of the following is the LEAST potent inhalational agent?
   A. Halothane
   B. Enflurane
   C. Isoflurane
   D. Nitrous oxide

Answer: D

Minimum alveolar concentration (MAC) is a measure of anesthetic potency. It is the ED_{50} of an inhaled agent (i.e., the dose required to block a response to a painful stimulus in 50% of subjects). The higher the MAC, the less potent an agent is. The potency and speed of induction of inhaled agents correlates with their lipid solubility and is known as the *Meyer-Overton rule*. Nitrous oxide has a low solubility and is a weak anesthetic agent, but has the most rapid onset and offset. The 'potent' gases (e.g., desflurane, sevoflurane, enflurane, and halothane) are more soluble in blood than nitrous oxide and can be given in lower concentrations, but have longer induction and emergence characteristics. (See Schwartz 9th ed., p 1739, and Table 47-2.)

TABLE 47-2 Advantages and disadvantages of common inhalational agents

Agent	MAC (%)	Advantages	Disadvantages
Nitrous oxide	105	Analgesia; minimal cardiac and respiratory depression	Sympathetic stimulation; expansion of closed air space
Halothane	0.75	Effective in low concentrations; minimal airway irritability; inexpensive	Cardiac depression and arrhythmia hepatic necrosis; slow elimination
Enflurane	1.68	Muscle relaxation No effect on cardiac rate or rhythm	Strong smell; seizures
Isoflurane	1.15	Muscle relaxation; no effect on cardiac rate or rhythm	Strong smell
Desflurane	6	Rapid induction and emergence	Coughing; high cost
Sevoflurane	1.71	Rapid induction and emergence; pleasant smell; ideal for mask induction	High cost; metabolized by liver

MAC = minimum alveolar concentration.
Source: Adapted with permission from Rutter TW, Tremper KK: Anesthesiology and pain management, in Greenfield LJ (eds): *Greenfield's Surgery: Scientific Principles and Practice*, 4th ed. Philadelphia: Lippincott & Williams, 2006, p 450.

5. Which of the following nerves are NOT blocked by spinal or epidural anesthesia?
   A. Motor
   B. Sensory
   C. Sympathetic
   D. Parasympathetic

Answer: D

As in spinal anesthesia, local anesthetic delivered to the epidural space bathes the spinal nerves as they exit the dura; the patient achieves analgesia from the sensory block, muscle relaxation from blockade of the motor nerves, and hypotension from blockade of the sympathetic nerves as they exit the spinal cord. (See Schwartz 9th ed., p 1737.)

6. The Mallampati classification is a risk stratification that evaluates a patient's
   A. Overall health
   B. Airway status
   C. Pulmonary status
   D. Circulatory status

Answer: B

The amount of the posterior pharynx one can visualize preoperatively is important and correlates with the difficulty of intubation. A large tongue (relative to the size of the mouth) that also interferes with visualization of the larynx on laryngoscopy will obscure visualization of the pharynx. The Mallampati classification (Fig. 47-1, Table 47-3) is based on the structures visualized with maximal mouth opening and tongue protrusion in the sitting position. (See Schwartz 9th ed., p 1740.)

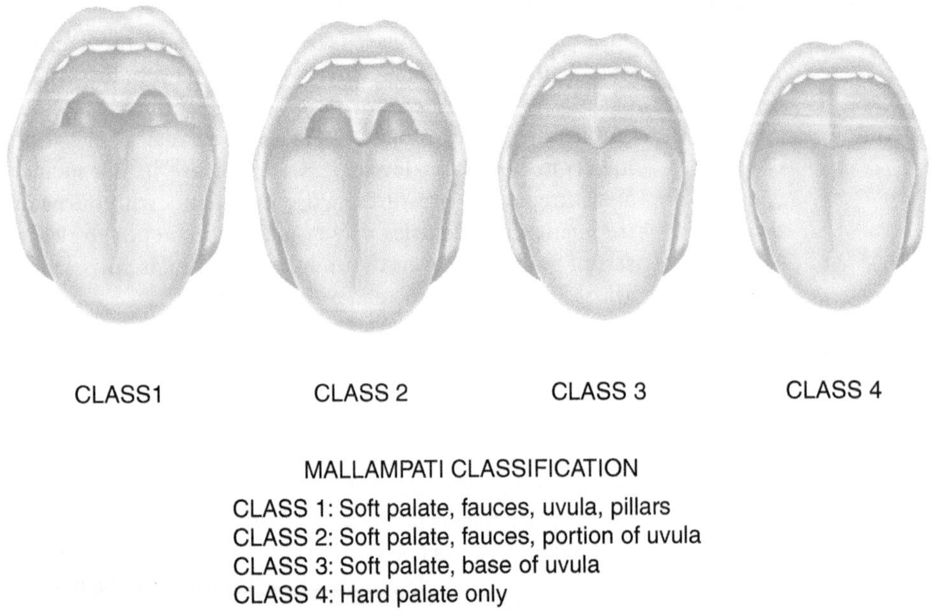

FIG. 47-1. The Mallampati classification.

TABLE 47-3 Mallampati classification
Class I: soft palate, fauces, uvula, pillars
Class II: soft palate, fauces, portion of uvula
Class III: soft palate, base of uvula
Class IV: hard palate only

7. The risk of "spinal headache" after a spinal anesthetic can be decreased by
   A. Using a small needle
   B. Slower injection of the anesthetic agent
   C. A traumatic lumbar puncture
   D. Increasing the narcotics instilled into the spinal fluid

Answer: A

Possible complications of spinal anesthesia include hypotension, especially if the patient is not adequately prehydrated; high spinal block requires immediate airway management; and postdural puncture headache sometimes occurs. Spinal headache is related to the diameter and configuration of the spinal needle, and can be reduced to approximately 1% with the use of a small 25- or 27-gauge needle. (See Schwartz 9th ed., p 1737.)

8. Which of the following is a potential triggering agent for malignant hyperthermia?
   A. Rocuronium
   B. Ketamine
   C. Propofol
   D. Isoflurane

Answer: D

Triggering agents for malignant hyperthermia include all volatile anesthetics (e.g., halothane, enflurane, isoflurane, sevoflurane, and desflurane), and the depolarizing muscle relaxant succinylcholine. (See Schwartz 9th ed., p 1750.)

9. Which of the following agents produces the least respiratory depression?
   A. Fentanyl
   B. Sufentanil
   C. Remifentanil
   D. None of the above

Answer: D

Although opioids have differing potencies required for effective analgesia, *equianalgesic doses of opioids result in equal degrees of respiratory depression*. Thus, there is no completely safe opioid analgesic. (See Schwartz 9th ed., p 1738.)

10. A 55-year-old man is scheduled to undergo an elective resection of a sessile polyp of the colon. He has chronic obstructive pulmonary disease and coronary artery disease, both of which are relatively well controlled by medication. He would be classified as
    A. ASA Class 2
    B. ASA Class 3
    C. ASA Class 4
    D. ASA Class 5

Answer: B

Research into quantifying preoperative factors that correlate with the development of postoperative morbidity and mortality has recently gained great interest. Originally designed as a simple classification of a patient's physical status immediately before surgery, the ASA physical status scale is one of the few prospective scales that correlate with the risk of anesthesia and surgery (Table 47-4). (See Schwartz 9th ed., p 1740.)

TABLE 47-4	American Society of Anesthesiologists physical status classification system
P1	A normal healthy patient
P2	A patient with mild systemic disease
P3	A patient with severe systemic disease
P4	A patient with severe systemic disease that is a constant threat to life
P5	A moribund patient who is not expected to survive without the operation
P6	A declared brain-dead patient whose organs are being removed for donor purposes

11. Inhalational anesthetic agents
    A. Dilate the airways
    B. Constrict the airways
    C. Increase the production of sputum
    D. Decrease the production of sputum

Answer: A

General anesthesia can be performed safely in patients with pulmonary disease. Inhaled anesthetics are often used due to their bronchodilating properties. (See Schwartz 9th ed., p 1741.)

12. Which of the following techniques for induction of general anesthesia is most commonly used in children?
    A. Intravenous induction
    B. Rapid sequence induction
    C. Inhalational induction
    D. Combined induction

Answer: C

Patients undergoing *inhalation induction* progress through three stages: (a) awake, (b) excitement, and (c) surgical level of anesthesia. Adult patients are not good candidates for this type of induction, as the smell of the inhalation agent is unpleasant and the excitement stage can last for several minutes, which may cause hypertension, tachycardia, laryngospasm, vomiting, and aspiration. Children, however, progress through stage 2 quickly and are highly motivated for inhalation induction as an alternative to the IV route. The benefit of postinduction IV cannulation is the avoidance of many presurgical anxieties, and inhalation induction is the most common technique for pediatric surgery. (See Schwartz 9th ed., p 1743, and Fig. 47-2.)

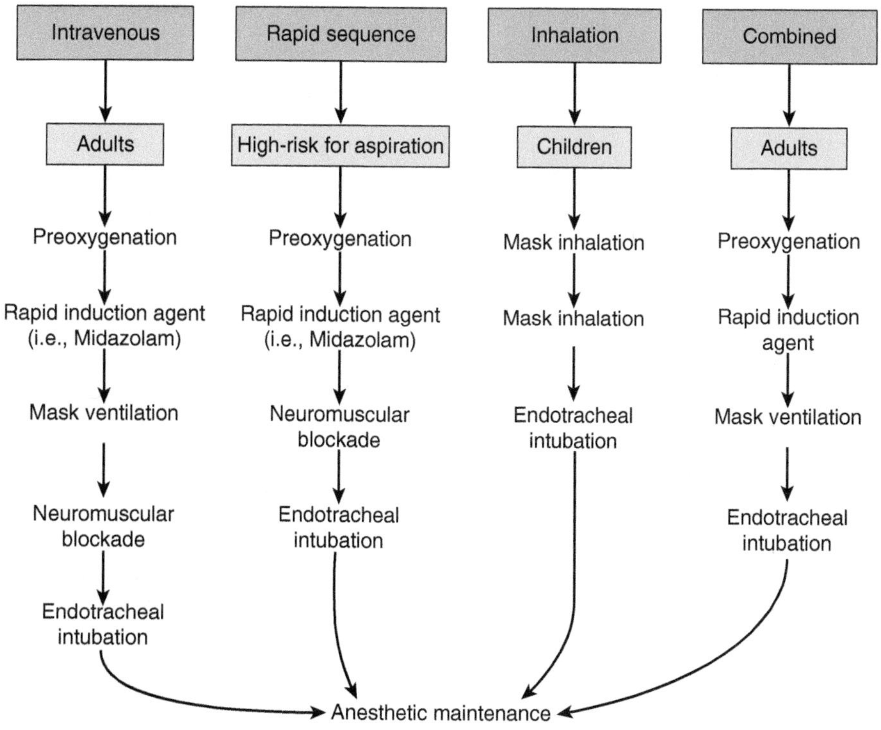

FIG. 47-2. Techniques for the induction of general anesthesia.

13. Patients with inherited atypical pseudocholinesterase should be advised to avoid
    A. Mivacurium
    B. Methohexitol
    C. Propofol
    D. Ketamine

Answer: A

Some patients have a genetic disorder manifesting as atypical plasma cholinesterase; the atypical enzyme has less-than-normal activity, and/or the patient has extremely low levels of the enzyme. The incidence of the homozygous form is approximately one in 3000; the effects of a single dose of succinylcholine may last several hours instead of several minutes. Two separate blood tests must be drawn: *pseudocholinesterase level* to determine the amount of enzyme present, and *dibucaine number*, which indicates the quality of the enzyme. Patients with laboratory-confirmed abnormal pseudocholinesterase levels and/or dibucaine numbers should be counseled to avoid succinylcholine as well as mivacurium, which is also hydrolyzed by pseudocholinesterase. First-degree family members should also be tested. (See Schwartz 9th ed., p 1738.)

14. Which of the following nondepolarizing neuromuscular blockers has the longest duration of action?
    A. Mivacurium
    B. Vecuronium
    C. Rocuronium
    D. Pancuronium

Answer: D

There are several competitive *nondepolarizing* agents available for clinical use. The longest acting is *pancuronium*, which is excreted almost completely unchanged by the kidney. Intermediate duration neuromuscular blockers include *vecuronium* and *rocuronium*, which are metabolized by both the kidneys and liver, and *atracurium* and cis-*atracurium*, which undergo breakdown in plasma known as *Hofmann elimination*. The agent with shortest duration is *mivacurium*, the only nondepolarizer that is metabolized by plasma cholinesterase, and like succinylcholine, is subject to the same prolonged blockade in patients with plasma cholinesterase deficiency. (See Schwartz 9th ed., p 1738, and Table 47-5.)

TABLE 47-5 Advantages and disadvantages to common nondepolarizing neuromuscular blocking agents

Agent	Duration (h)	Advantages	Disadvantages
Pancuronium	>1	No histamine release	Tachycardia; slow onset; long duration
Vecuronium	<1	No cardiovascular effects	Intermediate onset
Rocuronium	<1	Fast onset; no cardiovascular effects	—
Mivacurium	<1	Fast onset; short duration & histamine release	—

Source: Adapted with permission from Rutter TW, Tremper KK: Anesthesiology and pain management, in Greenfield LJ (ed): *Greenfield's Surgery: Scientific Principles and Practice*, 4th ed. Philadelphia: Lippincott & Williams, 2006, p 452.

15. Which of the following inhalational agents would be the best choice for a patient with chronic liver disease?
    A. Halothane
    B. Isoflurane
    C. Desflurane
    D. Sevoflurane

Answer: D

Halothane, enflurane, isoflurane, and desflurane all yield a reactive oxidative trifluoroacetyl halide and may be cross-reactive, but the magnitude of metabolism of the volatile anesthetics is a probable factor in the ability to cause hepatitis. Halothane is metabolized 20%, enflurane 2%, isoflurane 0.2%, and desflurane 0.02%; desflurane probably has the least potential for liver injury. Sevoflurane does not yield any trifluoroacetylated metabolites and is unlikely to cause hepatitis. (See Schwartz 9th ed., p 1742.)

16. Inhalational agents provide all of the following EXCEPT
    A. Unconsciousness
    B. Analgesia
    C. Amnesia
    D. Muscle relaxation

Answer: C

Unlike the IV agents, the inhalational agents provide all three characteristics of general anesthesia: unconsciousness, analgesia, and muscle relaxation. However, it would be impractical to use an inhalational technique in larger surgical procedures, because the doses required would cause unacceptable side effects, so IV adjuncts such as opioid analgesics and neuromuscular blockers are added to optimize the anesthetic. (See Schwartz 9th ed., p 1739.)

CHAPTER 48

Ethics, Palliative Care, and Care at the End of Life

BASIC SCIENCE QUESTIONS

1. Which of the following is one of the four guiding principles of bioethics in the principlist approach?
   A. Adherence to the law
   B. Autonomy
   C. Good communication
   D. Obtaining all information before making a decision

Answer: B

Biomedical ethics is the system of analysis and deliberation dedicated to guiding surgeons toward the 'good' in the practice of surgery. One of the most influential ethical 'systems' in the field of biomedical ethics is the principlist approach as articulated by Beauchamp and Childress. In this approach to ethical issues, moral dilemmas are deliberated by using four guiding principles: autonomy, beneficence, nonmaleficence, and justice. (See Schwartz 9th ed., p 1753, 55, and Fig. 48-1.)

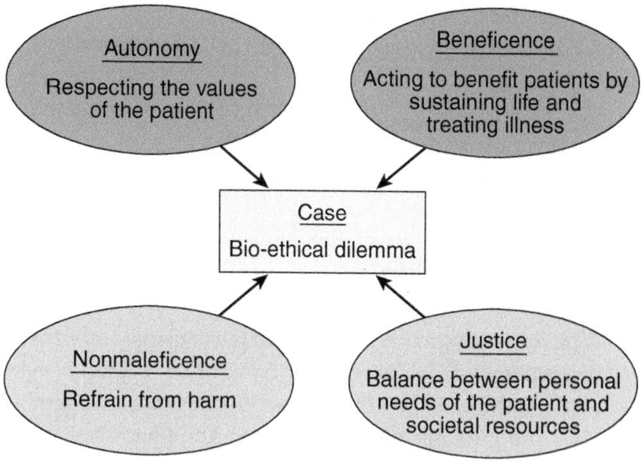

FIG. 48-1. The four principles of the care-based paradigm.

2. Which of the following is one of the four elements of informed consent?
   A. All family members must be informed of the options available
   B. The physician must document that the patient has the capacity to decide
   C. The patient must sign a legal consent form
   D. The legal consent form must be signed by a witness

Answer: B

Adequate informed consent entails at least four basic elements: a) The physician documents that the patient or surrogate has the capacity to make a medical decision; (b) The surgeon discloses to the patient details regarding the diagnosis and treatment options sufficiently for the patient to make an informed choice; (c) The patient demonstrates understanding of the disclosed information before (d) authorizing freely a specific treatment plan without undue influence.

The patient or the patient's surrogate is the only one who must be informed of the options available.

Although signing a legal consent form has become standard, it is not required to document informed consent. (See Schwartz 9th ed., p 1756.)

1. An unconscious accident victim is hypotensive from intra-abdominal hemorrhage and needs an emergency laparotomy. His identity is unknown and, therefore, no family is available. Which of the following should be done?
   A. Nothing; it is illegal to operate on a patient without consent
   B. The surgeon should document the need for the surgery in the chart and proceed
   C. Three doctors should document the need for the surgery in the chart and the surgeon should then proceed
   D. A court order for surgery should be obtained prior to proceeding

Answer: B

Emergency consent requires the surgeon to consider if and how possible interventions might save a patient's life, and if successful, what kind of disability might be anticipated. Surgical emergencies are one of the few instances where the limits of patient autonomy are freely acknowledged, and surgeons are empowered by law and ethics to act promptly in the best interests of their patients according to the surgeon's judgment. Most applicable medical laws require physicians to provide the standard of care to incapacitated patients, even if it entails invasive procedures without the explicit consent of the patient or surrogate. If at all possible, surgeons should seek the permission of their patients to provide treatment, but when emergency medical conditions render patients unable to grant that permission, and when delay is likely to have grave consequences, surgeons are legally and ethically justified in providing whatever surgical treatment the surgeon judges necessary to preserve life and restore health.

It would be unethical to withhold surgery from this patient. The concept of a "three doctor" documentation is not legally or ethically required in this situation, nor is a court order. (See Schwartz 9th ed., p 1756.)

2. A 3-year-old patient with a severe splenic injury is admitted to the ICU. Clinically, a transfusion is indicated. The parents are adamant that their religion forbids transfusions and threaten to sue the doctor if blood is transfused. The best course of action is
   A. Do not transfuse the patient, but use alternatives if available
   B. Try to reason with the family and obtain permission for transfusion
   C. Contact the hospital legal counsel and proceed with transfusion
   D. Proceed with transfusion after documenting the indication in the chart

Answer: C

Certain religious practices can present difficulties in treating minor children in need of life-saving blood transfusions; however, case law has made clear the precedent that parents, regardless of their held beliefs, may not place their minor children at mortal risk. In such a circumstance, the physician should seek counsel from the hospital medicolegal team, as well as from the institutional ethics team. Legal precedent has, in general, established that the hospital or physician can proceed with providing all necessary care for the child. (See Schwartz 9th ed., p 1757.)

3. A patient with carcinomatosis is requiring large amounts of morphine by PCA (averaging 15 mg/hr). Her pain is very poorly controlled and the pain service feels she will need at least 20mg/hr for adequate control. The pharmacy questions the dose since it is high enough to cause respiratory arrest. The appropriate course of action is
   A. Cancel the order and continue with her previous dose
   B. Compromise by increasing the dose, but not as much as planned
   C. Keep the order for 20 mg/hr
   D. Change to bolus morphine from the PCA

Answer: C

In deliberating the issue of withdrawing vs. withholding life-sustaining therapies, the principle of 'double effect' is often mentioned. According to the principle of 'double effect,' a treatment (e.g., opioid administration in the terminally ill) that is intended to help and not harm the patient (i.e., relieve pain) is ethically acceptable even if an unintended consequence (side effect) of its administration is to shorten the life of the patient (e.g., by respiratory depression). Under the principle of double effect, a physician may withhold or withdraw a life-sustaining therapy if the surgeon's *intent* is to relieve suffering, not to hasten death. The classic formulation of double effect has four elements (Fig. 48-2). (See Schwartz 9th ed., p 1758.)

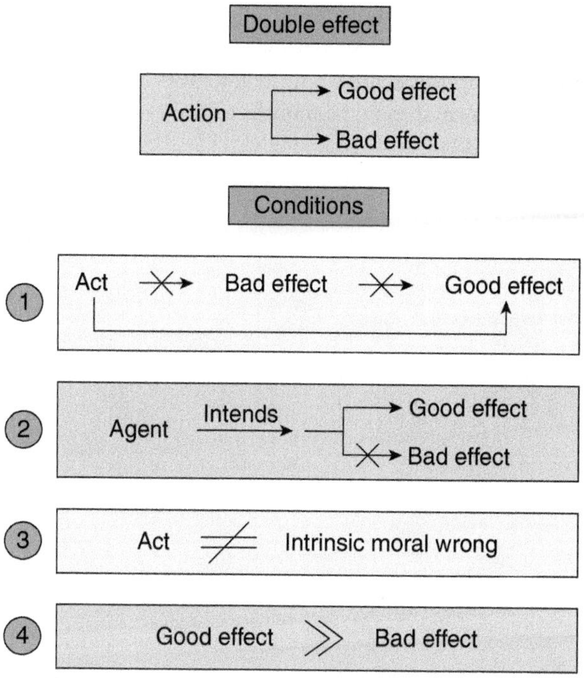

FIG. 48-2. The four elements of the double effect principle: 1) The good effect is produced directly by the action and not by the bad effect. 2) The person must intend only the good effect, even though the bad effect may be foreseen. 3) The act itself must not be intrinsically wrong, or needs to be at least neutral. 4) The good effect is sufficiently desirable to compensate for allowing the bad effect.

4. Which of the following is an indication for palliative care consultation?
   A. Any patient with a life-threatening diagnosis
   B. Counseling of physicians and staff after losing a colleague under their care
   C. Anticipation of painful procedures or other therapies
   D. Psychologic distress

Answer: B

Although not often used, palliative care teams provide bereavement support for physicians and staff after losing a patient.

Palliative care is primarily focused on end of life care. The diagnosis of a disease, anticipation of pain, or psychologic stress are not *per se* indications for a palliative care consultation.

Nathan Cherny, another pioneer of palliative care, echoes these themes in his definition of palliative care: '[it] is concerned with three things: the quality of life, the value of life, and the meaning of life.' Therefore, it is *existence*, not death, that is the focus of palliative care. (See Schwartz 9th ed., p 1759, and Table 48-1.)

TABLE 48-1 Indications for palliative care consultation

Patients with conditions that are progressive and life-limiting, especially if characterized by burdensome symptoms, functional decline, and progressive cognitive deficits
Assistance in clarification or reorientation of patient/family goals of care
Assistance in resolution of ethical dilemmas
Situations in which patient/surrogate declines further invasive or curative treatments with stated preference for comfort measures only
Patients who are expected to die imminently or shortly after hospital discharge
Provision of bereavement support for patient care staff, particularly after loss of a colleague under care

5. A patient with terminal cancer who is sleeping >50% of the day and requires some assistance with activities of daily living has approximately how long to live?
   A. Unknown, it could be months to years
   B. Months
   C. Weeks
   D. Days

Answer: C

For example, patients with advanced metastatic cancer who are resting/sleeping for 50% or more of normal waking hours and require some assistance with activities of daily living (ADL) have a projected survival of weeks, and patients who are essentially bedfast and dependent for ADL have a projected survival of days to a week or two at best. Table 48-2 shows a simple prognostic tool to aid clinicians in recognizing patients nearing the end of life. (See Schwartz 9th ed., p 1762.)

TABLE 48-2 Simple prognostication tool in advanced illness (especially cancer)

Functional Level	Performance Status (ECOG)	Prognosis
Able to perform all basic ADLs independently and some IADLs	2	Months
Resting/sleeping up to 50% or more of waking hours and requiring some assistance with basic ADLs	3	Weeks to a few months
Dependent for basic ADLs and bed to chair existence	4	Days to a few weeks at most

These observations apply to patients with advanced, progressive, incurable illnesses (e.g., metastatic cancer refractory to treatment). Basic ADL = activities of daily living (e.g., transferring, toileting, bathing, dressing, and feeding oneself); IADL = instrumental activities of daily living (e.g., more complex activities such as meal preparation, performing household chores, balancing a checkbook, shopping, etc.); ECOG = Eastern Cooperative Oncology Group functional (performance) status.

6. The primary treatment for dyspnea ("air hunger") in a dying patient is
   A. Supplemental oxygen by a non-rebreather mask
   B. Cooling the room
   C. Opioids
   D. Anxiolytic agents

Answer: C

The primary treatment of dyspnea (air hunger) in the dying is opioids, which should be cautiously titrated to increase comfort and reduce tachypnea to a range of 15 to 20 breaths/min. Air movement across the face generated by a fan can sometimes be quite helpful. If this is not effective, empiric use of supplemental O_2 by nasal cannula (2 to 3 L/min) may bring some subjective relief, independent of observable changes in pulse oximetry. Supplemental O_2 should be humidified to avoid exacerbation of dry mouth. Typical starting doses of an immediate release opioid for breathlessness should be one half to two thirds of a starting dose of the same agent for cancer pain. For patients already on opioids for pain, a 25 to 50% increment in the dose of the current immediate release agent for breakthrough pain often will be effective in relieving breathlessness. (See Schwartz 9th ed., p 1762, 63.)

INDEX

Note: Page numbers followed by *t* indicate tables; those followed by *f* indicate figures.

R

Transjugular intrahepatic portosystemic shunt (TIPS), 268, 328
Transperitoneal laparoscopic inguinal hernia repair, contraindications, 390
Transplantation, risk for Kaposi's sarcoma, 106
Transurethral resection, 436
Transvaginal ultrasound (TVUS), 445
Transverse rectus abdominus myocutaneous (TRAM) flap, 487
Traube's space, 388
Trauma
  cricothyroidotomy, 50
  intubation, indication for, 50
  renal injury scale, 431*t*
Traumatic brain injury (TBI)
  CT scan, 121
  Glasgow coma scale (GCS) score, 121
Traumatic injuries, to facial nerve, 490
Traumatic pericardial tamponade, acute treatment for, 52
Treacher Collins syndrome, 490
Triamcinolone acetonide, 481
Tricuspid atresia, 195
Trigger finger (TF), 481
Triggering agents, for malignant hyperthermia, 502
Trisomy 21, 428
Truncus arteriosus, 191
Trypsin, 282
Trypsinogen, 358
Trypsinogen inhibitor, 358
Tuberculosis, chronic infection with, 180
Tubular adenomas, 306
Tubulovillous adenomas, 306
Tumor, node, and metastasis (TNM) staging system, 96, 167
Tumorigenesis, field effect, 84, 85
Tumor marker, sensitivity/specificity, 96*t*
Tumor marker-disease associations, 96
Tumor necrosis factor alpha (TNF-α), 5, 6, 33, 34, 41, 71, 323
Tumor of peripheral nerves, 452
Tumors arising from LOH pathway, 301
Tumor-suppressor genes, 84, 300
  implicated in thyroid tumorigenesis, 400*t*
Tumor thrombus embolization, 432
Turcot's syndrome, 311
Turner's syndrome, 146
Twin pregnancy, 374
Type 1 and Type 11 aortoiliac disease, 225
Type E (H-type) tracheoesophageal fistula, 423
Type II choledochal cyst, 345
Type III, sphincterotomy, 345
Type III aortoiliac occlusive disease, 225
Type III (mixed) hiatal hernia, treatment for, 251
Typhlitis, 317

U
Ulcerative colitis, 305, 315
Ultrasonic energy, 123
Ultrasound, 103, 151
Umbilical hernia repair, 375
Unfractionated heparin (UFH) therapy, 231, 234
Unilateral inguinal hernia, 388
University of Wisconsin preservation solution, component of, 100
Unstable coronary syndromes, major predictors, 206
Upper eyelid, defect, 489
Upper gastrointestinal hemorrhage
  risk-stratification tools for, 264*t*
Urinary bladder, 429
Urinary metanephrines, 413
Urinary retention, 310
Urolithiasis, 432
Uterine myomas, types of, 445*f*

V
VACTERL complex, 423
VACTERL syndrome, 419
Vagal nerves, 257
Vagal stimulation, 337
Vaginitis, 440
  features of common causes of, 441*t*
Vagolytic agents, administration, 124
Vagotomy, 263
Vagovagal reflex arc, 257
Vagus nerve, 5
Variceal bleeding, 330
Vascular endothelial growth factor (VEGF), 70
Vascular malformations, 488
Vasoactive intestinal peptidesecreting tumor (VIPoma) syndrome, 357–358
Vasoconstriction, physiologic responses, 32
Vasopressin, 284, 330
VATS lobectomy, 174
Venous gangrene, 233
Venous insufficiency, chronic, initial therapy, 235
Venous occlusion, sign of, 491
Venous stasis ulcers, compression therapy, 78
Venous thoracic outlet syndrome, acute
  initial therapy, 236
Venous thromboembolism (VTE), 232, 236
Ventricular septal defect (VSD), 192
Very-low calorie diets, 271
Videoassisted thoracic surgery (VATS), 173
Viral carcinogens, 94*t*
Viral transmission rate, in blood product transfusions, 114*t*
Vitamin A
  daily dose of, 87
  deficiency, 87
Vitamin B_{12}
  deficiency, 256
  malabsorption, 286
Vitamin C
  daily dose of, 87
  deficiency, 87
Vitamin D, 279
Vitamin K antagonists, 231
Vitelline duct, 283
Vo_2 max, as determined by preoperative exercise testing, 186*t*
von Graefe's sign, 406
von Willebrand's disease (vWD), 23
  type 1, 23
von Willebrand's factor (vWF), 21

W
Wallenberg's syndrome, 455
Warfarin, 231, 233, 237
  thearpy, medications, 27*t*
Water, body weight percentage, 13
Watermelon stomach, 268
WDHA syndrome, 357
Wedged hepatic venous pressure (WHVP), 329
Weight loss, 257, 271, 272
Western blotting, 132
Western diet, 283
Whiff test, 440
Whipple resection, 362
Wilms' tumor, 421
Wilson's disease, 105, 326
Wound healing
  comparison of, 74*t*
  cytokine mediator, 72
  fibroblasts in, 69
  GI, diagrammatic representation, 75*f*
  growth factors, 72*t*
  infections, 114
  macrophages functiion, 70, 71*t*
  phases of, 69*f*, 70*f*
  protein calorie malnutrition, 77
  re-epithelialization, 71
  tensile strength, 71
Wrist at midcarpal level, cross-section, 482*f*
Wrong site surgery
  cause of, 109
  risk of, 111

Y
Yersinia species, 291

Z
Zinc deficiency, 73, 74
Zollinger–Ellison syndrome, 353
Z-plasty, 492
Zuska's disease, 146